Indopathy for Neuroprotection: Recent Advances

Edited by

Surya Pratap Singh
Department of Biochemistry
Institute of Science, Banaras Hindu University
Varanasi-221005, India

Hagera Dilnashin
Department of Biochemistry
Institute of Science, Banaras Hindu University
Varanasi-221005, India

Hareram Birla
Department of Biochemistry
Institute of Science, Banaras Hindu University
Varanasi-221005, India

&

Chetan Keswani
Department of Biochemistry
Institute of Science, Banaras Hindu University
Varanasi-221005, India

Indopathy for Neuroprotection: Recent Advances

Editors: Surya Pratap Singh, Hagera Dilnashin, Hareram Birla and Chetan Keswani

ISBN (Online): 978-981-5050-86-8

ISBN (Print): 978-981-5050-87-5

ISBN (Paperback): 978-981-5050-88-2

First published in 2022.

need for a court order if at any point you breach any terms of this License Agreement. In no event will any delay or failure by Bentham Science Publishers in enforcing your compliance with this License Agreement constitute a waiver of any of its rights.

3. You acknowledge that you have read this License Agreement, and agree to be bound by its terms and conditions. To the extent that any other terms and conditions presented on any website of Bentham Science Publishers conflict with, or are inconsistent with, the terms and conditions set out in this License Agreement, you acknowledge that the terms and conditions set out in this License Agreement shall prevail.

Bentham Science Publishers Pte. Ltd.
80 Robinson Road #02-00
Singapore 068898
Singapore
Email: subscriptions@benthamscience.net

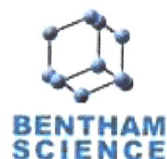

BENTHAM SCIENCE

CONTENTS

FOREWORD

Exposure to plant-based phytochemicals can promote health and prevent chronic neurodegenerative diseases. Most traditional treatment prescriptions consist of a combination of several drugs. The combination of multiple drugs is thought to maximize therapeutic effectiveness by promoting synergies and improving or preventing potential side effects while targeting multiple goals.

Indopathy is a valuable source of information for discovering new remedies for a variety of human illnesses. The complex etiology of neurodegenerative diseases and the multifactorial effects of Indopathy and its active ingredients may give a broad perspective on traditional indian medicine in neuroprotection. Some indian medicinal plants and their active ingredients have shown promising results for oxidative stress, inflammation, apoptosis, and neurodegeneration in laboratory studies. Indopathy has excellent prospects for the treatment of neurodegenerative diseases and is considered to be effective in neuroprotection.

Combining modern molecular medicine principles with some ideas of traditional indian empirical medicine may be beneficial to translation medicine.

The proposed book focuses on indopathy for the treatment of neurodegenerative diseases. This book reviews a subset of traditional indian medicines and highlights their neuroprotective active ingredients for their antioxidant, anti-inflammatory, and cognitive-enhancing effects. This volume provides a comprehensive introduction to therapeutic options for some popular plant-derived neuroprotective agents. I congratulate the editor for synchronizing with global authorities on the subject to underline the upcoming challenges and present the most viable options for translating commercially viable ideas into easily affordable products and technologies.

I wish all the editors great success with the launch of this book and thank them for their dedication to plant-based neuroprotection around the world.

Dr. Amulya K. Panda
Former Director
National Institute of Immunology
New Delhi
India

PREFACE

With the rapid increase in life expectancy and the proportion of the elderly population, the global prevalence of various neurodegenerative diseases, including Alzheimer's disease, Parkinson's disease and Huntington's disease, is rising dramatically. The demographic trend of the aged population has attracted people's attention to the discovery and treatment of new drugs for age-related diseases. Currently, there are various drugs and treatments available for the treatment of neurodegenerative diseases, but side effects or insufficient drug efficacy have been reported. With a long history of herbs or natural compounds used in the treatment of age-related diseases, new evidence has been reported to support the pharmacological effects of Indopathy in ameliorating symptoms or interfering with the pathogenesis of neurodegenerative diseases.

Many indian medicinal plants have been used for thousands of years in indopathy. Amongst these are plants used for the management of neurodegenerative diseases, such as Parkinson's, Alzheimer's, loss of memory, degeneration of nerves, and other neuronal disorders by Ayurvedic practitioners. Though the etiology of neurodegenerative diseases remains enigmatic, there is evidence indicating that defective energy metabolism, excitotoxicity, and oxidative damage may be crucial factors.

This book summarizes the new therapeutic leads from herbal sources for various types of neurodegenerative diseases. Based on recent research, this book makes an effort to utilize existing knowledge of some popular medicinal plants, and their biologically active components have been discussed, especially those used in indopathy. Several promising plants such as *Withania somnifera, Bacopa monnieri, Centella asiatica*, and *Mucuna pruriens* are worth exploring for the development of neuroprotective drugs.

Surya Pratap Singh
Department of Biochemistry
Institute of Science, Banaras Hindu University
Varanasi-221005, India

Hagera Dilnashin
Department of Biochemistry
Institute of Science, Banaras Hindu University
Varanasi-221005
India
Hareram Birla
Department of Biochemistry
Institute of Science, Banaras Hindu University
Varanasi-221005
India
&

Chetan Keswani
Department of Biochemistry
Institute of Science, Banaras Hindu University
Varanasi-221005, India

ABBREVIATIONS

6-OHDA 6-Hydroxydopamine

ABC ATP-Binding-Cassette

AP-1 Activator Protein 1

ADP Adenosine Dinucleotide Phosphate

α-Syn Alpha-Synuclein

AD Alzheimer Disease

Aβ Amyloid-Beta

APP Amyloid-Beta Precursor Protein

ApoE Apolipoprotein E

ASC Apoptosis-associated Speck-like Protein comprising a Caspase Recruitment Domain

AIF Apoptosis-Inducing Factor

AI Artificial Intelligence

Bcl-2 B-Cell Lymphoma 2

Bax Bcl-2 Associated X

BACE1 Beta-Site Amyloid Precursor Protein Cleaving Enzyme 1

HEXA Beta Hexosaminidase A

HEXB Beta Hexosaminidase B

BBB Blood-Brain Barrier

BDNF Brain-derived Neurotrophic Factor

JNK c-Jun N-Terminal Kinase

CLR C-Type Lectin Receptor

Iba1 Calcium-Binding Adaptor Molecule 1

CAT Catalase

CNS Central Nervous System

CSF Cerebrospinal Fluid

CVD Cerebrovascular Disease

COPD Chronic Obstructive Pulmonary Disease

CELA3A Chymotrypsin-Like Elastase Family Member 3A

COX-2 Cyclooxygenase-2

CBG Cytosolic Beta Glucosidase

DAT DA Transporter

DAMP Damage-Associated Molecular Pattern

DMC	Demethoxycurcumin
DA	Dopamine
Daergic	Dopaminergic
ERAD	Endoplasmic Reticulum Associated Degradation
EDS	Excessive Daytime Somnolence
EXOtic	Exosomal Transfer into Cells
ERK	Extracellular Signal-Regulated Kinases
FAD	Familial AD
FDG-PET	Fluorodeoxyglucose Positron Emission Tomography
fMRI	Functional Magnetic Resonance Imaging
NG2	Glial Antigen-2
GDNF	Glial-derived Neurotrophic Factor
GFAP	Glial Fibrillary Acidic Protein
GBA	Glucocerebrosidase
GSH	Glutathione
HO1	Hemeoxygenase 1
HD	Huntington's Disease
iPD	Idiopathic PD
IGLV1-33	Immunoglobulin Lambda Variable 1-33
iNOS	Induced Nitric Oxide Synthase
IRF3	Interferon Regulatory Factor 3
IL-1β	Interleukin-1 Beta
IL-2	Interleukin2
KMO	Kynurenine 3-Monooxygenase
LPH	Lactase Phlorizin Hydrolase
LTF	Lactoferrin
LRRK-2	Leucine Rich Repeat Kinase 2
LRR	Leucin Rich Repeats
L-Dopa	Levodopa
LBs	Lewy Bodies
LRP-1	Low-Density Lipoprotein Receptor-Related Peptide 1
LSD	Lysergic Acid Diethylamide
MRI	Magnetic Resonance Imaging
mTOR	Mammalian Target of Rapamycin
MPTP	1-Methyl-4-Phenyl-1, 2, 3, 6-Tetrahydroxypyridiine

MPP⁺	1-Methyl-4-phenylpyridinium
MCAO	Middle Cerebral Artery Occlusion
MCI	Mild Cognitive Impairment
MAPK	Mitogen-Activated Protein Kinase
MAO-B	Monoamine Oxidase B
MSA	Multiple System Atrophy
NLR	NOD-LRR-Containing Receptor
NEP	Neprilysin Protease
NCAM	Neural Cell Adhesion Molecule
NFTs	Neurofibrillary Tangles
NADH	Nicotinamide Adenine Dinucleotide
NO	Nitric Oxide
NOS	Nitric Oxide Synthase
Nrf2	Nuclear Factor Erythroid 2–Related Factor 2
NF-κB	Nuclear Factor Kappa B
NOD	Nucleotide-Binding Oligomerization Domain
OPC	Oligodendrocyte Precursor Cell
PRKN	Parkin
PD	Parkinson's Disease
PAMP	Pathogen-Associated Molecular Pattern
PRR	Pattern Recognition Receptor
PNS	Peripheral Nervous System
pMCAO	Permanent Distal Middle Cerebral Artery Occlusion
PPARγ	Peroxisome Proliferator-Activated Receptor Gamma
PI3K	Phosphoinositide 3-Kinase
PARP1	Poly (ADP-Ribose) Polymerase-1
PET	Positron Emission Tomography
PSEN	Presenilin
PSP	Progressive Supranuclear Palsy
PKB	Protein Kinase B
PINK	PTEN-induced Putative Kinase 1
REM	Rapid Eye Movement
ROS	Reactive Oxygen Species
RAGE	Receptor For Advanced Glycation End Products
REM8	Receptor-Mediated Endocytosis 8

RBD	REM Sleep Behaviour Disorder
RIG1	Retinoic Acid-Inducible Gene 1
RXR	Retinoid X Receptor
RLH	RIG1-Like Helicase
RLR	RIG1-Like Receptor
HTRA2	Serine Protease
Sema3A	Semaphorin-3A
SA-β-GAL	Senescence-Associated Beta Galactosidase
SASP	Senescence-Associated Secretory Phenotype
SNPs	Single Nucleotide Polymorphisms
SPECT	Single-photon Emission Tomography
SN	Substantia Nigra
SNpc	Substantia Nigra Pars Compacta
SOD	Superoxide Dismutase
SOCS	Suppressor of Cytokine Signaling Proteins
TLRs	Toll-Like Receptors
TCM	Traditional Chinese Medicine
TBI	Traumatic Brain Injury
TCS	Transcranial Sonography
TGF-β	Transforming Growth Factor Beta
TUBB4B	Tubulin Beta 4B Class IVb
TNF-α	Tumor Necrosis Factor Alpha
TNFR1	Tumor Necrosis Factor Receptor 1
TH	Tyrosine Hydroxylase
UCHL-1	Ubiquitin Carboxy-Terminal Hydrolase 1
UPR	Unfolded Protein Response
VPS35	Vacuolar Protein Sorting 35
VCI	Vascular Cognitive Impairment
VaD	Vascular Dementia
VHM	Venous Hypertensive Microangiopathy
WHO	World Health Organization

List of Contributors

Abhishek Mishra   Department of Pharmacology, Post Graduate Institute of Medical Education & Research, Chandigarh-160012 (Punjab), India

Ambarish Kumar Sinha   Department of Clinical Research, School of Biosciences and Biomedical Engineering, Galgotias University, Greater Noida, Uttar Pradesh, India

Anil Kumar Singh   Department of Dravyguna, Faculty of Ayurveda, Institute of Medical Sciences, Banaras Hindu University, Varanasi-221005 (U.P.), India

Anindita Bhattacharjee   Neuroimaging Laboratory, School of Bio-Medical Engineering, Indian Institute of Technology, Banaras Hindu University, Varanasi-221005 (U.P.), India

Aparna Mishra   Department of Bioscience and Biotechnology, Banasthali Vidyapith University, Banasthali-304022 (Rajasthan), India

Archana Dwivedi   Department of Neurology, Institute of Medical Sciences, Banaras Hindu University, Varanasi-221005 (U.P.), India

Ashutosh Kumar   Department of Pharmacology, Faculty of Medicine, Institute of Medical Sciences, Banaras Hindu University, Varanasi-221005 (U.P.), India

Atul Kabra   School of Pharmacy, Raffles University, Neemrana, Alwar-301020 (Rajasthan), India

Bikash Medhi   Department of Pharmacology, Post Graduate Institute of Medical Education & Research, Chandigarh-160012 (Punjab), India

Bipin Maurya   Laboratory of Morphogenesis, Centre of Advance Study in Botany, Institute of Science, Banaras Hindu University, Varanasi-221005 (U.P.), India

Caridad Ivette Fernandez Verdecia   International Center of Neurological Restoration (CIREN), Basic Division, La Habana, Cuba

Chetan Keswani   Department of Biochemistry, Institute of Science, Banaras Hindu University, Varanasi-221005 (U.P.), India

Christophe Hano   Laboratoire de Biologie des Ligneux et des Grandes Cultures, INRAUSC1328, Universitéd'Orléans, 45100 Orléans, France

Darshi Attanayake   Interdisciplinary Centre for Innovation in Biotechnology and Neurosciences, Faculty of Medical Sciences, University of Sri Jayewardenepura, Sri Jayewardenepura Kotte, Sri Lanka

Deepika Joshi   Department of Neurology, Institute of Medical Sciences, Banaras Hindu University, Varanasi-221005 (U.P.), India

Divya Raj Prasad   Department of Genetics and Plant Breeding, Institute of Agricultural Sciences, Banaras Hindu University, Varanasi-221005 (U.P.), India

Gaurav Kumar   Department of Clinical Research, School of Biosciences and Biomedical Engineering, Galgotias University, Greater Noida, Uttar Pradesh, India

Hagera Dilnashin   Department of Biochemistry, Institute of Science, Banaras Hindu University, Varanasi-221005 (U.P.), India

Hardik Koria   Department of Pharmacology, Ramanbhai Patel College of Pharmacy, Charotar University of Science and Technology, Charusat Campus, Changa-388421, (Gujarat), India

Hareram Birla   Department of Biochemistry, Institute of Science, Banaras Hindu University, Varanasi-221005 (U.P.), India

Héctor Eduardo López-Valdés   Departamento de Fisiología, Facultad de Medicina, Universidad Nacional Autónoma de México (UNAM), Ciudad de México, México

Hilda Martínez-Coria   Departamento de Fisiología, Facultad de Medicina, Universidad Nacional Autónoma de México (UNAM), Ciudad de México, México

Himanshu Verma   Department of Pharmaceutical Engineering and Technology, Indian Institute of Technology, Banaras Hindu University, Varanasi-221005 (U.P.), India

Kamal Uddin   Aligarh College of Pharmacy, Aligarh-202002 (U.P), India

K. Ranil D. de Silva   Interdisciplinary Centre for Innovation in Biotechnology and Neurosciences, Faculty of Medical Sciences, University of Sri Jayewardenepura, Sri Jayewardenepura Kotte, Sri Lanka
Institute for Combinatorial Advanced Research & Education (KDU-CARE), General Sir John Kotelawala Defence University, Colombo, Sri Lanka
European Graduate School of Neuroscience, Maastricht University, Maastricht, The Netherlands

Lakmal Gonawala   Interdisciplinary Centre for Innovation in Biotechnology and Neurosciences, Faculty of Medical Sciences, University of Sri Jayewardenepura, Sri Jayewardenepura Kotte, Sri Lanka
European Graduate School of Neuroscience, Maastricht University, Maastricht, The Netherlands,

Nalaka Wijekoon   Interdisciplinary Centre for Innovation in Biotechnology and Neurosciences, Faculty of Medical Sciences, University of Sri Jayewardenepura, Sri Jayewardenepura Kotte, Sri Lanka
European Graduate School of Neuroscience, Maastricht University, Maastricht, The Netherlands

Natália Cruz-Martins   Faculty of Medicine, University of Porto, Porto, Portugal
Institute for Research and Innovation in Health (i3S), University of Porto, Porto, Portugal,
Institute of Research and Advanced Training in Health Sciences and Technologies (CESPU), Rua Central de Gandra, 1317, 4585-116 Gandra PRD, Portugal

Naveen Shivavedi   Shri Ram Group of Institutions, Faculty of Pharmacy, Jabalpur-482002 (M.P.), India

Nilay Solanki   Department of Pharmacology, Ramanbhai Patel College of Pharmacy, Charotar University of Science and Technology, Charusat Campus, Changa-388421 (Gujarat), India

Phulen Sarma   Department of Pharmacology, Post Graduate Institute of Medical Education & Research, Chandigarh-160012 (Punjab), India

Prasanta Kumar Nayak   Department of Pharmaceutical Engineering and Technology, Indian Institute of Technology, Banaras Hindu University, Varanasi-221005 (U.P.), India

Prasun Kumar Roy Neuroimaging Laboratory, School of Bio-Medical Engineering, Indian Institute of Technology Banaras Hindu University, Varanasi-221005 (U.P.), India
Centre for Tissue Engineering, Indian Institute of Technology, Banaras Hindu University, Varanasi-221005 (U.P.), India

Pratibha Thakur Department of Bioscience, Endocrinology Unit, Barkatullah University, Bhopal- 462026 (M.P.), India

Pratistha Singh Department of Dravyguna, Faculty of Ayurveda, Institute of Medical Sciences, Banaras Hindu University, Varanasi-221005 (U.P.), India

Raffaele Capasso Universita Degli Studi di Napoli Federico II, Naples, Italy

Rohit Sharma Department of Rasa Shastra and Bhaishjya Kalpana, Faculty of Ayurveda, IMS, Banaras Hindu University, Varanasi-221005 (U.P), India

Rubal Singla Department of Pharmacology, Post Graduate Institute of Medical Education & Research, Chandigarh-160012 (Punjab), India

Ruchika Kabra School of Pharmacy, Raffles University, Neemrana, Alwar-301020 (Rajasthan), India

Rupa Joshi Department of Pharmacology, Post Graduate Institute of Medical Education & Research, Chandigarh-160012 (Punjab), India

Sarika Singh Department of Neuroscience and Ageing Biology and Division of Toxicology and Experimental Medicine, CSIR-Central Drug Research Institute, Lucknow-226031, (U.P.), India

Shilpa Negi Department of Neuroscience and Ageing Biology and Division of Toxicology and Experimental Medicine, CSIR-Central Drug Research Institute, Lucknow-226031, (U.P.), India

Sukala Prasad Biochemistry & Molecular Biology Laboratory, Department of Zoology, Brain Research Centre, Banaras Hindu University, Varanasi-221001 (U.P.), India

Surya Pratap Singh Department of Biochemistry, Institute of Science, Banaras Hindu University, Varanasi-221005 (U.P.), India

Uttam Singh Baghel Department of Pharmacy, University of Kota, Kota-324005 (Rajasthan), India

Vartika Gupta Biochemistry & Molecular Biology Laboratory, Department of Zoology, Brain Research Centre, Banaras Hindu University, Varanasi-221005 (U.P.), India

Yoonus Imran Interdisciplinary Centre for Innovation in Biotechnology and Neurosciences, Faculty of Medical Sciences, University of Sri Jayewardenepura, Sri Jayewardenepura Kotte, Sri Lanka

CHAPTER 1

Globalizing Traditional Knowledge of Indian Medicine: Evidence-based Therapeutics

Hagera Dilnashin[1,*], **Hareram Birla**[1], **Chetan Keswani**[1] and **Surya Pratap Singh**[1,*]

[1] *Department of Biochemistry, Institute of Science, Banaras Hindu University, Varanasi-221005 (U.P.), India*

Abstract: With the advent of modern medicine, the use of medicinal plants is an ancient therapeutic strategy used by traditional healers and is very useful in traditional medicine. Medicinal plants are compatible with human physiology, which has been adapted for centuries.

Keywords: Indopathy, Medicinal plants, Therapeutic strategy, Therapeutics, Traditional medicine.

INTRODUCTION

In today's scenario, scientists need to focus on finding the compounds of herbs involved in the cure, alleviation, and cure of the disease. Traditional medicine includes long-term treatments that people inherit and practice to prevent and treat illness. Plants have formed the basis of traditional medicinal systems. It consists of several medicinal systems from different parts of the world, which include Chinese herbal medicine (China), Indian herbal medicine (India), Kampo medicine (Japan), Native American medicine (US), Tibetan medicine (Tibetan), Jamu Genndong (Indonesia), traditional African medicine (Africa), and traditional Hawaiian medicine (Hawaii) [1, 2].

India has an ancient heritage of traditional medicine. *Materia medica* of India provides a wealth of information on the folklore practices and traditional aspects of therapeutically important natural products. Each of these traditional systems has unique aspects, but there is a common thread among their fundamental principles and practices in the use of natural products, mostly herbs [3 - 5].

* **Corresponding authors Hagera Dilnashin and Surya Pratap Singh:** Department of Biochemistry, Institute of Science, Banaras Hindu University, Varanasi-221005 (U.P.), India; E-mails: hagera.dilnashin10@bhu.ac.in and suryasinghbhu16@gmail.com

Indopathy is a traditional Indian medicinal system that includes Ayurveda, Yoga, and Naturopathy, Unani, Siddha, and Homeopathy (AYUSH). It is a well-known medication system because of its various pharmacological effects that are beneficial to human health [6]. In addition to its strong neuroprotective potential, many studies have also described the significant therapeutic effects of herbal medicine against several central nervous system diseases [4, 7 - 9]. The biological effects of herbal plants have been generally attributed to ancient science's major protective effect. The results of studies with different mechanisms indicate the neuroprotective effects of plants, most of which mention positive effects on oxidative stress and other assessment parameters [5, 10 - 13]. The modulatory role of the alternative medicinal system will not only bring new drug discoveries [14] but also treat central nervous system diseases and help understand the complex pathophysiology of neurodegenerative diseases [3, 15 - 18].

CONCLUSION

Over time, Indopathy has been tested, and people have used it for their medical care for a long time. Before British rule, these were the main treatments in India but later changed under the influence of western culture. So Indopathy are well-rooted with a profound clinical basis, where scientific validation is sometimes the major constraint for their development. Despite these setbacks, Indopathy remains in India and continues to grow in the global market [19]. As the Western world pays more and more attention to herbal drugs, especially Indopathy, it is necessary to examine these systems and take appropriate measures to restore the concept of traditional medicine as the main therapeutic medicinal system [20, 21].

CONSENT FOR PUBLICATION

Not applicable.

CONFLICT OF INTEREST

The author declares no conflict of interest, financial or otherwise.

ACKNOWLEDGEMENTS

Declared none.

REFERENCES

[1]   Mukherjee PK, Maiti K, Mukherjee K, Houghton PJ. Leads from Indian medicinal plants with hypoglycemic potentials. J Ethnopharmacol 2006; 106(1): 1-28.
[http://dx.doi.org/10.1016/j.jep.2006.03.021] [PMID: 16678368]

[2]   Law BYK, Wu AG, Wang MJ, Zhu YZ. Chinese medicine: a hope for neurodegenerative diseases? J Alzheimers Dis 2017; 60(s1): S151-60.
[http://dx.doi.org/10.3233/JAD-170374] [PMID: 28671133]

[3]   Singh SS, Rai SN, Birla H, *et al.* Neuroprotective effect of chlorogenic acid on mitochondrial dysfunction-mediated apoptotic death of DA neurons in a Parkinsonian mouse model. Oxid Med Cell Longev 2020; 2020: 1-14.
[http://dx.doi.org/10.1155/2020/6571484] [PMID: 32566093]

[4]   Birla H, Keswani C, Singh SS, *et al.* Unraveling the neuroprotective effect of tinospora *cordifolia* in parkinsonian mouse model through proteomics approach. ACS Chem Neurosci 2021; 12(22): 4319-35.

[5]   Birla H, Keswani C, Rai SN, *et al.* Neuroprotective effects of *Withania somnifera* in BPA induced-cognitive dysfunction and oxidative stress in mice. Behav Brain Funct 2019; 15(1): 9.
[http://dx.doi.org/10.1186/s12993-019-0160-4] [PMID: 31064381]

[6]   Gitler AD, Dhillon P, Shorter J. Neurodegenerative disease: models, mechanisms, and new hope. The Company of Biologists Ltd Dis Model Mech 2017; 10: pp. (5)499-502.

[7]   Zahra W, Rai SN, Birla H, *et al.* The global economic impact of neurodegenerative diseases: Opportunities and challenges. Bioeconomy for Sustainable Development 2020; pp. 333-45.

[8]   Rai SN, Birla H, Singh SS, *et al.* Pathophysiology of the Disease Causing Physical Disability. Biomedical Engineering and its Applications in Healthcare. Springer 2019; pp. 573-95.

[9]   Rai SN, Singh BK, Rathore AS, *et al.* Quality control in huntington's disease: a therapeutic target. Neurotox Res 2019; 36(3): 612-26.
[http://dx.doi.org/10.1007/s12640-019-00087-x] [PMID: 31297710]

[10]   Rathore AS, Birla H, Singh SS, *et al.* Epigenetic modulation in parkinson's disease and potential treatment therapies. neurochem res 2021; 46(7): 1618-26.
[http://dx.doi.org/10.1007/s11064-021-03334-w] [PMID: 33900517]

[11]   Singh S, Rai S, Birla H, Eds., *et al.* Chlorogenic acid protects against MPTP induced neurotoxicity in parkinsonian mice model *via* its anti-apoptotic activity. Journal of Neurochemistry. Hoboken 07030-5774, NJ USA: Wiley 111 River St 2019.

[12]   Rai SN, Dilnashin H, Birla H, *et al.* The role of PI3K/Akt and ERK in neurodegenerative disorders. Neurotox Res 2019; 35(3): 775-95.
[http://dx.doi.org/10.1007/s12640-019-0003-y] [PMID: 30707354]

[13]   Beal MF. Aging, energy, and oxidative stress in neurodegenerative diseases. Ann Neurol 1995; 38(3): 357-66.
[http://dx.doi.org/10.1002/ana.410380304] [PMID: 7668820]

[14]   Bhatnagar M. Novel leads from herbal drugs for neurodegenerative diseases. Herbal drugs: Ethnomedicine to modern medicine. Springer 2009; pp. 221-38.
[http://dx.doi.org/10.1007/978-3-540-79116-4_14]

[15]   Hassan MAG, Balasubramanian R, Masoud AD, Burkan ZE, Sughir A, Kumar RS. Role of medicinal plants in neurodegenerative diseases with special emphasis to alzheimer's. International Journal of Phytopharmacology 2014; 5(6): 454-62.

[16]   Zahra W, Rai SN, Birla H, *et al.* Neuroprotection of rotenone-induced Parkinsonism by ursolic acid in PD mouse model. CNS & Neurological Disorders-Drug Targets. CNS Neurol Disord Drug Targets 2020; 19: pp. (7)527-40.

[17]   Rai SN, Zahra W, Singh SS, *et al.* Anti-inflammatory activity of ursolic acid in MPTP-induced parkinsonian mouse model. Neurotox Res 2019; 36(3): 452-62.
[http://dx.doi.org/10.1007/s12640-019-00038-6] [PMID: 31016688]

[18]   Zahra W, Rai SN, Birla H, *et al.* Economic Importance of Medicinal Plants in Asian Countries. Bioeconomy for Sustainable Development. Springer 2020; pp. 359-77. [http://dx.doi.org/10.1007/978-981-13-9431-7_19]

[19]   Mukherjee PK, Bahadur S, Harwansh RK, Nema NK, Bhadra S. Development of traditional medicines: globalizing local knowledge or localizing global technologies. Pharma Times 2013; 45(9): 39-42.

[20]   Mukherjee P, Wahile A. Perspectives of safety for natural health products. Herbal Drugs-A Twenty first Century Perspectives 2006; 50-9.

[21]   Orhan IE. Urban: from traditional medicine to modern medicine with neuroprotective potential. Evidence-based complementary and alternative medicine 2012.

CHAPTER 2

Naturally-occurring Bioactive Molecules with Anti-Parkinson Disease Potential

Atul Kabra[1,*]**, Kamal Uddin**[2]**, Rohit Sharma**[3]**, Ruchika Kabra**[1]**, Raffaele Capasso**[4]**, Caridad Ivette Fernandez Verdecia**[5]**, Christophe Hano**[6,*]**, Natália Cruz-Martins**[7,8,9,*] **and Uttam Singh Baghel**[10,*]

[1] *School of Pharmacy, Raffles University, Neemrana, Alwar-301020 (Rajasthan), India*

[2] *Aligarh College of Pharmacy, Aligarh-202002 (U.P), India*

[3] *Department of Rasa Shastra and Bhaishjya Kalpana, Faculty of Ayurveda, IMS, Banaras Hindu University, Varanasi, 221005 (U.P) India*

[4] *Universita Degli Studi di Napoli Federico II, Naples, Italy*

[5] *International Center of Neurological Restoration (CIREN), Basic Division, La Habana, Cuba*

[6] *Laboratoire de Biologie des Ligneux et des Grandes Cultures, INRAUSC 1328, Université d' Orléans, 45100 Orléans, France*

[7] *Faculty of Medicine, University of Porto, Porto, Portugal*

[8] *Institute for Research and Innovation in Health (i3S), University of Porto, Porto, Portugal*

[9] *Institute of Research and Advanced Training in Health Sciences and Technologies (CESPU), Rua Central de Gandra, 1317, 4585-116 Gandra PRD, Portugal*

[10] *Department of Pharmacy, University of Kota, Kota-324005 (Rajasthan), India*

Abstract: Parkinson's disease (PD) is a complex limiting neurodegenerative disorder, with a rising incidence. Current therapeutic options for PD have multiple limitations, and naturally occurring biomolecules, often known as phytochemicals, with potent neuroprotective activities, have been searched to meet the need. Thus, this chapter encompasses in-depth information on reported anti-PD activities of medicinal plants in light of available pre-clinical and clinical studies and shares the mechanisms of action proposed in fighting PD. Published information from PubMed, Scopus, Science Direct, Springer, Google Scholar, and other allied databases was analyzed. There is rising interest among researchers in investigating medicinal plants and their isolated compounds for their anti-PD efficacy. Scattered information about the anti-PD potential of *plants* and bioactive compounds is reported in the scientific domain. A total of 92 medicinal plants belonging to 63 families, exhibiting anti-PD activity were

---

[*] **Corresponding authors Atul Kabra, Christophe Hano, Natália Cruz-Martins & Uttam Singh Baghel:** School of Pharmacy, Raffles University, Neemrana, Alwar-301020 (Rajasthan), India, Laboratoire de Biologie des Ligneux et des Grandes Cultures, INRAUSC1328, Universitéd'Orléans, 45100 Orléans, France, Faculty of Medicine, University of Porto, Porto, Portugal & Department of Pharmacy, University of Kota, Kota-324005 (Rajasthan), India; E-mails: ruchika.p88@gmail.com, drusb1985@yahoo.com, ncmartins@med.up.pt & hano@univ-orleans.fr

Surya Pratap Singh, Hagera Dilnashin, Hareram Birla & Chetan Keswani (Eds.)

discussed. Botanical species have revealed an extreme potential, encouraging future examination. Data discussed here can be used for further research and clinical purposes.

Keywords: Bioactive molecules, Dopamine, Lewy bodies, Medicinal plant extracts, Parkinson's disease, Substantia nigra.

INTRODUCTION

Despite presenting a pathological mark of slowness, the manifestation and progression of Parkinson's Disease (PD) are insinuated [1], featured by the progressive loss of dopaminergic neurons in the pars compacta of substantia nigra and by the decline in dopamine levels in the basal ganglia striatum [2, 3]. Consequently, the cholinergic neurons' activity becomes comparatively dominant, while the nigrostriatal dopaminergic neuronal activity is decreased, which results in the advancement of movement disorder [4 - 6]. In the human system, PD is categorized by symptoms of motor neurons, *viz.* bradykinesia, resting tremors, rigidity, and postural instability [7], besides non-motor manifestations, such as neuropsychiatric abnormalities, disturbed sleep, dysautonomia, gastrointestinal disturbances, and sensory problems [8 - 12].

At the molecular level, although the pathophysiology of the disease still remains unclear, several pathways have been proposed to be involved in dopaminergic neuronal death, such as oxidative stress, mitochondrial injury, excitatory amino acid toxicity, ubiquitin-proteasome system damage, proteolytic stress, immune disorders, inflammatory reactions, dopamine transporter (DAT) inactivation, abnormal deposition of α-synuclein, and cell apoptosis through c-Abl activation [1, 13 - 15]. In this context, environmental factors, like permethrin pesticide exposure during brain development, have been associated with genetic and epigenetic changes leading to PD in rats, as well as in their untreated offspring (Fig. **1**) [16 - 19].

For several decades, the therapeutic gold standard for PD has been based on the use of levodopa, in combination with a peripheral decarboxylase inhibitor. However, the long-term use of these drugs often leads to multiple secondary effects, including gastrointestinal, respiratory, and neurological symptoms [20 - 22]. More recently, several drugs were approved by FDA for treating PD, but they also have various side effects, as summarized in Table **1** [23 - 27]. Hence, the search for natural products with anti-PD activity has largely increased in these years owing to their safer approach and cost-effectiveness. Though plentiful research has been carried out during the past decades on the anti-PD potential of several botanical preparations, extracts, and isolated phytocompounds, only scattered information exploring their activity is accessible. Besides, earlier reports did not provide complete information apropos plant extract doses, animals used, and their possible anti-PD mechanism.

Considering this, the present chapter attempts to provide a comprehensive report on the anti-PD potential of several botanicals in light of available experimental and clinical studies.

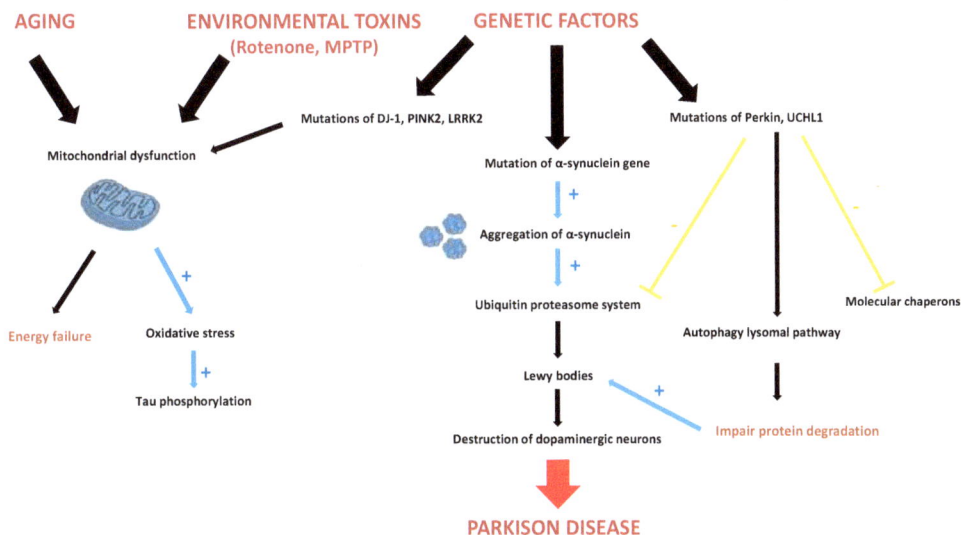

Fig. (1). Genetic, environmental, and lifestyle factors leading to PD.

Table 1. Recently FDA-approved anti-PD drugs.

S. No.	Drug	Brand Name	Mechanism of Action	Use	Side Effects	Approval Year	Company Name
1.	Safinamide	Xadago	MAO-B inhibitor	Adjunctive treatment to levodopa/carbidopa in patients with PD	Dyskinesia, fall, Nausea, Insomnia	2017	Newron Pharmaceuticals
2.	Amantadine	Gocovri	An uncompetitive antagonist of the NMDA receptor	PD dyskinesia	Hallucination, Dizziness, Dry Mouth, Peripheral Edema, Orthostatic, Hypotension	2017	Adamas Pharmaceuticals

(Table 1) cont.....

S. No.	Drug	Brand Name	Mechanism of Action	Use	Side Effects	Approval Year	Company Name
3.	Pimavanserin	Nuplazid	Inverse agonist and antagonist activity at serotonin 5-HT$_2$A receptors	Hallucinations and delusions associated with PD	Peripheral edema, confusional state	2016	Acadia Pharmaceuticals
4.	Carbidopa and levodopa	Duopa	Inhibits the peripheral levodopa decarboxylation	Motor fluctuations in patients with advanced PD	Hypertension, Peripheral Edema, Erythema, Upper Respiratory Tract Infection, Oropharyngeal Pain	2015	Abbvie Pharmaceuticals
5.	Carbidopa and levodopa	Rytary	-	-	Hypotension, Insomnia, Abnormal Dreams, Dry Mouth, Dyskinesia, Anxiety	2015	Impax Labs

NEUROPROTECTIVE POTENTIAL OF BOTANICALS

Available reports reveal that functional foods, such as green legumes, condiments, cereals, different medicinal plant parts, phytoconstituents obtained from leaves, bark, fruits, flowers and seeds, crude extractives and active phytocompounds are being investigated in experimental studies, while meagre attempts are found at clinical levels. These botanicals were found to exhibit significant neuroprotective activities and have been used as potent remedies for PD. Macroscopic features of common anti-PD plants and their bioactive compounds are mentioned in Fig. (**2**).

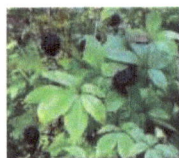

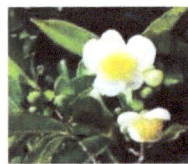

Acanthopanax senticosus   Sesamine   Camellia sinensis   Epigallocatechin-3-gallate

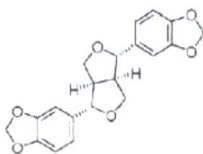

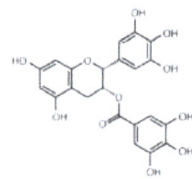

(Fig. 2) contd.....

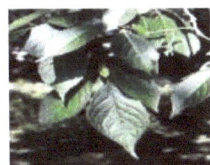
Eucommia ulmoides

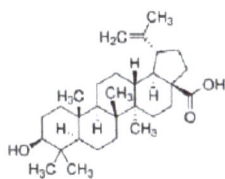
Betulinic acid

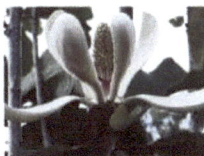
Magnolia officinalis

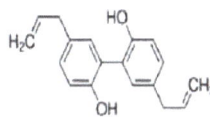
Magnolol

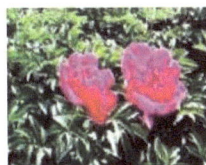
Paeonia lactiflora

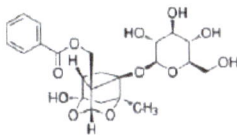
Paeoniflorin

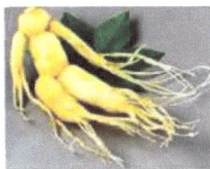
Panax ginseng

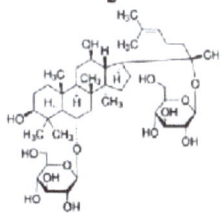
Ginsenoside Rg1

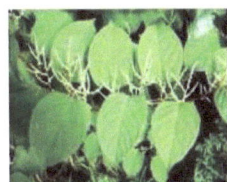
Polygonum cuspidatum

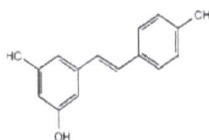
Resveratrol

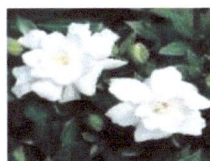
Gardenia jasminoides

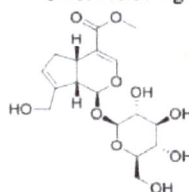
Geniposide

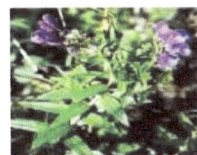
Scutellaria baicalensis

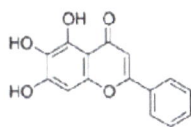
Baicalein

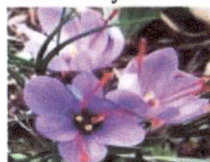
Crocus sativus

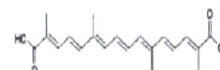
Crocetin

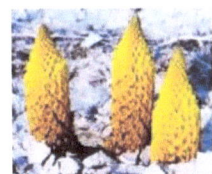
Cistanche deserticola

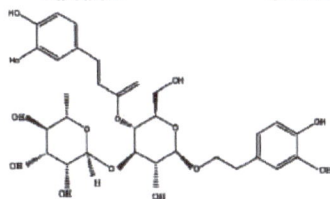
Acetoside

Fig. (2). Macroscopic features and bioactive compounds of medicinal plants with anti-PD potential.

In-vitro Studies

The majority of available *in-vitro* studies were carried out on neuronal PC-12 and SH-SY5Y cell lines, while some studies were carried out on SK-N-SH, MN9D,

BV-2 microglial, D8, HT22 murine hippocampal, N9 and EOC20 microglial cell lines (Table **2**). Sesamine isolated from *Acanthopanax senticosus* was able to decrease CAT activity, increase SOD as well as protein expression at a dose of 1 pM on PC-12 cells [28]. Protocatechuic acid isolated from kernels of *Alpinia oxyphylla* at a dose of 0.06-2.4 mM on PC-12 cells increases SOD, CAT, and GSH-Px levels [28], besides its ethanolic extract from ripe seeds also inhibits NO and iNOS production [29]. Aqueous and ethanol extracts from *Bacopa monnieri* at 50 and 10 µg/ml decreased ROS and mitochondrial superoxide levels and increased GSH levels [30, 31]. Polyphenolic catechins obtained from *Camellia sinensis* leaves were shown to decrease the accumulation of ROS and intracellular free Ca^{2+} ions, nNOS, and iNOS at a dose of 50, 100, and 200 µM [32]. EGCG, ECG isolated from *Camellia sinensis* exhibited anti-PD potential on PC-12 cells by activating MAPK and potentiating the ability of the cellular antioxidant defense system at a dose of 50-200 µM [33]. In PC-12 cells, EGCG also modulated DAT internalization by exerting an inhibitory effect on DAT at a dose of 1-100 µM [34]. Dried GT and BT extracts of *Camellia sinensis* attenuated NF-κB activation on SH-SY5Y cell and PC-12 cell at a dose of 0.6-3 µM [35].

Table 2. *In vitro* **anti-PD activity of medicinal plants.**

Plant Name	Family	Part Used	Extract/Fraction/Compound	Dose	*In-vitro*	Experimental Models	Result	References
Acantho panaxsenticosus (Rupr. et Maxim.) Harms.	Araliaceae	Seeds	Sesamine	1 pM	PC12 cells	MPP⁺ induced	↑SOD, ↑protein expression, ↓CAT	[51, 52]
			Eleutheroside B	---			↑ ERK ½ phosphorylation and ↓ c-fos and c-jun expressions	-
Ajuga ciliate Bungeciliate	Labiatae	Whole plant	Clerodane diterpenes	3-30 µM	SH-SY5Y cells	MPP⁺-induced	↑ Cell viability	[53]
Alpinia oxyphylla Miq.	Zingiberaceae	Ripe seeds	Ethanol extract	---	Neuronal PC12 cells	6-OHDA induced	↓IL-1β and TNF-α gene expression and inhibit NO production and iNOS expression	[29, 54]
		Kernels	Protocatechuic acid	0.06-2.4 mM	PC12 cells	H₂O₂ induced cell death	↑SOD, CAT, GSH-Px	-
Anemo paegmamirandum (Catuaba)	Bignoniaceae	---	Commercial Extract	0.312, 0.625 and 1.250 mg/ml	SH-SY5Y cells	Rotenone induced	↑ Cell viability	[28]
Apium graveolens L.	Apiaceae	Seed	DL-3-n-butylphthalide (NBP)	0.1-100 µM	SH-SY5Y cells	Rotenone induced	↑Mitochondrial membrane potential, ↓ROS, ↑Cell viability	[55]
Astragalus membranaceus (Fisch.) Bge.	Leguminosae	Roots	Astragaloside IV	---	SH-SY5Y cells	MPP+ induced	Inhibit ROS production and ↑ Bax/Bcl-2 ratio and activity of caspase-3	[56]
Bacopa monnieri (L.) Wettst.	Plantaginaceae	Whole plant	Aqueous extract	50 µg/ml	SH-SY5Y cells	MPTP and Paraquat induced	↑GSH, ↓ROS, mitochondrial superoxide level	[30, 31]
			Ethanol extract	10 µg/ml	PC-12 Cells	Rotenone induced	↑GSH, ↓ROS	-

(Table 2) cont.....

Plant Name	Family	Part Used	Extract/Fraction/Compound	Dose	*In-vitro*	Experimental Models	Result	References
Buddleja officinalis Maxim	Scrophulariaceae	---	Verbascoside	0.1, 1 or 10 µg/ml	PC-12 Cells	MPTP induced	↓Caspase-3 activation and collapse of mitochondrial membrane	[57]
Camellia sinensis (L.) Kuntze	Theaceae	Leaves	Polyphenolic catechins	50, 100, 200 µM	SH-SY5Y cells	6-OHDA induced	↓ ROS and intracellular free Ca^{-2}, nNOS and iNOS	[32 - 34, 36, 58]
			EGCG, ECG, EC, C, EGC	50-200 µM	PC12 cells	*In-vitro*	Activation of MAPK, ↑antioxidant enzymes	-
			EGCG	(1–100 µM)	PC12 cells	MPP$^+$ induced neurotoxicity	Modulation of DAT internalization	-
			Dried GT and BT extracts	0.6–3 µM	SH-SY5Y cells and PC-12 cell	6-OHDA induced	↓ NF-κB activation	-
				1, 3, and 10 µM	SH-SY5Y cells	DDT-induced	PAINS	-
Carthamus tinctorius L.	Compositae	---	kaempferol 3-O-β-rutinoside and 6-hydroxykaempferol 3,6-di-O-β-D-glucoside	1 µM	PC-12 cells	H$_2$O$_2$ induced	Bind DJ-1 (protein associated with PD); ↓Levels of H$_2$O$_2$ induced ROS and restore TH activity	[36]
Cassia obtusifolia L.	Leguminosae	Ripe seed	Ethanol extract	0.1–10 mg/ml	PC-12 cells	6-OHDA induced	Inhibit ROS overproduction, glutathione depletion, mitochondrial membrane depolarization, and caspase-3 activation	[37]
Chrysanthemum morifolium Ramat	Compositae	---	Aqueous extract	-	SH-SY5Y cells	MPP$^+$ induced	Inhibit mitochondrial apoptotic pathway and ↓ROS accumulation and ↑ cell viability.	[59, 60]
Chrysanthemum indicum Linn.		Seed	Methanolic extract	1, 10, and 100 µg	SH-SY5Y cells	MPP$^+$ induced	↓ROS production, inhibit PARP proteolysis	
					BV-2 cells	LPS induced	↓Production of PGE_2 COX-2, blocked IκB-α degradation and ↓activation of NF-κB	
Cistanche deserticola Y. C. Ma	Orobanchaceae	---	Acteoside	10, 20 or 40 mg/l	SH-SY5Y cells	Rotenone induced	Inhibit the aggregation of α-Syn	[38, 39]
			Tubuloside B	-	PC12 cells	MPP$^+$ induced	↓ROS, DNA fragmentation	-
Citrus aurantium L., *Citrus sinensis* (L.) Osbeck and Citrus unshiu (Yu. Tanaka ex Swingle) Marcow.	Rutaceae	Citrus Fruit flavanol	Hesperidin	2.5, 5, 10, 20, and 40 □g	SK-N-SH cells	Rotenone induced	↓ROS formation by ↓levels of TBARS and restored antioxidant enzyme activity and GSH	[61, 62]
		--	Hesperetin	--	PC12 cells	Oxidative stress-induced	Triggers ER- and TrkA-mediated parallel pathways	-
Clausena lansium (Lour.) Skeels	Rutaceae	Leaves	Bu-7	0.1 and 10 µmol/L	PC12 cells	Rotenone induced	Inhibit the phosphorylation of both JNK and p38 and ↓p53 levels.	[63]
Coptis chinensis Franch.	Ranunculaceae	Rhizome	Aqueous extract	---	SH-SY5Y cells	MPP+ induced	↑cell viability, ↑intracellular ATP concentration, and ↑TH	[64]
Curcuma longa L.	Zingiberaceae	Rhizome	Aqueous extract	0.001, 0.01, 0.05, 0.1, 0.2 and 0.4 mg/ml	SH-SY5Y cells	Salsolinol induced toxicity	Inhibition of apoptosis and ↓Gene expression levels of apoptosis markers (p53, Bax, and caspase 3)	[65]

(Table 2) cont.....

Plant Name	Family	Part Used	Extract/Fraction/Compound	Dose	In-vitro	Experimental Models	Result	References
Cuscuta australis R. Br. or Cuscuta chinensis Lam.	Convolvulaceae	Ripe seeds	Aqueous extract	0.001, 0.01, 5, and 10 μg	PC12 cells	MPP+ induced	↓GPx, ↓ROS	[66, 67]
			Flavonoid	0.001, 0.01, 5, and 10 μg	PC12 cells	H_2O_2 induced apoptosis	↓ROS, ↑Antioxidant enzymes	
Eucommia ulmoides Oliv.	Eucommiaceae	Bark	Betulinic acid, betulin, wogonin, oroxylin A, genipin, geniposidic, and aucubin	10 μM	SH-SY5Y cells	MPP+ induced	↑ Proteasome activity, ↑Cell viability	[68]
Fraxinus sieboldiana Blume	Oleaceae	-----	Esculin, 6,7-Di-O-glucopyrano-yl-esculetin and liriodendrin	10^{-7}, 10^{-6}, and 10^{-5} M	SH-SY5Y cells	-	↓ROS level, ↑Mitochondrion membrane potential, ↑SOD activity, and ↓glutathione GSH and regulate P53, Bax, and Bcl-2 expression; inhibit the release of cytochrome-c, apoptosis-inducing factor, and caspase 3 activation	[69]
Gardenia jasminoides J. Ellis	Rubiaceae	Fruit	Geniposide	5 and 50 μg/ml	SH-SY5Y cells	Corticosterone induced	Inhibit cell apoptosis, ↓P21, and P53 protein expression	[70]
Gastrodiaelata Blume	Orchidaceae	Rhizome	Ethanolic extract	10, 100, 200 g/mL	SH-SY5Y cells	MPP+ induced	↓ROS, ↓Caspase-3 activity, ↓Bax/Bcl-2 ratio	[71, 72]
		Rhizome	Vanillyl alcohol	---	MN9D cells	MPP+ induced	Inhibiting ROS levels, ↓Bax/Bcl-2 ratio, ↓caspase-3, and PARP proteolysis	-
Ginkgo biloba L	Ginkgoaceae	Leaves	EGb 761	10, 20, and 40 μg/mL	PC12 cells	Paraquat (PQ) induced	↓caspase-3 activation through a mitochondria-dependent pathway	[73]
Hypericum perforatum L.	Hypericaceae	Aerial part	Methanolic extract	10-100 μg/ml	PC12 cells	H_2O_2 induced	Inhibiting ROS	[40, 41]
		Ethyl acetate fraction	Hyperoside	10-180 μg/ml	PC12 cells	H_2O_2 induced	↓LDH level, ↑Cell viability	-
Lonicera japonica Thunb.	Caprifoliaceae	Flower buds	Aqueous extract	0.5, 5, 2.5, 5, and 10 μg/mL	BV-2 microglial cells	Lipopolysaccharide (LPS) induced	Inhibit proinflammatory cytokines and chemokines, TNF-α IL-1β, monocyte chemoattractant protein-1, ↓ROS production	[42]
Lycium chinense Mill.	Solanaceae	-	Extract	-	PC12 cells	Rotenone induced	↑Cell viability, ATP level, ↓caspase activation, ↓mitochondrial membrane depolarization, ↓mitochondrial superoxide production.	[74]
Magnolia officinalis Rehder & E. H. Wilson	Magnoliaceae	Stem bark	Magnolol	30 mg/kg	SH-SY5Y cells	MPP+ induced	↓ROS production	[75]
Morus alba L.	Moraceae	Fruit	70% ethanol extract	1, 10 and 100 μg/ml	SH-SY5Y cells	6-OHDA	Antioxidant and antiapoptotic effects	[43]
Murraya koenigii (L.) Spreng.	Rutaceae	Leaves	Aqueous extract	----	PC12 cells	6-OHDA	↓antioxidant enzymes	[45]
Paeonia lactiflora Pall.	Paeoniaceae	Root	Paeoniflorin	20-200 μg/ml	PC12 cells	MPP+ induced	↑expression of HATs, ↑H3K9ac and H3K27ac of Histone H3	[76]

(Table 2) cont.....

Plant Name	Family	Part Used	Extract/Fraction/Compound	Dose	*In-vitro*	Experimental Models	Result	References
Panax ginseng C. A. Mey.	Araliaceae	Rhizome	Aqueous extract	0.001, 0.01, 0.1 or 0.2 mg/mL	SH-SY5Y cells	MPP⁻ induced	↓ROS production, ↓Bax/Bcl-2 ratio, ↓activation of caspase-3	[45 - 47]
		Root	Ginsenoside Rg1	0.1-10 μM	PC12 cells	H_2O_2 induced	↓DA-induced apoptosis by suppressing oxidative stress and NF-κB activation	-
			Ginsenoside Rb1	---	SH-SY5Y cells	6-OHDA induced	Induction of NrF2 nuclear translocation and PI3K activation	-
Panax notoginseng (Burkill) F.H.Chen	Araliaceae	Root	Ethanolic extract	25, 50 and 100 μg/ml	N9 and EOC20 microglial cell lines	*In-vitro*	↓Production of inflammatory mediators (IL-6 and TNF-α) ↓NO	[75, 77]
			Panaxatriol saponins	0.5 mg/ml	PC12 cells	MPP⁺ induce	Induce thioredoxin-I	-
Polygala tenuifolia Willd.	Polygalaceae	Root	Aqueous extract	0.5-1 μg/ml	PC12 cells	6-OHDA induced	↓ROS, ↓NO, ↓Caspase-3 activity	[78, 79]
			Tenuigenin	1.0-10 μM	SH-SY5Y cells	6-OHDA induced	↓Caspase-3 activity, ↑TH, ↑SOD,	-
Polygonum cuspidatum Willd. ex Spreng.	Polygonaceae	Rhizome	Resveratrol	12.5, 25, and 50 μM	SH-SY5Y cells	Rotenone induced	↑degradation of α-synucleins	[48, 49, 80, 81]
			Resveratrol and Quercetin	----	PC12 cells	MPP+ induced	↑mRNA level	-
			Naphthoquinone, 2-methox-6acetyl-7-methyljuglone	2.5 μM	PC12 cells	Tert-butyl hydroperoxide induced	Induce the phosphorylation of ERK 1/2, JNK, and p38 MAPK,	-
			Pinostilbene	1-10 μM	SH-SY5Y cells	6-OHDA induced	↓Phosphorylation of JNK and c-jun	-
Psoralea corylifolia L.	Leguminosae	Seed	Petroleum ether extract	0.1, 1 and 10 μg/ml	SK-N-SH cell line	MPP+ induced	The extract has inhibitory effects on the DA transporter and NA transporter.	[82]
				1, 10 and 100 μg/ml	D8 cell line			
Pueraria lobata (Willd.) Ohwi	Fabaceae	Root	Puerarin	50 μM	SH-SY5Y cells	MPP+ induced	Activate PI3K/Akt pathway	[83]
				50 μM	PC12 cells	MPP+ induced	Inhibit the activation of caspase-9 and caspase-3	
Pueraria thomsonii Benth.	Fabaceae	Root	Daidzein and genistein	100 μM	PC12 cells	6-OHDA induced	Inhibit caspase-8 and partially inhibit caspase-3 activation	[84]
Rehmannia glutinosa (Gaertn.) DC.	Plantaginaceae	Root	Catalpol	----	PC12 cells	LPS induced	↓ROS, ↓ LPS-induced the expression of iNOS	[85]
Rhodiola crenulata (Hook. f. & Thomson) H.Ohba and Rhodiola rosea L.	Crassulaceae	Root	Salidroside	1, 10 and 30 μM	PC12 cells	MPP+ induced	inhibiting the NO pathway and activating PI3K/Akt pathway	[86]
Salvia miltiorrhiza Bunge	Lamiaceae	Root	Salvianic acid B	0.1–10 μM	SH-SY5Y cells	6-OHDA induced	↓Caspase-3 activity, ↓ cytochrome C translocation into the cytosol from mitochondria	[87 - 89]
				10-100 μM	SH-SY5Y cells	MPP⁻-induced	↓Caspase-3 activity, ↓ Ros ↓Bax/Bcl-2 ratio	-
				0.1-10 μM	PC12 cells	H_2O_2 induced	↓ intracellular Ca^{2+} elevation and ↓caspase-3	-
Schisandra chinensis (Turcz.) Baill.	Schisandraceae	Fruit	Schisantherin A	---	SH-SY5Y cells	MPP⁺ induced	↑CREB-mediated Bcl-2 expression and activating PI3K/Akt survival signalling	[90]

(Table 2) cont.....

Plant Name	Family	Part Used	Extract/Fraction/Compound	Dose	*In-vitro*	Experimental Models	Result	References
Scutellaria baicalensis Georgi	Lamiaceae	Root	Baicalein	0.05, 0.5 and 5 µg/mL	PC12 cells	6-OHDA	↓ROS, ↑ mitochondrial membrane potential, ↓ caspase-3/7 activation	[91, 92]
				10-50 µM	HT22 murine hippocampal neuronal cells	TG and BFA induced cell death	↓ROS and C/EBP homologous protein induction	-
Thuja orientalis L.	Cupressaceae	Leaf	Ethanolic extract	10 µg/mL	SH-SY5Y cells	6-OHDA induced	↓ROS	[93]
Toxicodendron vernicifluum (Stokes) F.A.Barkley	Anacardiaceae	Leaf	Extract	---	SH-SY5Y cells	Rotenone induced	↑TH level	[94]
Uncaria rhynchophylla (Miq.) Miq. ex Havil.	Rubiaceae	Hook	Aqueous extract	0.1, 0.5 and 1.0 µg	PC12 cells	6-OHDA induced	↑GSH, ↓ROS, and inhibited caspase-3 activity	[95]
Valeriana jatamansi Jones	Caprifoliaceae	Roots	Bakkenolidesvalerilactones A (1), and B (2), and two known analogues, bakkenolide-H (3)	-	SH-SY5Y cells	MPP⁺-induced neuronal cell death	↓NO production	[50]
Valeriana offcinalis subsp. collina (Wallr.) Nyman	Caprifoliaceae	-	Aqueous extract	0.049, 0.098 and 0.195 mg/mL	SH-SY5Y cells	Rotenone induced	↓NO production, ↑Cell viability	[96]

PD: Parkinson's disease; CAT: Catalase; DA: Dopamine, H_2O_2: Hydrogen peroxide; LPS: Lipopolysaccharide; NO: Nitrogen Monoxide; iNOS: inducible Nitric Oxide Synthase; ROS: Reactive Oxygen Species; MPTP: 1-Methyl-4-phenyl-1,2,3,6-tetrahydropyridine; NA: Noradrenaline; NF-κB: Nuclear factor-κB; 6- OHDA: 6-Hydroxydopamine; MPP⁺: 1-methyl-4-phenyl-pyridinium iodide; PI3K: Phosphoinositide 3-kinase; TH: Tyrosine hydroxylase; DAT: Dopamine transporter; MAO-B: Monoamine oxidase B; MDA: Malondialdehyde; SNpc: Substantia nigra pars compacta; SOD: Superoxide dismutase; GSH-Px: Glutathione Peroxidase; BFA: Brefeldin A; COX: Cyclooxygenase; CHOP: C/EBP Homologous Protein; PRAP: Poly (ADP-ribose) Polymerase; PI: Propidium Iodide; TG: Thapsigargin; MAPK: Mitogen Activated Protein Kinase; LDH: Lactate Dehydrogenase; LPO: Lipid Peroxidation ; CTG: Cistanche Total Glycosides; T-AOC: Total Antioxidant Capacity; GFAP: Glial Fibrillary Acidic Protein; P53: Tumor protein p53; EGCG: Epigallocatechin gallate; ECG: (−)-epicatechin-3-gallate; EGC: (−)-epigallocatechin; EC: (−)-epicatechin; GT: Green Tea; BT: Black Tea; *EGb 761*: Extract of *Ginkgo biloba* 761; PC12: Pheochromocytoma 12.

K3R and AYB, two bioactive compounds obtained from *Carthamus tinctorius* belonging to the *Asteraceae* family, at 1 µM increased cell viability on PC12 cells by Bind DJ-1 and decreased the H_2O_2-induced ROS levels [36]. Ripe seed ethanol extract of *Cassia obtusifolia* inhibited ROS overproduction, glutathione depletion, mitochondrial membrane depolarization, and caspase-3 activation in PC-12 cells at 0.1-10 µg/ml [37]. Acetosoide isolated from *Cistanche deserticola* at a dose of 10, 20 and 40 mg/l inhibited α-Synuclein protein aggregation in the brain [38]; tubuloside-B also obtained from its stem decreased ROS production and attenuated DNA fragmentation in PC12 cell against MPP⁺ induced Parkinson [39]. EGb 761, a standardized extract from *Ginkgo biloba*, at a dose of 10, 20, and 40 µg/ml, decreased caspase-3 activation in PC-12 cells against paraquat-induced PD [40]. *Hypericum perforatum* aerial part methanolic extract at 10-100 µg/ml decreased ROS level in PC-12 cells [41], as well as hyperoside isolated from the ethylacetate fraction, and at 10-180 µg/ml raised cell viability against hydrogen peroxide-induced PD [42].

Magnolol isolated from *Magnolia officinalis* stem bark at 30 mg/kg inhibited ROS production in SH-SY5Y cells [43]. *Morus alba* fruits ethanolic extract at 70% exerted antioxidant and antiapoptotic effects in SH-SY5Y cells against MPP+ induced PD at a dose of 1, 10, and 100 µg/ml [44]. Paeoniflorin, a bioactive compound isolated from *Paeonia lactiflora* roots, increased Hats, H3K9ac, and H3K27ac expression of Histone H3 [45]. *Panax ginseng* aqueous extract from rhizomes at 0.001, 0.01, 0.1 or 0.2 mg/ml decreased ROS production, Bax/Bcl-2 ratio and caspase-3 expression [46]. Ginsenoside Rg1, a bioactive compound isolated from *Panax ginseng* roots at a dose of 0.1-10 µM, increased cell viability by inhibiting apoptosis and oxidative stress and inhibiting NF-κB activation [47]. Resveratrol isolated from *Polygonum cuspidatum* rhizomes increased α-synucleins degradation in SH-SY5Y cells and PC-12 cells at a dose of 12.5, 25, and 50 µM [48]. Napthaquinone, 2-methoxy-6-acetyl-7methyljuglone is another compound isolated from *P. cuspidatum* that increases PC12 cell viability by inhibiting apoptotic pathways and increasing the level of antioxidant enzymes at 2.5 µM [49]. *Uncaria rhynchophylla* aqueous extract at 0.1, 0.5 and 1.0 µg also decreased ROS and caspase-3 activity in PC-12 cells [50].

Most aforesaid studies examined the effect of extracts, fractions, and their active compounds on SOD, GSH, CAT, DA, LDH, TH, and ROS levels; Bax/Bcl-2 ratio; caspase-3 activity; α-synuclein protein aggregation, mitochondrial activity, and NF-κB activity.

In-vivo Studies

Based on the outcomes from *in-vitro* reports, a few potent anti-PD botanicals were further subjected to *in-vivo* studies by using various neurotoxin and drug-induced anti-PD models, like 6-OHDA, rotenone, MPP+, MPTP, haloperidol, and reserpine (Table **3**). *Acanthopanax senticosus* root and rhizome ethanolic extract at 80%, at doses of 182 and 45.5 mg/kg increased DA level in C57BL/6 mice, while 100% and 50% ethanol extract and hot water extract at 250 mg/kg also raised the DA level in Male rat of Lewis strain. Sesamin isolated from *A. senticosus* stem bark increased DA levels at 3 and 30 mg/kg in male rats [97]. *Alpinia oxyphylla* ripe seed ethanol extract at 80% decreased IL-1β, TNF-α, and NO levels and activated the PI3K-AKT pathway in zebrafish [97]. Standard extract of *Bacopa monnieri* at 200 mg/kg decreased NOS, MDA and HP levels in the paraquat-induced mice model; its acetone extract at 0.25, 0.50 and 1.0 µl/ml and standardized extract at 0.01, 0.025, 0.05, and 0.1% decreased NOS, MDA, HP, and oxidative stress levels and apoptosis in *Drosophila melanogaster*.

Concentrated mother tincture of *B. monnieri* decreased α-synuclein aggregation and prevented dopaminergic neurodegeneration in the NL5901 strain of *Caenorhabditis elegans* of nematodes [98].

EGCG, a bioactive compound obtained from *Camellia sinensis* leaves, reduced NOS levels at 25 mg/kg and increased TH, DA, HVA, and 3,4-dihydroxyphenylacetic acid [98]. Flavonoid-rich dried flower petals extract of *Carthamus tinctorius* at 70 mg/kg in SD rats reduced α-synuclein aggregation and suppressed reactive astrogliosis [99 - 101]. Ripe seeds ethanol extract of *Cassia obtusifolia* at 50 mg/kg increased DA, GSH levels and decreased ROS levels in C57BL/6 mice [97]. CTG (100, 200, 400 mg/kg) and acetoside (30 mg/kg) isolated from *Cistanche deserticola* stem increased TH and DA levels in SD rat and C57BL/6 mice [95]. *Eucommia almoidea* bark at 100, 300, and 600 mg/kg increased DA, DOPAC, and HVA levels in mice [68]. Geniposide isolated from fruits of *Gardenia jasminoides* at 100 mg/kg in mice increased TH and decreased Bcl-2 and caspase-3 [71]. EGb 761, a bioactive compound from *Ginkgo biloba* leaves at 50, 100, and 150 mg/kg in rats, augmented the level of antioxidants enzymes and reduced the level of thiobarbituric acid reactive substances (TBARS) [97]. The methanol extract from *Hypericum perforatum* aerial part at 300 mg/kg inhibited MAO-B activity and reduced astrocytes activation in the striatal area in swiss albino mice; the standardized extract at 4 mg/kg increased antioxidant enzymes levels and decreased MDA level [97]. Fucoidan, a sulfated polysaccharide from *Laminaria japonica* seaweeds, augmented the level of antioxidant enzymes and decreased the level of LPO at 12.5 and 25 mg/kg in C57BL/6 mice [102]. Magnolol isolated from *Magnolia officinalis* bark at 30 mg/kg inhibited MAO-B and decreased the level of ROS and TBARS while increasing the AKT phosphorylation in C57BL/6 mice [43]. *Morus alba* fruits ethanol extract at 70%, at 500 mg/kg decreased NO, ROS and Bcl-2, and caspase-3 levels [97]. Paeoniflorin isolated from *Paeonia lactiflora* roots inhibited neuroinflammation by activating A1AR (adenosine A1 receptor) in mice and SD rats [97]. Ginseng extract G115 in SD rats at 100 mg/kg suppressed oxidative stress and blocked JNK signalling activation and protected dopaminergic neurons [97]. Ginsenoside Re isolated from *Panax ginseng,* at 6.5, 13, and 26 mg/kg in mice decreased Bax, Bax mRNA and iNOS expression and caspase-3 activation. Aqueous extract from *P. ginseng* at 37.5, 75 and 150 mg/kg in C57BL/6 mice led to inhibition of MAPKs and NF-κB pathways [103].

Table 3. Medicinal plants tested *in-vivo* for anti-PD activity.

Plant Name	Family	Part Used	Extract/Fraction/Compound	Dose	*in-vivo*	Experimental Models	Mechanism of Action	Reference
Acanthopanax senticosus (Rupr. et Maxim) Harms	Araliaceae	Roots and rhizomes	80% ethanolic extract	182, 45.5 mg/kg	C57BL/6 mice	MPTP induced	↑ DA	[112]
		Stem bark	100% ethanol, 50% ethanol, and hot water	250 mg/kg	Male rats of the Lewis strain	MPTP induced	↑DA	
		Stem bark	Sesamin	3, 30 mg/kg	Male rats of the Lewis strain	Rotenone-induced	↑DA	
Albizia adianthifolia (Schum.) W. Wight	Leguminosae	Leaves	Aqueous extract	150, 300 mg/kg	Male Wistar rats	6-OHDA induced	↑SOD, GPX, and GSH ↓MDA and protein carbonyl	[97]
Allium sativum L.	Amaryllidaceae	Cloves	Ethanol extract	200, 400 mg/kg	Female Swiss Albino Mice	Haloperidol induced	↑ SOD, GPX, and GSH	[113 - 115]
		---	S-allylcysteine	120 mg/kg	Mice	MPTP induced	↓TNF-α, iNOS, GFAP, ↑DA	-
				125 mg/kg	C57BL/6J mice	MPP⁺ induced	↑DA, LPO	-
Aloe arborescens Mill.	Xanthorrhoeaceae	Fresh Leaves	Gel	200 mg/kg	Rat	Copper induced	DA	[116]
Alpinia oxyphylla Miq.	Zingiberaceae	Ripe seeds	80% ethanolic extract	--	Zebrafish	6-OHDA induced	↓IL-1β, TNF-α, NO activation of PI3K/AKT pathway	[112]
		--	Protocatechuic acid	--	C58BL/6J mice	MPTP induced	DA	
Alternanthera sesilis (L.) R.Br. ex DC.	Amaranthaceae	Whole plant	Ethanolic extract	200 mg/kg	Male Wistar albino rat	Rotenone induced	↑GSH, ↓ LPO	[117]
Bacopa monnieri (L.) Wettst.	Plantaginaceae	--	Concentrated mother tincture	50 μM	NL5901 strain of *Caenorhabditis elegans*	6-OHDA induced	↓α-synuclein aggregation prevents dopaminergic neurodegeneration restores the lipid content in nematodes	[118]
		---	Standard extract	200 mg/kg	Mice	Paraquat-induced	↓NOS, MDA, HP	-
		---	Standard extract	---	Mice	Rotenone induced	↓NOS, MDA, HP	-
		Leaf	Acetone extract	0.25, 0.50 and 1.0 μl/ml	*Drosophila melanogaster*	Rotenone model	↓Oxidative stress and apoptosis	-
		--	standardized extract	0.01, 0.025, 0.05 and 0.1%	*Drosophila melanogaster*	Rotenone model	↓NOS, MDA, HP	-
		Whole plant	--	40 mg/kg	Swiss albino mice	MPTP model	↑TH, caspase-3 and expression of neurogenic gene in the SN	-
		Whole plant	Ethanolic extract	180 mg/kg	Rat	Rotenone Induced Model	↓ Glutamine content, GDH and GS ↑Glutaminase	-
Berberis aristata DC.	Berberidaceae	Roots	Methanolic extract	100, 300 and 500 mg/kg	Sprague dawley rats Rat	6-OHDA	↑SOD, CAT, GSH, and total thiol ↓LPO	[98]
Beta vulgaris L.	Amaranthaceae	Leaves	Methanolic extract	100, 200 and 300 mg/kg	Wistar Rats	Reserpine, Haloperidol and tacrine induced	↑SOD, CAT ↓LPO	[119]
Bougainvillea spectabilis Willd.	Nyctaginaceae	Flower	Methanolic extract	25 and 50 mg/kg	SD Rat	Rotenone induced	↓LPO, inhibit (butyrylcholinesterase) BChE, (paraoxonase-1) PON-1 activity and increased brain Il-1β	[120]
Brassica oleracea L.	Brassicaceae	Powder	Hydroalcoholic extract	250 and 500 mg/kg	Wistar albino rats	Haloperidol induced	↑GSH and ↓LPO	[121]
Camellia sinensis (L.) Kuntze	Theaceae	Leaves	GTP	-	Rat	6-OHDA induced	Inhibition of ROS-NO pathway	[118]
		Leaves	EGCG	25 mg/kg	C57B6 mice	MPTP induced	↓NOS expression ↑TH, DA, HVA, 3,4-dihydroxyphenylacetic acid	-
Carthamus tinctorius L.	Compositae	Dried flower petals	Flavonoid extract	70 mg/kg	SD Rat	MPTP and 6-OHDA induced	↓α-synuclein aggregation, suppression of reactive astrogliosis	[122]

(Table 3) cont.....

Plant Name	Family	Part Used	Extract/Fraction/Compound	Dose	*in-vivo*	Experimental Models	Mechanism of Action	Reference
Cassia obtusifolia L.	Leguminosae	Ripe seed	Ethanolic extract	50 mg/kg	C57BL/6Mice	MPTP and 6-OHDA induced	↑ DA, GSH, ↓ROS	[112]
Chaenomeles speciosa (Sweet) Nakai	Rosaceae	Dried fruit	Aqueous extract	0.5 gm/kg	SD Rat	6-OHDA induced	Inhibit DAT, ↑DA	[99]
					C57BL/6 Mice	MPTP induced		
Cistanche deserticola Y.C.Ma	Orobanchaceae	Stem	CTG	100, 200 and 400 mg/kg	C57BL/6 Mice	MPTP induced	↑TH and nigral dopaminergic neurons	[112]
			Acetoside	30 mg/kg				
Cistanche salsa (C.A.Mey.) Beck		Stem	Echinacoside	30 mg/kg	C57Bl/6 Mice	MPTP induced	↑expression of GDNF and BDNF mRNA and protein inducer of NTFs and inhibitor of apoptosis	-
				3.5 and 7.0 mg/kg	Wistar rat	6-OHDA induced	↑DA, DOPAC, and HVA	-
Citrus	Rutaceae	Peel, seed	Tangerine peel, grape seeds, cocoa, and red clover	35, 100, 100 and 200 mg/kg	Rat	6-OHDA induced	↑DA, DOPAC, and HVA	[123]
Combretum leprosum Mart.	Combretaceae	Flower	Ethanolic extract	100 mg/kg	C57Bl/6	MPTP induced	↑DA	[124]
Crocus sativus L.	Iridaceae	Fruit and flower	----	0.01% w/v	BALB/c mice	MPTP model	Protect dopaminergic cells of SN and retina	[125]
			Crocetin	25, 50 and 75 μg/kg	Wistar rats	6-OHDA Model	↑GSH, DA ↓TBARS	
Cynodon dactylon (L.) Pers.	Poaceae	Whole plant	Aqueous extract	150 and 300 mg/kg	Rat	Rotenone induced	↑GSH, SOD, and CAT ↓TBARS, MDA, and NO	[112]
					Swiss albino mice	Reserpine induced		
Decalepis hamiltonii Wight &Arn.	Apocynaceae	Root	Aqueous extract	0.1%, 0.5% w/v	Flies	Ethanol-induced toxicity	↓ROS, LPO ↑SOD, CAT	[126]
Dimocarpus longan Lour.	Sapindaceae	Flower	Aqueous extract	125-500 mg/kg	Rat	MPP⁺ induced	Antioxidant, anti-inflammatory, and anti-apoptotic activity	[127]
Elaeocarpus ganitrus Roxb. ex G.Don	*Elaeocarpaceae*	Seed	Ethanolic extract	200 and 400 mg/kg	Mice	Haloperidol induced	↓MDA, ↑GSH	[128]
Eucommia almoidea Oliv.	*Eucommiaceae*	Bark	Ethanolic extract	100, 300 and 600 mg/kg	Mice	MPTP induced	↑DA, DOPAC, HVA	[68]
Evolvulus alsinoides (L.) L.	Convolvulaceae	Root	Methanolic extract	200,400mg/kg	Rat	Reserpine induced	↓ROS, LPO ↑SOD, CAT	[129]
Ficus religiosa L.	Moraceae	Leaves	Petroleum ether extract	100, 200, and 400 mg/kg	Wistar rat	Haloperidol and 6-OHDA induced	↓MDA, ↑SOD, CAT, and GSH	[130]
Gardenia jasminoides J. Ellis	Rubiaceae	Fruit	Geniposide	100 mg/kg	Mice	MPTP induced	↑TH, Bax, ↓Bcl-2, Caspase 3 (enhancing growth factor signalling and the reduction of apoptosis)	[70]
Ginkgo biloba L	Ginkgoaceae	Leaves	EGb 761	50, 100, and 150 mg/kg EGb	Rat	6-OHDA induced	↑GSH, SOD, GPX, CAT ↓TBARS	-
Gynostemma pentaphyllum (Thunb.) Makino	Cucurbitaceae	Whole herb	Ethanolic extract	10, 30 mg/kg	Rat	6-OHDA induced	↑DA, DOPAC, HVA, NA	[112]
		Whole herb	Gypenosides	100, 200 mg/kg	C57BL/6 Mice	MPTP induced	↑GSH, SOD, GPX	-
Hyoscyamus niger L.	Solanaceae	Seeds	Methanolic extract	125-500 mg/kg	Rat	Rotenone induced	↑GPX, SOD, AND CAT ↓TBARS	[131]
Hypericum perforatum L.	Hypericaceae	Aerial part	Methanolic extract	300 mg/kg	Swiss albino mice	MPTP induced	Inhibit monoamine oxidase-B (MAO-B) and reduce astrocyte activation in striatal area induced by MPTP	[112]
		---	Standardized extract of *Hypericum perforatum* (SHP)	4 mg/kg	albino rats	Rotenone induced	↑GSH, SOD, GPX ↓MDA,	-
Juniperus communis L.	Cupressaceae	Leave	Methanolic extract	100, 200 mg/kg	Wistar rats	Chlorpromazine induced	↑GSH, total protein ↓TBARS, nitrate	[132]
						Reserpine induced		
Laminaria japonica	Laminariaceae	Seaweed	Fucoidan	12.5, 25 mg/kg	C57BL/6 mice	MPTP induced	↑GSH, SOD, GPX, CAT ↓LPO	[133]

(Table 3) cont.....

Plant Name	Family	Part Used	Extract/Fraction/Compound	Dose	*in-vivo*	Experimental Models	Mechanism of Action	Reference
*Leucas lanata*Benth.	Lamiaceae	Whole plant	Ethyl acetate fraction of ethanolic extract	100, 200 and 300 mg/kg	Mice	Rotenone induced	↓α-synuclein aggregation and free radicals' production	[102]
Ligusticum chuanxiong S.H. Qiu	Apiaceae	Rhizome	Tetramethylpyrazine	--	Mice	MPTP induced	↑Dopaminergic neurons and the neurite length	[112]
Lomatia oblique (Ruiz & Pav.) R. Br.	Proteaceae	---	Naphthazarin	---	Mice	MPTP induced	suppression of astroglial activation	[134]
Magnolia officinalis Rehder&E.H.Wilson	Magnoliaceae	Bark	Magnolol	30 mg/kg	C57BL/6 mice	MPTP and 6-OHDA induced	Inhibit monoamine oxidase-B (MAO-B), ↑Akt phosphorylation, ↓ROS, TBARS	[135]
Morus alba L.	Moraceae	Fruit	70% ethanol extract	500 mg/kg	C57BL/6 mice	MPTP induced	Block ROS and NO generation, regulate Bcl-2 family protein, stabilize mitochondrial membrane and inhibit caspase-3	[112]
Mucunapruriens (L.) DC.	Fabaceae	Cotyledon	Powder	100 mg/kg	Rat	6-OHDA induced	↑DA, NA and serotonin, ↑Brain mitochondrial-I complex activity	[118]
		Seed + estrogen	Ethanolic extract	100 mg/kg	Swiss albino mice	MPTP induced	↑DA, DOPAC, HVA	-
Murrayakoenigii(L.) Spreng.	Rutaceae	Leaf	Methanolic extract	30,100,200 mg/kg	Albino Mice	Reserpine induced	↑SOD, GSH, CAT ↓LPO	[135]
				100 and 300 mg/kg	Rat	Haloperidol induced		
Nardosta chysjatamansi (D.Don) DC.	Caprifoliaceae	Root	Ethanolic extract	200, 400, and 600 mg/kg	Rat	6-OHDA induced	↑GSH, SOD, TH-IR fibers in the ipsilateral striatum	[135]
Nigella sativa L.	Ranunculaceae	Seed	Thymoquinone	5, 10 mg/kg	Wistar Rat	6-OHDA induced	↓MDA, NO ↑SOD	[103]
Ocimum sanctum Linn	Lamiaceae	Leaves	Ethanolic extract	1.75, 4.25 and 8.5 mg/kg	Albino Mice	Haloperidol induced	↑DA	[135]
			Hydroalcoholic extract	100, 200 mg/kg	Wistar Rat	Rotenone induced	↓MDA, ↑SOD, GSH	-
			Aqueous extract	100, 200, 300 and 600 mg/kg		Haloepridol induced	↑DA	-
Paeonia lactiflora Pall.	Paeoniaceae	Root	Paeoniflorin	2.5 and 5 mg kg	Mice	6-OHDA induced	Inhibit neuroinflammation by A1AR activation	[112]
		Root	Paeoniflorin	2.5, 5 and 10 mg/kg	SD Rat	6-OHDA induced		
Panax ginseng C. A. Mey.	Araliaceae	Root	Ginseng extract G115	100 mg/kg	SD Rat	*β*-sitosterol *β*-D-glucoside (BSSG) induced	Suppress oxidative stress and block JNK signaling activation, activate insulin-like growth factor receptors	[112, 135]
		Root	Aqueous extract (KRGE)	37.5, 75 and 150 mg/kg	C57BL/6J mice	MPTP induced	Activate Nrf2 pathway, inhibit MAPKs and NF-kB pathways, and maintains BBB integrity	-
		Root	Ginsenoside Re	6.5, 13, 26 mg kg	Mice	MPTP induced	↑ Bcl-2 protein and Bcl-2 mRNA, ↓ Bax, Bax mRNA, and iNOS, inhibit caspase-3	-
		Root	Ginsenoside Rg1	2.5, 5.0 and 10.0 mg/kg	C57B1 male mice	MPTP induced	↑Bcl-2 and Bcl-xl, ↓Bax and iNOS, and inhibit caspase-3	-
				5mg/kg	C57BL6 mice		↑DA, TH, FP1 expression, and ↓DMT1 expression in the SN.	-
		Root	Ginsenoside Rg1	10 mg/kg	Wistar rats	6-OHDA induced	↑Bcl-2 protein expression Activation of the IGF-IR signalling pathway	-
Panax notoginseng (Burkill) F.H.Chen		Root	Panaxatriol saponin	100 mg/kg	Kunming mice	MPTP induced	↑Trx1 expression, ↓ COX-2 and inhibit mitochondria-mediated apoptosis pathway	-
Passiflora incarnata L.	Passifloraceae	Flowers	n-butanol	150 and 300 mg/kg	SD rat	Haloperoidol induced	-	[136]

(Table 3) cont.....

Plant Name	Family	Part Used	Extract/Fraction/Compound	Dose	*in-vivo*	Experimental Models	Mechanism of Action	Reference
Piper longum L.	Piperaceae	Seed	Piperine and piperlonguminine alkaloids	30, 60, and 120 mg/kg	C57BL/6 mice	MPTP induced	↑DA, DOPAC, GSH, SOD, ↓MDA	[137]
Plumbago scandens L.	Plumbaginaceae	whole plant	Ethanol extract and total acetate fraction	500,1000 and 2000 mg/kg	Swiss albino mice	Tremorine induced tremors	↑DA	[135]
Portulaca oleracea L.	Portulaceae	Weed	Purslane aqueous juice	1.5 mL/Kg	Rat	Rotenone induced	↑DA	[135]
Polygonum cuspidatum Siebold &Zucc.	Polygonaceae	Rhizome	Resveratrol	20 mg/kg	Wistar rats	6-OHDA induced	↑ T-AOC, DA, ↓ROS	[135]
			Resveratrol	10, 20, or 40 mg/kg	SD rat	6-OHDA model	↓COX-2 and TNF-α mRNA	-
Pueraria lobate (Willd.) Ohwi	Leguminosae	Root	Puerarin	0.12 mg/kg	Rat	6-OHDA model	↑DA, TH, ↓Bax	[112]
Scutellaria baicalensis Georgi	Lamiaceae	Root	Baicalein	0.05, 0.5, 5 µg/mL	Rat	6-OHDA induced	↑Th, GFAP	[112]
		Root	Baicalein	280 and 560 mg/kg	C57BL/6Mice	MPTP induced	↑DA	-
Selaginella delicatula (Desv. ex Poir.) Alston	Selaginellaceae	Whole plant	Aqueous extract	100 mg/kg	Drosophila melanogaster	Rotenone induced	↑ mitochondrial electron transport chain enzymes (complex I/II)	[135]
Sida cordifolia L.	Malvaceae	Whole plant	Aqueous extract	50, 100, 250 mg/kg	SD Rat	Rotenone induced	↑GSH, CAT ↓TBARS, SAG	[138]
Stereospermum suaveolens (Roxb.) DC.	Bignoniaceae	Stem barks	Methanolic extract	125, 250 and 500 mg/kg	SD Rat	6-OHDA induced	↑SOD, CAT, GSH, total thiol, ↓LPO	[139]
Tinospora cordifolia Willd.	Menispermaceae	Aerial Part	Ethanolic extract	200 and 400 mg/kg	Rat	6-OHDA induced	↑DA, mitochondrial complex-I activity	[140, 141]
Trifolium pratenseL.	Leguminosae	--	--	200 mg/kg	SD Rat	6-OHDA induced	↑DA, DOPAC, HVA	[135]
Tripterygium wilfordii Hook. F.	Celastraceae	Root	Triptolide	---	Rat	MPP⁺ induced	inhibit microglial activation, ↑DA	[142]
Uncaria rhynchophylla (Miq.) Miq. ex Havil.	Rubiaceae	Hook	Aqueous extract	5 mg/kg	Rat	6-OHDA induced	↑GSH, DA, ↓ROS and inhibit caspase-3	[95]
Vitis vinifera L.	Vitaceae	Fruit	Fruit Juice	50% GJ	Wistar Rat	6-OHDA induced	↑SOD, CAT, GSH, ↓LPO	[143]
Withania somnifera (L.) Dunal	Solanaceae	Root	Ethanolic extract	---	Rat	Paraquat induced	↑SOD, CAT ↓TBARS, ROS, MDA, HP, LPO	[118, 144]
			Powder	100-400 mg/ kg	Mice	Rotenone induced		
			Extract	100, 200 and 300 mg/kg	Rat Albino mice	6-OHDA induced MPTP induced		
			Aqueous extract	100 mg/kg	Mice	----		

PD: Parkinson's disease; CAT: Catalase; DA: Dopamine, H_2O_2: Hydrogen peroxide; LPS: Lipopolysaccharide; NO: Nitrogen Monoxide; iNOS: inducible Nitric Oxide Synthase; ROS:Reactive Oxygen Species; MPTP: 1-Methyl-4-phenyl-1,2,3,6-tetrahydropyridine; NA: Noradrenaline; NF-κB: Nnuclear factor-κB; 6-OHDA: 6-Hydroxydopamine; MPP⁺: 1-methyl-4-phenyl-pyridinium iodide; PI3K: Phosphoinositide 3-kinase; TH:Tyrosine hydroxylase; DAT: Dopamine transporter; MAO-B: Monoamine oxidase B; MDA: Malondialdehyde; SNpc: Substantia nigra pars compacta; SOD: Superoxide dismutase; GSH-Px: Glutathione Peroxidase; BFA: Brefeldin A; COX:Cyclooxygenase; CHOP: C/EBP Homologous Protein; PRAP: Poly (ADP-ribose) Polymerase; PI: Propidium Iodide; TG: Thapsigargin; MAPK: Mitogen Activated Protein Kinase; LDH: Lactate Dehydrogenase; LPO: Lipid Peroxidation ; CTG: Cistanche Total Glycosides; T-AOC: Total Antioxidant Capacity; GFAP: Glial Fibrillary Acidic Protein; P53: Tumor protein *p53;* EGCG: Epigallocatechin gallate; ECG: (−)-epicatechin-3-gallate; EGC: (−)-epigallocatechin; EC: (−)-epicatechin; GT: Green Tea; BT: Black Tea; *EGb 761*: Extract of *Ginkgo biloba* 761; GJ: Grape Juice; K3R: kaempferol 3-O-beta-rutinoside 6-hydroxykaempferol 3,6-di-O-beta-D-glucoside.

Resveratrol isolated from *Polygonum cuspidatum* rhizomes at 10, 20, and 40 mg/kg reduced COX-2, TNF-α mRNA, and ROS and raised DA and T-AOC levels [103]. Aqueous extract from *Uncaria rhyncphophylla* hooks increased GSH and DA levels and decreased ROS level and caspase-3 activity [50].

Several plant extracts are being investigated for their potential against drug-induced PD in animal models, *viz. Allium sativum, Brassica oleracea, Ficus religiosa, Ocimum sanctum,* and *Passiflora incarnata* against haloperidol-induced PD; *Cynodon dactylon, Evolvulu salsinoides, Elaecocarpus ganitrus* against reserpine-induced PD; *Beta vulgaris, Murraya koenigii* against haloperidol- and reserpine-induced PD and *Juniperus communis* against reserpine- and chlorpromazine-induced PD.

Recent experimental studies on herbal medicines have been consistent with their ancient and traditional uses in PD. Most of the plants studied belong to Leguminosae, Rutaceae, Fabaceae, and Araliaceae families. Very few clinical reports assessing the effect of herbal medicines against PD are available, as detailed in Table **4**. The current chapter outlines various *in-vivo, in-vitro,* and clinical evidence which indicates that the number of Chinese and Indian herbs possess significant anti-PD efficacy and rejuvenating effects, thus imperative to provide a better quality of life in geriatric patients. They possess multiple target actions and mechanisms obliterating the complex pathology of PD. Available reports indicate that oxidative stress, mitochondrial membrane dysfunction, and the formation of Lewy bodies are the common key culprit for PD [104 - 107].

Table 4. Randomized controlled clinical trials using herbal medicines against PD.

Plant/Extract/ Compounds	N° of Patients	Effect	Reference
Mucuna pruriens	18	Produce anti-PD effect with fewer dyskinesias and adverse effects	[145, 146]
Bu Shen Ping Chan Fang	52 (M31/F21)	UPDRS, Clinical symptoms, Adverse effect	
Zi Yin Xi Feng HuoXue Tang	20 (M11/F9)	UPDRS, Tremble function	
Zi Bu Gan Shen	40 (M26/F14)	UPDRSII, III, Webster scale	
Pa Bing I Hao	22 (M18/F4)	UPDRS	
Jun Fu Kang Jiao	14 (M8/F6)	UPDRS, Adverse effect, Clinical symptom	[147 - 149]
Xi Feng Ding Chan	20 (M12/F8)	UPDRS	
Ding Zhen Tang	34 (M23/F11)	UPDRS	
Gui Ling Pa An Jiao Nang	75 (M46/F29)	UPDRSII, III, total; Levodopa dosage, Clinical effect	
Jia Wei Liu Jun Zi Tang	22 (M14/F8)	PDQ-39; UPDRS; GDS; SF-36; DSQS	
Bu Shen HuoXue	45 (M29/F26)	UPDRS III; Movement experiment; 10 m re-entry run, Muscular tension	

(Table 4) cont.....

Plant/Extract/ Compounds	N° of Patients	Effect	Reference
Jia Wei Liu Jun Zi Tang (JWLJZT)	55 patients	Relieve some non-motor conventional drugs complications and raise communication ability	[150]
Cannabinoid (CBD) and tetrahydrocannabinol (THC)	119 patients	CBD improved quality of life measures in PD patients without psychiatric comorbidities	[151]

UPDRS: Unified Parkinson's Disease Rating Scale; M: Male; F: Female; PDQ-39: Parkinson's Disease Questionnaire 39; GDS: Geriatric Depression Scale; SF 36: Short-Form-36; DSQS: Deficiency of Splenic Qi Scale.

Most plants have been found to exert their anti-PD potential by enhancing the levels of SOD, GSH, CAT, DA, DOPAC, HVA LPO, and TH; preventing mitochondrial membrane potential; reducing caspase-3, -8, and -9 activity; reducing Bax/Bcl-2 ratio; inhibiting α-synuclein aggregation; attenuating NF-κB activation; and inhibiting NO, iNOS, nNOS, and ROS production. The remaining plants exert mechanisms such as inhibiting the PI3K/AKT pathway; inhibiting PARP proteolysis; reducing c-fos and c-jun expression; decreasing the production of anti-inflammatory mediators, such as IL-6, TNF-α; inhibiting JK and p38 phosphorylation; decreasing the level of p53; reducing the level of TBARS, MDA; decreasing the gene expression level of apoptosis markers; suppressing intracellular Ca^{2+} level and inhibiting MAO-B. In *in-vitro* studies, PC12 cells and SH-SY5Y cells are the most commonly used, while *in-vivo* are C57BL/6 mice and SD rat models [12, 101, 108].

Additionally, it has been observed that herbal therapies are comparatively safer than synthetic chemical agents; therefore, their concomitant use with conventional drugs, *viz.* Levodopa, Carbidopa, or Safinamide should be further explored to find out whether it helps to reduce drug dose and/or frequency of use or whether prevent the common and often severe side effects. Several potent botanicals having proven efficacy in PD are incorporated as an active ingredient in traditional Chinese and Ayurvedic formulations (Table **5**).

Table 5. Chinese and Ayurvedic formulations in the market for PD.

Formulation	Ingredients	Company Name
Chinese Formulations [118, 148]		
Ban xia bai zhu tian ma tang	Pinellia rhizome, Gastrodia rhizome, White atractylodes rhizome, Outermost citrus peel, tangerine peel, and orange peel, Sclerotium of tuckahoe, China Root, poria, hoelen, Licorice root, Fresh ginger rhizome, Fructus *Zizyphi jujubae*	Min Tong Pharmaceutical Co., Ltd.

(Table 5) cont.....

Formulation	Ingredients	Company Name
Si wu-tang	Processed Radix rehmanniae, Radix *Albus paeoniae* lactiflorae, Radix Angelicae sinensis, Rhizoma Ligustici chuanxiong	Bio-essence
Gui bi tang	Radix Ginseng, Radix Astragali Membranacei, *Atractylodes macrocephala*, *Wolfiporia extensa*, Semen Zizyphi Spinosae, Arilluslongan, Radix aucklandiae, Radix Glycyrrhizae, *Angelica sinensis*, Radix Polygalae	Evergreen herbs
Tian ma gouteng yin	Gastrodia Rhizome, Gambir Vine Stems and Thorns, Abalone Shell, Gardenia, Cape Jasmine Fruit, Baical Skullcap Root, Chinese Motherwort, Cyathula Root, Eucommia Bark, Mulberry Mistletoe Stems, Fleece flower Vine, Polygonum Vine, Poria Spirit	Sun Ten Pharmaceutical Co., Ltd.
Da Cheng Qi Tang	Rhubarb Root and Rhizome, Sodium Sulfate, Mirabilite, Glauber's Salt, Immature Fruit of the Bitter Orange, Magnolia Bark	Sun Ten Pharmaceutical Co., Ltd.
Chong paesagan tang	Radix Puerariae, Radix Scutellariae Baicalensis, Rhizoma Ligustici, Semen Raphani, Radix Platycodi, Rhizoma Cimicifugae, Radix Angelicaedahuricae, Rheum palmatum	Korean Sasang Medicine
Jia Wei Liu Jun Zi Tang	The dried root of *Codonopsis pilosula*, Dried root tuber of *Rehmannia glutinosa*Libosch., Dried sclerotium of the fungus, *Poriacocos* (Schw.) Wolf., Dried hook-bearing stem branch of *Uncaria rhynchophylla* (Miq.) Jacks., Rhizome of *Atractylodes macrocephala*Koidz., Dried root of *Angelica sinensis* (Oliv) Diels., the dried tuber of *Pinelliae ternate* (Thunb.) Breit., the Dried rhizome of *Ligusticum chuanxiong* Hort., the dried pericarp of the ripe fruit of *Citrus reticulata* Blanco., Dried root and rhizome of *Glycyrrhiza uralensis* Fisch.	Sun Ten Pharmaceutical Co., Ltd.
BanXiaHouPo Tang	*Pinellia ternate*, *Poriacocos*, *Magnolia obovata*, Thunberg, *Perilla frutescens*, *Zingiber officcinale*	Evergreen Herbs & Medical Supplies
BushenYangganXifeng Decoction	*Radix Rehmanniae*, *Rehmannia glutinosa*, *Uncaria eramulus*, *Paeonia lactiflora*, Radix polygoni Multiflori	Sun Ten Pharmaceutical Co., Ltd.

(Table 5) cont.....

Formulation	Ingredients	Company Name
Chuanxiong Chatiaopulvis	*Ligusticum striatum, Schizonepeta tenuifolia,* Angelica dahurica, *Notopterygii Rhizoma* Et Radix, Radix Glycyrrhizae, Asari Radix Et Rhizoma, *Saposhnikovia*divaricata (Turcz.) Schischk., *Mentha haplocalyx* Briq., Green Tea	nuherbs Co.
Huang-Lian-Jie-Du decoction	*Coptis chinensis* Franch, *Scutellaria baicalensis* Georgi, *Phellodendron amurense* Rupr, *Gardenia jasminoides* Ellis	Sun Ten Pharmaceutical Co., Ltd.
Kami-shoyo-san	*Bupleurum falcatum, Paeonia lactiflora* Pall., *Atractylodes lancea, Angelica acutiloba, Poriacocos* (Schw.) Wolf, *Gardenia jasminoides* Ellis, *Paeonia suffruticosa* Andr., *Glycyrrhiza uralensis* Fisch., *Zingiber officcinale* Roscoc, *Menthae arvensis*	Honso Pharmaceutical Co., Ltd.
LiuWeiDihuang Pill	Radix Rehmanniae Preparata, Corni fructus Praeparata, *Paeonia suffruticosa* Andr., *Dioscorea opposita* Thunb., *Poriacocos* (Schw.) Wolf, *Alisma orientalis* (Sam.) Juzep.	Lanzhou Foci Pharmaceutical Co. Ltd.
San-Huang-Xie-Xin-Tang	*Coptis chinesis* Franch, *Scutellaria baicalensis* Georgi, *Rheum officinale* Baill.	Evergreen Herbs and Medical Supplier
TianmaGouteng Yin	*Gastrodia elata* Bl., *Uncariae Ramulus* Cum Uncis, *Haliotidis Concha, Gardenia jasminoides* Ellis, *Cyathula officinalis* Kuan, *Eucommia ulmoides* Oliv., *Taxillus chinensis* (DC.), *Polygoni Multiflori* Caulis, Fulingshen, *Leonurus japonicas* Houtt.	TCMzone
Yeoldahanso-tang	*Pueraria lobata* (Willd.) Ohwi, *Angelica tenuissima* Nakai, *Scutellaria baicalensis* Georgi, *Platycodon grandiflorum* (Jacq), *Angelica dahurica, Cimicifuga heracleifolia* Kom, *Raphanus sativa* L., *Polygala tenuifolia* (Willd.), *Acorus gramineus* Soland., *Dimocarpus longan* Lour	Jilin Zhen'ao Pharmaceutical Co. Ltd.
Zhen-wu-tang	*Paeonia lactiflora* Pall., *Atractylodes macrocephala* Koidz, *Typhonium giganteum* Engl., *Poriacocos* (Schw.) Wolf, *Zingiber officcinale* Roscoc	Sun Ten Pharmaceutical Co., Ltd.
Zhichan Soup	*Astragalus mongholicus, Salvia*miltiorrhiza Bge., *Gastrodia elata* Bl., *Uncaria rhynchophylla* (Miq.) Miq. ex Havil, *Paeonia lactiflora* Pall., *Cimicifugae Rhizoma, Anemarrhena asphodeloides* Bge	TCMzone
Ayurvedic formulations [10, 12, 100, 108 - 110, 118, 152 - 154]		

(Table 5) cont.....

Formulation	Ingredients	Company Name
Ekangveerras	Herbal purified Mercury, Herbal purified Sulphur, Manganese calx, Tin calx, Lead calx, Bhasma prepared from Copper, Purified and processed Mica, Bhasma prepared from Iron, *Zingiber officinalis*, *Piper nigrum*, *Piper longum*	Baidyanath, Patanjali Ayurved Limited
Moti pishti	Purified Pearl, Rosewater	Baidyanath, Patanjali Ayurved Limited
Yogendra ras	Purified and processed Mercury, Purified and processed sulphur, Iron Bhasma, Gold Bhasma, Purified and processed Silica, Purified and processed Pearl, Bhasma of tin	Dabur,PatanjaliAyurved Limited
Rasrajras	Purified and processed Mercury, Purified and processed Silica, Gold Bhasma, Iron Bhasma, Silver Bhasma, Tin Bhasma	Patanjali Ayurved Limited
Pravalpishti	Purified Coral, Rosewater	Patanjali Ayurved Limited
Giloy sat	*Tinospora cordifolia*, water	Patanjali Ayurved Limited
Medhavati	*Centella asiatica, Convolvulus pluricaulis, Acorus calamus, Lavandula stoechas, Withania somnifera, Celastrus paniculatus, Foeniculum vulgare, Onosma bracteatum,* Mukta Pishti	Patanjali Ayurved Limited
Trayodashanggguggul	*Commiphora mukul*, Babool Seed pods and stem *Withania somnifera, Juniperus communis, Tinospora cordifolia, Asparagus racemosus, Tribulus terrestris, Operculina turpethum, Foeniculum vulgare, Pluchea lanceolata, Curcuma zedoaria, Trachysper mumammi, Zingiber officinale,* Clarified butter	Dhootapapeshwar, Baidyanath, Dabur, Patanjali Ayurved Limited
Ashwagandha churna	*Withania somnifera*	Baidyanath, Patanjali Ayurved Limited
Ashwagandha oil	*Withania somnifera, Phyllanthus emblica, Terminalia chebula, Terminalia bellirica, Santalum albu, Boerhaaviadiffusa, Solanum surattense*	Patanjali Ayurved Limited
Swarna maksikaBhasm	Chalcopyrite or copper iron sulphide, Horse gram, castor oil, buttermilk	Patanjali Ayurved Limited
Makaradhwaj	Purified and processed Sulphur, Purified and processed Mercury Gold Bhasma	Dhootapapeshwar, Uma AyurvedicsPvt. Ltd., Baidyanath, Dabur, Zandu

(Table 5) cont.....

Formulation	Ingredients	Company Name
Chandraprabhavati	*Cinnamomum camphora, Acorus calamus, Cyperus rotundus, Andrographis paniculata, Tinospora cordifolia, Cedrus deodara, Curcuma longa, Aconitum heterophyllum, Berberis aristata, Piper longum, Plumbago zeylanica, Coriandrum sativum, Terminalia chebula, Terminalia bellirica, Emblica officinalis, Piper chaba, Embeliaribes, Piper chaba, Zingiber officinalis, Piper nigrum, Piper longum,* Purified Copper Iron Sulphate, *Hordeum vulgare,* Rock salt, Sochal salt, Vida salt, *Operculina turpethum, Baliospermum montanum, Cinnamomum tamala, Cinnamomum zeylanicum, Elettaria cardamomum, Bambusa bambos,* Iron Bhasma Sugar, Asphaltum, *Commiphora mukul*	Patanjali Ayurved Limited, Baidyanath, Dabur
Shilajit sat	Shilajeet	Patanjali Ayurved Limited
Zandopa	*Mucuna pruriens*	Zandu Pharma

When the scientific names of reported anti-PD plants were compared with the plant list some variations in the taxonomy of plants species were observed. The old scientific names mentioned in published reports are *Acanthopanax senticosus*; *Ajuga ciliate*; *Albiziaa dianthifolia*; *Alternanthera sesilis*; *Anemopaegma mirandum*; *Apium graveolens*; *Astragalus membranaceus*; *Bacopa monnieri*; *Buddleja lindleyana*; *Clausena lansium*; *Fructus psoraleae L.*; *Magnolia officinalis*; *Panax notoginseng*; *Rehmannia glutinosa*; *Rhodiola crenulata*; *Schisandra chinensis*; *Toxicodendron vernicifluum*; *Uncaria rhynchophylla*; *Valeriana offcinalis*. The new scientific names are presented in Tables **2** and **3**. This reflects that special attention needs to be taken while explaining any plant taxonomically.

In the present chapter, 77 different bioactive compounds (catechol, stilbenoids, flavonoids, phenylpropanoid, lignans, phenylethanoid glycoside, phenolics, and saponins) were identified and analysed for their antioxidant, anti-apoptotic, anti-inflammatory, and adaptogenic activities conceivably valuable for PD.

Several other plants and bioactive compounds, such as *Cuscuta chinensis* [66, 67], *Gastroia eleta* [72], and *Hypericum perforatum* L [41]. *Murraya koenigii* [76], herperetin [62], geniposide [71], and hyperoside [42] have shown their rich antioxidant potential in various *in-vitro* investigations, which could be of interest to manage the intricate pathophysiology of PD, though further investigations are warranted.

It is also noteworthy that aforesaid botanical extracts upgrade the working of mitochondria and consequently give insurance to dopaminergic neurons in SN. Be that as it may, additional ponders are needed to investigate involved fundamental mechanisms and pathways. In addition, every herb should be investigated up to each constituent level to obtain data with respect to their individual and in-combination adequacy in PD. Furthermore, the majority of the examinations are attempted in cell lines or on rodent models, notwithstanding, clinical investigations are rare. Along these lines, future investigations on botanicals are warranted to develop new chemical moieties with anti-PD potential. Detailed investigations should also be done to further exploit the impact of Ayurvedic nootropic herbs and holistic therapies in quest of novel drug development for effective PD management [51, 109 - 111].

CONCLUSION

Although the various therapeutic options for PD are available, they have limited efficacy and are unable to avert the gradual dopaminergic neuronal damage among PD patients. Therefore, options from alternative herbal therapies are being searched, and have been revealed to be comparatively safer, having low side effects and high efficacy. It is evident from the present report that medicinal plant extracts and fractions, such as *Acanthopanax senticosus*, *Bacopa monnieri*, *Camellia sinensis*, *Cistanche deserticola*, *Hypericum perforatum*, *Mucuna pruriens*, *Panax ginseng,* and *Polygonum cuspidatum* exhibit potential anti-PD activity by improving the level of several antioxidant enzymes, *viz.* GSH, SOD, GPX, CAT, DA, HVA, NA; PI3K/AKT pathway activation and decreasing the level of TBARS, MDA, ROS, NO, iNOS, Bcl-2, Caspase-3, IL-1β, TNF-α, and α-synuclein aggression and suppressing astrogliosis. Hence, further studies are warranted to thoroughly investigate the anti-PD potential of aforesaid botanicals in various pre-clinical experiments. Though the anti-PD role of plant extracts and their isolated compounds have been targeted of extreme interest in experimental studies, adequate clinical evidence is limited to understanding their bioefficacies in humans. Thus, medicinal plants can be conceived as a complementary and effective cradle for anti-PD drug development and the evolution of new functional moieties to manage PD. Data discussed here will boost further research as well as clinical investigations.

CONSENT FOR PUBLICATION

Not applicable.

CONFLICT OF INTEREST

The author declares no conflict of interest, financial or otherwise.

ACKNOWLEDGEMENTS

The authors are thankful to Dr. A.P. Singh, Dean RIC, I. K Gujral Punjab Technical University and members of staff in the department of RIC, I. K Gujral Punjab Technical University for support and encouragement in this work. N.C.-M. acknowledges the Portuguese Foundation for Science and Technology under the Horizon 2020 Program (PTDC/PSI-GER/28076/2017).

REFERENCES

[1]   Kabra A, Sharma R, Kabra R, Baghel US. Emerging and alternative therapies for Parkinson disease: an updated review. Curr Pharm Des 2018; 24(22): 2573-82.
[http://dx.doi.org/10.2174/1381612824666180820150150] [PMID: 30124146]

[2]   Lees A, Hardy J, Revesz T. Parkinson's disease. Lancet 2009; 373(9680): 2055-66.

[3]   Dauer W, Przedborski S. Parkinson's Disease. Neuron 2003; 39(6): 889-909.
[http://dx.doi.org/10.1016/S0896-6273(03)00568-3] [PMID: 12971891]

[4]   Phani S, Loike JD, Przedborski S. Neurodegeneration and inflammation in Parkinson's disease. Parkinsonism Relat Disord 2012; 18 (Suppl. 1): S207-9.
[http://dx.doi.org/10.1016/S1353-8020(11)70064-5] [PMID: 22166436]

[5]   Pringsheim T, Jette N, Frolkis A, Steeves TDL. The prevalence of Parkinson's disease: A systematic review and meta-analysis. Mov Disord 2014; 29(13): 1583-90.
[http://dx.doi.org/10.1002/mds.25945] [PMID: 24976103]

[6]   Hughes AJ, Daniel SE, Ben-Shlomo Y, Lees AJ. The accuracy of diagnosis of parkinsonian syndromes in a specialist movement disorder service. Brain 2002; 125(4): 861-70.
[http://dx.doi.org/10.1093/brain/awf080] [PMID: 11912118]

[7]   Lill CM. Genetics of Parkinson's disease. Mol Cell Probes 2016; 30(6): 386-96.
[http://dx.doi.org/10.1016/j.mcp.2016.11.001] [PMID: 27818248]

[8]   Tysnes OB, Storstein A. Epidemiology of Parkinson's disease. J Neural Transm (Vienna) 2017; 124(8): 901-5.
[http://dx.doi.org/10.1007/s00702-017-1686-y] [PMID: 28150045]

[9]   Rai SN, Birla H, Singh SS, *et al.* Biomedical Engineering and its Applications in Healthcare. Pathophysiology of the Disease Causing Physical Disability. Springer 2019; pp. 573-95.

[10]   Rai SN, Singh BK, Rathore AS, *et al.* Quality control in huntington's disease: a therapeutic target. Neurotox Res 2019; 36(3): 612-26.
[http://dx.doi.org/10.1007/s12640-019-00087-x] [PMID: 31297710]

[11]   Singh S, Rai S, Birla H, Eds., *et al.* Chlorogenic acid protects against MPTP induced neurotoxicity in parkinsonian mice model *via* its anti-apoptotic activity. Journal of Neurochemistry. NJ USA: Wiley 111 River St, Hoboken 2019.

[12]   Zahra W, Rai SN, Birla H, *et al.* Neuroprotection of rotenone-induced Parkinsonism by ursolic acid in PD mouse model. CNS & Neurological Disorders-Drug Targets 2020; 527-40.
[http://dx.doi.org/10.2174/1871527319666200812224457]

[13]   Diederich NJ, Fénelon G, Stebbins G, Goetz CG. Hallucinations in Parkinson disease. Nat Rev Neurol 2009; 5(6): 331-42.
[http://dx.doi.org/10.1038/nrneurol.2009.62] [PMID: 19498436]

[14]   Chaudhuri KR, Odin P, Antonini A, Martinez-Martin P. Parkinson's disease: The non-motor issues. Parkinsonism Relat Disord 2011; 17(10): 717-23.
[http://dx.doi.org/10.1016/j.parkreldis.2011.02.018] [PMID: 21741874]

[15]   Urwyler P, Nef T, Killen A, *et al.* Visual complaints and visual hallucinations in Parkinson's disease. Parkinsonism Relat Disord 2014; 20(3): 318-22.
[http://dx.doi.org/10.1016/j.parkreldis.2013.12.009] [PMID: 24405755]

[16]   Nasuti C, Brunori G, Eusepi P, Marinelli L, Ciccocioppo R, Gabbianelli R. Early life exposure to permethrin: a progressive animal model of Parkinson's disease. J Pharmacol Toxicol Methods 2017; 83: 80-6.
[http://dx.doi.org/10.1016/j.vascn.2016.10.003] [PMID: 27756609]

[17]   Bordoni L, Nasuti C, Di Stefano A, Marinelli L, Gabbianelli R. Epigenetic memory of early-life parental perturbation: Dopamine decrease and DNA methylation changes in offspring. Oxidative medicine and cellular longevity 2019.

[18]   Fedeli D, Montani M, Bordoni L, *et al. In vivo* and *in silico* studies to identify mechanisms associated with Nurr1 modulation following early life exposure to permethrin in rats. Neuroscience 2017; 340: 411-23.
[http://dx.doi.org/10.1016/j.neuroscience.2016.10.071] [PMID: 27826104]

[19]   Bordoni L, Nasuti C, Mirto M, Caradonna F, Gabbianelli R. Intergenerational effect of early life exposure to permethrin: changes in global DNA methylation and in Nurr1 gene expression. Toxics 2015; 3(4): 451-61.
[http://dx.doi.org/10.3390/toxics3040451] [PMID: 29051472]

[20]   Lee Mosley R, Benner EJ, Kadiu I, *et al.* Neuroinflammation, oxidative stress, and the pathogenesis of Parkinson's disease. Clin Neurosci Res 2006; 6(5): 261-81.
[http://dx.doi.org/10.1016/j.cnr.2006.09.006] [PMID: 18060039]

[21]   Abushouk AI, Negida A, Elshenawy RA, *et al.* C-Abl inhibition; a novel therapeutic target for Parkinson's disease. CNS & Neurological Disorders-Drug Targets 2018; 17(1): 14-21.

[22]   Rascol O, Brooks DJ, Korczyn AD, De Deyn PP, Clarke CE, Lang AE. A five-year study of the incidence of dyskinesia in patients with early Parkinson's disease who were treated with ropinirole or levodopa. N Engl J Med 2000; 342(20): 1484-91.
[http://dx.doi.org/10.1056/NEJM200005183422004] [PMID: 10816186]

[23]   Kurlan R. "Levodopa phobia": A new iatrogenic cause of disability in Parkinson disease. Neurology 2005; 64(5): 923.2-4.
[http://dx.doi.org/10.1212/01.WNL.0000152880.77812.5B] [PMID: 15753443]

[24]   Mopuri R, Islam MS. Medicinal plants and phytochemicals with anti-obesogenic potentials: A review. Biomed Pharmacother 2017; 89: 1442-52.
[http://dx.doi.org/10.1016/j.biopha.2017.02.108] [PMID: 28372259]

[25]   Teixeira FG, Gago MF, Marques P, *et al.* Safinamide: a new hope for Parkinson's disease? Drug Discov Today 2018; 23(3): 736-44.
[http://dx.doi.org/10.1016/j.drudis.2018.01.033] [PMID: 29339106]

[26]   Lee EQ, Chukwueke UN, Hervey-Jumper SL, *et al.* Barriers to accrual and enrollment in brain tumor trials. Neuro-oncol 2019; 21(9): 1100-17.
[PMID: 31175826]

[27]   Kennedy DO, Wightman EL. Herbal extracts and phytochemicals: plant secondary metabolites and the enhancement of human brain function. Adv Nutr 2011; 2(1): 32-50.
[http://dx.doi.org/10.3945/an.110.000117] [PMID: 22211188]

[28]   De Andrade DVG, Madureira de Oliveria D, Barreto G, *et al.* Effects of the extract of *Anemopaegma mirandum* (Catuaba) on Rotenone-induced apoptosis in human neuroblastomas SH-SY5Y cells. Brain Res 2008; 1198: 188-96.
[http://dx.doi.org/10.1016/j.brainres.2008.01.006] [PMID: 18241847]

[29]   Shui Guan , Bao YM, Bo Jiang , An LJ. Protective effect of protocatechuic acid from *Alpinia oxyphylla* on hydrogen peroxide-induced oxidative PC12 cell death. Eur J Pharmacol 2006; 538(1-3):

73-9.
[http://dx.doi.org/10.1016/j.ejphar.2006.03.065] [PMID: 16678817]

[30]   Singh M, Murthy V, Ramassamy C. Standardized extracts of *Bacopa monniera* protect against MPP+-
        and paraquat-induced toxicity by modulating mitochondrial activities, proteasomal functions, and
        redox pathways. Toxicol Sci 2012; 125(1): 219-32.
        [http://dx.doi.org/10.1093/toxsci/kfr255] [PMID: 21972102]

[31]   Swathi G, Ramaiah CV, Rajendra W. Protective role of *Bacopa monnieri* against Rotenone- induced
        Parkinson's disease in PC 12 cell lines. Int J Phytomed 2017; 9(2): 219-22.
        [http://dx.doi.org/10.5138/09750185.2008]

[32]   Guo S, Yan J, Yang T, Yang X, Bezard E, Zhao B. Protective effects of green tea polyphenols in the
        6-OHDA rat model of Parkinson's disease through inhibition of ROS-NO pathway. Biol Psychiatry
        2007; 62(12): 1353-62.
        [http://dx.doi.org/10.1016/j.biopsych.2007.04.020] [PMID: 17624318]

[33]   Nie G, Jin C, Cao Y, Shen S, Zhao B. Distinct effects of tea catechins on 6-hydroxydopamine-induced
        apoptosis in PC12 cells. Arch Biochem Biophys 2002; 397(1): 84-90.
        [http://dx.doi.org/10.1006/abbi.2001.2636] [PMID: 11747313]

[34]   Li R, Peng N, Li X, Le W. (−)-Epigallocatechin gallate regulates dopamine transporter internalization
        via protein kinase C-dependent pathway. Brain Res 2006; 1097(1): 85-9.
        [http://dx.doi.org/10.1016/j.brainres.2006.04.071] [PMID: 16733047]

[35]   Levites Y, Youdim MB, Maor G, Mandel S. Attenuation of 6-hydroxydopamine (6-OHDA)-induced
        nuclear factor-kappaB (NF-kappaB) activation and cell death by tea extracts in neuronal cultures.
        Biochem Pharmacol 2002; 63(1): 21-9.
        [http://dx.doi.org/10.1016/S0006-2952(01)00813-9] [PMID: 11754870]

[36]   Qu W, Fan L, Kim Y, *et al.* Kaempferol derivatives prevent oxidative stress-induced cell death in a
        DJ-1-dependent manner. J Pharmacol Sci 2009; 110(2): 191-200.
        [http://dx.doi.org/10.1254/jphs.09045FP] [PMID: 19498271]

[37]   Ju MS, Kim HG, Choi JG, *et al.* Cassiae semen, a seed of *Cassia obtusifolia*, has neuroprotective
        effects in Parkinson's disease models. Food Chem Toxicol 2010; 48(8-9): 2037-44.
        [http://dx.doi.org/10.1016/j.fct.2010.05.002] [PMID: 20457209]

[38]   Gao Y, Xiaoping P. Neuroprotective effect of acteoside against rotenone-induced damage of SH-
        SY5Y cells and its possible mechanism. Chinese Pharmacological Bulletin 1987.

[39]   Sheng G, Pu X, Lei L, Tu P, Li C. Tubuloside B from *Cistanche salsa* rescues the PC12 neuronal cells
        from 1-methyl-4-phenylpyridinium ion-induced apoptosis and oxidative stress. Planta Med 2002;
        68(11): 966-70.
        [http://dx.doi.org/10.1055/s-2002-35667] [PMID: 12451484]

[40]   Zou YP, Lu YH, Wei DZ. Protective effects of a flavonoid-rich extract of *Hypericum perforatum* L.
        against hydrogen peroxide-induced apoptosis in PC12 cells. Phytother Res 2010; 24(S1) (Suppl. 1):
        S6-S10.
        [http://dx.doi.org/10.1002/ptr.2852] [PMID: 19548287]

[41]   Liu Z, Tao X, Zhang C, Lu Y, Wei D. Protective effects of hyperoside (quercetin-3-o-galactoside) to
        PC12 cells against cytotoxicity induced by hydrogen peroxide and tert-butyl hydroperoxide. Biomed
        Pharmacother 2005; 59(9): 481-90.
        [http://dx.doi.org/10.1016/j.biopha.2005.06.009] [PMID: 16271843]

[42]   Ma CJ, Weon JB, Lee B, *et al.* Neuroprotective activity of the methanolic extract of Lonicera japonica
        in glutamate-injured primary rat cortical cells. Pharmacogn Mag 2011; 7(28): 284-8.
        [http://dx.doi.org/10.4103/0973-1296.90404] [PMID: 22262930]

[43]   Kim HG, Ju MS, Shim JS, *et al.* Mulberry fruit protects dopaminergic neurons in toxin-induced
        Parkinson's disease models. Br J Nutr 2010; 104(1): 8-16.

[http://dx.doi.org/10.1017/S0007114510000218] [PMID: 20187987]

[44]   Sinha N, Sharma S, Haroon R. Antioxidant profiling of leaf extracts of *Murraya koenigii* (L.) Spreng (Curry Leaf) in PC-12 cells exposed to neurotoxic shock. Indian J Agric Biochem 2010; 23(2): 91-6.

[45]   Hu S, Han R, Mak S, Han Y. Protection against 1-methyl-4-phenylpyridinium ion (MPP+)-induced apoptosis by water extract of ginseng (*Panax ginseng* C.A. Meyer) in SH-SY5Y cells. J Ethnopharmacol 2011; 135(1): 34-42.
[http://dx.doi.org/10.1016/j.jep.2011.02.017] [PMID: 21349320]

[46]   Chen X, Zhu YG, Zhu LA, *et al.* Ginsenoside Rg1 attenuates dopamine-induced apoptosis in PC12 cells by suppressing oxidative stress. Eur J Pharmacol 2003; 473(1): 1-7.
[http://dx.doi.org/10.1016/S0014-2999(03)01945-9] [PMID: 12877931]

[47]   Hwang YP, Jeong HG. Ginsenoside Rb1 protects against 6-hydroxydopamine-induced oxidative stress by increasing heme oxygenase-1 expression through an estrogen receptor-related PI3K/Akt/Nrf2-dependent pathway in human dopaminergic cells. Toxicol Appl Pharmacol 2010; 242(1): 18-28.
[http://dx.doi.org/10.1016/j.taap.2009.09.009] [PMID: 19781563]

[48]   Bournival J, Quessy P, Martinoli MG. Protective effects of resveratrol and quercetin against MPP+ -induced oxidative stress act by modulating markers of apoptotic death in dopaminergic neurons. Cell Mol Neurobiol 2009; 29(8): 1169-80.
[http://dx.doi.org/10.1007/s10571-009-9411-5] [PMID: 19466539]

[49]   Chao J, Li H, Cheng KW, Yu MS, Chang RCC, Wang M. Protective effects of pinostilbene, a resveratrol methylated derivative, against 6-hydroxydopamine-induced neurotoxicity in SH-SY5Y cells. J Nutr Biochem 2010; 21(6): 482-9.
[http://dx.doi.org/10.1016/j.jnutbio.2009.02.004] [PMID: 19443200]

[50]   Sadras SR, Sridharan S, Jeepipalli S. *In vitro* neuroprotective effect of *Valeriana wallichii* extract against neurotoxin and endoplasmic reticulum stress induced cell death in SH-SY5Y cells. Advanced Journal of Phytomedicine and Clinical Therapeutics 2014; 2(4): 509-23.

[51]   Lahaie-Collins V, Bournival J, Plouffe M, Carange J, Martinoli MG. Sesamin modulates tyrosine hydroxylase, superoxide dismutase, catalase, inducible NO synthase and interleukin-6 expression in dopaminergic cells under MPP+-induced oxidative stress. Oxid Med Cell Longev 2008; 1(1): 54-62.
[http://dx.doi.org/10.4161/oxim.1.1.6958] [PMID: 19794909]

[52]   Dong Y, Liu S, An L, Lu F, Tang B, Zhou S. The effect of Eleutheroside B on ERK1/2 of MPP+-induced PC12 cells. J Mol Diagn Ther 2011; 3: 155-8.

[53]   Guo P, Li Y, Xu J, *et al.* neo-Clerodane diterpenes from *Ajuga ciliata* Bunge and their neuroprotective activities. Fitoterapia 2011; 82(7): 1123-7.
[http://dx.doi.org/10.1016/j.fitote.2011.07.010] [PMID: 21807075]

[54]   Zhang ZJ, Cheang LCV, Wang MW, *et al.* Ethanolic extract of fructus *Alpinia oxyphylla* protects against 6-hydroxydopamine-induced damage of PC12 cells *in-vitro* and dopaminergic neurons in zebrafish. Cell Mol Neurobiol 2012; 32(1): 27-40.
[http://dx.doi.org/10.1007/s10571-011-9731-0] [PMID: 21744117]

[55]   Xiong N, Huang J, Chen C, *et al.* Dl-3-n-butylphthalide, a natural antioxidant, protects dopamine neurons in rotenone models for Parkinson's disease. Neurobiol Aging 2012; 33(8): 1777-91.
[http://dx.doi.org/10.1016/j.neurobiolaging.2011.03.007] [PMID: 21524431]

[56]   Zhang Z, Wu L, Wang J, *et al.* Astragaloside IV prevents MPP+-induced SH-SY5Y cell death *via*the inhibition of Bax-mediated pathways and ROS production. Mol Cell Biochem 2012; 364(1-2): 209-16.
[http://dx.doi.org/10.1007/s11010-011-1219-1] [PMID: 22278385]

[57]   Sheng GQ, Zhang JR, Pu XP, Ma J, Li CL. Protective effect of verbascoside on 1-methyl-4-phenylpyridinium ion-induced neurotoxicity in PC12 cells. Eur J Pharmacol 2002; 451(2): 119-24.
[http://dx.doi.org/10.1016/S0014-2999(02)02240-9] [PMID: 12231380]

[58]   Tai KK, Truong DD. (−)-Epigallocatechin-3-gallate (EGCG), a green tea polyphenol, reduces

dichlorodiphenyl-trichloroethane (DDT)-induced cell death in dopaminergic SHSY-5Y cells. Neurosci Lett 2010; 482(3): 183-7.
[http://dx.doi.org/10.1016/j.neulet.2010.06.018] [PMID: 20542083]

[59]   Kim IS, Ko HM, Koppula S, Kim BW, Choi DK. Protective effect of *Chrysanthemum indicum* Linne against 1-methyl-4-phenylpridinium ion and lipopolysaccharide-induced cytotoxicity in cellular model of Parkinson's disease. Food Chem Toxicol 2011; 49(4): 963-73.
[http://dx.doi.org/10.1016/j.fct.2011.01.002] [PMID: 21219959]

[60]   Kim IS, Koppula S, Park PJ, *et al. Chrysanthemum morifolium* Ramat (CM) extract protects human neuroblastoma SH-SY5Y cells against MPP+-induced cytotoxicity. J Ethnopharmacol 2009; 126(3): 447-54.
[http://dx.doi.org/10.1016/j.jep.2009.09.017] [PMID: 19770030]

[61]   Tamilselvam K, Braidy N, Manivasagam T, *et al.* Neuroprotective effects of hesperidin, a plant flavanone, on rotenone-induced oxidative stress and apoptosis in a cellular model for Parkinson's disease. Oxid Med Cell Longev 2013; 2013: 1-11.
[http://dx.doi.org/10.1155/2013/102741] [PMID: 24205431]

[62]   Hwang SL, Lin JA, Shih PH, Yeh CT, Yen GC. Pro-cellular survival and neuroprotection of citrus flavonoid: the actions of hesperetin in PC12 cells. Food Funct 2012; 3(10): 1082-90.
[http://dx.doi.org/10.1039/c2fo30100h] [PMID: 22767158]

[63]   Li B, Yuan Y, Hu J, Zhao Q, Zhang D, Chen N. Protective effect of Bu-7, a flavonoid extracted from Clausena lansium, against rotenone injury in PC12 cells. Acta Pharmacol Sin 2011; 32(11): 1321-6.
[http://dx.doi.org/10.1038/aps.2011.119] [PMID: 21963892]

[64]   Friedemann T, Ying Y, Wang W, *et al.* Neuroprotective effect of coptis chinensis in MPP+ and MPTP-induced Parkinson's disease models. Am J Chin Med 2016; 44(5): 907-25.
[http://dx.doi.org/10.1142/S0192415X16500506] [PMID: 27430912]

[65]   Ma XW, Guo RY. Dose-dependent effect of *Curcuma longa* for the treatment of Parkinson's disease. Exp Ther Med 2017; 13(5): 1799-805.
[http://dx.doi.org/10.3892/etm.2017.4225] [PMID: 28565770]

[66]   Li Z, Jiang B, Bao Y, An L. Protection of Semen Cuscuta extracts from apoptosis PC12 cell of induced by1-methyl-4-phenylpyridinium. Zhongchengyao 2006; 28: 219-21.

[67]   Zhen GH, Jiang B, Bao YM, Li DX, An LJ. [The protect effect of flavonoids from Cuscuta chinensis in PC12 cells from damage induced by H2O2]. Zhong Yao Cai 2006; 29(10): 1051-5.
[PMID: 17326406]

[68]   Guo H, Shi F, Li M, Liu Q, Yu B, Hu L. Neuroprotective effects of Eucommia ulmoides Oliv. and its bioactive constituent work *via*ameliorating the ubiquitin-proteasome system. BMC Complement Altern Med 2015; 15(1): 151.
[http://dx.doi.org/10.1186/s12906-015-0675-7] [PMID: 25994206]

[69]   Zhao DL, Zou LB, Lin S, Shi JG, Zhu HB. Anti-apoptotic effect of esculin on dopamine-induced cytotoxicity in the human neuroblastoma SH-SY5Y cell line. Neuropharmacology 2007; 53(6): 724-32.
[http://dx.doi.org/10.1016/j.neuropharm.2007.07.017] [PMID: 17904593]

[70]   Chen L, Wang F, Geng M, Chen H, Duan D. Geniposide protects human neuroblastoma SH-SY5Y cells against corticosterone-induced injury. Neural Regen Res 2011; 6(21): 1618-22.

[71]   An H, Kim IS, Koppula S, *et al.* Protective effects of *Gastrodia elata* Blume on MPP+-induced cytotoxicity in human dopaminergic SH-SY5Y cells. J Ethnopharmacol 2010; 130(2): 290-8.
[http://dx.doi.org/10.1016/j.jep.2010.05.006] [PMID: 20470875]

[72]   Kim IS, Choi DK, Jung HJ. Neuroprotective effects of vanillyl alcohol in *Gastrodia elata* Blume through suppression of oxidative stress and anti-apoptotic activity in toxin-induced dopaminergic MN9D cells. Molecules 2011; 16(7): 5349-61.

[http://dx.doi.org/10.3390/molecules16075349] [PMID: 21705974]

[73]   Kang X, Chen J, Xu Z, Li H, Wang B. Protective effects of *Ginkgo biloba* extract on paraquat-induced apoptosis of PC12 cells. Toxicol in-vitro 2007; 21(6): 1003-9.
[http://dx.doi.org/10.1016/j.tiv.2007.02.004] [PMID: 17509817]

[74]   Im AR, Kim YH, Uddin MR, *et al.* Neuroprotective effects of *Lycium chinense* Miller against rotenone-induced neurotoxicity in PC12 cells. Am J Chin Med 2013; 41(6): 1343-59.
[http://dx.doi.org/10.1142/S0192415X13500900] [PMID: 24228605]

[75]   Beamer CA, Shepherd DM. Inhibition of TLR ligand- and interferon gamma-induced murine microglial activation by *Panax notoginseng.* J Neuroimmune Pharmacol 2012; 7(2): 465-76.
[http://dx.doi.org/10.1007/s11481-011-9333-0] [PMID: 22183805]

[76]   Cao BY, Yang YP, Luo WF, *et al.* Paeoniflorin, a potent natural compound, protects PC12 cells from MPP+ and acidic damage *via* autophagic pathway. J Ethnopharmacol 2010; 131(1): 122-9.
[http://dx.doi.org/10.1016/j.jep.2010.06.009] [PMID: 20558269]

[77]   Luo FC, Wang SD, Li K, Nakamura H, Yodoi J, Bai J. Panaxatriol saponins extracted from *Panax notoginseng* induces thioredoxin-1 and prevents 1-methyl-4-phenylpyridinium ion-induced neurotoxicity. J Ethnopharmacol 2010; 127(2): 419-23.
[http://dx.doi.org/10.1016/j.jep.2009.10.023] [PMID: 19857566]

[78]   Choi JG, Kim HG, Kim MC, *et al.* Polygalae radix inhibits toxin-induced neuronal death in the Parkinson's disease models. J Ethnopharmacol 2011; 134(2): 414-21.
[http://dx.doi.org/10.1016/j.jep.2010.12.030] [PMID: 21195155]

[79]   Liang Z, Shi F, Wang Y, *et al.* Neuroprotective effects of tenuigenin in a SH-SY5Y cell model with 6-OHDA-induced injury. Neurosci Lett 2011; 497(2): 104-9.
[http://dx.doi.org/10.1016/j.neulet.2011.04.041] [PMID: 21536104]

[80]   Wu Y, Li X, Zhu JX, *et al.* Resveratrol-activated AMPK/SIRT1/autophagy in cellular models of Parkinson's disease. Neurosignals 2011; 19(3): 163-74.
[http://dx.doi.org/10.1159/000328516] [PMID: 21778691]

[81]   Li Y, Lin Z, Zhang Z, *et al.* Protective, antioxidative and antiapoptotic effects of 2-methoxy-6-ace-yl-7-methyljuglone from Polygonum cuspidatum in PC12 cells. Planta Med 2011; 77(4): 354-61.
[http://dx.doi.org/10.1055/s-0030-1250385] [PMID: 20922651]

[82]   Zhao G, Li S, Qin GW, Fei J, Guo LH. Inhibitive effects of *Fructus Psoraleae* extract on dopamine transporter and noradrenaline transporter. J Ethnopharmacol 2007; 112(3): 498-506.
[http://dx.doi.org/10.1016/j.jep.2007.04.013] [PMID: 17555897]

[83]   Zhu G, Wang X, Wu S, Li Q. Involvement of activation of PI3K/Akt pathway in the protective effects of puerarin against MPP+-induced human neuroblastoma SH-SY5Y cell death. Neurochem Int 2012; 60(4): 400-8.
[http://dx.doi.org/10.1016/j.neuint.2012.01.003] [PMID: 22265823]

[84]   Lin CM, Lin RD, Chen ST, *et al.* Neurocytoprotective effects of the bioactive constituents of *Pueraria thomsonii* in 6-hydroxydopamine (6-OHDA)-treated nerve growth factor (NGF)-differentiated PC12 cells. Phytochemistry 2010; 71(17-18): 2147-56.
[http://dx.doi.org/10.1016/j.phytochem.2010.08.015] [PMID: 20832831]

[85]   Tian YY, An LJ, Jiang L, Duan YL, Chen J, Jiang B. Catalpol protects dopaminergic neurons from LPS-induced neurotoxicity in mesencephalic neuron-glia cultures. Life Sci 2006; 80(3): 193-9.
[http://dx.doi.org/10.1016/j.lfs.2006.09.010] [PMID: 17049947]

[86]   Li X, Ye X, Li X, *et al.* Salidroside protects against MPP+-induced apoptosis in PC12 cells by inhibiting the NO pathway. Brain Res 2011; 1382: 9-18.
[http://dx.doi.org/10.1016/j.brainres.2011.01.015] [PMID: 21241673]

[87]   Tian LL, Wang XJ, Sun YN, *et al.* Salvianolic acid B, an antioxidant from *Salvia*miltiorrhiza, prevents 6-hydroxydopamine induced apoptosis in SH-SY5Y cells. Int J Biochem Cell Biol 2008; 40(3): 409-

22.
[http://dx.doi.org/10.1016/j.biocel.2007.08.005] [PMID: 17884684]

[88]   Zeng G, Tang T, Wu HJ, *et al.* Salvianolic acid B protects SH-SY5Y neuroblastoma cells from 1-methyl-4-phenylpyridinium-induced apoptosis. Biol Pharm Bull 2010; 33(8): 1337-42.
[http://dx.doi.org/10.1248/bpb.33.1337] [PMID: 20686228]

[89]   Liu CS, Chen NH, Zhang JT. Protection of PC12 cells from hydrogen peroxide-induced cytotoxicity by salvianolic acid B, a new compound isolated from *Radix Salviae miltiorrhizae.* Phytomedicine 2007; 14(7-8): 492-7.
[http://dx.doi.org/10.1016/j.phymed.2006.11.002] [PMID: 17175150]

[90]   Sa F, Zhang LQ, Chong CM, *et al.* Discovery of novel anti-parkinsonian effect of schisantherin A in *in-vitro* and *in-vivo.* Neurosci Lett 2015; 593: 7-12.
[http://dx.doi.org/10.1016/j.neulet.2015.03.016] [PMID: 25770828]

[91]   Li X, He G, Mu X, *et al.* Protective effects of baicalein against rotenone-induced neurotoxicity in PC12 cells and isolated rat brain mitochondria. Eur J Pharmacol 2012; 674(2-3): 227-33.
[http://dx.doi.org/10.1016/j.ejphar.2011.09.181] [PMID: 21996316]

[92]   Choi JH, Choi AY, Yoon H, *et al.* Baicalein protects HT22 murine hippocampal neuronal cells against endoplasmic reticulum stress-induced apoptosis through inhibition of reactive oxygen species production and CHOP induction. Exp Mol Med 2010; 42(12): 811-22.
[http://dx.doi.org/10.3858/emm.2010.42.12.084] [PMID: 20959717]

[93]   Saravanan R. Neuroprotective effect of *Thuja orientalis* in haloperidol induced animal model of Parkinson's Disease. IJPR 2016; 6(10): 308.

[94]   Essa MM, Akbar M, Guillemin G. The benefits of natural products for neurodegenerative diseases. Springer 2016.
[http://dx.doi.org/10.1007/978-3-319-28383-8]

[95]   Shim JS, Kim HG, Ju MS, Choi JG, Jeong SY, Oh MS. Effects of the hook of *Uncaria rhynchophylla* on neurotoxicity in the 6-hydroxydopamine model of Parkinson's disease. J Ethnopharmacol 2009; 126(2): 361-5.
[http://dx.doi.org/10.1016/j.jep.2009.08.023] [PMID: 19703534]

[96]   de Oliveria DM, Barreto G, De Andrade DVG, *et al.* Cytoprotective effect of *Valeriana officinalis* extract on an *in-vitro* experimental model of Parkinson disease. Neurochem Res 2009; 34(2): 215-20.
[http://dx.doi.org/10.1007/s11064-008-9749-y] [PMID: 18512151]

[97]   Beppe GJ, Dongmo AB, Foyet HS, Dimo T, Mihasan M, Hritcu L. The aqueous extract of *Albizia adianthifolia* leaves attenuates 6-hydroxydopamine-induced anxiety, depression and oxidative stress in rat amygdala. BMC Complement Altern Med 2015; 15(1): 374.
[http://dx.doi.org/10.1186/s12906-015-0912-0] [PMID: 26481946]

[98]   Magnnavar CV, Panji AS, Chinnam S. Neuroprotective Activity of Berberis aristata against 6-OHDA Induced Parkinson's Disease Model. Wiley Online Library 2013.

[99]   Zhang SY, Han LY, Zhang H, Xin HL. *Chaenomeles speciosa*: A review of chemistry and pharmacology. Biomed Rep 2014; 2(1): 12-8.
[http://dx.doi.org/10.3892/br.2013.193] [PMID: 24649061]

[100] Keswani C, Dilnashin H, Birla H, Singh SP. Unravelling efficient applications of agriculturally important microorganisms for alleviation of induced inter-cellular oxidative stress in crops. Acta Agric Slov 2019; 114(1): 121-30.
[http://dx.doi.org/10.14720/aas.2019.114.1.14]

[101] Singh SS, Rai SN, Birla H, *et al.* Neuroprotective effect of chlorogenic acid on mitochondrial dysfunction-mediated apoptotic death of DA neurons in a Parkinsonian mouse model. Oxid Med Cell Longev 2020; 2020: 1-14.
[http://dx.doi.org/10.1155/2020/6571484] [PMID: 32566093]

[102] Ramani R, Anisetti RN, Boddupalli BM, Malothu N, Arumugam BS. Antiparkinson's and free radical scavenging study of ethyl acetate fraction of ethanolic extract of *Leucas lanata*. Drug Invention Today 2013; 5(3): 251-5.
[http://dx.doi.org/10.1016/j.dit.2013.07.001]

[103] Sedaghat R, Roghani M, Khalili M. Neuroprotective effect of thymoquinone, the nigella sativa bioactive compound, in 6-hydroxydopamine-induced hemi-parkinsonian rat model. Iran J Pharm Res 2014; 13(1): 227-34.
[PMID: 24734075]

[104] Keswani C. Agri-based Bioeconomy: Reintegrating Trans-disciplinary Research and Sustainable Development Goals. CRC Press 2021.
[http://dx.doi.org/10.1201/9781003033394]

[105] Keswani C, Bisen K, Singh S, Singh H. Traditional knowledge and medicinal plants of India in intellectual property landscape. Med Plants Int J Phytomed Relat Ind 2017.
[http://dx.doi.org/10.5958/0975-6892.2017.00001.6]

[106] Keswani C, Mishra S, Sarma BK, Singh SP, Singh HB. Unraveling the efficient applications of secondary metabolites of various *Trichoderma spp.* Appl Microbiol Biotechnol 2014; 98(2): 533-44.
[http://dx.doi.org/10.1007/s00253-013-5344-5] [PMID: 24276619]

[107] Keswani C, Singh HB, Hermosa R, *et al.* Antimicrobial secondary metabolites from agriculturally important fungi as next biocontrol agents. Appl Microbiol Biotechnol 2019; 103(23-24): 9287-303.
[http://dx.doi.org/10.1007/s00253-019-10209-2] [PMID: 31707442]

[108] Birla H, Keswani C, Singh SS, *et al.* Unraveling the Neuroprotective Effect of tinospora cordifolia in Parkinsonian Mouse Model Through Proteomics Approach 2021; 527-40.
[http://dx.doi.org/10.1021/acschemneuro.1c00481]

[109] Sharma R, Kuca K, Nepovimova E, Kabra A, Rao MM, Prajapati PK. Traditional Ayurvedic and herbal remedies for Alzheimer's disease: from bench to bedside. Expert Rev Neurother 2019; 19(5): 359-74.
[http://dx.doi.org/10.1080/14737175.2019.1596803] [PMID: 30884983]

[110] Sharma R, Kabra A, Rao MM, Prajapati PK. Herbal and Holistic Solutions for Neurodegenerative and Depressive Disorders: Leads from Ayurveda. Curr Pharm Des 2018; 24(22): 2597-608.
[http://dx.doi.org/10.2174/1381612824666180821165741] [PMID: 30147009]

[111] Keswani C. Bioeconomy for Sustainable Development. Springer 2020.
[http://dx.doi.org/10.1007/978-981-13-9431-7]

[112] Li X, Zhang S, Liu S, Lu F. Recent advances in herbal medicines treating Parkinson's disease. Fitoterapia 2013; 84: 273-85.
[http://dx.doi.org/10.1016/j.fitote.2012.12.009] [PMID: 23266574]

[113] Banu Z, Fatima SJ, Fatima A, Fatima S, Zohra SF, Sultana T. Phytochemical Evaluation and Pharmacological Screening of Antiparkinson's Activity of *Allium sativum* In Swiss/Albino Mice. IOSR J Pharm 2016; 6(6): 1-12.

[114] García E, Villeda-Hernández J, Pedraza-Chaverrí J, Maldonado PD, Santamaría A. S-allylcysteine reduces the MPTP-induced striatal cell damage *via* inhibition of pro-inflammatory cytokine tumor necrosis factor-α and inducible nitric oxide synthase expressions in mice. Phytomedicine 2010; 18(1): 65-73.
[http://dx.doi.org/10.1016/j.phymed.2010.04.004] [PMID: 20576415]

[115] Rojas P, Serrano-García N, Medina-Campos ON, Pedraza-Chaverri J, Maldonado PD, Ruiz-Sánchez E. S-Allylcysteine, a garlic compound, protects against oxidative stress in 1-methyl-4-phenylpyridinium-induced parkinsonism in mice. J Nutr Biochem 2011; 22(10): 937-44.
[http://dx.doi.org/10.1016/j.jnutbio.2010.08.005] [PMID: 21190833]

[116] Abbaoui A, Hiba OE, Gamrani H. Neuroprotective potential of Aloe arborescens against copper

induced neurobehavioral features of Parkinson's disease in rat. Acta Histochem 2017; 119(5): 592-601.
[http://dx.doi.org/10.1016/j.acthis.2017.06.003] [PMID: 28619286]

[117] Ittiyavirah SP, Hameed J. Protective Role of *Alternanthera sessilis* (Linn.) Silver Nanoparticles and Its Ethanolic Extract against Rotenone Induced Parkinsonism.

[118] Srivastav S, Fatima M, Mondal AC. Important medicinal herbs in Parkinson's disease pharmacotherapy. Biomed Pharmacother 2017; 92: 856-63.
[http://dx.doi.org/10.1016/j.biopha.2017.05.137] [PMID: 28599249]

[119] Nade V, Kapure AB, Kawale LA, Zambre SS. Neuroprotective potential of *Beta vulgaris* L. in Parkinson's disease. Indian J Pharmacol 2015; 47(4): 403-8.
[http://dx.doi.org/10.4103/0253-7613.161263] [PMID: 26288473]

[120] Abdel-Salam OME, Youness ER, Ahmed NA, *et al. Bougainvillea spectabilis* flowers extract protects against the rotenone-induced toxicity. Asian Pac J Trop Med 2017; 10(5): 478-90.
[http://dx.doi.org/10.1016/j.apjtm.2017.05.013] [PMID: 28647186]

[121] Nagarjuna S, Reddy YP, Arifullah M, Kumar AS, Srinath B, Reddy KS. Evaluation of antioxidant and antiparkinsonian activities of *Brassica oleracea* in haloperidol-induced tardive dyskinesia. International Journal of Green Pharmacy 2015; 9(3): 143-9. [IJGP].
[http://dx.doi.org/10.4103/0973-8258.161230]

[122] Ren R, Shi C, Cao J, *et al.* Neuroprotective effects of a standardized flavonoid extract of safflower against neurotoxin-induced cellular and animal models of Parkinson's disease. Sci Rep 2016; 6(1): 22135.
[http://dx.doi.org/10.1038/srep22135] [PMID: 26906725]

[123] Datla KP, Zbarsky V, Rai D, *et al.* Short-term supplementation with plant extracts rich in flavonoids protect nigrostriatal dopaminergic neurons in a rat model of Parkinson's disease. J Am Coll Nutr 2007; 26(4): 341-9.
[http://dx.doi.org/10.1080/07315724.2007.10719621] [PMID: 17906186]

[124] Moraes LS, Rohor BZ, Areal LB, *et al.* Medicinal plant *Combretum leprosum* mart ameliorates motor, biochemical and molecular alterations in a Parkinson's disease model induced by MPTP. J Ethnopharmacol 2016; 185: 68-76.
[http://dx.doi.org/10.1016/j.jep.2016.03.041] [PMID: 26994817]

[125] Ahmad AS, Ansari MA, Ahmad M, *et al.* Neuroprotection by crocetin in a hemi-parkinsonian rat model. Pharmacol Biochem Behav 2005; 81(4): 805-13.
[http://dx.doi.org/10.1016/j.pbb.2005.06.007] [PMID: 16005057]

[126] Jahromi SR, Haddadi M, Shivanandappa T, Ramesh SR. Modulatory effect of *Decalepis hamiltonii* on ethanol-induced toxicity in transgenic Drosophila model of Parkinson's disease. Neurochem Int 2015; 80: 1-6.
[http://dx.doi.org/10.1016/j.neuint.2014.10.010] [PMID: 25451756]

[127] Lin AMY, Wu LY, Hung KC, *et al.* Neuroprotective effects of longan (*Dimocarpus longan* Lour.) flower water extract on MPP+-induced neurotoxicity in rat brain. J Agric Food Chem 2012; 60(36): 9188-94.
[http://dx.doi.org/10.1021/jf302792t] [PMID: 22920583]

[128] Bagewadi HG, Afzal Khan A. Evaluation of anti-parkinsonian activity of *Elaeocarpus ganitruson* haloperidol induced Parkinson's disease in mice. Int J Basic Clin Pharmacol 2015; 4: 102-6.

[129] Sathish K, Rahman A, Buvanendran R, Obeth D, Panneerselvam U. Effect of *Evolvulus alsinoides* root extracts on acute reserpine induced orofacial d yskinesia. International Journal of Pharmacy and Pharmaceutical Sciences 2010.

[130] Bhangale JO, Acharya SR. Anti-Parkinson activity of petroleum ether extract of *Ficus religiosa* (L.) leaves. Advances in pharmacological sciences 2016.

[131] Sengupta T, Vinayagam J, Nagashayana N, Gowda B, Jaisankar P, Mohanakumar KP. Antiparkinsonian effects of aqueous methanolic extract of *Hyoscyamus niger* seeds result from its monoamine oxidase inhibitory and hydroxyl radical scavenging potency. Neurochem Res 2011; 36(1): 177-86.
[http://dx.doi.org/10.1007/s11064-010-0289-x] [PMID: 20972705]

[132] Bais S, Gill NS, Rana N. Effect of *Juniperus communis* extract on reserpine induced catalepsy. Inventi Impact: Ethnopharmacol 2014; 2014: 117-20.

[133] Luo D, Zhang Q, Wang H, *et al.* Fucoidan protects against dopaminergic neuron death *in-vivo* and *in-vitro*. Eur J Pharmacol 2009; 617(1-3): 33-40.
[http://dx.doi.org/10.1016/j.ejphar.2009.06.015] [PMID: 19545563]

[134] Choi SY, Son TG, Park HR, *et al.* Naphthazarin has a protective effect on the 1-methyl-4-phe-yl-1,2,3,4-tetrahydropyridine-induced Parkinson's disease model. J Neurosci Res 2012; 90(9): 1842-9.
[http://dx.doi.org/10.1002/jnr.23061] [PMID: 22513651]

[135] Ittiyavirah SP, Hameed J. Herbs treating Parkinson's disease. Biomed Aging Pathol 2014; 4(4): 369-76.
[http://dx.doi.org/10.1016/j.biomag.2014.08.003]

[136] Ingale S, Kasture S. Protective effect of standardized extract of *Passiflora incarnata* flower in parkinson's and alzheimer's disease. Anc Sci Life 2017; 36(4): 200-6.
[http://dx.doi.org/10.4103/asl.ASL_231_16] [PMID: 29269972]

[137] Bi Y, Qu PC, Wang QS, *et al.* Neuroprotective effects of alkaloids from *Piper longum* in a MPTP-induced mouse model of Parkinson's disease. Pharm Biol 2015; 53(10): 1516-24.
[http://dx.doi.org/10.3109/13880209.2014.991835] [PMID: 25857256]

[138] Khurana N, Gajbhiye A. Ameliorative effect of *Sida cordifolia* in rotenone induced oxidative stress model of Parkinson's disease. Neurotoxicology 2013; 39: 57-64.
[http://dx.doi.org/10.1016/j.neuro.2013.08.005] [PMID: 23994302]

[139] Chandrashekhar VM, Avinash SP, Sowmya C, Ramkishan A, Shalavadi MH. Neuroprotective activity of *Stereospermum suaveolens* DC against 6-OHDA induced Parkinson's disease model. Indian J Pharmacol 2012; 44(6): 737-43.
[http://dx.doi.org/10.4103/0253-7613.103275] [PMID: 23248404]

[140] Kosaraju J, Chinni S, Roy P, Kannan E, Antony AS, Kumar MNS. Neuroprotective effect of *Tinospora cordifolia* ethanol extract on 6-hydroxy dopamine induced Parkinsonism. Indian J Pharmacol 2014; 46(2): 176-80.
[http://dx.doi.org/10.4103/0253-7613.129312] [PMID: 24741189]

[141] Birla H, Rai SN, Singh SS, Zahra W, Rawat A, Tiwari N. *Tinospora cordifolia* suppresses neuroinflammation in parkinsonian mouse model. NeuroMol Med 2019.

[142] Li FQ, Cheng XX, Liang XB, *et al.* Neurotrophic and neuroprotective effects of tripchlorolide, an extract of Chinese herb *Tripterygium wilfordii* Hook F, on dopaminergic neurons. Exp Neurol 2003; 179(1): 28-37.
[http://dx.doi.org/10.1006/exnr.2002.8049] [PMID: 12504865]

[143] Cilia R, Laguna J, Cassani E, *et al.* *Mucuna pruriens* in Parkinson disease. Neurology 2017; 89(5): 432-8.
[http://dx.doi.org/10.1212/WNL.0000000000004175] [PMID: 28679598]

[144] Birla H, Keswani C, Rai SN, *et al.* Neuroprotective effects of *Withania somnifera* in BPA induced-cognitive dysfunction and oxidative stress in mice. Behav Brain Funct 2019; 15(1): 9.
[http://dx.doi.org/10.1186/s12993-019-0160-4] [PMID: 31064381]

[145] Rai SN, Birla H, Singh SS, Zahra W, Patil RR, Jadhav JP. *Mucuna pruriens* protects against MPTP Intoxicated neuroinflammation in Parkinson's disease through NF-κB/pAKT signaling pathways. Front Aging Neurosci 2017.

[146] Sathiyanarayanan L, Arulmozhi S. *Mucuna pruriens* Linn.-A comprehensive review. Pharmacogn Rev 2007; 1(1): 157-62.

[147] Wang Y, Xie CL, Lu L, Fu DL, Zheng GQ. Chinese herbal medicine paratherapy for Parkinson's disease: a meta-analysis of 19 randomized controlled trials. Evidence-based Complementary and Alternative Medicine 2012.
[http://dx.doi.org/10.1155/2012/534861]

[148] Zahra W, Rai SN, Birla H, *et al.* The global economic impact of neurodegenerative diseases: Opportunities and challenges. Bioeconomy for Sustainable Development 2020; pp. 333-45.

[149] Zahra W, Rai SN, Birla H, *et al.* Economic Importance of Medicinal Plants in Asian Countries. Bioeconomy for Sustainable Development. Springer 2020; pp. 359-77.
[http://dx.doi.org/10.1007/978-981-13-9431-7_19]

[150] Kum WF, Durairajan SSK, Bian ZX, *et al.* Treatment of idiopathic Parkinson's disease with traditional chinese herbal medicine: a randomized placebo-controlled pilot clinical study. Evidence-Based Complementary and Alternative Medicine 2011.
[http://dx.doi.org/10.1093/ecam/nep116]

[151] Lotan I, Treves TA, Roditi Y, Djaldetti R. *Cannabis* (medical marijuana) treatment for motor and non-motor symptoms of Parkinson disease: an open-label observational study. Clin Neuropharmacol 2014; 37(2): 41-4.
[http://dx.doi.org/10.1097/WNF.0000000000000016] [PMID: 24614667]

[152] Rai SN, Dilnashin H, Birla H, *et al.* The role of PI3K/Akt and ERK in neurodegenerative disorders. Neurotox Res 2019; 35(3): 775-95.
[http://dx.doi.org/10.1007/s12640-019-0003-y] [PMID: 30707354]

[153] Rathore AS, Birla H, Singh SS, *et al.* Epigenetic Modulation in Parkinson's Disease and Potential Treatment Therapies. Neurochem Res 2021; 46(7): 1618-26.
[http://dx.doi.org/10.1007/s11064-021-03334-w] [PMID: 33900517]

[154] Raina AP, Khatri R. Quantitative determination of L-DOPA in seeds of *Mucuna pruriens* germplasm by high performance thin layer chromatography. Indian J Pharm Sci 2011; 73(4): 459-62.
[PMID: 22707835]

CHAPTER 3

Indopathy for Neuroprotection in Parkinson's Disease

Archana Dwivedi[1] and **Deepika Joshi**[1,*]

[1] *Department of Neurology, Institute of Medical Sciences, Banaras Hindu University, Varanasi-221005 (U.P.), India*

Abstract: Parkinson's disease (PD) is a chronic, multi-system, complex neurodegenerative disorder pathologically characterized by motor dysfunctions caused mainly due to the loss of dopamine (DA) neurotransmitters producing dopaminergic (DAergic) neurons. In Ayurveda, which is an indigenous medicine system of India, various medicinal herbs have been used for the treatment of PD since ancient times. A growing number of studies have proven that these Ayurvedic herbs can protect DAergic neurons from neuronal degeneration and hence can increase the level of DA. Phytochemicals or active ingredients present in these Ayurvedic herbs can target oxidative stress, mitochondrial dysfunction, neuroinflammation, apoptosis, and autophagy and can reduce α-synuclein (α-syn) protein aggregation, which are the basic pathological causes of neurodegeneration and can improve the motor ability and sometimes longevity in animal models of PD. The mainstay of treatment of PD is levodopa (L-Dopa), a precursor of DA, used for achieving the optimal level of DA. But its long-term use has debilitating side effects. Ayurvedic herbs have provided relief in PD with no or minimal side-effect even after long-term administration. Some plants, such as *M. pruriens,* are a natural source of L-Dopa. Here, we have discussed the major classes of phytochemicals found in Ayurvedic medicines and the pathogenic mechanisms of PD targeted by them. After that, we have discussed the recent advances in experimental and clinical data that support the neuroprotective properties of these phytochemicals used in Ayurveda and their potential to be developed as a therapeutic intervention for the prevention of PD.

Keywords: Ayurveda, *B. monnieri, C. Asiatica, C. Longa, C. sinensis, M. pruriens*, Neuroprotection, Parkinson's disease, Phytochemicals, *V. vinifera, W. somnifera.*

* **Corresponding author Deepika Joshi:** Department of Neurology, Institute of Medical Sciences, Banaras Hindu University, Varanasi-221005 (U.P.), India; E-mail: drdeepikajoshi73@gmail.com

Surya Pratap Singh, Hagera Dilnashin, Hareram Birla & Chetan Keswani (Eds.)

INTRODUCTION

Parkinson's disease (PD) is the second most common and the major age-related neurodegenerative disorder affecting more than 10 million people worldwide, with an estimated annual incidence of 1.5 per 100,000 to 346 per 100,000 in different parts of the world and a prevalence of 41/100000 in the age of 40s to 1900/100000 in the age of 80s, equally affecting males and females [1 - 6]. It is a most common extrapyramidal neurodegenerative disorder primarily affecting voluntary movements and characterized by progressive degeneration of dopaminergic neurons in substantia nigra pars compacta (SNpc). The pathological hallmarks of PD manifesting due to DA deficiency are bradykinesia, rigidity, resting tremor, and postural instability [7]. PD also involves a broad range of non-motor symptoms, such as cognitive deficits, autonomic dysfunctions, and mood disorders [8]. Another important feature of PD is the abnormal aggregation of phosphorylated α-synuclein (α-syn) protein within Lewy bodies (LB). PD is a complex multifactorial disorder, and the exact etiology of PD is not yet clear. The following are considered risk factors for the development of PD- genetic factors, aging, environmental toxins, drugs, infections, and ethnicity. Many of the pathogenic processes in PD are in parallel to aging shifts [2, 9 - 12].

Pharmacological treatment of PD can be accomplished with L-Dopa, DA agonists, catechol-O-Methyl transferase (COMT) inhibitors, monoamino oxidase-B (MAO-B) inhibitors, antimuscarinics, or amantadine. The mainstay of treatment and the most effective symptomatic therapy remains the use of dopamine precursor L-Dopa [13]. Other strategies of PD treatment are deep brain stimulation and stem cell transplantation into the striatum [14]. Although there is no cure for PD presently, attempts to slow or stop the neuronal cell loss in the disease have failed [15]. Also, with the advancement of disease duration, the effectiveness in relieving symptoms reduces, so higher doses of L-Dopa are required, leading to the development of drug-induced motor complications [16 - 19].

Ayurveda (Ayu: life, the combined state of body, senses, mind, and soul; Veda: science. Ayurveda: the science of life, Sanskrit) is an ancient Indian medical system and is the oldest functional science-based system of medicine in the world. There are three dynamic principles of humor according to Ayurveda, namely, "doshas", "dhatus", and "malas". "Doshas" governs the body's physiological and physicochemical activities. It can be of three types, namely, "Vata" (responsible for movement), "Pitta" (responsible for transformation), and "Kapha" (responsible for anabolic activities). In Ayurveda, Physiology is the situation of harmony in the functioning of these "Doshas", and pathology is the situation of the discordance in their functions affecting the "Dhatu" (structural element) and the "Mala" (elimination of wastes). So "Vata doshas" is responsible for all the movements and sensations, including motor actions [20, 21].

In Ayurvedic literature, Paralysis agitans/ PD are called "Kampa Vata" (Kampa: tremor). "Charaka Samhita", "Madhavanidana" and other Ayurvedic literature contain and describe various signs and symptoms of "Kampa Vata", such as no inclination for movement (akinesia), drooling of saliva, love of solitude (depression), constant drowsy feeling, and fixation and whiteness of eyes (probable reptilian stare), "Pravepana" (excessive tremor), "Sirahkampa" (skull tremor), "Cestapranasa" (loss of movement), "Stabdhagatratva" (stiffness of the body), and "Anukirna svara" (stammering), "Cittanasa" (loss of mind or dementia), "Buddhi pramaha" (Mental confusion) [21]. Ayurveda stresses an inherently holistic approach to health and disease, and treatment is focused on modifying the pathophysiology of the disease and symptom management.

This Ayurvedic health management system may be complementary or alternative to the existing medical system being used, especially in the case of chronic conditions. A number of plants with therapeutic benefits are used in Ayurveda for the treatment of neurodegenerative diseases. These Ayurvedic medicines are used as concoctions or concentrated plant extracts without isolation of active compounds or after the isolation and purification of one or two active compounds. But sometimes, the isolation of the "active compound" has made the compound ineffective. Therefore, while using the plant-based drug, one must start with a combinatorial approach when evaluating candidate compounds. A reverse pharmacology approach, based on traditional medicine as Ayurveda, can be exploited as a smart strategy for discovering new drug candidates and also for the development of better synergistic herbal formulations with enhanced performance in terms of safety, efficacy, and cost [16, 17, 22 - 24]. These pharmacological approaches involving herbal extracts from medicinal plants or nutraceuticals have been shown to impart at least three clinical beneficial effects for better management of PD:

a. Affecting the neurodegenerative process from the prodromal stage onward.
b. Reducing the incidence and severity of the side effects of the conventional therapy.
c. Improving non-motor symptoms [25].

CLASSIFICATION OF NEUROPROTECTIVE PHYTOCHEMICALS USED IN AYURVEDIC HERBAL FORMULATIONS

Phytochemicals are non-nutritive secondary metabolites used for drug discovery and development. Depending upon the chemical structures and characteristics, phytochemicals can be broadly classified into polyphenols, terpenes, alkaloids, and other nitrogen-containing compounds (*e.g.*, glucosinolates and polyamines), carbohydrates, lipids, and steroids [26]. The main classes of phytochemicals found in Ayurvedic medicinal herbs are taken into account here.

Polyphenols

Polyphenols are a large group of naturally occurring plant chemicals, widely found in fruits and vegetables [27]. A number of nutritional studies have shown significant neuroprotective potential and cognitive benefits of polyphenols [28]. Polyphenol-rich plants used in Ayurveda for the treatment of PD include *Curcuma longa*, (turmeric) containing curcumin, *Camellia sinensis* (green tea) containing catechins, and flavonoids, *Centella asiatica* (Gotu kola) containing gallic acids and flavonoids, and *Vitis vinifera* (common grape vine) containing resveratrol. Polyphenols consist of multiple hydroxyl groups on aromatic rings, and depending upon the number of phenol rings present and their properties, these compounds are broadly classified into two groups:

Flavonoids

Flavonoids are the most common bioactive polyphenols, and they are characterized by a structure consisting of two benzene rings - A and C-linked by a heterocyclic "pyran" or "pyrone" B ring, each bearing at least one hydroxyl group, and connected with a three-carbon bridge. Flavonoids are divided into subgroups based on the degree of the C ring oxidation, the ring's hydroxylation pattern, and substitution at position 3 in the C ring. The six subgroups are - flavonols (found mainly in broccoli, onion, kale, and fruit peels), flavones (found in apple skins, parsley, and celery), flavanols (*e.g.*, catechins, ECGC [epicatechin (EC), epicatechin-3-gallate (ECG), epigallocatechin-3-gallate (EGCG)] in green tea, red wine, and chocolate,), flavanones (found in citrus food, and tomatoes), anthocyanidins (found in red wine cherries, grapes, and berry fruits), and isoflavonoids (found in soybeans, and legumes).

Non-flavonoids

Stilbenes (*e.g.*, reseveratrol), phenolic acids (derivatives of cinnamic acid *e.g.*, curcumin, and derivatives of benzoic acid *e.g.*, gallic acid), and lignans (sesamin, sesaminol, and sesamonil found in sesame).

Terpenes

Another very important group of phytochemicals in PD treatment is terpenes. Terpenes are a diverse family of organic compounds categorized based on the number of carbon atoms in the carbon skeleton and isoprene units present in the structure [29]. Nearly 50 000 terpene molecules have been discovered so far, and based on the number of carbon atoms, they are classified into hemiterpenes (C5), monoterpenes (C10), sesquiterpenes (C15), diterpenes (C20), sesterterpenes (C25), triterpenes (C30) and tetraterpenes or carotenoids (C40) [29]. Asiatic Acid is a triperpene found in *C. asiatica* (gotu kola). Two other major bioactive compounds used in ayurvedic treatment for PD are bacosides/bacopasides found in *Bacopa monnieri* (Brahmi) and withanolides found in *Withania somnifera* (Ashwagandha). These two compounds are triterpenes and steroidal, known as triterpenoid saponins [26].

Alkaloids

Alkaloids are naturally occurring compounds containing carbon, hydrogen, nitrogen, and usually oxygen and are primarily found in plants; important plant families highly rich in several kinds of alkaloids are Papaveraceae (poppies family), Solanaceae (nightshades), Amaryllidaceae (amaryllis), and Ranunculaceae (buttercups). Alkaloids are divided into different classes based on their sources, pharmacokinetics, and chemical structures. Alkaloid phytochemicals found beneficial in different PD models are berberine, piperine, and caffeine [30].

Other Nitrogen-Containing Phytochemicals

This group of naturally occurring compounds found in cruciferous vegetables (*i.e.*, broccoli, cabbage, brussels sprouts, watercress, and cauliflower) has PD preventive and therapeutic potential. The most important phytochemicals of this group are sulforaphane (glucosinolate group), and spermine/ spermidine, which is a polyamine found in soybean seeds [29, 31].

MECHANISTIC ACTION OF PHYTOCHEMICALS IN NEUROPROTECTION

Phytochemicals can exert their neuroprotective effect by following molecular mechanisms (Fig. **1**).

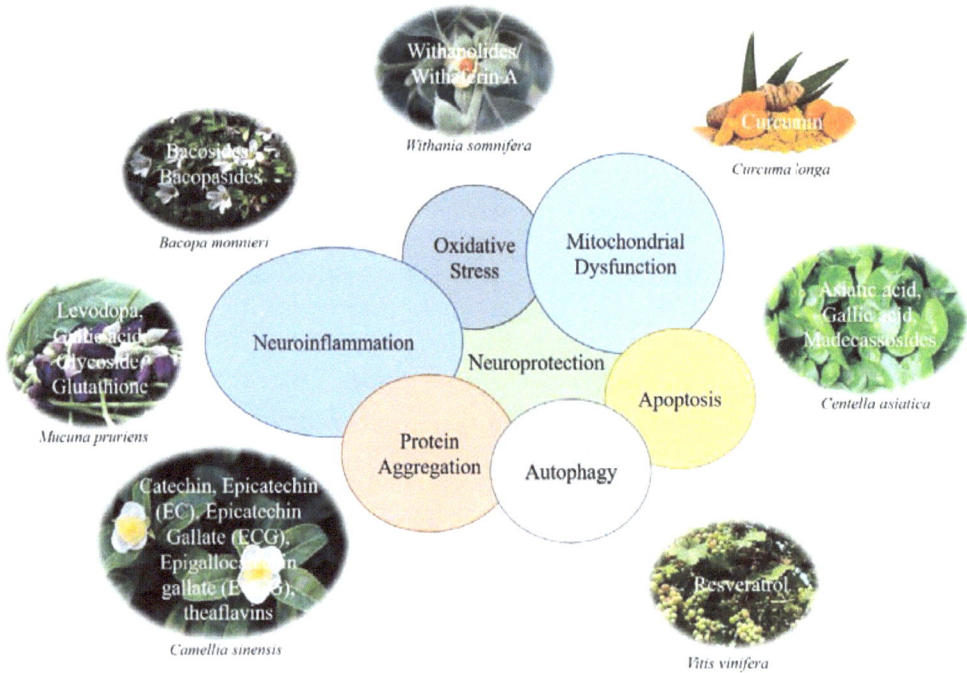

Fig. (1). Neuroprotective effect of various phytochemicals of plants used in Ayurveda.

Reactive Oxygen Species (ROS) Regulation

Oxidative stress is a significant PD-related phenomenon occurring due to imbalanced redox homeostasis due to increased production of ROS or reduced cellular antioxidant activity of a cell. Oxidative stress can be generated due to DA metabolism, mitochondrial dysfunction, neuroinflammation, iron, calcium, and aging [32]. DA metabolism can itself increase ROS through DA quinines which can modify several PD-related proteins, such as α-syn, parkin, DJ-1, superoxide dismutase-2 (SOD2), and ubiquitin carboxy-terminal hydrolase-L1 (UCH-L1), can cause inactivation of the DA transporter (DAT) and the tyrosine hydroxylase (TH) enzyme, leading to dysfunction in mitochondrial complex I activity. Complex I further is a primary source of ROS in PD. Reduction in complex I activity in the SNpc of PD patients is very well described [33].

The antioxidant mechanisms of phytochemicals consist of:

a. Promoting ROS scavenging and suppressing intracellular ROS accumulation;
b. Activation of antioxidant activity of cell- Nuclear factor erythroid 2-related factor 2/ antioxidant responsive element (Nrf2/ ARE), which induces the expression of various ROS-dissipating and antioxidant enzymes. These include heme oxygenase-1 (HO-1), NADPH quinone oxidoreductase (NQO1) and γ-glutamyl-cysteine synthetase (GCS), which promotes the synthesis of glutathione (GSH), GSH synthetase (GSS), GSH reductase (GSR), GSH peroxidase (GPx), superoxide dismutase (SOD), catalase (CAT), thioredoxin (THx), and glutamate-cysteine ligase (GCL);
c. Metal ion chelating ability like copper (II) and iron (III);
d. ROS-mediated lipid peroxidation (LPO).

Mitochondrial Dysfunction

In neurodegenerative diseases, oxidative stress and mitochondrial dysfunction form a vicious cycle, ultimately leading to apoptosis. Mitochondria are the main source of adenosine triphosphate (ATP) generation in neurons, but damaged mitochondria are the main intracellular source of ROS and pro-apoptotic caspases. Defects of the electron transport chain (*etc.*) complexes, such as lower complex I activity in mitochondria and increased oxidative damage, are consistent features of the parkinsonian brain [34]. Complex I dysfunction increases ROS/ RNS, inflammatory cytokines, and vice versa. This triggers the mutation, damage, and fragmentation of mitochondrial DNA (mtDNA). Mutation and deletion in different genes encoded by mtDNA are significantly elevated in DAergic neurons of aging, and early PD patients' brains [35]. Oxidative stress and mitochondrial dysfunction in PD are associated with the accumulation of α-syn oligomers and fibrils in mitochondria, accelerating its dysfunction. Oxidative stress due to ROS/ RNS, reduced ATP production, presence of neurotoxins, excitotoxicity, and reduced level of neurotrophic factors (NTFs) initiates mitochondrial apoptosis cascade and formation of the mitochondrial permeability transition pore (mPTP) [36]. Phytochemicals in Ayurvedic herbs can improve mitochondrial functions, especially the *etc.* activity, and modulate the redox state [34].

Anti-Neuroinflammatory Pathways

Abnormal aggregation of α-syn in neurons in PD gets released in extracellular space and can be transmitted from cell to cell. Also, there is oxidation and glycation of different proteins, which form danger-associated molecular patterns

(DAMPs), including advanced glycation end products (AGE), AGE-modified proteins, and high mobility group box 1 (HMGB1), depolarized mitochondria leaking ROS, and also fragments of mtDNA. If there is a failure of a cell clearing system like the proteasomal pathway and the autophagy-lysosome pathway, in an unconventional solution to overcome DAMPs, cells release them extracellularly as free compounds or exosomes. These DAMPs can bind to toll-like receptors (TLRs), and AGE receptors (RAGEs), in neighboring cells (including neurons, and glia), and as a consequence, downstream oxidative and inflammatory signaling pathways are activated. TLRs- and RAGEs-induced activation of protein kinase C (PKC), Janus kinase 2/signal transducer and activators of transcription 1 (JAK2/STAT1), Protein Kinase B (also known as AKT)/Mammalian Target of Rapamycin (AKT/mTOR) and NF-kB pathways converge in promoting neuroinflammation through NF-kB-related inflammasome (NLRP3) activation within neurons, microglia, and astrocytes and hence cause an increase in proinflammatory cytokines and chemokines and enzymes like iNOS and COX-2. This way, indigested DAMPs can propagate oxidative and inflammatory damage in the surrounding neuronal microenvironment. Phytochemicals have anti-inflammatory action mechanisms that alleviate neuroinflammatory pathways, such as AGE/RAGEs, HMGB1/TLR-4, and NF-kB/NLRP3, and up-regulation of AMPK/SIRT1/PGC-1α and Nrf2. Various phytochemicals can attenuate neuroinflammatory processes by inhibiting the inflammatory signaling pathway and various factors involved [37 - 39].

Modulating Cell Signaling Pathways

Several phytochemicals can interact with cell survival signaling pathways and apoptotic pathways, for example, polyphenols activate cell-survival signaling pathways, including phosphoinositide 3-kinase (PI3K), Akt/protein kinase B (Akt/PKB), tyrosine kinases, protein kinase C (PKC), and mitogen-activated protein kinase (MAPK) signaling cascades [40]. PKC is activated by phospholipids and Ca^{2+} and mediates normal cell function. MAPK signal pathways mediate the expression of pro-survival genes, including antioxidant enzymes, Neurotrophic Factors (NTFs), and cytokines. MAPKs are classified into ERK, JNK, and p38. ERK1/2 phosphorylate CREB and upregulate Bcl-2 and Bcl-xL, and JNK regulates the transcription-dependent apoptotic signals, whereas p38 is implicated in cell death and cell cycle [41, 42].

Apoptosis

An increase in mitochondrial membrane permeability transition (MPT), leads to loss of mitochondrial membrane potential ($\Delta\Psi m$), followed by the opening of the non-specific channel called the mitochondrial permeability transition pore (mPTP), and release of apoptosis-executing molecules, such as cytochrome c (Cytc), an activator of caspases (Smac)/Diablo, apoptosis-inducing factor (AIF) is the key event in apoptosis. The major components of the mPTP are Voltage-Dependent Anion Channel (VDAC), adenine nucleotide translocator (ANT), and cyclophilin D (CypD). In addition, anti- and pro-apoptotic Bcl-2 protein family, TSPO, hexokinase (HK)-I and -II are associated with VDAC and creatine kinases (CK). Glycogen synthase kinase-3β (GSK-3β) phosphorylates VDAC and inhibits the interaction of VDAC with HK [35, 36].

Autophagy

Three signaling complexes and pathways are involved in autophagic response during neurodegeneration- a) the mTOR signaling pathway, b) the ATG1 complex (indirect involvement of mTOR), and c) the Vps34-beclin 1/class III PI3K complex [43]. Complex machinery of more than 30 autophagy-related genes (Atg) regulates the whole autophagy process. In normal non-stress condition, mTOR complex1 (mTORC1) hyperphosphorylation Atg13, which further inhibit Atg1 or Vps34 along with Vps15, activates the PI3K pathway, both causing negative regulation of autophagy. Atg3 to Atg7 help in the conversion of Atg8 to LC3II isoform during autophagosome maturation. Other than Akt/mTOR, other pathways involved in autophagy are 5' AMP-activated Protein Kinases (AMPK) activation or inhibition of Glycogen Synthase Kinase3-β (GSK3-β), activation of NAD-dependent deacetylase Sirtuin-1 (Sirt-1), which causes deacetylation of Atg5, Atg7, LC3, and transcription factor Forkhead box O3 (FOXO3), which in turn controls expression of several pro-autophagic proteins. Alteration in autophagy has been documented in the PD patient brain, and various PD mutations such as α-Syn, LRRK2, UCH-L1, DJ-1, PINK-1, and Parkin. It has been found that α-Syn co-accumulation with LC3-II, increased level of mTOR and decreased level of Atg7, α-Syn binding with Lysosomal-associated membrane protein type 2A and inhibiting its own and other autophagy substrates by lysosome in PD [44 - 46]. Phytochemicals cause neuroprotection by modulation of autophagy by Beclin-1 dependent (canonical) and Beclin-1 independent (non-canonical) pathways [47].

Hypoxia Inducible Factor 1 Alpha (HIF-1 α) Pathway

PD caused due to Phosphatase and tensin (PTEN) induced kinase 1 (PINK1); Deglycase (DJ-1) deficiencies exhibited significantly reduced induction of HIF-1α level. The activation of hypoxia signal transduction pathways through which the hypoxic condition is sensed and appropriate genes are activated and expressed is important to mediate compensatory survival conditions for the cells. A high percentage of hypoxic responses in cells is controlled by hypoxia-inducible transcription factor-1. Phytochemicals can induce neuroprotection through induction of the HIF-1 [48, 49].

α- Synuclein Aggregation

α-Synuclein is a 140 amino acid long protein that plays a key role in synaptic vesicle trafficking and fusion and also in the release of dopamine at presynaptic terminals. In native condition, it exists as a monomer, and upon binding with lipid vesicle, attains an α-helical structure. In PD, cytoplasmic inclusions called Lewy bodies are formed, in which large aggregates with β sheet-rich α-Syn fibrils are found. α-Syn has three distinct domains, in which the central hydrophobic non-amyloid-β component (NAC) domain is responsible for aggregation. Several theories describe the role of α-Syn in PD neurodegeneration as impaired synaptic vesicle trafficking and fusion, free radical generation, mitochondrial stress, endoplasmic reticulum stress, and impaired autophagy lysosomal pathway. Phytochemicals have been found to inhibit oligomerization and fibrillation and disaggregation of preformed fibrils of α-Syn [50].

NEUROPROTECTIVE PLANTS IN AYURVEDA FOR PARKINSON'S DISEASE MANAGEMENT (TABLE 2)

Table 2. Neuroprotective effect of various phytochemicals of plants used in Ayurveda for Parkinson's disease management in various experimental models of Parkinson's disease.

Botanical name/ Common name [Phytochemical or Active agent]	Neuroprotective Mechanism		Refs.
	Cell-based models PD model	*In vivo* PD models	
Bacopa monnieri/ **Brahmi** [Bacosides/ Bacopasides]	*B.monnieri* in SH-SY5Y cells ↓toxicity and morphologic alterations ↑mitochondrial functions, MMP, NADH dehydrogenase, mitochondrial complex I activity ↓ROS and superoxide anion levels	*B. monnieri* in mice and rat ↓Parkinsonian motor abnormalities ↓behavioral alterations ↓TH-positive cell loss ↓neurotransmitter alterations ↑DA and its metabolite levels ↑cholinergic enzymes activity ↑neurogenic genes in the SNc ↓oxidative stress, mitochondrial dysfunctions, and ↑anti-oxidant enzymes CAT, GR, GPx and SDH ↓ROS, MDA and H2O2 levels ↑ and mitochondrial complex enzymes activities ↓lipid peroxidation, nitrite levels and protein carbonyl content ↓apoptotic enzymes caspase-3 and Bax ↑anti-apoptotic enzyme Bcl-2 *B.*	[51 - 62]

(Table 2) cont.....

Botanical name/ Common name [Phytochemical or Active agent]	Neuroprotective Mechanism		Refs.
	Cell-based models PD model	*In vivo* **PD models**	
	↑GSH and antioxidant enzymes levels ↑proteasome activity ↑pAkt/total Akt ratio, and activation of Nrf2 *B. monnieri* in PC12 cells ↓toxicity ↑TH levels ↓ROS, superoxide anion, MMP ↑anti-oxidant systems, (GCS) and Trx1 levels ↓activation of Akt and HSP90 *B. monnieri* in N27 DA-cells ↓toxicity ↓ROS and H2O2 levels ↑GSH levels	*monnieri* in *Drosophila* ↑climbing ability ↓motor alterations and lethality and toxicity ↑ striatal DA levels and cholinergic enzymes activity↓oxidative stress, mitochondrial dysfunctions ↑survival and locomotor activity ↓MDA, ROS, H2O2, lipid peroxidation and protein carbonyl content ↓apoptosis-associated genes and proteins JNK, caspase-3 ↑SDH, mitochondrial complex I-III, and II-III enzymes, CAT, and ATP *B. monnieri* in *C. elegans* ↓loss of DA neurons ↓α-syn aggregation ↑lipid content *B. monnieri* in zebrafish ↓Parkinsonian motor symptoms ↑DA and its metabolites levels ↑GSH, GPx, CAT, SOD, and mitochondrial complex-I ↓lipid peroxidation, MDA levels	
***Mucuna pruriens*/ Velvet beans** [Levodopa, Gallic acid, Glycoside, glutathione]	Microglia BV-2 cells ↓H2O2 cytotoxicity ↓ROS, Nitric oxide, IL-1β, IL-6, TNF-α, and nuclear translocation of NF-κB. ↓apoptosis *M. pruriens* in SH-SY5Y cells ↓apoptosis	*M. pruriens* in mice and rat ↓motor abnormalities, behavioral alterations ↑DA and its metabolite levels ↑TH-positive neurons ↓GFAP, iNOS, ICAM, TNF-α, NF-κB ↑pAkt1 activity, ↑GSH Catalase ↓apoptosis ↓apoptotic enzymes caspase-3 and Bax ↑anti-apoptotic enzyme Bcl-2 *M. Pruriens* in Drosophila ↑climbing ability, ↑lifespan ↓neurotoxicity *M. Pruriens* in *C. elegans* ↑survival	[63 - 71]

(Table 2) cont.....

Botanical name/ Common name [Phytochemical or Active agent]	Neuroprotective Mechanism		Refs.
	Cell-based models PD model	***In vivo* PD models**	
***Withania somnifera*/ Ashwagandha** or Indian ginseng [Withanolides/ Withaferin A]		Ashwagandha in mice and rat ↓Parkinsonian motor abnormalities ↓behavioral alterations and TH loss ↑TH expression ↑DA and its metabolite levels, DA D2 receptor binding ↑GSH, GPx, GR, GST, SOD, and CAT ↓lipid peroxidation and thiobarbituric acid reactive substance (TBARS) ↑Bcl-2 Ashwagandha in *Drosophila* ↓toxicity and motor alterations ↑lifespan, locomotor activity, muscle electrophysiological response to stimuli ↑climbing ability ↑striatal DA levels ↓mitochondria degeneration ↓ROS, lipid peroxidation, and H2O4 ↑GSH, GST, SOD, and CAT ↑SDH, mitochondrial complex-I-III and complex-II-III	[72 - 80]
***Curcuma longa*/ Turmeric** [Curcumin]	Curcumin in SH-SY5Y ↓cytotoxicity ↑DA and tyrosine hydroxylase (TH) levels ↓loss of TH ↓α-syn protein and mRNA levels aggregation ↓toxic quinone formation ↓ROS ↑anti-oxidant enzyme levels and MMP ↓Nuclear Factor K Beta (NF-kβ) nuclear translocation ↓p38-Mitogen-Activated Protein Kinase (MAPK) ↓mTOR ↑LAMP2, LC3II, co-localization of LC3-α-syn puncta and TFEB	Curcumin in mice and rat ↓loss of TH-positive neurons ↑stimulates DA neurogenesis through HDAC inhibition ↓Parkinsonian motor symptoms ↑locomotor activity ↓behavioral alterations ↓L-DOP--induced dyskinesia, depletion of DA levels and dopamine transporter (DAT)-positive fibers in the striatum ↑TH and DAT expression ↓α-syn aggregation ↓α-syn positive Lewy Bodie's ↓neurotoxicity ↓ROS ↑anti-oxidant markers SOD, Catalase, GSH, SDH activity, NADPH oxidase complex and mitochondrial enzyme complex activity ↓MDA, Hsp70 and (NADPH): quinone oxidoreductase 1 level ↓lipid peroxidation nitrite levels ↓iron deposition ↑Nrf2 pathway	[81 - 101]

(Table 2) cont.....

Botanical name/ Common name [Phytochemical or Active agent]	Neuroprotective Mechanism		Refs.
	Cell-based models PD model	*In vivo* **PD models**	
	↓c-Jun, c-Jun N-Terminal Kinase (JNK) ↓necrotic-like morphologic alterations ↓p53-mediated apoptosis ↓proapoptotic proteins Bax, BAD, caspase-3, -6, -8, -9 in cytochrome-c in ↑MMP ↑anti-apoptotic markers Bcl-2, Bcl-xL, and Cyt-c in mitochondria curcumin in PC12 cells ↑neuronal differentiation ↓α-sy--induced cytotoxicity ↑ DAT and TH expression ↓ROS, mitochondrial depolarization and Cyt-c release, caspase-9 and -3 activation ↓pro-inflammatory cytokine release ↓NO and iNOS levels ↓apoptosis Curcumin in HEK293T cells and primary neurons ↓combined cytotoxicity ↓LRRK2 kinase activity Curcumin in deutocerebrum primary cells ↑survival, anti-oxidant defense, and adhesive ability ↑Wnt/β-catenin signaling pathway	↓GFAP, NF-kβ, TNF-α, IL-1β and 1α, iNOS and tyrosine receptor kinase A (TrkA) expression ↓JNK and caspase-related apoptotic pathways ↓Bax, Caspase 3, and Caspase 9 ↓c-Fos, Fra, FosB, and c-Jun ↑regeneration of neuroblasts in the subventricular zone (SVZ) ↑Wnt3/b-catenin pathway ↑GDNF, NGF and TGF-β1 Curcumin in *Drosophila* models ↑lifespan, survival, and activity pattern ↓locomotor defects ↓loss of TH-positive neurons and DA levels ↓oxidized protein levels and LRRK2 kinase activity ↓oxidative stress, ↓ROS apoptosis, lipid peroxidation protein carbonyl overload	
Centella asiatica/ **Gotu kola** [Asiatic acid, Gallic acid, Madecassosides]	*C. asiatica* in SH-SY5Y cells ↓cytotoxicity and DNA damage ↓ROS, ↑MPP, ↓apoptosis, ↑ Bcl-2 ↓Bax, Cyt-c, caspases-3, -6, -8, and -9	*C. asiatica* in mice and rat ↓motor abnormalities ↓loss of TH cells ↑DA levels and its metabolite levels ↑DAT and VMAT2) in the SN and striatum ↑mitochondrial complex I activity ↑GSH, ↑SOD, CAT, GPx, and GSH ↓lipid peroxidation, and protein carbonyl content ↓MDA,↑Brain-Derived and Vascular-Endothelial Growth Factors (BDNF, VEGF), GDNF, and TrKB ↓MAPK-P38 related activation of JNK and ERK *C. asiatica* in rats ↓motor abnormalities ↑GSH, Bcl-2/Bax ratio, BDNF *C. asiatica* in *Drosophila* ↑climbing ability and activity pattern ↑GSH ↓MDA, ↓lipid peroxidation, and protein carbonyl content	[102 - 107]

(Table 2) cont.....

Botanical name/ Common name [Phytochemical or Active agent]	Neuroprotective Mechanism		Refs.
	Cell-based models PD model	*In vivo* **PD models**	
Camellia sinensis/ **Green tea,** [Catechin, Epicatechin (EC), Epicatechin Gallate (ECG), Epigallocatechin gallate (EGCG), theaflavins]	EGCG in PC12 cells ↓cytotoxicity ↓ROS production ↑SOD1 and GPx ↑SIRT1/ Peroxisome PGC-1α pathway ↓NF-kβ nuclear translocation and binding activity EGCG in PC12 ↓toxicity ↓Nf-kβ nuclear translocation and binding activity EGCG in RGC-5 ↓toxicity ↓lipid peroxidation ↓MAPK, c-Jun, JNK, and p38	EGCG in mice and rat ↓motor abnormalities ↓behavioral alterations ↓loss of TH-positive neurons ↑striatal DA levels, ↑TH activity ↓α-syn accumulation ↑Protein Kinase C alpha (PKC-α) overexpression ↓oxidative stress and protein carbonyl content [72] ↓lipid peroxidation, nitrite levels ↑ iron-export protein ferroportin ↓mTOR, AKT, and GSK3β levels ↑COX-2 ↓the ratio of CD3+CD4+ to CD3+CD8+ T lymphocytes in the peripheral blood [73] ↓iNOS ↓TNF-α and IL-6 in the serum ↑Bcl-2 ↓Bax Catechins (EGCG and propyl gallate, PG) in Drosophila ↑life-span ↑climbing and locomotor ability ↓loss of DA neurons ↓degeneration of TH-positive neurons ↑mitochondrial integrity ↓lipid peroxidation ↑activation of AMPK ↓apoptosis	[68, 108 - 117]
Vitis vinifera/ Red grapevine [Resveratrol]	Resveratrol in SH-SY5Y and PC12 cells ↓α-syn mRNA levels ↓α-syn aggregation ↓cytotoxicity ↓mitochondrial damage ↓ROS and apoptosis [104 - 106] ↓histone-associated DNA fragmentation ↑p-ERK1/2/ERK1/2 ratio	Resveratrol in mice and rat ↓Parkinsonian motor symptoms ↓behavioral alterations ↓cognitive deficits ↓nigral histopathology ↓loss of TH-positive neurons and striatal DA depletion ↓α-syn levels ↓neurotoxicity ↓total α-syn aggregation ↓oxidative stress ↑SDH, GSH, CAT, GPx citrate synthase, aconitase, and mitochondrial complex I activity ↓lipid peroxidation, MDA ↓ protein carbonyl content ↓ER stress markers CHOP and GRP78 ↓apoptosis, Bax and Caspase 3	[118 - 123]

(Table 2) cont.....

Botanical name/ Common name [Phytochemical or Active agent]	Neuroprotective Mechanism		Refs.
	Cell-based models PD model	***In vivo* PD models**	
	↓cleaved Poly ADP-ribose Polymerase (PARP) ↑autophagy ↑Heme Oxygenase-1-dependent autophagy [104, 105] ↑SIRT1 pathway and autophagy Resveratrol in SK-N-BE cells ↓cytotoxicity ↓ROS ↑SIRT1-dependent autophagy	↓MALAT1 and miR-129 expression ↓neuroinflammation ↓proinflammatory cytokine IL-1β and GFAP ↓COX-2 and TNF-α ↑Nrf2 DNA-binding activity ↑pAkt/Akt ratio ↓p62 levels ↑SIRT1 and autophagy ↓chromatin condensation and clumping, ↓mitochondrial tumefaction, and vacuolization. Resveratrol in *Drosophila* ↑survival rate and lifespan ↑locomotor activity, and muscle ATP production ↓behavioral deficits and brain histopathology ↓DA neuron loss and abnormal wing posture ↓mitochondrial aggregates ↓H2O2 and nitric oxide (NO) ↑GST and CAT ↑ mitophagy ↑autophagy	

Bacopa monnieri (Brahmi)

Bacopa monnieri (L.) – (Common names: Brahmi, Waterhyssop) (BM), is a perennial creeping herb of the family Scrophulariaceae, and a well-known nootropic plant. In Ayurveda, it is well known as a "Medhya Rasayana", a herb that sharpens the mind and the intellect [124], commonly used to improve cognitive function of the brain, promote longevity, and effective in inflammatory conditions, possess anticholinesterase activity and anti-depressant activity [124]. Phytochemical studies on "Brahmi" have shown that it contains many active constituents found in BM phytochemical studies, including alkaloids, brahmine, herpestine, D-mannitol, betulinic acid, β-sitosterol, stigmasterols, and the major and most important one is saponins (bacosides A, A3, and B and bacopasaponin A to F) [125]. BM has proven its anti-parkinsonism efficiency, in both, *in vitro* and *in vivo*; toxin-induced and transgenic experimental conditions are attributed to its neuroprotective, anti-oxidative, anti-apoptotic, and anti-inflammatory properties [62]. In accordance with it, BM Extract (BME) provides protection against Paraquat (PQ) and rotenone-induced toxicity by reducing oxidative stress markers level, including ROS, malondialdehyde (MDA), Hydroperoxide (HP), improved redox homeostasis, diminutive mitochondrial dysfunction, and restored striatal DA in PQ mice model [62] rotenone-induced mouse model [60] and Rotenone-treated *Drosophila* model and PQ induced *Drosophila* model [59] of PD and BM diminished the mortality induced by PQ also PQ induced *Drosophila* model of PD [59] and reduced the cytotoxicity in DAergic neurons due to rotenone treatment

[61]. Besides, BME supplementation in the transgenic PD model of *Drosophila* expressing wild-type human α-syn showed a reduction of oxidative stress and apoptosis and delayed the loss of climbing ability [58]. Further, BM supplementation reduces the α-syn aggregation and prevents the degeneration of DAergic neurons, increased longevity, and restored lipid content in two transgenic PD models of *C. elegans* overexpressing human α-syn, and a 6-OHDA induced PD model expressing green fluorescent protein (GFP) specifically in DA neurons [57]. Besides, BME supplementation in MPP+ and PQ-induced SK-N-SH cell line improves mitochondrial functioning by improving Mitochondrial membrane potential, restoring normal electron transport chain (*etc.*) complexes activity, increasing GSH level, and proteasome activity, and increasing activation of Nrf2 [55, 56]. Further, BME also increased DA and its metabolite level and rescued the loss of the tyrosine hydroxylase (TH)-positive cell, inhibited lipid peroxidation, enhanced the level of the anti-oxidant enzyme, such as Catalase, Glutathione reductase, GPx, and anti-apoptotic Bcl-2 activity in MPTP induced PD mice model [1, 58]. BM supplementation rescued the reduction of exploratory behaviour, gait abnormalities and motor impairment in MATP and PQ-induced PD mouse model, increased dopamine levels, and reversed cholinergic activity striatum [53, 54]. BM supplementation improved locomotor abilities in *Drosophila* PD model having PINK1 mutation [52]. BME significantly rescued the locomotory behaviour in the MPTP-induced mouse model of PD. BME improved the dopaminergic cell survival, and activated Akt and Hsp90 in PQ induced PC12 cell model of PD [51]. BME phytochemical coated platinum nanoparticle BmE-PtNPs showed neuroprotective potentials as it significantly increased the level of DA and its metabolites, GSH, GPx, catalase, SOD, and complex I, reduced MDA and improved the locomotor activity in MPTP induced PD model in zebrafish [126]. Therefore, the anti-parkinsonism potential of BME is evident, and BME seems to have significant potential as an herbal drug. However, more studies are required for a clearer understanding of the molecular mechanism utilized for using BM as a potential drug against PD.

Mucuna pruriens (Velvet Beans)

Mucuna pruriens (Mp), also referred to as velvet beans (Atmagupta: Sanskrit), is a tropical climbing type legume plant from the family Fabaceae, known for its medicinal importance. Mp seeds possess anti-inflammatory, anti-oxidant, anti-microbial, anti-diabetic, and anti-epileptic properties and treat ulcers, helminthiasis, and nephropathy [127]. In Ayurveda, the importance of Mp has been well known since ancient times and is used for the treatment of PD [128]. Mp seed contains 6-9% of levodopa by weight and is the best source of natural levodopa, but it also contains gallic acid, phytic acid, quercetin, catechin equivalents, triterpenes, and sterols [3, 129]. Ursolic acid (UA) is a triterpenoid discovered in MP recently [3]. In a study of treatment of 60 PD patients (about half of them being L-DOPA naïve) over 12 weeks with MP, preparations showed a significant improvement in both UPDRS score and the H and Y stage, after which *Mucuna* preparation (Zandopa™) was registered as a PD treatment in India [130]. A similar type of result was found in another study, including 18 PD patients in India [131]. A clinical trial comparing the efficacy of MP with levodopa/carbidopa (L/C) in single-dose shows that MP has quicker action onset, last longer, and without worsening dyskinesia, but the result was not so positive when MP was given for a longer duration of 16 weeks mainly due to gastrointestinal disturbances and worse motor symptom [132 - 134]. When MP is used along with carbidopa, it has better outcomes [135]. Studies in human subjects and animal models have shown that supplementation of Mp seed improved locomotor behaviour after MP seed supplementation [70, 71]. Studies show that Mp improves redox status by attenuating oxidative stress, inhibiting lipid peroxidation and nitrite level [10, 11, 70]. Mp, through its anti-oxidant property, improves catalase and glutathione activity, and the metal-chelating property improves synaptic and mitochondrial functions, hence increasing neuronal survival [67]. MP extract shows anti-neuroinflammatory action in the MPTP-induced mice model and anti-apoptotic activity in the PQ-induced mice model and improves TH expression in *Drosophila* and a mouse model of PD [67]. In a comparative analysis of the BME and Mp seed extract effect in a mouse model of PD, BME is more effective than Mp seed extract [66]. More research is needed for a better understanding of the comparison of the herbal drugs for their potential efficiency in PD management. A silver-velvet bean nanoparticle (AgMPn) at the best dose was 5 mg/kg body weight and magnetite -*M. pruriens* nanoparticle (FeMPn) at the best dose of 10 mg/kg body weight, significantly lowered the catalepsy symptoms in the PD mice model [64, 65]. While *M. pruriens* Gold nanoparticles (MPGNPs) improved the behavioral changes in the MPTP-induced mice PD model [63].

Withania somnifera (Ashwagandha or Indian Ginseng)

Withania somnifera (Ws) or Ashwagandha (Solanaceae family) is an important ayurvedic medicinal plant and has been used as a medicine for over 3000 years [136]. The main constituents of ashwagandha are Withanoloid and withaferin A; others are Withanine, alanine, somnine, somniferine, and somniferinine. Ws have various medicinal potentials, such as an aphrodisiac, sedative, a potential nerve tonic, rejuvenating, and life-prolonging properties [137]. The roots of Ws are also useful for depression, anxiety, constipation, general and senile debility, rheumatism, loss of muscular energy, and spermatorrhea (Singh and Kumar

1998). Ws roots show anti-oxidant, anti-inflammatory, anti-carcinogenic, and memory-enhancing properties [138 - 140]. Therefore, it can be useful in treating several disorders, including neurodegenerative diseases like PD [79, 80]. Ws root extract tends to improve motor functions by elevating DA levels in the striatum MPTP mouse model of PD [78]. Studies have shown the anti-oxidant property of Ws, as in the MPTP-induced mouse model of PD Ws root extract, can normalize oxidative stress by increasing antioxidant enzyme glutathione (GSH) and glutathione peroxidase (GPx) levels [77, 79]. It reduces oxidative stress in 6-Hydroxydopamine (6-OHDA) and induces the rat model of PD by reducing lipid peroxidation and increasing the antioxidant enzyme level, increasing TH expression, and increasing the level of dopamine and its metabolites, binding dopamine with DA D2 receptor [80]. Another study on ethanolic extract of Ws shows that Ws causes the reduction in oxidative stress and pro-oxidants like nitrite and lipid peroxidation, iNOS expression, increases catalase enzyme level, and improves motor function in the Maneb-PQ mouse model of PD [76]. Therefore, studies on the rat and mouse model of PD favor the potential of Ws against PD, but the Ws effect on the *Drosophila* PD model shows contradictory findings. In the LRRK2 mutation PD model of *Drosophila,* Ws extract improved locomotor activity, muscle electrophysiological response to stimuli, and also reduced mitochondria degeneration; on the other hand, reduced the lifespan impaired with the endosomal function suggest that Ws extract supplementation is effective in rescuing PD phenotype [74, 75]. However, the other groups have shown that Ws administration in the PINK1 mutant model of PD did not improve the climbing ability of *Drosophila* and so cannot rescue the PD phenotype [73]. More studies will be required to test the potential of Ws in the *Drosophila* model of PD. In this milieu, Ws increased the anti-apoptotic Bcl-2 while reducing the level of pro-apoptotic Bax in the maneb-PQ mouse model of PD, thereby reducing the level of apoptosis [72]. Therefore, Ws, although they have drug potential against PD, more studies will be required for further validation.

Curcuma longa (Turmeric)

Curcuma longa (Cl), or turmeric from the ginger family (Zingiberaceae), is a perennial herb, the oldest cultivated spice, and its rhizome is used in traditional ayurvedic treatment of a large number of diseases [141]. Curcumin is the active ingredient of *Curcuma longa,* which possesses anti-oxidant, anti-apoptotic, anti-inflammatory, anti-depressant, anti-microbial, anti-diabetic, and anticancer properties. Cl also possesses properties such as neuroprotection against aging of the brain, neuronal death, damage to the blood-brain barrier (BBB), and behavioral deficits and can also be efficient in neurodegenerative disorders like PD [142, 143]. Research has shown Curcumin improves striatal DA level, can increase Tyrosine hydroxylase expression and activity increase level of Dopamine transporter in 6-OHDA and rotenone-induced rat PD model, MPTP induced SH-SY5Y cell model of PD [98 - 101]. Cl also causes a reduction in the α-syn protein and mRNA level as well as α-Syn aggregation in the LPS induced rat model and MPTP induced SH_SY5Y cell model [95 - 97, 101]. Cl can improve the motor function in MPTP, Rotenone and Copper induced PD rat model and climbing ability of dUCH and LRRK2 knock out Drosophila model of PD [89, 91 - 95, 98, 101]. Curcumin is a potent hydrogen-atom donor, and its anti-oxidant property by imparted due to the phenolic hydroxyl, β-diketo, and methylene group. Curcumin is lipophilic and can scavenge free radicals hydrogen peroxide, hydroxyl radical, and peroxynitrite, which cause ROS/RNS oxidative stress and prevent lipid peroxidation *in vivo* and *in vitro* [54]. Curcumin can cause ferric ion (Fe^{3+}) reduction and ferrous ion (Fe^{2+}) chelation. Further, curcumin treatment to MPTP, Rotenone, 6-OHDA, and LPS induced mouse model tends to improve the level of anti-oxidant enzymes such as GSH, SOD, GPx, SDH, and Catalase and reduces ROS lipid peroxidation and MDA, thereby protecting proteins from oxidation [88, 93, 99, 100]. It also maintains mitochondrial complex I activity [109], reducing nitrosative stress and mitochondrial damage *in vitro* and *in vivo* PD models [87]. DA and ACh levels upregulation was also observed [99]. Cl can reduce neuroinflammation as evident by a reduction in reduction in TNF-α, IL-1β, GFAP, NF-κB, NO, and iNOS in LPS-induced Rat and 6-OHDA induced SH-SY5Y cell and MPTP-induced PC-12 cell model of PD [85, 86, 90, 95]. Besides, memory ability was also found to be improved substantially [99]. An increase in LAMP2, LC3II, and TFEB shows improved autophagy in the MPTP-induced SH-SY5Y cell model of PD after Cl treatment. Cl also reduces the level of pro-apoptotic protein as Bax, Bad, Caspase 3, -6, -8, and -9 and increases the level of anti-apoptotic proteins Bcl-2 and Bcl-xl in α-Syn overexpressing, MPTP, and rotenone-induced SH-SY5Y cell models of PD and LPS induced rat PD model [84, 88, 95, 96, 98]. Further, a synthetic derivative of curcumin referred to as curcumin-glucoside is also capable of binding with α-syn oligomeric form and prevents further fibrillization of α-syn [83]. Therefore, indicating the potential of Curcumin as a targeted therapy for PD and synucleinopathies. Hence to improve the bioavailability of Curcumin, research has now focused on nanoformulations as amine-functionalized mesoporous silica nanoparticle of curcumin reduces α-syn fibrillization [82], another with lactoferrin sol-oil chemistry reduces neurotoxicity in DA cell model due to rotenone toxicity [81], and further Curcumin loaded polysorbate 80-modified cerasome nanoparticles promote α-syn clearance, confer neuroprotection and alleviate motor deficits [101]. Moreover, curcumin does not show any side effects or toxicity, further improving its importance in PD therapy. Therefore, it seems evident that Cl has immense potential as a candidate drug development for PD

Centella asiatica (Gotu Kola)

Centella asiatica (L.), commonly known as Indian pennywort and Gotu kola and as Mandukaparni in Ayurveda, belonging Apiaceae family, is a perennial creeper plant. For thousands of years, it has been used in Indian ayurvedic medicine as a nootropic herb that enhances memory and cognitive function and is neuroprotective. It is also used for treating skin problems, wounds healing, asthma, revitalizing nerves and brain cells, increasing attention span and concentration, and also acts on gastric mucosa, lymphatic system, and heart. It is used to treat neurodegenerative disease and combat aging [144]. *C. asiatica* contains a wide variety of phytochemicals, including triterpenoids, Asiatic acid, Polyphenol Gallic acid, and madecassoside as major ones, and also contains flavonoids, alkaloids, tannins, volatile fatty acids, and glycosides [145]. *C. asiatica* possesses anxiolytic, anti-depressant, mood enhancer, anti-inflammatory, anti-oxidant, and anti-apoptotic properties, which probably makes it beneficial in neurodegenerative diseases as PD same is indicated by various *in vitro* and *in vivo* experimental studies also. Asiatic acid treatment in MPTP-induced mice model of PD can significantly reduce motor abnormalities, and increased expression of DA and Neurotrophic factors inhibited phosphorylation of JNK and ERK (MAPK/p38 related proteins) and enhanced phosphorylation of PI3K, Akt, and Gsk3β and hence activating PI3K/Akt/mTOR pathway which is important autophagy inducing pathway ultimately causing neuroprotection of DAergic neurons [107]. *C. asiatica* extract is found to reduce motor abnormality induced by MPTP in mice and also reduces Oxidative stress by increasing SOD, Catalase, GPx, and GSH and by reducing lipid peroxidation [105]. Asiatic Acid and madecassoside also have a similar effect as *C. asiatica* extract on MPTP toxicity in mice by reducing oxidative stress (reduced lipid peroxidation, MDA, and protein carbonyl content) and can also reduce apoptosis by increasing the Bcl-2/Bax ratio [103, 104]. Further reduction in mitochondrial dysfunction (improved Mitochondrial complex I activity) and apoptosis is observed in the rotenone-induced rat and SH-SY5Y cell model of PD [102, 106]. *C. asiatica* extracts given to Drosophila overexpressing human α-syn can significantly delay the loss of the climbing ability and improve the activity pattern, further, it also reduces the redox imbalance in this PD model of the fly. So, *C. asiatica* can reduce α-syn aggregation and increase disintegration of oligomers and fibrils of α-syn, reducing oxidative stress and Ca^{2+} overload while rescuing mitochondrial dysfunction through activation of autophagy. So, *C. asiatica* is very effective in neuroprotection in PD both *in vitro* and *in vivo*.

Camellia sinensis (Tea Plant)

Camellia sinensis (Cs) (Shyamaparni in Ayurveda) are known for a variety of tea like green tea, black tea, and oolong tea. It is an evergreen shrub from the family Theaceae. The main active compound in *C. sinensis* is Catechin - Epigallocatechin gallate (EGCG), which also contains another catechin [Epicatechin (EC), Epicatechin Gallate (ECG), theaflavins] and caffeine. The medicinal property of *C. sinensis* is different flavonoids and other antioxidant constituents [105]. In Ayurveda, it is used for the treatment of various conditions such as vitiate vata, pitta, fatigue, nervine tension, migraine, gas trouble, urinary retention, piles, inflammations, fever, and fatigue. It possesses anti-inflammatory, antioxidant, anti-cancer, anti-diabetic, anti-aging, anti-bacterial, anti-allergic, and anti-hair fall properties and is very useful in neurodegenerative disorders like PD. Green tea catechin, EGCG is remarkably efficient against α-syn aggregation and fibrillization [66]. EGCG can reduce the α-syn toxicity by disaggregating α-syn fibrils into small amorphous aggregates, so conformational changes required to form a larger aggregate are inhibited [117]. In the 6-OHDA-induced PD rat Model, EGCG effectively provides neuroprotection and reduces motor abnormalities, which is again due to reduced α-syn expression and decreased mTOR, AKT, and GSK3-β levels, hence upregulating autophagy [116]. Hence another possible mechanism for α-syn aggregation and level reduction could be the induction of autophagy-dependent protein clearance. The autophagic property of EGCG is dependent on dose, stress level and experimental model used. A low to moderate dose of EGCG increases autophagy, reduces apoptosis, and causes cell survival, while a higher concentration may reduce autophagy and hence induction of apoptosis [114, 115]. EGCG can also modulation of the hypoxia-inducible factor (HIF)-1 signaling pathway, leading to reduced oxidative stress and iron homeostasis maintenance [112, 113]. EGCG improved motor function, reduced oxidative stress, increased the iron export protein ferroportin in substantia nigra, and increased dopamine levels causing neuroprotection against MPTP-induced toxicity in mice [110, 111]. So EGCG possesses antioxidant and metal chelating ability in dopaminergic neurons. Further, EGCG inhibits the ROS-NO pathway improving redox homeostasis in the 6-OHDA-induced rat model of PD and inhibits iNOS in the MPTP-induced mouse model of PD [108, 109]. EGCG from *C. sinensis* has significant neuroprotection properties in PD models and holds the potential to be used as a future therapeutic strategy against PD.

Vitis vinifera (Common Grapevine)

Vitis vinifera or common grapevine (Angoor or munakka) is a deciduous climber of the family Vitaceae, Resveratrol a stilbene (polyphenol) is the main active component of *V. vinifera,* others being catechin, epicatechin, B-sitosterol, Ergosterol, and jasmonic acid. Resveratrol is present in the skin of red grapes, blueberries, raspberries, red wine, and Japanese knotweed. Resveratrol is water-soluble and can cross the blood-brain barrier (BBB). It has multiple biological and medicinal properties: neuroprotective, anti-oxidant, anti-inflammatory, antimicrobial, anti-aging, cardio-protective, and anti-tumor activities [146 - 149]. Resveratrol can also promote stem cell neural differentiation, as evidenced by elevated expression of neuro-progenitor markers Nestin, Musashi, and CD133 [149]. Resveratrol confers neuroprotection and rescues the loss of TH-positive dopaminergic neurons, increases the level of striatal DA, reduces the parkinsonian motor dysfunction, and improves behavioral abnormalities by activation of SIRT1-dependent autophagy in MPTP-induced mice model of parkinsonism [121, 122]. Further, Resveratrol can modulate the MALAT1/miR-129/SNCA signaling pathway, negatively regulating the SNCA gene hence reducing the mRNA expression level of α-syn and can also reduce α-Syn aggregation in MPTP-induced mice and SH-SY5Y cell model of PD [122]. This is recapitulated in MPTP-induced mice models of PD, where resveratrol can reduce the loss of DA neurons, increases TH and DA levels reduce α-syn aggregation and apoptosis as the level of pro-apoptotic signaling molecule Bax decreases while increasing the level of anti-apoptotic signaling molecule Bcl-2, reduces proinflammatory cytokines level as IL-1β and GFAP hence provide protection from cytotoxicity in both cell-based and animal models of parkinsonism. Remarkably, in the MPTP Mouse model of PD, a co-administration of resveratrol and L-DOPA reduces the dose of L-DOPA, which is required to produce positive effects and also reduces the side effects of L-DOPA, which may be due to an increased pAkt/Akt ratio and activation of autophagy through mTOR and Beclin-1 dependent pathways [120]. Indeed, it has been reported that Resveratrol can cause neuroprotection by activating autophagy through the AMPK/SIRT1 signaling pathway in rotenone-induced SH-SY5Y cells and α-syn overexpressing PC-12 cell model of PD and *via* the SIRT1-dependent LC3 de-acetylation pathway in MPTP-induced mice model of PD which ultimately degrades the α-syn [121, 123]. Reduction in the neuroprotective effect of Resveratrol after using an inhibitor of SIRT1 further strengthens the concept that autophagy induction and reduced degradation of α-Syn is the main neuroprotective mechanism of Resveratrol [121]. Hydroxyl group of Resveratrol helps it in scavenging hydroxyl radicals *in vitro* although, *in vivo*, the antioxidant potency is quite low, and this antioxidant property is mainly due to activation of Nrf2/ARE pathway and activation of antioxidants GSH, CAT, HO-1, and SOD and mitochondrial complex I activity [119]. Further, resveratrol nanoparticles (NRSV) prepared by temperature-controlled anti-solvent precipitation method, can improve the motor behaviour; reduce oxidative stress (reduced lipid peroxidation and increase GSH and CAT), and mitochondrial damage induced by rotenone treatment of mice model of PD. In this study, NRSV presented better efficiency than Resveratrol treatment of PD mice model [118]. Taken together, it is evident that Resveratrol is beneficial in the cell and animal model of parkinsonism, as it has the disease-modifying capability through induction of autophagy and α-syn degradation being the main mechanism.

CONCLUSION

All these experimental results suggest that phytochemicals have significant neuroprotective properties targeting disease-causing factors in PD in the experimental condition. Although some clinical trials have yielded inclusive results due to suboptimal doses formulation and timing affecting their bioavailability in the brain and accumulation at the desired concentration to produce therapeutic effects, more clinical trials with well-defined parameters are highly needed. The use of nanoparticles-based formulations and phytochemical supplementation with bioavailability-enhancing compounds like piperine should be the strategy of choice. As ayurvedic formulations have no or very minimal side effects and are great in efficacy and cost, research should be promoted to use them for drug discovery.

CONSENT FOR PUBLICATION

Not applicable.

CONFLICT OF INTEREST

The author declares no conflict of interest, financial or otherwise.

ACKNOWLEDGEMENTS

Declared none.

REFERENCES

[1]   Cacabelos R. Parkinson's disease: from pathogenesis to pharmacogenomics. Int J Mol Sci 2017; 18(3): 551.
        [http://dx.doi.org/10.3390/ijms18030551] [PMID: 28273839]

[2]   Singh SS, *et al.* Neuroprotective effect of chlorogenic acid on mitochondrial dysfunction-mediated apoptotic death of DA neurons in a Parkinsonian mouse model 2020.
        [http://dx.doi.org/10.1155/2020/6571484]

[3]   Rai SN, Zahra W, Singh SS, *et al.* Anti-inflammatory activity of ursolic acid in MPTP-induced parkinsonian mouse model. Neurotox Res 2019; 36(3): 452-62.
        [http://dx.doi.org/10.1007/s12640-019-00038-6] [PMID: 31016688]

[4]   Rai SN, *et al.* Pathophysiology of the Disease Causing Physical Disability.Biomedical Engineering and its Applications in Healthcare. Springer 2019; pp. 573-95.
        [http://dx.doi.org/10.1007/978-981-13-3705-5_23]

[5]   Birla H, Keswani C, Singh SS, *et al.* Unraveling the Neuroprotective Effect of *Tinospora cordifolia* in a Parkinsonian Mouse Model through the Proteomics Approach. ACS Chem Neurosci 2021; 12(22): 4319-35.
        [http://dx.doi.org/10.1021/acschemneuro.1c00481] [PMID: 34747594]

[6]   Zhao C, Wang Y, Zhang B, Yue Y, Zhang J. Genetic variations in catechol-O-methyltransferase gene are associated with levodopa response variability in Chinese patients with Parkinson's disease. Sci Rep 2020; 10(1): 9521.
        [http://dx.doi.org/10.1038/s41598-020-65332-2] [PMID: 32533012]

[7]   Greffard S, Verny M, Bonnet AM, *et al.* Motor score of the Unified Parkinson Disease Rating Scale as a good predictor of Lewy body-associated neuronal loss in the substantia nigra. Arch Neurol 2006; 63(4): 584-8.
        [http://dx.doi.org/10.1001/archneur.63.4.584] [PMID: 16606773]

[8]   Marras C, Chaudhuri KR. Nonmotor features of Parkinson's disease subtypes. Mov Disord 2016; 31(8): 1095-102.
        [http://dx.doi.org/10.1002/mds.26510] [PMID: 26861861]

[9]   Emamzadeh FN, Surguchov A. Parkinson's disease: biomarkers, treatment, and risk factors. Front Neurosci 2018; 12: 612.
        [http://dx.doi.org/10.3389/fnins.2018.00612] [PMID: 30214392]

[10]   Birla H, Keswani C, Rai SN, *et al.* Neuroprotective effects of Withania somnifera in BPA induced-cognitive dysfunction and oxidative stress in mice. Behav Brain Funct 2019; 15(1): 9.
        [http://dx.doi.org/10.1186/s12993-019-0160-4] [PMID: 31064381]

[11]   Rai SN, Dilnashin H, Birla H, *et al.* The role of PI3K/Akt and ERK in neurodegenerative disorders. Neurotox Res 2019; 35(3): 775-95.
        [http://dx.doi.org/10.1007/s12640-019-0003-y] [PMID: 30707354]

[12]   Zahra W, *et al.* Neuroprotection of rotenone-induced Parkinsonism by ursolic acid in PD mouse model 2020.
        [http://dx.doi.org/10.2174/1871527319666200812224457]

[13]   Buck K, Ferger B. The selective Î± ₁ adrenoceptor antagonist HEAT reduces L-DOPA-induced dyskinesia in a rat model of Parkinson's disease. Synapse 2010; 64(2): 117-26.
        [http://dx.doi.org/10.1002/syn.20709] [PMID: 19771592]

[14]   Fu W, Zhuang W, Zhou S, Wang X. Plant-derived neuroprotective agents in Parkinson's disease. Am J Transl Res 2015; 7(7): 1189-202.
        [PMID: 26328004]

[15]   Seidl SE, Potashkin JA. The promise of neuroprotective agents in Parkinson's disease. Front Neurol 2011; 2: 68.
        [http://dx.doi.org/10.3389/fneur.2011.00068] [PMID: 22125548]

[16]   Keswani C, *et al.* Re-addressing the commercialization and regulatory hurdles for biopesticides in India 2019.

[17]   Keswani C, Mishra S, Sarma BK, Singh SP, Singh HB. Unraveling the efficient applications of secondary metabolites of various Trichoderma spp. Appl Microbiol Biotechnol 2014; 98(2): 533-44.
        [http://dx.doi.org/10.1007/s00253-013-5344-5] [PMID: 24276619]

[18]   Zahra W, *et al.* Economic Importance of Medicinal Plants in Asian Countries 2020.
        [http://dx.doi.org/10.1007/978-981-13-9431-7_19]

[19]   Zahra W, *et al.* The global economic impact of neurodegenerative diseases: Opportunities and challenges. Bioeconomy for Sustainable Development 2020; pp. 333-45.

[20]   Manyam BV. Paralysis agitans and levodopa in? Ayurveda?: Ancient Indian medical treatise. Mov Disord 1990; 5(1): 47-8.

[http://dx.doi.org/10.1002/mds.870050112] [PMID: 2404203]

[21]   Essa MM, Akbar M, Guillemin G. The benefits of natural products for neurodegenerative diseases. Springer 2016; Vol. 232.
[http://dx.doi.org/10.1007/978-3-319-28383-8]

[22]   Thomford N, Senthebane D, Rowe A, *et al.* Natural products for drug discovery in the 21st century: innovations for novel drug discovery. Int J Mol Sci 2018; 19(6): 1578.
[http://dx.doi.org/10.3390/ijms19061578] [PMID: 29799486]

[23]   Patwardhan B, Mashelkar RA. Traditional medicine-inspired approaches to drug discovery: can Ayurveda show the way forward? Drug Discov Today 2009; 14(15-16): 804-11.
[http://dx.doi.org/10.1016/j.drudis.2009.05.009] [PMID: 19477288]

[24]   Keswani C. Bioeconomy for Sustainable Development. Springer 2020.
[http://dx.doi.org/10.1007/978-981-13-9431-7]

[25]   Pathak- Gandhi N, Vaidya ADB. Management of Parkinson's disease in Ayurveda: Medicinal plants and adjuvant measures. J Ethnopharmacol 2017; 197: 46-51.
[http://dx.doi.org/10.1016/j.jep.2016.08.020] [PMID: 27544001]

[26]   Limanaqi F, Biagioni F, Mastroiacovo F, Polzella M, Lazzeri G, Fornai F. Merging the multi-target effects of phytochemicals in neurodegeneration: From oxidative stress to protein aggregation and inflammation. Antioxidants 2020; 9(10): 1022.
[http://dx.doi.org/10.3390/antiox9101022] [PMID: 33092300]

[27]   Singh S, *et al.* Chlorogenic acid protects against MPTP induced neurotoxicity in parkinsonian mice model via its anti-apoptotic activity. 2019.

[28]   Figueira I, Garcia G, Pimpão RC, *et al.* Polyphenols journey through blood-brain barrier towards neuronal protection. Sci Rep 2017; 7(1): 11456.
[http://dx.doi.org/10.1038/s41598-017-11512-6] [PMID: 28904352]

[29]   Santín-Márquez R, Alarcón-Aguilar A, López-Diazguerrero NE, Chondrogianni N, Königsberg M. Sulforaphane - role in aging and neurodegeneration. Geroscience 2019; 41(5): 655-70.
[http://dx.doi.org/10.1007/s11357-019-00061-7] [PMID: 30941620]

[30]   Hussain G, Rasul A, Anwar H, *et al.* Role of plant derived alkaloids and their mechanism in neurodegenerative disorders. Int J Biol Sci 2018; 14(3): 341-57.
[http://dx.doi.org/10.7150/ijbs.23247] [PMID: 29559851]

[31]   Yang Y, Chen S, Zhang Y, *et al.* Induction of autophagy by spermidine is neuroprotective via inhibition of caspase 3-mediated Beclin 1 cleavage. Cell Death Dis 2017; 8(4): e2738-8.
[http://dx.doi.org/10.1038/cddis.2017.161] [PMID: 28383560]

[32]   Dias V, Junn E, Mouradian MM. The role of oxidative stress in Parkinson's disease. J Parkinsons Dis 2013; 3(4): 461-91.
[http://dx.doi.org/10.3233/JPD-130230] [PMID: 24252804]

[33]   Blesa J, Trigo-Damas I, Quiroga-Varela A, Jackson-Lewis VR. Oxidative stress and Parkinson's disease. Front Neuroanat 2015; 9: 91.
[http://dx.doi.org/10.3389/fnana.2015.00091] [PMID: 26217195]

[34]   Mizuno Y, Ikebe S, Hattori N, *et al.* Role of mitochondria in the etiology and pathogenesis of Parkinson's disease. Biochim Biophys Acta Mol Basis Dis 1995; 1271(1): 265-74.
[http://dx.doi.org/10.1016/0925-4439(95)00038-6] [PMID: 7599219]

[35]   Lin MT, Cantuti-Castelvetri I, Zheng K, *et al.* Somatic mitochondrial DNA mutations in early parkinson and incidental lewy body disease. Ann Neurol 2012; 71(6): 850-4.
[http://dx.doi.org/10.1002/ana.23568] [PMID: 22718549]

[36]   Vianello A, Casolo V, Petrussa E, *et al.* The mitochondrial permeability transition pore (PTP) — An example of multiple molecular exaptation? Biochim Biophys Acta Bioenerg 2012; 1817(11): 2072-86.

[http://dx.doi.org/10.1016/j.bbabio.2012.06.620] [PMID: 22771735]

[37] Lyman M, Lloyd DG, Ji X, Vizcaychipi MP, Ma D. Neuroinflammation: The role and consequences. Neurosci Res 2014; 79: 1-12.
[http://dx.doi.org/10.1016/j.neures.2013.10.004] [PMID: 24144733]

[38] Gambardella S, Limanaqi F, Ferese R, *et al.* ccf-mtDNA as a potential link between the brain and immune system in neuro-immunological disorders. Front Immunol 2019; 10: 1064.
[http://dx.doi.org/10.3389/fimmu.2019.01064] [PMID: 31143191]

[39] Grimm S, Ott C, Hörlacher M, Weber D, Höhn A, Grune T. Advanced-glycation-end-product-induced formation of immunoproteasomes: involvement of RAGE and Jak2/STAT1. Biochem J 2012; 448(1): 127-39.
[http://dx.doi.org/10.1042/BJ20120298] [PMID: 22892029]

[40] Ebrahimi A, Schluesener H. Natural polyphenols against neurodegenerative disorders: Potentials and pitfalls. Ageing Res Rev 2012; 11(2): 329-45.
[http://dx.doi.org/10.1016/j.arr.2012.01.006] [PMID: 22336470]

[41] Gupta S, Hussain T, Mukhtar H. Molecular pathway for (−)-epigallocatechin-3-gallate-induced cell cycle arrest and apoptosis of human prostate carcinoma cells. Arch Biochem Biophys 2003; 410(1): 177-85.
[http://dx.doi.org/10.1016/S0003-9861(02)00668-9] [PMID: 12559991]

[42] Mansuri ML, Parihar P, Solanki I, Parihar MS. Flavonoids in modulation of cell survival signalling pathways. Genes Nutr 2014; 9(3): 400.
[http://dx.doi.org/10.1007/s12263-014-0400-z] [PMID: 24682883]

[43] Naoi M, Wu Y, Shamoto-Nagai M, Maruyama W. Mitochondria in neuroprotection by phytochemicals: Bioactive polyphenols modulate mitochondrial apoptosis system, function and structure. Int J Mol Sci 2019; 20(10): 2451.
[http://dx.doi.org/10.3390/ijms20102451] [PMID: 31108962]

[44] Zhou J, Tan SH, Nicolas V, *et al.* Activation of lysosomal function in the course of autophagy via mTORC1 suppression and autophagosome-lysosome fusion. Cell Res 2013; 23(4): 508-23.
[http://dx.doi.org/10.1038/cr.2013.11] [PMID: 23337583]

[45] Yu L, Chen Y, Tooze SA. Autophagy pathway: Cellular and molecular mechanisms. Autophagy 2018; 14(2): 207-15.
[http://dx.doi.org/10.1080/15548627.2017.1378838] [PMID: 28933638]

[46] Xie Z, Klionsky DJ. Autophagosome formation: core machinery and adaptations. Nat Cell Biol 2007; 9(10): 1102-9.
[http://dx.doi.org/10.1038/ncb1007-1102] [PMID: 17909521]

[47] Hasima N, Ozpolat B. Regulation of autophagy by polyphenolic compounds as a potential therapeutic strategy for cancer. Cell Death Dis 2014; 5(11): e1509-9.
[http://dx.doi.org/10.1038/cddis.2014.467] [PMID: 25375374]

[48] Lin W, Wadlington NL, Chen L, Zhuang X, Brorson JR, Kang UJ. Loss of PINK1 attenuates HIF-1α induction by preventing 4E-BP1-dependent switch in protein translation under hypoxia. J Neurosci 2014; 34(8): 3079-89.
[http://dx.doi.org/10.1523/JNEUROSCI.2286-13.2014] [PMID: 24553947]

[49] Parsanejad M, Zhang Y, Qu D, *et al.* Regulation of the VHL/HIF-1 Pathway by DJ-1. J Neurosci 2014; 34(23): 8043-50.
[http://dx.doi.org/10.1523/JNEUROSCI.1244-13.2014] [PMID: 24899725]

[50] Javed H, Nagoor Meeran MF, Azimullah S, Adem A, Sadek B, Ojha SK. Plant extracts and phytochemicals targeting α-synuclein aggregation in Parkinson's disease models. Front Pharmacol 2019; 9: 1555.
[http://dx.doi.org/10.3389/fphar.2018.01555] [PMID: 30941047]

[51]   Singh M, Murthy V, Ramassamy C. Neuroprotective mechanisms of the standardized extract of Bacopa monniera in a paraquat/diquat-mediated acute toxicity. Neurochem Int 2013; 62(5): 530-9. [http://dx.doi.org/10.1016/j.neuint.2013.01.030] [PMID: 23402822]

[52]   Jansen RLM, Brogan B, Whitworth AJ, Okello EJ. Effects of five Ayurvedic herbs on locomotor behaviour in a Drosophila melanogaster Parkinson's disease model. Phytother Res 2014; 28(12): 1789-95. [http://dx.doi.org/10.1002/ptr.5199] [PMID: 25091506]

[53]   Krishna G, Hosamani R. Bacopa monnieri supplements offset paraquat-induced behavioral phenotype and brain oxidative pathways in mice 2019. [http://dx.doi.org/10.2174/1871524919666190115125900]

[54]   Singh B, Pandey S, Yadav SK, Verma R, Singh SP, Mahdi AA. Role of ethanolic extract of Bacopa monnieri against 1-methyl-4-phenyl-1,2,3,6-tetrahydropyridine (MPTP) induced mice model via inhibition of apoptotic pathways of dopaminergic neurons. Brain Res Bull 2017; 135: 120-8. [http://dx.doi.org/10.1016/j.brainresbull.2017.10.007] [PMID: 29032054]

[55]   Singh M, Murthy V, Ramassamy C. Standardized extracts of Bacopa monniera protect against MPP+- and paraquat-induced toxicity by modulating mitochondrial activities, proteasomal functions, and redox pathways. Toxicol Sci 2012; 125(1): 219-32. [http://dx.doi.org/10.1093/toxsci/kfr255] [PMID: 21972102]

[56]   Hosamani R. Prophylactic treatment with Bacopa monnieri leaf powder mitigates paraquat-induced oxidative perturbations and lethality in Drosophila melanogaster 2010.

[57]   Jadiya P, Khan A, Sammi SR, Kaur S, Mir SS, Nazir A. Anti-Parkinsonian effects of Bacopa monnieri: Insights from transgenic and pharmacological Caenorhabditis elegans models of Parkinson's disease. Biochem Biophys Res Commun 2011; 413(4): 605-10. [http://dx.doi.org/10.1016/j.bbrc.2011.09.010] [PMID: 21925152]

[58]   Siddique YH, Mujtaba SF, Faisal M, Jyoti S, Naz F. The effect of Bacopa monnieri leaf extract on dietary supplementation in transgenic Drosophila model of Parkinson's disease. Eur J Integr Med 2014; 6(5): 571-80. [http://dx.doi.org/10.1016/j.eujim.2014.05.007]

[59]   Hosamani R, Muralidhara . Neuroprotective efficacy of Bacopa monnieri against rotenone induced oxidative stress and neurotoxicity in Drosophila melanogaster. Neurotoxicology 2009; 30(6): 977-85. [http://dx.doi.org/10.1016/j.neuro.2009.08.012] [PMID: 19744517]

[60]   Hosamani R, Krishna G, Muralidhara . Standardized *Bacopa monnieri* extract ameliorates acute paraquat-induced oxidative stress, and neurotoxicity in prepubertal mice brain. Nutr Neurosci 2016; 19(10): 434-46. [http://dx.doi.org/10.1179/1476830514Y.0000000149] [PMID: 25153704]

[61]   Shinomol GK, Mythri RB, Srinivas Bharath MM, Muralidhara . Bacopa monnieri extract offsets rotenone-induced cytotoxicity in dopaminergic cells and oxidative impairments in mice brain. Cell Mol Neurobiol 2012; 32(3): 455-65. [http://dx.doi.org/10.1007/s10571-011-9776-0] [PMID: 22160863]

[62]   Sukumaran NP, Amalraj A, Gopi S. Neuropharmacological and cognitive effects of Bacopa monnieri (L.) Wettst – A review on its mechanistic aspects. Complement Ther Med 2019; 44: 68-82. [http://dx.doi.org/10.1016/j.ctim.2019.03.016] [PMID: 31126578]

[63]   Arulkumar S, Sabesan M. The behavioral performance tests of Mucuna pruriens gold nanoparticles in the 1-methyl 4-phenyl-1,2,3,6-tetrahydropyridine treated mouse model of Parkinsonism. Asian Pac J Trop Dis 2012; 2: S499-502. [http://dx.doi.org/10.1016/S2222-1808(12)60210-2]

[64]   Sardjono R, *et al.* Biosynthesis, characterization and anti-Parkinson activity of magnetite-Indonesian velvet beans (*Mucuna pruriens* L.) nanoparticles. J Eng Sci Technol 2018; 13(12): 4258-70.

[65]   Sardjono, R., *et al.* Synthesize, characterization, and anti-Parkinson activity of silver-Indonesian velvet beans (Mucuna pruriens) seed extract nanoparticles (AgMPn). Journal of Physics Conference Series. 2018.

[66]   Singh B, *et al.* Comparative evaluation of extract of Bacopa monnieri and Mucuna pruriens as neuroprotectant in MPTP model of Parkinson's disease 2016.

[67]   Dhanasekaran M, Tharakan B, Manyam BV. Antiparkinson drug - *Mucuna pruriens* shows antioxidant and metal chelating activity. Phytother Res 2008; 22(1): 6-11.
[http://dx.doi.org/10.1002/ptr.2109] [PMID: 18064727]

[68]   Rai SN, Birla H, Singh SS, *et al. Mucuna pruriens* Protects against MPTP Intoxicated Neuroinflammation in Parkinson's Disease through NF-κB/pAKT Signaling Pathways. Front Aging Neurosci 2017; 9: 421.
[http://dx.doi.org/10.3389/fnagi.2017.00421] [PMID: 29311905]

[69]   Yadav SK, Rai SN, Singh SP. Mucuna pruriens reduces inducible nitric oxide synthase expression in Parkinsonian mice model. J Chem Neuroanat 2017; 80: 1-10.
[http://dx.doi.org/10.1016/j.jchemneu.2016.11.009] [PMID: 27919828]

[70]   Poddighe S, De Rose F, Marotta R, *et al.* Mucuna pruriens (Velvet bean) rescues motor, olfactory, mitochondrial and synaptic impairment in PINK1B9 Drosophila melanogaster genetic model of Parkinson's disease. PLoS One 2014; 9(10)e110802
[http://dx.doi.org/10.1371/journal.pone.0110802] [PMID: 25340511]

[71]   Singhal B, Lalkaka J, Sankhla C. Epidemiology and treatment of Parkinson's disease in India. Parkinsonism Relat Disord 2003; 9 (Suppl. 2): 105-9.
[http://dx.doi.org/10.1016/S1353-8020(03)00024-5] [PMID: 12915075]

[72]   Prakash J, Chouhan S, Yadav SK, Westfall S, Rai SN, Singh SP. Withania somnifera alleviates parkinsonian phenotypes by inhibiting apoptotic pathways in dopaminergic neurons. Neurochem Res 2014; 39(12): 2527-36.
[http://dx.doi.org/10.1007/s11064-014-1443-7] [PMID: 25403619]

[73]   Siddique YH, *et al.* Effect of Withania somnifera leaf extract on the dietary supplementation in transgenic Drosophila model of Parkinson's disease. All Results J Biol 2015; 6(2): 16-23.

[74]   Manjunath MJ, Muralidhara . Standardized extract of Withania somnifera (Ashwagandha) markedly offsets rotenone-induced locomotor deficits, oxidative impairments and neurotoxicity in Drosophila melanogaster. J Food Sci Technol 2015; 52(4): 1971-81.
[http://dx.doi.org/10.1007/s13197-013-1219-0] [PMID: 25829577]

[75]   De Rose F. Drosophila melanogaster Genetic Model of Parkinson's Disease: phytotherapy approach for a new and more sustainable pre-clinical investigation 2016.

[76]   Prakash J, Yadav SK, Chouhan S, Singh SP. Neuroprotective role of Withania somnifera root extract in maneb-paraquat induced mouse model of parkinsonism. Neurochem Res 2013; 38(5): 972-80.
[http://dx.doi.org/10.1007/s11064-013-1005-4] [PMID: 23430469]

[77]   Sankar S, Manivasagam T, Krishnamurti A, Ramanathan M. The neuroprotective effect of Withania somnifera root extract in MPTP-intoxicated mice: An analysis of behavioral and biochemical varibles. Cell Mol Biol Lett 2007; 12(4): 473-81.
[http://dx.doi.org/10.2478/s11658-007-0015-0] [PMID: 17415533]

[78]   De Rose F, Marotta R, Poddighe S, *et al.* Functional and morphological correlates in the Drosophila LRRK2 loss-of-function model of Parkinson's disease: drug effects of Withania somnifera (Dunal) administration. PLoS One 2016; 11(1)e0146140
[http://dx.doi.org/10.1371/journal.pone.0146140] [PMID: 26727265]

[79]   RajaSankar S, Manivasagam T, Sankar V, *et al.* Withania somnifera root extract improves catecholamines and physiological abnormalities seen in a Parkinson's disease model mouse. J Ethnopharmacol 2009; 125(3): 369-73.

[http://dx.doi.org/10.1016/j.jep.2009.08.003] [PMID: 19666100]

[80] Ahmad M, Saleem S, Ahmad AS, *et al*. Neuroprotective effects of Withania somnifera on 6-hydroxydopamine induced Parkinsonism in rats. Hum Exp Toxicol 2005; 24(3): 137-47.
[http://dx.doi.org/10.1191/0960327105ht509oa] [PMID: 15901053]

[81] Bollimpelli VS, Kumar P, Kumari S, Kondapi AK. Neuroprotective effect of curcumin-loaded lactoferrin nano particles against rotenone induced neurotoxicity. Neurochem Int 2016; 95: 37-45.
[http://dx.doi.org/10.1016/j.neuint.2016.01.006] [PMID: 26826319]

[82] Taebnia N, Morshedi D, Yaghmaei S, Aliakbari F, Rahimi F, Arpanaei A. Curcumin-loaded amine-functionalized mesoporous silica nanoparticles inhibit α-synuclein fibrillation and reduce its cytotoxicity-associated effects. Langmuir 2016; 32(50): 13394-402.
[http://dx.doi.org/10.1021/acs.langmuir.6b02935] [PMID: 27993021]

[83] Gadad BS, Subramanya PK, Pullabhatla S, Shantharam IS, Rao KS. Curcumin-glucoside, a novel synthetic derivative of curcumin, inhibits α-synuclein oligomer formation: relevance to Parkinson's disease. Curr Pharm Des 2012; 18(1): 76-84.
[http://dx.doi.org/10.2174/138161212798919093] [PMID: 22211690]

[84] Ramkumar M, Rajasankar S, Gobi VV, *et al*. Neuroprotective effect of Demethoxycurcumin, a natural derivative of Curcumin on rotenone induced neurotoxicity in SH-SY 5Y Neuroblastoma cells. BMC Complement Altern Med 2017; 17(1): 217.
[http://dx.doi.org/10.1186/s12906-017-1720-5] [PMID: 28420370]

[85] Jaisin Y, Thampithak A, Meesarapee B, *et al*. Curcumin I protects the dopaminergic cell line SH-SY5Y from 6-hydroxydopamine-induced neurotoxicity through attenuation of p53-mediated apoptosis. Neurosci Lett 2011; 489(3): 192-6.
[http://dx.doi.org/10.1016/j.neulet.2010.12.014] [PMID: 21167259]

[86] Jinfeng, L., *et al*., Therapeutic effects of CUR-activated human umbilical cord mesenchymal stem cells on 1-methyl-4-phenylpyridine-induced Parkinson's disease cell model. BioMed Research International 2016.

[87] Mythri RB, Harish G, Dubey SK, Misra K, Srinivas Bharath MM. Glutamoyl diester of the dietary polyphenol curcumin offers improved protection against peroxynitrite-mediated nitrosative stress and damage of brain mitochondria *in vitro*: implications for Parkinson's disease. Mol Cell Biochem 2011; 347(1-2): 135-43.
[http://dx.doi.org/10.1007/s11010-010-0621-4] [PMID: 20972609]

[88] Khatri DK, Juvekar AR. Neuroprotective effect of curcumin as evinced by abrogation of rotenone-induced motor deficits, oxidative and mitochondrial dysfunctions in mouse model of Parkinson's disease. Pharmacol Biochem Behav 2016; 150-151: 39-47.
[http://dx.doi.org/10.1016/j.pbb.2016.09.002] [PMID: 27619637]

[89] Yang D, Li T, Liu Z, *et al*. LRRK2 kinase activity mediates toxic interactions between genetic mutation and oxidative stress in a Drosophila model: Suppression by curcumin. Neurobiol Dis 2012; 47(3): 385-92.
[http://dx.doi.org/10.1016/j.nbd.2012.05.020] [PMID: 22668778]

[90] Wang J, Du XX, Jiang H, Xie JX. Curcumin attenuates 6-hydroxydopamine-induced cytotoxicity by anti-oxidation and nuclear factor-kappaB modulation in MES23.5 cells. Biochem Pharmacol 2009; 78(2): 178-83.
[http://dx.doi.org/10.1016/j.bcp.2009.03.031] [PMID: 19464433]

[91] Abbaoui A, Gamrani H. Neuronal, astroglial and locomotor injuries in subchronic copper intoxicated rats are repaired by curcumin: A possible link with Parkinson's disease. Acta Histochem 2018; 120(6): 542-50.
[http://dx.doi.org/10.1016/j.acthis.2018.06.005] [PMID: 29954586]

[92] Abbaoui A, Hiba OE, Gamrani H. Neuroprotective potential of Aloe arborescens against copper induced neurobehavioral features of Parkinson's disease in rat. Acta Histochem 2017; 119(5): 592-

601.
[http://dx.doi.org/10.1016/j.acthis.2017.06.003] [PMID: 28619286]

[93] Xia X-J, *et al.* Curcumin protects from oxidative stress and inhibits α-synuclein aggregation in MPTP induced parkinsonian mice. Int J Clin Exp Med 2016; 9(2): 2654-65.

[94] Pan J, Li H, Ma JF, *et al.* Curcumin inhibition of JNKs prevents dopaminergic neuronal loss in a mouse model of Parkinson's disease through suppressing mitochondria dysfunction. Transl Neurodegener 2012; 1(1): 16.
[http://dx.doi.org/10.1186/2047-9158-1-16] [PMID: 23210631]

[95] Sharma N, Nehru B. Curcumin affords neuroprotection and inhibits α-synuclein aggregation in lipopolysaccharide-induced Parkinson's disease model. Inflammopharmacology 2018; 26(2): 349-60.
[http://dx.doi.org/10.1007/s10787-017-0402-8] [PMID: 29027056]

[96] Yu S, Zheng W, Xin N, *et al.* Curcumin prevents dopaminergic neuronal death through inhibition of the c-Jun N-terminal kinase pathway. Rejuvenation Res 2010; 13(1): 55-64.
[http://dx.doi.org/10.1089/rej.2009.0908] [PMID: 20230279]

[97] Wu Y, *et al. Protective effect of curcumin on dopamine neurons in Parkinson's disease and its mechanism.* Zhejiang da xue xue bao. Yi xue ban= Journal of Zhejiang University. Med Sci 2018; 47(5): 480-6.

[98] Cui Q, Li X, Zhu H. Curcumin ameliorates dopaminergic neuronal oxidative damage via activation of the Akt/Nrf2 pathway. Mol Med Rep 2016; 13(2): 1381-8.
[http://dx.doi.org/10.3892/mmr.2015.4657] [PMID: 26648392]

[99] Song S, Nie Q, Li Z, Du G. Curcumin improves neurofunctions of 6-OHDA-induced parkinsonian rats. Pathol Res Pract 2016; 212(4): 247-51.
[http://dx.doi.org/10.1016/j.prp.2015.11.012] [PMID: 26922613]

[100] Wang YL, Ju B, Zhang YZ, *et al.* Protective effect of curcumin against oxidative stress-induced injury in rats with Parkinson's disease through the Wnt/β-catenin signaling pathway. Cell Physiol Biochem 2017; 43(6): 2226-41.
[http://dx.doi.org/10.1159/000484302] [PMID: 29069652]

[101] Zhang N, Yan F, Liang X, *et al.* Localized delivery of curcumin into brain with polysorbate 80-modified cerasomes by ultrasound-targeted microbubble destruction for improved Parkinson's disease therapy. Theranostics 2018; 8(8): 2264-77.
[http://dx.doi.org/10.7150/thno.23734] [PMID: 29721078]

[102] Teerapattarakan N, Benya-aphikul H, Tansawat R, Wanakhachornkrai O, Tantisira MH, Rodsiri R. Neuroprotective effect of a standardized extract of Centella asiatica ECa233 in rotenone-induced parkinsonism rats. Phytomedicine 2018; 44: 65-73.
[http://dx.doi.org/10.1016/j.phymed.2018.04.028] [PMID: 29895494]

[103] Haleagrahara N, Ponnusamy K. Neuroprotective effect of Centella asiatica extract (CAE) on experimentally induced parkinsonism in aged Sprague-Dawley rats. J Toxicol Sci 2010; 35(1): 41-7.
[http://dx.doi.org/10.2131/jts.35.41] [PMID: 20118623]

[104] Xu CL, Qu R, Zhang J, Li LF, Ma SP. Neuroprotective effects of madecassoside in early stage of Parkinson's disease induced by MPTP in rats. Fitoterapia 2013; 90: 112-8.
[http://dx.doi.org/10.1016/j.fitote.2013.07.009] [PMID: 23876367]

[105] Sharangi AB. Medicinal and therapeutic potentialities of tea (Camellia sinensis L.) – A review. Food Res Int 2009; 42(5-6): 529-35.
[http://dx.doi.org/10.1016/j.foodres.2009.01.007]

[106] Nataraj J, Manivasagam T, Justin Thenmozhi A, Essa MM. Neuroprotective effect of asiatic acid on rotenone-induced mitochondrial dysfunction and oxidative stress-mediated apoptosis in differentiated SH-SYS5Y cells. Nutr Neurosci 2017; 20(6): 351-9.
[http://dx.doi.org/10.1080/1028415X.2015.1135559] [PMID: 26856988]

[107] Nataraj J, Manivasagam T, Justin Thenmozhi A, Essa MM. Neurotrophic effect of asiatic acid, a triterpene of Centella asiatica against chronic 1-methyl 4-phenyl 1, 2, 3, 6-tetrahydropyridine hydrochloride/probenecid mouse model of Parkinson's disease: The role of MAPK, PI3K-Akt-GSK3β and mTOR signalling pathways. Neurochem Res 2017; 42(5): 1354-65.
[http://dx.doi.org/10.1007/s11064-017-2183-2] [PMID: 28181071]

[108] Kim JS, Kim JM, O JJ, Jeon BS. Inhibition of inducible nitric oxide synthase expression and cell death by (−)-epigallocatechin-3-gallate, a green tea catechin, in the 1-methyl-4-phenyl-1,2-3,6-tetrahydropyridine mouse model of Parkinson's disease. J Clin Neurosci 2010; 17(9): 1165-8.
[http://dx.doi.org/10.1016/j.jocn.2010.01.042] [PMID: 20541420]

[109] Guo S, Yan J, Yang T, Yang X, Bezard E, Zhao B. Protective effects of green tea polyphenols in the 6-OHDA rat model of Parkinson's disease through inhibition of ROS-NO pathway. Biol Psychiatry 2007; 62(12): 1353-62.
[http://dx.doi.org/10.1016/j.biopsych.2007.04.020] [PMID: 17624318]

[110] Xu Q, Langley M, Kanthasamy AG, Reddy MB. Epigallocatechin gallate has a neurorescue effect in a mouse model of Parkinson disease. J Nutr 2017; 147(10): 1926-31.
[http://dx.doi.org/10.3945/jn.117.255034] [PMID: 28835392]

[111] Mandel S, Maor G, Youdim MBH. Iron and α-synuclein in the substantia nigra of MPTP-treated mice: effect of neuroprotective drugs R-apomorphine and green tea polyphenol (-)-epigallocatechi--3-gallate. J Mol Neurosci 2004; 24(3): 401-16.
[http://dx.doi.org/10.1385/JMN:24:3:401] [PMID: 15655262]

[112] Zhang H, Bosch-Marce M, Shimoda LA, et al. Mitochondrial autophagy is an HIF-1-dependent adaptive metabolic response to hypoxia. J Biol Chem 2008; 283(16): 10892-903.
[http://dx.doi.org/10.1074/jbc.M800102200] [PMID: 18281291]

[113] Weinreb O, Mandel S, Youdim MBH, Amit T. Targeting dysregulation of brain iron homeostasis in Parkinson's disease by iron chelators. Free Radic Biol Med 2013; 62: 52-64.
[http://dx.doi.org/10.1016/j.freeradbiomed.2013.01.017] [PMID: 23376471]

[114] Hashimoto K, Sakagami H. Induction of apoptosis by epigallocatechin gallate and autophagy inhibitors in a mouse macrophage-like cell line. Anticancer Res 2008; 28(3A): 1713-8.
[PMID: 18630530]

[115] Holczer, M., et al., Epigallocatechin-3-gallate (EGCG) promotes autophagy-dependent survival via influencing the balance of mTOR-AMPK pathways upon endoplasmic reticulum stress. Oxidative Medicine and Cellular Longevity 2018.

[116] Zhou W, Chen L, Hu X, Cao S, Yang J. Effects and mechanism of epigallocatechin-3-gallate on apoptosis and mTOR/AKT/GSK-3β pathway in substantia nigra neurons in Parkinson rats. Neuroreport 2019; 30(2): 60-5.
[http://dx.doi.org/10.1097/WNR.0000000000001149] [PMID: 30571663]

[117] Liu X, Zhou S, Shi D, Bai Q, Liu H, Yao X. Influence of EGCG on α-synuclein (αS) aggregation and identification of their possible binding mode: A computational study using molecular dynamics simulation. Chem Biol Drug Des 2018; 91(1): 162-71.
[http://dx.doi.org/10.1111/cbdd.13067] [PMID: 28667699]

[118] Palle S, Neerati P. Improved neuroprotective effect of resveratrol nanoparticles as evinced by abrogation of rotenone-induced behavioral deficits and oxidative and mitochondrial dysfunctions in rat model of Parkinson's disease. Naunyn Schmiedebergs Arch Pharmacol 2018; 391(4): 445-53.
[http://dx.doi.org/10.1007/s00210-018-1474-8] [PMID: 29411055]

[119] Gaballah HH, Zakaria SS, Elbatsh MM, Tahoon NM. Modulatory effects of resveratrol on endoplasmic reticulum stress-associated apoptosis and oxido-inflammatory markers in a rat model of rotenone-induced Parkinson's disease. Chem Biol Interact 2016; 251: 10-6.
[http://dx.doi.org/10.1016/j.cbi.2016.03.023] [PMID: 27016191]

[120]   Liu Q, Zhu D, Jiang P, *et al.* Resveratrol synergizes with low doses of L-DOPA to improve MPTP-induced Parkinson disease in mice. Behav Brain Res 2019; 367: 10-8.
[http://dx.doi.org/10.1016/j.bbr.2019.03.043] [PMID: 30922940]

[121]   Guo YJ, Dong SY, Cui XX, *et al.* Resveratrol alleviates MPTP-induced motor impairments and pathological changes by autophagic degradation of α-synuclein via SIRT1-deacetylated LC3. Mol Nutr Food Res 2016; 60(10): 2161-75.
[http://dx.doi.org/10.1002/mnfr.201600111] [PMID: 27296520]

[122]   Xia D, Sui R, Zhang Z. Administration of resveratrol improved Parkinson's disease□like phenotype by suppressing apoptosis of neurons via modulating the MALAT1/miR□129/SNCA signaling pathway. J Cell Biochem 2019; 120(4): 4942-51.
[http://dx.doi.org/10.1002/jcb.27769] [PMID: 30260025]

[123]   Wu Y, Li X, Zhu JX, *et al.* Resveratrol-activated AMPK/SIRT1/autophagy in cellular models of Parkinson's disease. Neurosignals 2011; 19(3): 163-74.
[http://dx.doi.org/10.1159/000328516] [PMID: 21778691]

[124]   Singh B, Pandey S, Rumman M, Mahdi AA. Neuroprotective effects of Bacopa monnieri in Parkinson's disease model. Metab Brain Dis 2020; 35(3): 517-25.
[http://dx.doi.org/10.1007/s11011-019-00526-w] [PMID: 31834548]

[125]   Sõukand R, Pieroni A, Biró M, *et al.* An ethnobotanical perspective on traditional fermented plant foods and beverages in Eastern Europe. J Ethnopharmacol 2015; 170: 284-96.
[http://dx.doi.org/10.1016/j.jep.2015.05.018] [PMID: 25985766]

[126]   Nellore, J., C. Pauline, and K. Amarnath, Bacopa monnieri phytochemicals mediated synthesis of platinum nanoparticles and its neurorescue effect on 1-methyl 4-phenyl 1, 2, 3, 6 tetrahydropyridine-induced experimental parkinsonism in zebrafish. Journal of Neurodegenerative Diseases 2013.

[127]   Verma D, Balakrishnan N, Dixit R. Flora of Madhya Pradesh Botanical Survey of India. Calcutta 1993; Vol. I.

[128]   Ovallath S, Deepa P. The history of parkinsonism: descriptions in ancient Indian medical literature. Wiley Online Library 2013; pp. 566-8.

[129]   Damodaran M, Ramaswamy R. Isolation of *l* -3:4-dihydroxyphenylalanine from the seeds of *Mucuna pruriens*. Biochem J 1937; 31(12): 2149-52.
[http://dx.doi.org/10.1042/bj0312149] [PMID: 16746556]

[130]   Group, H.-i.P.s.D.S., *An alternative medicine treatment for Parkinson's disease: results of a multicenter clinical trial.* J Altern Complement Med 1995; 1(3): 249-55.
[http://dx.doi.org/10.1089/acm.1995.1.249] [PMID: 9395621]

[131]   Nagashayana N, Sankarankutty P, Nampoothiri MRV, Mohan PK, Mohanakumar KP. Association of l-DOPA with recovery following Ayurveda medication in Parkinson's disease. J Neurol Sci 2000; 176(2): 124-7.
[http://dx.doi.org/10.1016/S0022-510X(00)00329-4] [PMID: 10930594]

[132]   Katzenschlager R, Evans A, Manson A, *et al.* Mucuna pruriens in Parkinson's disease: a double blind clinical and pharmacological study. J Neurol Neurosurg Psychiatry 2004; 75(12): 1672-7.
[http://dx.doi.org/10.1136/jnnp.2003.028761] [PMID: 15548480]

[133]   Cilia R, Laguna J, Cassani E, *et al. Mucuna pruriens* in Parkinson disease. Neurology 2017; 89(5): 432-8.
[http://dx.doi.org/10.1212/WNL.0000000000004175] [PMID: 28679598]

[134]   Cilia R, Laguna J, Cassani E, *et al.* Daily intake of Mucuna pruriens in advanced Parkinson's disease: A 16-week, noninferiority, randomized, crossover, pilot study. Parkinsonism Relat Disord 2018; 49: 60-6.
[http://dx.doi.org/10.1016/j.parkreldis.2018.01.014] [PMID: 29352722]

[135] Radder DLM, Tiel Groenestege AT, Boers I, Muilwijk EW, Bloem BR. Mucuna pruriens combined with carbidopa in Parkinson's disease: a case report. J Parkinsons Dis 2019; 9(2): 437-9.
[http://dx.doi.org/10.3233/JPD-181500] [PMID: 30856121]

[136] Mirjalili M, Moyano E, Bonfill M, Cusido R, Palazón J. Steroidal lactones from Withania somnifera, an ancient plant for novel medicine. Molecules 2009; 14(7): 2373-93.
[http://dx.doi.org/10.3390/molecules14072373] [PMID: 19633611]

[137] Williamson, E., Major Herbs of Ayurveda. Churchill Livingstone. Edimburgh: Elsevier Science Limited, 2002.

[138] Sun GY, Li R, Cui J, *et al.* Withania somnifera and its withanolides attenuate oxidative and inflammatory responses and up-regulate antioxidant responses in BV-2 microglial cells. Neuromolecular Med 2016; 18(3): 241-52.
[http://dx.doi.org/10.1007/s12017-016-8411-0] [PMID: 27209361]

[139] Rai M, Jogee PS, Agarkar G, Santos CA. Anticancer activities of *Withania somnifera* : Current research, formulations, and future perspectives. Pharm Biol 2016; 54(2): 189-97.
[http://dx.doi.org/10.3109/13880209.2015.1027778] [PMID: 25845640]

[140] Shivamurthy S, Manchukonda R, Ramadas D. Evaluation of learning and memory enhancing activities of protein extract of Withania somnifera (Ashwagandha) in Wistar albino rats. Int J Basic Clin Pharmacol 2016; 5(2): 453-7.
[http://dx.doi.org/10.18203/2319-2003.ijbcp20160761]

[141] Ammon H, Wahl M. Pharmacology of *Curcuma longa*. Planta Med 1991; 57(1): 1-7.
[http://dx.doi.org/10.1055/s-2006-960004] [PMID: 2062949]

[142] Zbarsky V, Datla KP, Parkar S, Rai DK, Aruoma OI, Dexter DT. Neuroprotective properties of the natural phenolic antioxidants curcumin and naringenin but not quercetin and fisetin in a 6-OHDA model of Parkinson's disease. Free Radic Res 2005; 39(10): 1119-25.
[http://dx.doi.org/10.1080/10715760500233113] [PMID: 16298737]

[143] Mythri RB, Bharath MM. Curcumin: a potential neuroprotective agent in Parkinson's disease. Curr Pharm Des 2012; 18(1): 91-9.
[http://dx.doi.org/10.2174/138161212798918995] [PMID: 22211691]

[144] Brinkhaus B, Lindner M, Schuppan D, Hahn EG. Chemical, pharmacological and clinical profile of the East Asian medical plant Centella aslatica. Phytomedicine 2000; 7(5): 427-48.
[http://dx.doi.org/10.1016/S0944-7113(00)80065-3] [PMID: 11081995]

[145] Das AJ. Review on nutritional, medicinal and pharmacological properties of Centella asiatica (Indian pennywort). Journal of Biologically Active Products from Nature 2011; 1(4): 216-28.
[http://dx.doi.org/10.1080/22311866.2011.10719089]

[146] Zhang F, Shi JS, Zhou H, Wilson B, Hong JS, Gao HM. Resveratrol protects dopamine neurons against lipopolysaccharide-induced neurotoxicity through its anti-inflammatory actions. Mol Pharmacol 2010; 78(3): 466-77.
[http://dx.doi.org/10.1124/mol.110.064535] [PMID: 20554604]

[147] Wight RD, Tull CA, Deel MW, *et al.* Resveratrol effects on astrocyte function: Relevance to neurodegenerative diseases. Biochem Biophys Res Commun 2012; 426(1): 112-5.
[http://dx.doi.org/10.1016/j.bbrc.2012.08.045] [PMID: 22917537]

[148] Zhang F, *et al.* Resveratrol produces neurotrophic effects on cultured dopaminergic neurons through prompting astroglial BDNF and GDNF release 2012.
[http://dx.doi.org/10.1155/2012/937605]

[149] Renaud J, Bournival J, Zottig X, Martinoli MG. Resveratrol protects DAergic PC12 cells from high glucose-induced oxidative stress and apoptosis: effect on p53 and GRP75 localization. Neurotox Res 2014; 25(1): 110-23.
[http://dx.doi.org/10.1007/s12640-013-9439-7] [PMID: 24218232]

CHAPTER 4

Neuroprotective Sri Lankan Plants: Back to the Future with Phytomedicine

Nalaka Wijekoon[1,3], Yoonus Imran[1], Darshi Attanayake[1], Lakmal Gonawala[1,3] and K. Ranil D. de Silva[1,2,3,*]

[1] *Interdisciplinary Centre for Innovation in Biotechnology and Neurosciences, Faculty of Medical Sciences, University of Sri Jayewardenepura, Sri Jayewardenepura Kotte, Sri Lanka*

[2] *Institute for Combinatorial Advanced Research & Education (KDU-CARE), General Sir John Kotelawala Defence University, Colombo, Sri Lanka*

[3] *European Graduate School of Neuroscience, Maastricht University, Maastricht, The Netherlands*

Abstract: Sri Lanka is listed as the top 34th biodiversity hotspot globally and has the highest biodiversity per unit area of terrestrial in the Asian continent. Intriguingly, it has been reported that 3771 flowering plant species are grown in Sri Lanka, of which 927 (24%) are endemic to the country, and 1430 species are considered medicinal plants. Surprisingly, it is reported that up to 40% of all new molecular entities submitted to the Food and Drug Administration (FDA) approval are either natural products or natural product-derived compounds. This chapter aims to explore the therapeutic potential of Sri Lankan plants/natural products in neuroprotection as possible synergistic targets of the nuclear factor erythroid (NF-E2)-related factor 2 (Nrf2) pathway. Nonetheless, the symptoms of neurological diseases are different; oxidative stress plays a central role in pathogenesis, thus, Nrf2 activation will counteract common pathogenic processes involved in neurodegener-ative/neuro-muscular disorders. Therefore, targeting Nrf2 signaling may provide a therapeutic option to delay onset, slow progression, and ameliorate symptoms of neurological disorders. However, when translating from the bench to the bedside, the knowledge of the timing of Nrf2 modulating compounds and dosage is crucial to define at which point should an Nrf2 activator be used versus an Nrf2 inhibitor. In this scenario, blends of natural products that synergize and provide multi-site action on Nrf2 regulation *via* different pathways are vital and will pave the way for the development of evidence-based effective neuro-nutraceuticals with a stride of innovation.

Keywords: Inhibitors, Keap1, Neurological disorders, Nrf2, PKC pathway.

* **Corresponding author K. Ranil D. de Silva:** Interdisciplinary Centre for Innovation in Biotechnology and Neurosciences, Faculty of Medical Sciences, University of Sri Jayewardenepura, Sri Jayawardenepura Kotte, Sri Lanka; Institute for Combinatorial

Advanced Research & Education (KDU-CARE), General Sir John Kotelawala Defence University, Colombo, Sri Lanka & European Graduate School of Neuroscience, Maastricht University, Maastricht, The Netherlands; E-mails: ranildesilva@kdu.ac.lk and ranil@sjp.ac.lk

INTRODUCTION

"Genetic error led humans to evolve bigger, but more vulnerable, brains", *Horizon; The EU Research And Innovation Magazine, 2018* [1].

The human brain is considered an "expensive tissue" that consumes an outstanding 20% of the total body energy budget despite the brain representing only 2% of body mass. Enhancing the brain activity and its functions was top in the research priorities, thus neuroprotection was among the forgotten and forsaken topics in the past. However, this trend has changed in the 21st century, with the argument that increased longevity is an opportunity or a threat to the stability of societies. The answer depends not only on whether populations are living longer but whether they are experiencing the negative health effects of aging [2 - 5].

"*Let food be thy medicine and medicine be thy food*", the popular quote by Hippocrates (400 BC), was further supported by Ibnu Sina or Avicenna, a Persian physician (981–1037 BCE), who stated that 'attention to the prevention of diseases rather than their treatment', which is an unmet need of current era of medicine [6 - 8]. The idea of "You are what you eat" was not novel to the 3 millennia-old indigenous medicinal systems in Sri Lanka, which are still in use and generally the first approach for disease control by the locals [9 - 11].

Typically, the herbs used for medicinal purposes are evergreen in nature, grown in the backyards of houses, and sometimes considered weeds. The traditional Sri Lankan education system centered on the temple, and the knowledge passed down by the ancestors made most Sri Lankans familiar and were even able to identify or administer the herbs growing within their area of residence even without the advice of a traditional medicinal practitioner [12, 13]. Sri Lanka was listed as the top 34th biodiversity hotspot globally and it has the highest biodiversity per unit area of terrestrial in the Asian continent [13]. Sri Lanka is gifted with many plant resources. It has been reported that there are 3771 flowering plant species grown in Sri Lanka. Out of them, about 927 (24%) are endemic to the country. Also, 1430 species are considered to have medicinal value. Of these medicinal plants, 174 (12%) are endemic to Sri Lanka. Also, it is reported that around 250 species are commonly used in traditional medicine [9, 14].

Nonetheless, the scientific explanation of the curative powers remained unsolved; natural products based on traditional remedies have been employed for thousands of years [15 - 19]. These time-tested natural remedies have long served as a chemical matter for the discovery and/or development of modern pharmaceuticals. Surprisingly, it is reported that up to 40% of all new molecular entities submitted to the Food and Drug Administration (FDA) approval are either natural products or natural product-derived compounds [18, 20 - 30]. The scientific identification of possible targets to natural products intriguingly has usually paved the way for new biology or opened entirely novel fields. This is the case for the nuclear factor erythroid (NF-E2)-related factor 2 (Nrf2) pathway and its relationship with natural products [21, 31 - 38].

NRF2 AS A POTENTIAL THERAPEUTIC TARGET

The Nrf2/ARE pathway is modulated by the Kelch-like ECH-associated protein 1 (Keap1). In basal conditions, Keap1 protein acts as an Nrf2 repressor, binding to Nrf2 and maintaining it in the cell cytoplasm [39 - 42]. Keap1 regulatory protein also directs Nrf2 to ubiquitination and degradation by proteasomes, thereby limiting its basal cellular levels [43, 44]. Considering that the Nrf2 signaling pathway can regulate at least 600 genes, of which 200 encode cytoprotective proteins involved in diseases and the dynamic connections between diseases and drugs, modulating Nrf2 activity is a promising pharmacological approach [45 - 48]. A central theme emerging from the identification of these target genes and their functions is resistance to oxidants and electrophiles. Notably, three major groups of Nrf2 target genes regulate drug metabolism and disposition, antioxidant defense, and oxidant signaling, respectively, to impact the response to oxidants and electrophiles (Fig. **1**). In addition, Nrf2 regulates proteasomal protein degradation [49, 50], cell proliferation [51 - 54] and metabolic reprogramming as well [55 - 63].

Nrf2 is ubiquitously expressed [64 - 66] and, in the brain, is an important defense against toxic insults in both glial cells as well as neurons [67 - 69]. In addition to upregulating numerous antioxidant enzymes, Nrf2 can also increase the expression of anti-inflammatory mediators, phase I and II drug-metabolizing enzymes as well as mitochondrial pathways [70 - 79].

NRF2 IN AGING/ NEURODEGENERATIVE DISORDERS

Developing a detailed understanding of the brain, which is commonly referred to as "the final frontier of science", is still in its relative infancy, but there are already several key observations that clearly attest to the power of the mind for proper coordination [80, 81]. Although ND has distinct pathologic features, there is considerable evidence to support oxidative stress as a common pathogenetic mechanism. Evidence of lipid peroxidation, protein nitration, and nucleic acid oxidation is abundant in affected brain regions of ND [82 - 84].

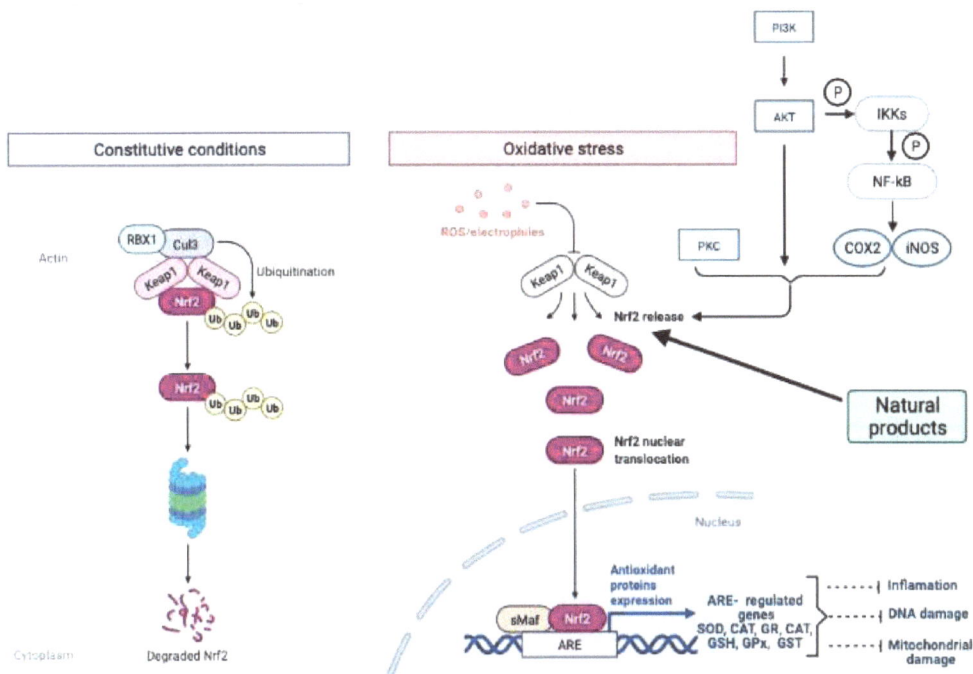

Fig. (1). In basal conditions, Keap1 protein acts as an Nrf2 repressor, binding to Nrf2 and is activated by oxidants and electrophiles *via* modification of critical cysteine thiols of Keap1 and Nrf2. Induction requires a common DNA sequence called antioxidant response element (ARE) that resembles the NFE2-binding motif. Nrf2 activation is regulated by P13K, NF-kB, and PKC pathways. The synergistic effect of the natural products offers significant neuroprotection by targeting Nrf2 pathway molecules.

Oxidative damage occurs early in the disease, suggesting that oxidative stress plays a role in ND progression [85, 86]. Increased antioxidant activity confers protection in mouse and culture models and has been reported to lower the risk of several ND [87 - 92]. However, how disease mechanisms affect endogenous antioxidant defenses is still not completely understood. By using etiologic descriptions of neurodegenerative disease, we can develop new therapeutic strategies to target specific cellular processes known to participate in neuronal death. Current research is uncovering several conditions, proving to be commonalities among neurodegenerative diseases. These include protein aggregation, proteasomal or autophagic dysfunction, inflammation, neuronal apoptosis, oxidative stress, mitochondrial dysfunction, and interactions between neurons and glia [40].

Aging leads to a gradual increase in brain oxidative stress, accompanied by reduced antioxidant defenses and lower levels of neurogenesis [86]. Aging is the main risk factor for neurodegenerative disorders [93, 94], which accounts for 12% of total deaths worldwide [95]. Aging is also associated with a progressive reduction in Nrf2 activity [96]. Interestingly, long-lived animal species have higher Nrf2 signaling levels, highlighting the importance of Nrf2 protection against aging and aging-related diseases [97]. Nrf2 is pivotal in the regulation of cellular redox status, modulating the expression of more than 200 downstream genes encoding Phase II response enzymes during an oxidative challenge, including HO-1, GST, CAT, SOD, and NQO1 [43, 98]. Nrf2 not only modulates antioxidant defense genes but also genes that have autophagic and anti-inflammatory properties as well as glucose and lipid metabolism effects [97, 99].

Oxidative stress, inflammation, and mitochondrial dysfunction are all features of the aging brain, and because aging is the primary risk factor for most neurodegenerative diseases, Nrf2 has emerged as an attractive target for clinical intervention. In fact, the Nrf2-activating compound dimethyl fumarate (DMF) is an existing FDA-approved therapy for use in Multiple Sclerosis (MS) [47].

Alzheimer's Disease (AD)

Multifactorial neurodegenerative disorder, Alzheimer's Disease (AD), affects more than 50 million people worldwide and is estimated to reach 150 million in 2050 [100, 101]. Since the pathogenesis of AD is partially understood due to the multifactorial nature of pathology, the treatment of AD is still a challenge and remains an unsolved problem [102 - 104]. In a context where numerous phase III clinical trials addressing Aβ production and aggregation in AD failed, and some trials on modern pharmaceuticals, Crenezumab (NCT03491150), lanabecestat (NCT02972658), and solanezumab (NCT01900665) were terminated due to lack of efficacy, scientists were motivated to explore novel multitarget strategies against AD [100].

AD has multiple pathological characteristics, inclusive of oxidized DNA, mitochondrial damage, lipid peroxidation, and elevated levels of Aβ [105 - 107]. However, all of these characteristics are found to be centered on free radicals or reactive oxygen species (ROS) [21, 108]. Under normal conditions, Oxidative stress is well maintained in the physiological cellular antioxidant defense network with the aid of heme oxygenase-1 (HO-1), superoxide dismutase (SOD), glutathione (GSH), catalase (CAT), thioredoxin (Trx), thioredoxin reductase (TrxR), glutathione peroxidase (Gpx) and quinone oxidoreductase 1 (NQO1) [109, 110]. Intriguingly, AD studies exploring the patient brain indicated reduced levels of Nrf2, SOD1, CAT, and Gpx, which may eventually lead AD brains to ROS leading to progressive and irreversible damage to the brains [109, 110].

In this scenario, nevertheless, direct targeting of known antioxidants, vitamin E, vitamin C, and estrogen may exert positive effects in AD, but the efficacy of such an approach dwindles when translated from bench to bedside [111 - 115]. Since Nrf2 was reported to induce over 250 genes [72, 98, 116, 117] related to antioxidant, cryoprotection, and detoxifying proteins, it was suggested that enhanced Nrf2 activity could ameliorate the damages caused by ROS and/or mitochondrial dysfunction in AD [118 - 121]. The role of Nrf2 on neuroprotection in AD achieved through regulation of antioxidant and detoxification proteins and Nrf2 interfering with the β-secretase enzyme (BACE1), Aβ, and p-tau were recently reported by Bahn *et al.*, 2019 [122], Kitaoka *et al.*, 2019 [123], Tang *et al.*, 2018 [124] and Sotolongo *et al.*, 2020 [125] in mouse models of AD and *in vitro,* respectively.

Intriguingly, the findings of the largest and the most comprehensive study for aging pathologies performed across two countries in South Asia; India and Sri Lanka, Wijesinghe *et al.*, 2016, a concluded that aging cytoskeletal pathologies are comparatively higher in elderly Sri Lankans, and this might be due to their genetic, dietary and/or environmental variations or a combination [126]. Moreover, it is reported that modification of lifestyle and health behaviors, such as a vegetarian diet (green-yellow vegetables) and consumption of black tea, is particularly effective in neurodegenerative diseases [127].

Since Nrf2 can simultaneously interfere with Aβ and p-tau in both direct and indirect pathways, it is well accepted that activation of Nrf2 is useful for several age-related diseases that share common pathogenetic features with AD [128 - 130]. Thus, activation of Nrf2 *via* natural or synthetic Nrf2 activators may be favorable in age-related diseases that share common pathogenetic features with AD, where such innovative approaches will reduce the associated cost, side effects and drug interactions [121, 131 - 136].

Parkinson's Disease (PD)

Parkinson's disease (PD) is a common neurodegenerative disease, and the major unmet needs of PD are the identification of reliable biomarkers and the development of successful disease-modifying treatments [137]. The multifactorial causes, including aging, environmental factors, and genetic variability, are key factors that trigger the progression of the disease [138, 139].

To date, treatments are available only for temporary symptomatic relief, and all the attempts to develop an effective disease-modifying therapy failed due to the rudimentary understanding of the targeted mechanisms of disease [137, 140]. Dopaminergic neurons produce ROS as a by-product of their metabolic activity, and these neuronal cells are vulnerable to oxidative changes because of their high oxygen consumption and enrichment in fatty acids [141 - 143].

As demonstrated in the literature, oxidative stress is highlighted as a major contributing factor in the accumulation of Lewy bodies and α-synuclein, which result in ROS imbalance, thereby tentatively implicating the "master regulator" of oxidative management, Nrf2, in the pathophysiological process. Oxidative stress and neuroinflammation processes are highly controlled by the transcription factor Nrf2, which is a master regulator of cellular defense in neurodegeneration [47, 144 - 148].

Even though Nrf2 has not yet been targeted in clinical interventions in PD, epidemiological evidence suggests that high levels of consumption of the Nrf2-activating vitamins E, C, and natural products, including tea and coffee, are associated with decreased risk of PD [149 - 151]. In addition, 4 weeks of treatment with N-acetyl cysteine, which also activates Nrf2, improved scores on the Unified Parkinson's Disease Rating Scale and increased peripheral markers for antioxidant activity [152], as did 12 weeks of intervention with omega 3 fatty acids and vitamin E [153].

However, to date, no studies have directly evaluated the efficacy of pharmacologically targeting Nrf2 as a modifying disease treatment strategy for PD. Nevertheless, this caveat, *in-vitro* and *in-vivo* models (Tables **1** and **2**) of PD provide compelling evidence that the synergistic effect of the natural products offers significant protection to neurons by targeting the Nrf2 pathway molecules.

Huntington's Disease (HD)

The toxicity due to the huntingtin protein aggregates in neurons promotes the generation of ROS [154]. Oxidative stress is particularly prominent in the neostriatum of HD brains [155] and is thought to be an important driver of neurodegeneration. In addition to reports of increased oxidative stress [156 - 160] and mitochondrial dysfunction [161 - 163], chronic inflammation is also evident in HD [164 - 167]. Plasma concentrations of inflammatory cytokines are likewise elevated prior to the onset of disease symptoms, and increased immune activity persists in the CSF of HD patients [166]. Thereby, Nrf2 has emerged as a promising therapeutic target in HD.

In humans, disrupted Nrf22 signaling has also been observed where compared to non-disease controls, the levels of Nrf2 targets, including glutathione peroxidase, catalase, and SOD1, are increased in human HD brains [168, 169], suggesting a partial activation of the Nrf2-dependent antioxidant defense. In addition, it has been reported that in striatal neurons, abnormal Huntington protein disturbs Nrf2 signaling, promoting mitochondrial dysfunction and increased oxidative stress [163]. Although Nrf2-activating compounds have not been tested in clinical trials in primary monocytes from HD patients, Nrf2 induction by the Keap1 modifying small molecule C151 repressed IL-1, IL-6, IL-8, and TNFα production [170]. Even though targeting of Nrf2 by phytochemical has not been studied in HD future *in-vitro*, *in-vivo* studies leading to clinical trials may provide a therapeutic option to delay onset, slow progression, and ameliorate symptoms.

Spinocerebellar Ataxias

The Nrf2 pathway is involved in the induction of autophagy which plays an important role in eliminating aggregation-prone proteins and is impaired in neurodegenerative disorders, including Spinocerebellar Ataxias. Studies of SCA3 have shown that polyQ mutant ataxin-3 contributes to decreased expression and transcriptional activity of Nrf2, which is involved in the impaired mitochondrial dynamics and increased oxidative stress in cells expressing mutant polyQ proteins [171, 172]. Moreover, over-expression and knockdown of Nrf2, respectively, reduce and augment the aggregation of mutant ataxin-3 in cells expressing mutant ataxin-3 with 75 glutamine repeats [171]. These findings strongly suggest that activation of the Nrf2 pathway may be an attractive treatment approach for SCA3 and other polyQ diseases.

A study by Wu *et al.*, 2018 showed for the first time that caffeic acid and resveratrol, through induction of Nrf2 activation, can correct disorders induced by mutant ataxin-3 in human neuroblastoma cell models of SCA3. Moreover, supplementation with caffeic acid and resveratrol improved life-span and climbing activity in SCA3 *Drosophila,* strengthening the therapeutic value [173]. These findings evident that increased consumption of polyphenols or polyphenol-rich foods is associated with decreased risk of neurodegenerative diseases through activation of the Nrf2 pathway.

Muscular Dystrophy

Although antioxidant systems and enzymes can limit the impact of Reactive Oxygen Species (ROS), the excess of ROS production in a dystrophic context might impair the cellular antioxidant defense, leading to irreversible oxidative damage. A study by Khairallah *et al.*, in 2012 [174], analyzing transcriptome on biopsies from Duchenne Muscular Dystrophy (DMD) patients indicated a link between an impaired antioxidant response and DMD progression through reduced expression of antioxidant enzymes including Catalase (CAT-1), Superoxide

Dismutase (SOD1/2), and thioredoxin, which was further supported by Petrillo *et al.*, 2017 [175]. Intriguingly, Pelosi *et al.*, 2017 [176] discussed the existence of an antioxidant compensatory mechanism in muscles of young MDX mice and DMD patients prior to the symptom onset (0-2 years). The same study further revealed a significant upregulation of Nrf2-dependent genes and enzymes to counteract the major source of ROS production in dystrophic muscles; induction of NOX2 (NADPH oxidase 2) expression. Furthermore, in symptomatic DMD patients (2–9 years of age), the progressive increase of NOX2 expression failed to activate the Nrf2-mediated antioxidant response, strongly indicating that the imbalance between oxidant and antioxidant systems is involved in DMD progression [176 - 178].

Nonetheless, DMD is a pathophysiologically complex disease with many druggable targets, including calcium (Ca^{2+}) regulation [179], mitochondria [180, 181], and antioxidant defense systems [182, 183]; most experimental therapeutics developed in the past focused on just one of these targets that limited the therapeutic benefit. Thus, a strategy that simultaneously modulates each of these targets to amplify remedial potential is crucial. The nuclear factor erythroid 2-related factor 2 (Nrf2) signaling pathway has this potential upon activation [184, 185].

Migraine

Migraine sufferers still have no effective and widely applicable drug treatment methods, thus, the development of more effective and safe anti-migraine agents is still a pressing task [186]. Oxidative stress has been implicated in various headache disorders because it arises an imbalance between the production of reactive oxygen species (ROS) and elimination by antioxidant defense mechanisms, consequently in endogenous ROS that can cause oxidative damage to DNA, lipids, and proteins [187 - 191]. Several studies have shown that oxidative stress plays a role in the central sensitization of migraine [192]. Further oxidative stress is transduced into a neural signal by the TRPA1 ion channel on meningeal pain receptors, eliciting neurogenic inflammation, a key event in migraine [193].

It has been documented that the Nrf-2/ARE pathway is the most important endogenous antioxidant defense system and plays a critical role in regulating cellular oxidation, cell defense, and protection; moreover, increasing data points out the protective role of Nrf2/ARE pathway activation in the brain [98]. Wei *et al.*, 2016 demonstrated that activation of the Nrf-2/ARE pathway by sulforaphane which is found in cruciferous vegetables, inhibited the activation of the trigeminovascular system (TGVS) and prevented the induction of hyperalgesia, however without specifying the underlying mechanisms of migraine [194].

Pro-nociceptive neuropeptide CGRP activates multiple signaling pathways, including protein kinase A (PKA) and protein kinase C (PKC), leading to sensitization of receptors transducing pain-producing stimuli in trigeminal neurons [195, 196]. Activation of PKC by polyphenols has been positively associated with direct Nrf2 phosphorylation and activity/abundance, contributing to elevated Nrf2 signaling [197, 198].

According to the systemic review by Lopresti *et al.*, 2020 [199], although herbal treatments for migraine are promising, definitive conclusions cannot be made due to inconsistency in clinical and biochemical outcome measures. Future clinical trials could utilize combinations of omics approaches to provide more integrated pictures of the actions of targeted Nrf2 activation by polyphenols.

Stroke

Stroke is a major cause of death and long-term disability worldwide; however, effective clinical and therapeutic approaches are still limited [200, 201]. In 1996, intravenous recombinant tissue plasminogen activator (rtPA) was introduced as a successful therapeutic strategy in combination with thrombectomy for salvaging ischemic brain tissue and promoting clinical outcomes by restoring blood flow in acute ischemic stroke [202, 203]. Unfortunately, nearly 95% of stroke patients do not benefit from rtPA due to the narrow therapeutic window (4.5 hours) [204 - 207].

In addition, to date, there is no efficacious treatment that shows long-term recovery improvement. Therefore, the development of new therapeutic strategies by targeting vital cellular and sub-cellular components of the ischemic cascade is urgently needed. As oxidative stress is a key factor in the pathogenesis of acute ischemic stroke, reactive oxygen species produced during ischemic and reperfusion phases attack the cerebral tissue. Recent findings concern the dynamic change of Nrf2 signaling, its functional importance, and its targeted intervention in cerebral ischemia due to oxidative stress and ROS [208, 209].

Following ischemic stroke, neuronal death occurs due to multiple cascades of events, leading to mitochondrial damage and the generation of free radicals, hence increasing oxidative stress [210, 211]. Free radicals initiate apoptosis through complex signaling pathways, which include activating p53 and p38 MAPK, and the Nrf2 pathway is activated following an ischemic insult [212, 213]. Studies done in mice models to study stroke penumbra found that Nrf2 expression was significantly higher in the penumbra than in the infarct core, moreover, astrocytic Nrf2 contributes to neuronal survival following brain ischemia, whereas this protection was absent in cultures from Nrf2 knockout animals [214]. Anti-inflammatory response by microglia and macrophages by upregulating pro-inflammatory cytokines, such as IL-1β and TNF-α and by releasing other factors, such as cyclooxygenase-2 (COX-2), NO, and MMPs prevent neuronal death [215, 216]. As a way of self-defense, endothelial cells equip themselves with the Nrf2 system, and Alfieri *et al.*, 2013 suggest that Nrf2 and its target enzymes protect endothelial cells from oxidative insults and sustain BBB integrity following brain ischemia [217, 218].

Consumption of plant-based food will reduce the risks of developing life-threatening neurodegenerative diseases, including stroke. Higher antioxidant and ant-inflammatory phytochemicals are more potent to act on oxidative stress molecules by regulating the Nrf2 pathway [117, 219 - 221].

This scientific evidence provides insights into when and how Nrf2 functions during brain injury. Accordingly, (1) what is the dynamic regulation of the Nrf2 signaling following cerebral ischemia? (2) Does the evidence from Nrf2 models support the functional importance of Nrf2 in ischemic injury? (3) Whether Nrf2 induction is protective against ischemic injury, and is it facilitative for recovery [222].

Precisely no studies are available on stroke patients based on Nrf2 even with the availability of the *in vivo* treatment evidence with natural products in different models of cerebral ischemia. Using various ischemic stroke rodent models, recent preclinical studies provide direct *in vivo* evidence revealing the contribution of the Nrf2 pathway in ischemic stroke pathogenesis and neuroprotection. The investigations of Nrf2 and natural products in stroke are still in the initial stages in humans; future research is expected to elucidate the natural properties of Nrf2 in stroke leading to the development of novel drugs that target Nrf2 [223 - 239].

TARGETING NRF2 BY NATURAL PRODUCTS FOR NEUROLOGICAL DISORDERS

Phytochemicals in natural products are biologically active compounds found in plants and are considered to be extraordinarily rich sources of Nrf2-activators (Fig. **3.2**) [240, 241].

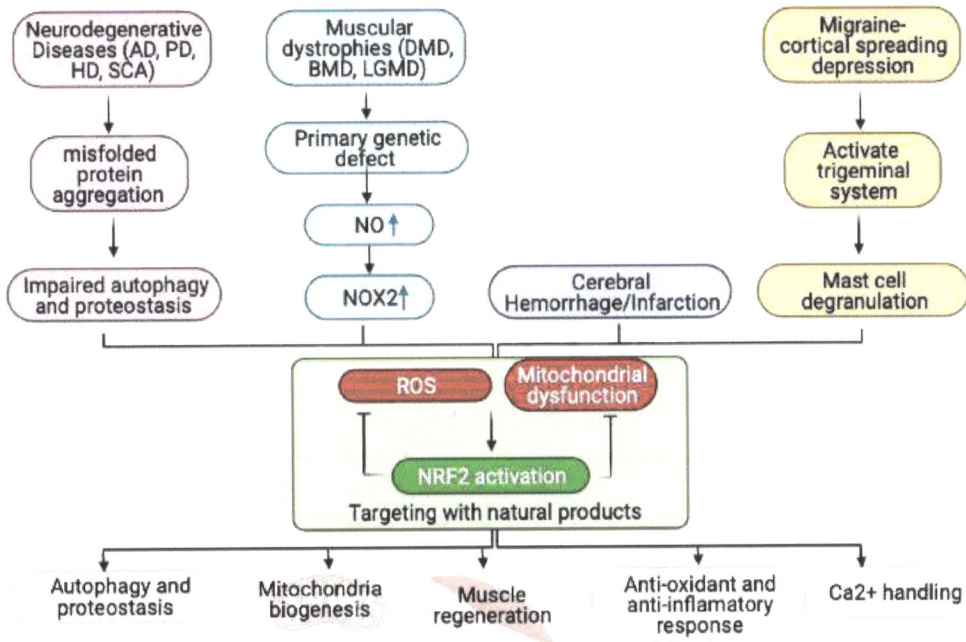

Fig. (2). Disease pathological pathways of neurodegenerative, muscular dystrophies, stroke, and migraine leading to activation of Nrf2 pathway. Activation of the Nrf2 pathway plays a vital role in autophagy, proteostasis, mitochondria biogenesis, muscle regeneration, Ca^{2+} handling, antioxidant and anti-inflammatory response.

Targeting Ca^{2+} Through Nrf2

Chronic increase of intracellular Ca^{2+} is commonly evident in neurodegenerative and neuromuscular disorders [242 - 246], which in turn impairs autophagy [247], and induces mitochondrial accumulation of Ca^{2+} [248] and apoptosis signaling [249]. A study by Ahn *et al.*, 2018 [122]on Nrf2 Knockout mice evident that Nrf2 facilitates Ca^{2+} handling as well as sarcoplasmic reticulum (SR) storage.

Moreover, two recent studies by Granatiereo *et al.*, 2019 [250] and Morciano *et al.*, 2018 [251] revealed that Probable glutathione peroxidase 8 (GPX8) protein which is regulated by Nrf2 selectively modulates Ca^{2+} storage and fluxes [252].

Targeting Inflammation by Nrf2

It is now evident in literature that strong activation of innate immune system components, including altered signaling *via* NF-KB, occurs prior to the clinical symptom onset in muscular dystrophies [253] and neurodegenerative disorders

[254 - 256]. Nrf2 activation modulates NF-κB attenuating inflammation [257 - 260]. Moreover, Nrf2 and NF-κB cross-talk to further amplify the levels of redox modulators under basal and disease conditions, thus maintaining redox homeostasis [45]. Activation of Heme Oxygenase-1 (HO-1) and its heme metabolism by Nrf2 also exerts an anti-inflammatory effect [185, 261, 262] which is further confirmed by a study on MDX mice by Pietraszek-Gremplewicz *et al.*, 2018 [263].

Targeting Mitochondria by Nrf2

The critical role of Nrf2 to maintain mitochondrial function *via* the modulation of substrate utilization during respiration is supported by increasing evidence [71, 264]. Studies on Nrf2 Knockout mice have shown elevated ROS production, depolarization of mitochondria, impaired respiration, and fatty acid oxidation, all of which can be repaired following Nrf2 activation [264] or knockout of Keap 1 [265, 266]. Further evidence was provided by Hayashi *et al.*, from a study on human fibroblasts of MS patients and wild-type mice that demonstrated the effect of the canonical Nrf2 activator Dimethyl fumarate (DMF); in increasing mitochondrial DNA and mitochondrial complex mRNA expression [73]. Mitochondrial integrity is pivotal for mitochondrial function and cell survival, whereas Murata *et al.*, demonstrated that stress-damaged mitochondria induce Nrf2-dependant transcription of the PINK1 gene; PTEN-induced kinase 1 (PINK1)/Parkinson juvenile disease protein 2 (Parkin) pathway, indicating that PINK1 expression is positively regulated by Nrf2 [267, 268].

Targeting Proteostasis by Nrf2

The damage caused to proteins by ROS consequently affects the protein assembly/reassembly and function, leading to protein aggregation and protein conformational diseases [269, 270]. Playing a role in the regulation of antioxidant response, Nrf2 amplifies the cellular protein quality control measures preparing the cell for the toxic insult by ROS [184]. As the first line of defense for proteostasis, Nrf2 induces molecular chaperons to unfold the misfolded proteins. However, degradation and disposal are the only possible solutions for proteins that are terminally misfolded and aggregated which is achieved through either the calpain and ubiquitin-proteasome systems (UPS) or autophagy [271]. Intriguingly, a non-canonical Nrf2 activation mechanism induced by autophagy deregulation has been described [272], where autophagy maintains the integrity of the Nrf2/Keap1 pathway by governing Keap1 turnover, which is different from the Nrf2 canonical pathway [273].

Targeting Muscle Regeneration by Nrf2

It is reported that Nrf2 plays a vital role as a regulator of tissue repair and regeneration, in addition to its role in cellular protection [66]. The skeletal muscle possesses a population of "satellite" stem cells (SCs) that will undergo proliferation, differentiation, fusion, and maturation, facilitating muscle repair under the influence of myogenic program factors MyoD and Myogenin [274, 275]. In this scenario, it is reported that Nrf2 prolongs SC proliferation *via* the upregulation of MyoD and suppresses SC differentiation by downregulating myogenin thus, Nrf2 ablation reduces MyoD mRNA and protein expression, delaying muscle regeneration following injury [274, 276]. Intriguingly, several studies on mdx mice demonstrated that injection of freshly isolated SC subsets renews the endogenous stem cell pool and contributes to improving the efficiency of subsequent injury repair [277 - 279]. These findings pave the way for alternative therapies for DMD that enhance muscle SC activity, where modulation of Nrf2 will play a crucial role.

NATURAL PRODUCTS BASED CLINICAL TRIALS FOR NEUROLOGICAL DISORDERS (TABLES 1, 2 AND 3)

Table 1. Clinical trials based on Nrf2 pathway.

Natural Product	Disease	Nrf2-related Outcome Measure	Clinical Outcome	Refs
Green Tea.	PD.	Increase in the antioxidant enzymes catalase, SOD, and reduced the oxidation of proteins.	No change in total UPDRS scores, total PDQ-39 scores, or PD non-motor symptom measure.	[280].
Green tea.	Healthy Individual.	Reduction in serum levels of oxidative stress.	Healthy Individuals.	[281].
Cinnamomum zeylanicum.	Migraine.	Serum concentrations of IL-6 and NO were significantly reduced.	Reduced frequency, severity, and duration of the headache.	[282].
Beetroot juice.	BMD.	Increasing NO.	Improved blood flow. Corrected deficient sympatholytic.	[283].

Table 2. Clinical trials for neuroprotection: Nrf2 treatment strategies should be considered in future studies.

Natural Product	Disease	Outcome	Ref
Cinnamomum zeylanicum.	PD.	Clinical improvement in the "on-time" administered along with oral pharmacological medicine.	[284].
Turmeric.	AD.	Improvement in the behavioral symptoms and quality of life.	[285].
Cinnamomum zelanicum.	Migraine.	Cinnamon supplementation reduced inflammation as well as frequency, severity, and duration of headache in patients with migraine.	[282].
Coconut oil-enriched Mediterranean diet.	AD.	Improved the cognitive functions.	[286].
Huperzine A.	AD.	Improvement in memory, cognitive, and behavior functions.	[287].
Ginkgo biloba special extract EGb 761.	Dementia.	Efficacy is confirmed. The investigational drug was found to be well tolerated.	[288].
Bacopa monnieri extract.	AD.	significant improvement in mental control, logical memory.	[289].
Tea.	PD.	Regular tea drinking habit was found to be a protective factor.	[290].
Tea.	PD.	Reduced risks were observed for consumption of 2 cups/day or more of tea.	[291].
Tea.	PD.	More tea drinking is associated with a lower risk of PD.	[292].
Tea.	PD.	Consumption of tea more than 3 cups per day delayed age of motor symptoms.	[293].
Coffee.	PD.	Coffee consumption exceeding 3 cups per day advanced the age of PD onset by 4.8 years.	[293].
Tea.	DMD.	Results not yet published.	NCT01183767.
Epicatechin (Tea).	DMD.	Results not yet published.	NCT02964377.
Epigallocatechin-Gallate (EGCg).	DMD.	Results not yet published.	NCT01183767.
(-)- Epicatechin.	BMD.	Results not yet published.	NCT03236662.
(-)-Epicatechin.	BMD.	Results not yet published.	NCT01856868.
Epigallocatechin Gallate.	HD.	Results not yet published.	NCT01357681.

Table 3. Sri Lankan native herbs; potential targets for dementia, cognition, and AD.

Herbs Local name English Scientific name	Dementia Treatment Outcome	Cholinesterase Activity	Ref
Ekaveriya Indian snakeroot *Rauvolfia serpentina.*	Therapeutic effects in the treatment of schizophrenia and traditional use in dementia and insanity.	Enzyme inhibitory activity of both (AChE) and (BuChE) enzymes.	[294 - 297].
Jaatamansa Indian spikenard *Nardostachys jatamansi.*	Improvement of cognition Significantly improved learning and memory in young mice.	*in-vitro*-derived plants showed significant inhibitory potential AChE and BuChE enzymes as compared to standard inhibitor galanthamine. Showed neuroprotective activity by inhibition of AChE and antioxidant activity, which enhances memory.	[298 - 302].
Duhudu Black oil plant, Jyotishmati *Celastrus paniculatus.*	Significantly and reversibly inhibited whole-cell currents activated by NMDA Reduces the concentration of monoamine neurotransmitters (noradrenaline, dopamine, and serotonin) and their metabolites in the brain - decreases the turnover of central monoamines.	Significantly decreased AChE activity as compared with control respectively by improved the memory of rats. *Celastrus paniculatus* seed has dose-dependent cholinergic activity.	[303 - 305].
Gotu Kola Mandukaparni *Hydrocotyle asiatica L Centella asiatica.*	Improvement was observed in memory-related behaviors in rats A high dose of *C. asiatica* extract tested in this study possessed a cognitive enhancing effect. Gotu kola was shown to be more effective than folic acid in improving the memory domain Cognition enhanced in the Mild Cognitive Impairment.	AChE inhibitory potential of extracts against AChE, BChE, and tyrosinase Extract administration resulted in an increase in AChE activity and dendritic arborization in CA3 neurons located in the hippocampus Decrease in malondialdehyde (MDA) and an increase in glutathione and CAT levels were recorded,.	[306 - 310].
Ela nitul Chitrak / Ceylon leadwort / Doctor-bush *Plumbago zeylanica.*	Significantly improved learning and memory of mice.	Significantly decreases the cholinesterase level in the brain.	[311, 312].

(Table 3) cont.....

Herbs Local name English Scientific name	Dementia Treatment Outcome	Cholinesterase Activity	Ref
Lunuwila Bacopa *B. monnieri.*	*B. monnieri* treated healthy adults group showed improved working memory. There was little evidence of enhancement in any other cognitive domains.	*B. monnieri* inhibited AChE differentially in various brain regions. *B. monnieri* similarly elicited higher AChE inhibition in the cerebral cortex. The suppression of plasma AChE activity was also observed.	[313 - 315].
Vacha Sweet flag *Acorus calamus.*	*Acorous calamus* has the ability to reduce the prognosis of Alzheimer's disease in rats.	*A. calamus* has potential effects against scopolamine-induced Alzheimer's by regulating AchE activity, free radical scavenging activity.	[316 - 319].
Nil Vishnukranthi Shankhapushpi *Evolvulus alsinoides.*	The amnesiac effects of scopolamine were greatly attenuated relative to control rats Clinical studies in Unani and Ayurveda are warranted for the potential use of *E. alsinoides* in treating dementia, pre-clinical research has justified the ancient claim of brain-tonic.	Inhibit the acetylcholinesterase enzyme Inhibit catechol-o-methyltransferase (COMT) Improved the cholinergic neurotransmission and reduced the cholinergic deficits produced by Scopolamine administration resulting in an enhanced neuroprotective effect.	[320 - 322].
Kalu wellangiriya Grudhra-nakha / Indian caper *Capparis zeylanica* Linn.	Showed that extracts significantly enhanced memory Significantly increased the time spent in the target quadrant during the probe trial, indicating retention of spatial memory.	Inhibit AChE activity, whereas these extracts did not alter MAO activity. Improves scopolamine-induced memory deficits through inhibition of AChE activity.	[319, 323].
Sakmal Daakuni / Shankhapushpi *Canscora decussate.*	Showed significant effect on learning behavior & memory enhancement as evidenced by the experimental performance.	Showed the highest acetylcholinesterase (AChE) inhibitory activity.	[324, 325].

BIOFUNCTIONS OF SRI LANKAN PHYTOCHEMICALS IN MODULATING THE NRF2/KEAP1 SYSTEM

Cinnamon

Cinnamon is a common spice used by different cultures around the world for several centuries. *Cinnamomum zeylanicum* is an indigenous tree of Sri Lanka [326, 327]. Trans-cinnamaldehyde activated the Nrf2 [328] and restored levels of downstream antioxidant enzymes superoxide dismutase and glutathione---transferase (GST) in the hippocampus of lipopolysaccharide (LPS)-induced neuroinflammation in mice. It attenuated an LPS-induced increase in hippocampal contents of interleukin-1β (IL-1β), malondialdehyde, and caspase-3. Immuno-histochemistry results of the same study showed that Trans-cinnamaldehyde reduced Aβ1-42 protein accumulation in the brain of mice. This study demonstrates the memory-enhancing effects of Trans-cinnamaldehyde through modulation of Nrf2 antioxidant defense in the hippocampus, inhibition of neuroinflammation, apoptosis, and amyloid protein burden [329 - 331].

A study by Liao 2008 examined the effects of both cinnamaldehyde and extracts of C. cassia on cytokine-induced monocyte/human endothelial cell interactions and showed in the short term, the NF- B inhibition by cinnamaldehyde was the result of the obstruction of IkB degradation, whereas, over a long term pretreatments, the inhibitory effect occurred *via* the induction of Nrf2 related path-way mainly involved in the regulation of the intracellular thiol redox state [332]. Moreover, it is shown that cinnamaldehyde devotes a protective effect toward endothelial dysfunction *in vivo* models under hyperglycemic conditions, and this phenomenon was mediated by Nrf2 activation and up-regulation of downstream target proteins [333] Cinnamaldehyde has a Michael acceptor in the form of an α,β-unsaturated carbonyl group and thus the main mechanism by which it activates Nrf2 is by alkylating a protein thiol on the Keap-1-Nrf2 binding complex, which allows Nrf2 to translocate to the nucleus to initiate antioxidant gene expression changes [334]. Moreover, Cinnamaldehyde acts on the upstream kinases such as Akt, ERK, and JNK, causing the release of Nrf2 from Keap1 [335].

Emblica officinalis (Nelli)

The major polyphenols in Amla include gallic and ellagic acid [336]. A study by Yamamoto *et al*., 2016, observed that Amla treatment protected mitochondrial function in C2C12 myotubes, a murine skeletal muscle cell model cell, against t-BHP-induced cell death, likely by reducing ROS levels through activation of the Nrf2 pathway. Amla treatment stimulated mitochondrial biogenesis and antioxidant systems along with activation of the AMPKα and Nrf2 pathways [337]. Studies showed that both mitochondrial biogenesis and antioxidant systems could regulate mitochondrial spare respiratory capacity. Increased mitochondrial biogenesis and energy production caused by thyroid hormone treatment leads to stimulation of mitochondrial spare respiratory capacity in skeletal muscle [338]. Ellagic acid consumption improved oxidant-induced endothelial dysfunction through Nrf2 activation [339]. *E. officinalis* tannins exhibited good affinity to Nrf2 receptors in *in silico* studies, significantly reversed the changes in the biomarkers of oxidative stress which were altered in the model group, as well as improved the performance of rats in the Morris water maze task indicating the potential use in the treatment of cognitive impairment [340].

In another study by Ding *et al.*, 2017 in an *in vivo* rat model, Corilagin was found in *E. officinalis* post-treatment with Corilagin reduced infarct volume and apoptosis and improved neurologic score. Corilagin treatment-induced also angiogenesis and increased the vascular endothelial growth factor (VEGF) and VEGFR2 expression. Corilagin also exerted an antioxidant action, shown by the reduction of MDA levels and the increase of SOD and GPx activities, together with nuclear Nrf2 and HO-1 levels. Interestingly, the protective actions exerted by Corilagin were Nrf2 dependent, indeed, Nrf2 silencing suppressed Corilagin protection. Also, in *in vitro,* neurons were exposed to OGD, CL increased cell *via*bility in a dose-dependent manner and also increased Nrf2 levels, but these effects were blocked by Nrf2 knockdown [341].

Bacopa monnieri (Brahmi)

A study by Leung *et al.*, 2017 [342] used deep sequencing (RNA-Seq) to identify the transcriptome changes upon *B. monnieri* treatment on SH-SY5Y human neuroblastoma cells. Biostatistical analysis of the RNA-Seq data identified biological pathways and molecular functions that were regulated by *B. monnieri,* including regulation of mRNA translation and transmembrane transport, responses to oxidative stress, and protein misfolding. *B. monnieri* activates ATF4 and Nrf2, while it inhibits the function of FOXO3. Activation of Nrf2 by *B. monnieri* plays a critical role in neuroprotection [343, 344].

Annona muricata (Katu Anoda)

Annona muricata leaves-derived polysaccharide extracts (ALPs) treatment was shown to induce concentration-dependent antioxidant activity in HT22 cells, and to increase cell *via*bility in H_2O_2-treated HT22 cells. These effects were correlated with a decrease in major components of oxidation, including Ca^{2+}, ROS, and malondialdehyde (MDA). Mediators of the intracellular response to oxidation, including Bax, cytochrome *c*, and cleaved caspases-3, -8, -9, MAPKs, and NF-κB, were positively influenced by ALP treatment under conditions of H_2O_2-mediated oxidative stress. In addition, ALP restored the expression of superoxide dismutase (SOD) and associated signaling pathways (PARP, PI3K/AKT, and Nrf2-mediated HO-1/NQO-1) following H_2O_2 treatment [345]. Another study by Ola-Davies *et al.*, 2019 in $K_2Cr_2O_7$-induced hypertension rats showed that the antioxidant capacity of *A. muricata* extract was demonstrated by the increased expressions of

Nrf2, indicating that its antioxidant property might be through the Nrf2/ARE signaling pathway [346].

Centella asiatica (Gotu Kola)

C. asiatica, widely recognized as "Gotu kola" is native to wetland areas of tropical countries, including Sri Lanka. In Sri Lanka. *C. asiatica* is utilized as a leafy vegetable. It is recognized for its traditional use as a memory enhancer [306] and is also believed to exert diverse pharmacological activities such as neuroprotective, nerve regenerative, immunomodulatory, anti-depressive, and antioxidative properties [347, 348]. It is reported that bioactive compounds of *C. asiatica,* including asiaticoside, madecassoside, and asiatic acid demonstrated high capability to cross the BBB, comparable to central nervous system drugs, and therefore warrant further development as therapeutics for the treatment of neurodegenerative diseases [348]. Recently Matthews *et al.*, 2019 [349] demonstrated that *C. asiatica* water extract (CAW) treatment increased Nrf2 and ARE gene expression in the hippocampus of the aged 5XFAD model of AD in a dose-dependent manner. Qi *et al.*, 2017 [350] performed a study to investigate the antioxidative effect of Asiatic Acid against oxidative stress and the antioxidative mechanism in tert-butyl hydroperoxide (t-BHP) -stimulated the HepG2 cells. Surprisingly, the findings of Qi *et al.*, 2017 [350] indicated that Asiatic Acid activates Nrf2 nuclear translocation, reduction in the expression of Keap1 and upregulation of ARE activity leads to the activation of a variety of antioxidant genes such as heme oxygenase-1(HO-1), NAD(P)H quinone oxidase(NQO-1), and glutamyl cysteine ligase catalytic (GCLC) through Akt, ERK activation.

Green Tea

Epigallocatechin-3-gallate (EGCG), a catechin found in green tea [351], has been widely investigated for its neuroprotective effects [352, 353]. Previous studies demonstrated that EGCG exerts its protective effects, possibly through the activation of the Nrf2/ARE signaling pathway [354, 355] by disruption of Nrf2/Keap1 interaction [356, 357]. In addition, it has been proved that EGCG can effectively pass through BBB and reach the functional parts of the brain even at very low concentrations [358]. Moreover, EGCG appears to be safe even when administered at a relatively high dose [359]. A study by Romeo *et al.*, 2009 [355] showed that pre-incubating rat hippocampal neurons with 25 µM EGCG for 12 hours before exposing them to 50 mU/mL glucose oxidase maintained cell *via*bility due to the induction of HO-1 (heme oxygenase) expression through Nrf2. Moreover, it is reported that EGCG is also involved in the activation of different kinases, including PI3K/AKT MAPK and PKC activating Nrf2 [238, 360, 361], and is also capable to inhibit GSK3β activity [362].

Allium sativum (Garlic)

Garlic is a widely consumed spice globally. Kohda *et al.*, 2013 [363] revealed that aged garlic has the potential to protect cells from ROS-induced damage through both capturing ROS directly and stimulating antioxidant gene expression *via* the Nrf2-ARE pathway. Moreover, it is reported that Allicin, from garlic, possesses pharmacological properties, including anti-oxidation, neuroprotection, and anti-inflammation [364, 365]. Recently Gao *et al.*, 2020 [366] revealed that Allicin attenuates depressive-like behaviors triggered by long-term high fat diet consumption by inhibiting ROS production and oxidative stress, improving mitochondrial function, regulating autophagy, and reducing insulin resistance in the hippocampus *via* decreasing NADPH oxidase (NOX2 and NOX4) levels and activating Nrf2 pathway.

Zingiber officinale (Ginger)

Since ancient times Ginger has been commonly consumed both as a spice and a herb [367]. It is reported in the literature that Ginger possesses various types of therapeutic effects, including anti-inflammatory, antioxidant, and neuroprotective activities [368 - 370]. Gingerol and 6-shogaol (6-S) are the primary bioactive compounds in ginger. 6-dehydrogingerdione (6-DG) is also one of the phenolic compounds found in ginger (Tanaka *et al.*, 2015).

Intriguingly it has been highlighted that the phenolic compound found in ginger; 6-dehydrogingerdione (6-DG) and 6-shogaol (6-S), exert cytoprotection against oxidative stress-induced neuronal cell damage in the neuron-like rat pheochromocytoma cell line, PC12 cells *via* promoting the activation of Nrf2 and up-regulation of phase II antioxidant molecules including glutathione, heme oxygenase, NAD(P)H: quinone oxidoreductase and thioredoxin reductase. Furthermore, it has been revealed that activation of the Keap1-Nrf2-ARE pathway is the molecular basis for the cytoprotection of 6-DG and 6-S that, increases the expression of Nrf2 target genes by modifying Keap1 and preventing Nrf2 from proteasomal degradation [135, 136, 371 - 373].

Piper nigrum (Black Pepper)

Piperine is the main alkaloid of black pepper which is being used for various therapeutic purposes in traditional medicine. Piperine is a potent Nrf2 activator [374] and has a wide range of pharmacological properties, including anti-inflammatory, antioxidant, antidepressant, anticonvulsant, and cognitive-enhancing effects [375]. In addition, Piperine is best known for enhancing the bioavailability of drugs and nutraceuticals, where it was reported recently by Roshanbakhsh *et al.*, 2020 [376] that piperine treatment enhanced the total antioxidant capacity Nrf2 and HO1 in the rat hippocampus.

THE DARK SIDE OF NRF2 ACTIVATION

Regulation of Nrf2 is reported to be a "Double-Edged Sword" since it is consequently accepted that even though there are numerous benefits of enhancing the Nrf2 activity, high levels of Nrf2 promote tumor progression, metastasis, chemoresistance, and poor prognosis [21, 39, 377 - 382]. Moreover, it is also reported that oncogenes, including KRAS, BRAF, and MYC, play a role in promoting the transcription of Nrf2 through the modulation of signaling pathways [383 - 385].

It is noteworthy that survival of non-cancerous cells and their protection against carcinogenesis can be achieved *via* temporary activation of Nrf2, which is critical [386]. However, constant activation of this pathway is detrimental, especially in a cancerous context [378]. Several lines of evidence state that Nrf2 leads to diminished apoptosis [387, 388] and increased drug resistance in Cancer [389], thus inhibition of Nrf2 signaling enhances apoptosis in response to oxidative insults [390, 391]

PLANT-BASED INHIBITORS OF NRF2

With the identification of the dark side in Nrf2 activation leading to cancer and chemotherapy resistance, even though it was urged to expand the research towards the development of Nrf2 inhibitors, no selective Nrf2 inhibitors have been developed or evaluated under clinical trials to date [392 - 394]. Yet, natural product-based alternative approaches are being investigated as potential Nrf2 inhibitors [390].

In this scenario, ample studies have been conducted on the plant *Brucea javanica* (Local Sri Lankan Name: Titta Kohomba or Kaputu Gedi; Native to Sri Lanka), its metabolite Brusatol and the derivatives in tumors evaluating the inhibition of proliferation and the disruption of antioxidant defenses caused by Nrf2 depletion [59, 114, 229, 395 - 398]. Halofuginone from the plant *Dichroa febrifuga,* one of the fundamental herbs in traditional Chinese medicine, is an emerging Nrf2 inhibitor [399 - 402]. Intriguingly a study by Tsuchida *et al.*, 2017 [403] revealed that Halofuginone has a similar mechanism of action to that of Brusatol, highlighting the utility of protein synthesis inhibition as a strategy to block Nrf2 signaling.

Moreover, it is reported that Chrysin; a flavone found in blue passion flowers and honey, has anticancer potential against various tumors [404, 405]. Intriguingly, Gao *et al.*, 2013 revealed that on BEL-7402 human HCC cells, Chrysin significantly reduced Nrf2 expression both at the mRNA and protein levels, by interfering with PI3K/AKT and ERK pathways [366]. The findings were further supported by Wang *et al.*, 2018 [406] by his study on human T98, U251, and U87 glioblastoma (GBM) cells and BALB/c mice identified that Chrysin impaired Nrf2 nuclear translocation, by decreasing the protein levels of phospho-extracellular signal-regulated kinase-1/2 (ERK1/2) and antioxidant enzymes HO-1 and NQO-1 respectively. A diterpenoid Oridonin found in *Rabdosia rubescens*; a popular Chinese herb, was found to be with potent anti-tumor effects on Breast Cancer [407], Colorectal Cancer [408], and Leukemia [409]. A recent study by Lu *et al.*, 2018 [103] on osteosarcoma cells revealed that Oridonin suppresses both NF-κB and Nrf2 pathways preventing Nrf2 nuclear translocation.

Intriguingly a natural naphthoquinone; Plumbagin which is highly abundant in a native Sri Lankan herb *Plumbago zeylanica* (Local Sri Lankan Name: Ela Nitul; English Name: Chitrak), has been extensively studied as a potent inducer for apoptosis [410, 411]. A recent study by Kapur *et al.*, in 2018 [412] revealed that Plumbagin promotes ROS generation and synergizes with Brusatol (found in *B. javanica*; a native Sri Lankan plant) to block the Nrf2 pathway, triggering cell death. Such possible synergistic activities are crucial for pharmaceutical/nutraceutical development. A study by Pan *et al.*, 2015 [413] concluded that Plumbagin decreases the Nrf2 nuclear translocation and suppresses the induction of its target genes, thus promoting an unbalanced ROS overproduction leading to cell cycle arrest and triggering apoptosis.

CONCLUSION AND FUTURE DIRECTION

Nonetheless, the symptoms of neurological diseases are different; oxidative stress plays a central role in pathogenesis. Nrf2 activation will counteract common pathogenic processes involved in neurodegenerative/neuromuscular disorders through upregulation of antioxidant defense [414], improvement of mitochondrial function, protein homeostasis, and inhibition of inflammation. Therefore, targeting Nrf2 signaling may provide a therapeutic option to delay onset, slow progression, and ameliorate symptoms of neurological disorders.

However, it is noteworthy that even though Nrf2 activation is reported to be novel and attractive, the Nrf2 pathway is complicated since numerous biomolecules are involved in Nrf2 regulation thus, Nrf2 can be activated with different mechanisms. In this scenario, the importance of natural products as chemical/ biological tools in the regulation of Nrf2 has been revealed in the case of the Nrf2-ARE cellular protective axis. However, as highlighted by Cuadrado *et al.*, 2019, a suitable dosing regimen should be inferred due to the short half-life of Nrf2 compared with its target genes [415].

Even though it is evident that Nrf2 activation is effective against neurological diseases, it is crucial to further investigate whether chronic, long-term Nrf2 activation therapy increases the risk of cancer development, since pleiotropic effects of Nrf2 modulating compounds have added some confusion. In this scenario, the knowledge of the timing of Nrf2 modulating compounds and dosage is crucial to define at which point should an Nrf2 activator be used versus an Nrf2 inhibitor? And which outcome measures are truly Nrf2 related and which are due to off-target or different target effects? In this scenario, the knowledge of blends of natural products that synergize and provide multi-site action on Nrf2 regulation *via* different pathways is vital. Moreover, the identification of the optimum ratio for Nrf2 agonist and Nrf2 antagonist natural products and evaluation of the exact effect of Nrf2 by utilizing serum/urine proteomic, metabolomic, and transcriptomic biomarkers [416] will pave the way for the development of evidence-based effective neuro-nutraceuticals with a stride of innovation.

CONSENT FOR PUBLICATION

Not applicable.

CONFLICT OF INTEREST

The author declares no conflict of interest, financial or otherwise.

ACKNOWLEDGMENTS

The authors greatly appreciate the financial support received from the Ministry of Primary Industries, through National Science Foundation Grant Number SP/CIN/2016/02 and the University of Sri Jayewardenepura (WCUP/Ph.D./19, WCUP/Ph.D./19B, ASP/01/RE/MED/2019/47). We would like to acknowledge Ms. Shamali Wasala, Ms. Dilukshi Shashikaran, and Dr. Gayathri Wijeweera of the Interdisciplinary Centre for Innovation in Biotechnology and Neuroscience, University of Sri Jayewardenepura, Sri Lanka, for their contribution to writing this chapter.

REFERENCES

[1]   Jiang LF, Yao TM, Zhu ZL, Wang C, Ji LN. Impacts of Cd(II) on the conformation and self-aggregation of Alzheimer's tau fragment corresponding to the third repeat of microtubule-binding domain. Biochim Biophys Acta Proteins Proteomics 2007; 1774(11): 1414-21.
[http://dx.doi.org/10.1016/j.bbapap.2007.08.014] [PMID: 17920001]

[2]   Chang AY, Skirbekk VF, Tyrovolas S, Kassebaum NJ, Dieleman JL. Measuring population ageing: an analysis of the Global Burden of Disease Study 2017. Lancet Public Health 2019; 4(3): e159-67.
[http://dx.doi.org/10.1016/S2468-2667(19)30019-2] [PMID: 30851869]

[3]   Beard JR, Officer AM, Cassels AK. The world report on ageing and health. Oxford University Press US 2016.
[http://dx.doi.org/10.1093/geront/gnw037]

[4]   López-Otín C, Blasco MA, Partridge L, Serrano M, Kroemer G. The hallmarks of aging. Cell 2013; 153(6): 1194-217.
[http://dx.doi.org/10.1016/j.cell.2013.05.039] [PMID: 23746838]

[5]   Herculano-Houzel S. The remarkable, yet not extraordinary, human brain as a scaled-up primate brain and its associated cost. Proc Natl Acad Sci USA 2012; 109 (Suppl. 1): 10661-8.
[http://dx.doi.org/10.1073/pnas.1201895109] [PMID: 22723358]

[6]   Dzhusupov KO, Sulaimanova CT, Toguzbayeva KK, *et al.* The State of Higher Education in Occupational Health and Safety in Central Asian Countries. Ann Glob Health 2018; 84(3): 397-407.
[http://dx.doi.org/10.29024/aogh.2322] [PMID: 30835393]

[7]   Buranova DD. The value of Avicenna's heritage in development of modern integrative medicine in Uzbekistan. Integr Med Res 2015; 4(4): 220-4.
[http://dx.doi.org/10.1016/j.imr.2015.06.002] [PMID: 28664128]

[8]   Hajar R. The air of history (part V) Ibn Sina (Avicenna): the great physician and philosopher. Heart views: the official journal of the Gulf Heart Association 2013; 14(4): 196.

[9]   Kankanamalage TNM, Dharmadasa RM, Abeysinghe DC, Wijesekara RGS. A survey on medicinal materials used in traditional systems of medicine in Sri Lanka. J Ethnopharmacol 2014; 155(1): 679-91.
[http://dx.doi.org/10.1016/j.jep.2014.06.016] [PMID: 24933220]

[10]   Imran Y, Wijekoon N, Gonawala L, Chiang YC, De Silva KRD. Biopiracy: Abolish Corporate Hijacking of Indigenous Medicinal Entities. The Scientific World Journal 2021.

[11]   Ediriweera E, Ratnasooriya W. A review on herbs used in treatment of diabetes mellitus by Sri Lankan ayurvedic and traditional physicians. Ayu 2009; 30(4): 373-91.

[12]   Tissera M, Thabrew M. Medicinal plants and Ayurvedic preparations used in Sri Lanka for the control of diabetes mellitus. Sri Lanka: A publication of the Department of Ayurveda, Ministry of Health and Indigenous Medicine 2001.

[13]   Waisundara VY, Watawana MI. The classification of sri lankan medicinal herbs: an extensive comparison of the antioxidant activities. J Tradit Complement Med 2014; 4(3): 196-202.
[http://dx.doi.org/10.4103/2225-4110.126175] [PMID: 25161925]

[14]   Gunawardana S, Jayasuriya W. Medicinally important herbal flowers in Sri Lanka. Evidence-Based Complementary and Alternative Medicine 2019.
[http://dx.doi.org/10.1155/2019/2321961]

[15]   Bernardini S, Tiezzi A, Laghezza Masci V, Ovidi E. Natural products for human health: an historical overview of the drug discovery approaches. Nat Prod Res 2018; 32(16): 1926-50.
       [http://dx.doi.org/10.1080/14786419.2017.1356838] [PMID: 28748726]

[16]   Yuan H, Ma Q, Ye L, Piao G. The traditional medicine and modern medicine from natural products. Molecules 2016; 21(5): 559.
       [http://dx.doi.org/10.3390/molecules21050559] [PMID: 27136524]

[17]   Shen B. A new golden age of natural products drug discovery. Cell 2015; 163(6): 1297-300.
       [http://dx.doi.org/10.1016/j.cell.2015.11.031] [PMID: 26638061]

[18]   Chen J, Li W, Yao H, Xu J. Insights into drug discovery from natural products through structural modification. Fitoterapia 2015; 103: 231-41.
       [http://dx.doi.org/10.1016/j.fitote.2015.04.012] [PMID: 25917513]

[19]   Dias DA, Urban S, Roessner U. A historical overview of natural products in drug discovery. Metabolites 2012; 2(2): 303-36.
       [http://dx.doi.org/10.3390/metabo2020303] [PMID: 24957513]

[20]   Atanasov AG, Zotchev SB, Dirsch VM, Supuran CT. International Natural Product Sciences Taskforce. Natural products in drug discovery: advances and opportunities. Nat Rev Drug Discov 2021; 20(3): 200-16.
       [http://dx.doi.org/10.1038/s41573-020-00114-z] [PMID: 33510482]

[21]   Zhang J, Duan D, Song ZL, Liu T, Hou Y, Fang J. Small molecules regulating reactive oxygen species homeostasis for cancer therapy. Med Res Rev 2021; 41(1): 342-94.
       [http://dx.doi.org/10.1002/med.21734] [PMID: 32981100]

[22]   Newman DJ, Cragg GM. Natural products as sources of new drugs over the nearly four decades from 01/1981 to 09/2019. J Nat Prod 2020; 83(3): 770-803.
       [http://dx.doi.org/10.1021/acs.jnatprod.9b01285] [PMID: 32162523]

[23]   Newman DJ, Cragg GM. Natural product scaffolds as leads to drugs. Future Med Chem 2009; 1(8): 1415-27.
       [http://dx.doi.org/10.4155/fmc.09.113] [PMID: 21426057]

[24]   Newman DJ, Giddings LA. Natural products as leads to antitumor drugs. Phytochem Rev 2014; 13(1): 123-37.
       [http://dx.doi.org/10.1007/s11101-013-9292-6]

[25]   Newman DJ, Cragg GM. Natural products as sources of new drugs over the 30 years from 1981 to 2010. J Nat Prod 2012; 75(3): 311-35.
       [http://dx.doi.org/10.1021/np200906s] [PMID: 22316239]

[26]   Newman DJ. Developing natural product drugs: Supply problems and how they have been overcome. Pharmacol Ther 2016; 162: 1-9.
       [http://dx.doi.org/10.1016/j.pharmthera.2015.12.002] [PMID: 26706239]

[27]   Newman D. Screening and identification of novel biologically active natural compounds. F1000 Res 2017; 6: 783.
       [http://dx.doi.org/10.12688/f1000research.11221.1] [PMID: 28649374]

[28]   Guo Z. The modification of natural products for medical use. Acta Pharm Sin B 2017; 7(2): 119-36.
       [http://dx.doi.org/10.1016/j.apsb.2016.06.003] [PMID: 28303218]

[29]   Brown DG, Lister T, May-Dracka TL. New natural products as new leads for antibacterial drug discovery. Bioorg Med Chem Lett 2014; 24(2): 413-8.
       [http://dx.doi.org/10.1016/j.bmcl.2013.12.059] [PMID: 24388805]

[30]   Cragg GM, Pezzuto JM. Natural products as a vital source for the discovery of cancer chemotherapeutic and chemopreventive agents. Med Princ Pract 2016; 25 (Suppl. 2): 41-59.
       [http://dx.doi.org/10.1159/000443404] [PMID: 26679767]

[31] Itoh K, Tong KI, Yamamoto M. Molecular mechanism activating Nrf2–keap1 pathway in regulation of adaptive response to electrophiles. Free Radic Biol Med 2004; 36(10): 1208-13.
[http://dx.doi.org/10.1016/j.freeradbiomed.2004.02.075] [PMID: 15110385]

[32] Kobayashi M, Yamamoto M. Molecular mechanisms activating the Nrf2-Keap1 pathway of antioxidant gene regulation. Antioxid Redox Signal 2005; 7(3-4): 385-94.
[http://dx.doi.org/10.1089/ars.2005.7.385] [PMID: 15706085]

[33] Suzuki T, Motohashi H, Yamamoto M. Toward clinical application of the Keap1–Nrf2 pathway. Trends Pharmacol Sci 2013; 34(6): 340-6.
[http://dx.doi.org/10.1016/j.tips.2013.04.005] [PMID: 23664668]

[34] Zhang DD. Mechanistic studies of the Nrf2-Keap1 signaling pathway. Drug Metab Rev 2006; 38(4): 769-89.
[http://dx.doi.org/10.1080/03602530600971974] [PMID: 17145701]

[35] Keswani C, Dilnashin H, Birla H, Singh S. Re-addressing the commercialization and regulatory hurdles for biopesticides in India. Rhizosphere 2019; 11(100155): 10.1016.

[36] Rathore AS, Birla H, Singh SS, *et al.* Epigenetic Modulation in Parkinson's Disease and Potential Treatment Therapies. Neurochem Res 2021; 46(7): 1618-26.
[http://dx.doi.org/10.1007/s11064-021-03334-w] [PMID: 33900517]

[37] Singh SS, Rai SN, Birla H, *et al.* Application of Biomedical Engineering in NeuroscienceTechniques Related to Disease Diagnosis and Therapeutics. Application of Biomedical Engineering in Neuroscience. Springer 2019; pp. 437-56.
[http://dx.doi.org/10.1007/978-981-13-7142-4_22]

[38] Zahra W, Rai SN, Birla H, *et al.* The global economic impact of neurodegenerative diseases: Opportunities and challenges. Bioeconomy for Sustainable Development 2020; pp. 333-45.

[39] Satoh H, Moriguchi T, Saigusa D, *et al.* Nrf2 intensifies host defense systems to prevent lung carcinogenesis, but after tumor initiation accelerates malignant cell growth. Cancer Res 2016; 76(10): 3088-96.
[http://dx.doi.org/10.1158/0008-5472.CAN-15-1584] [PMID: 27020858]

[40] Calkins MJ, Johnson DA, Townsend JA, *et al.* The Nrf2/ARE pathway as a potential therapeutic target in neurodegenerative disease. Antioxid Redox Signal 2009; 11(3): 497-508.
[http://dx.doi.org/10.1089/ars.2008.2242] [PMID: 18717629]

[41] Joshi G, Johnson JA. The Nrf2-ARE pathway: a valuable therapeutic target for the treatment of neurodegenerative diseases. Recent Patents on CNS Drug Discovery (Discontinued) 2012; 7(3): 218-29.
[http://dx.doi.org/10.2174/157488912803252023] [PMID: 22742419]

[42] Keswani C. Bioeconomy for Sustainable Development. Springer 2020.
[http://dx.doi.org/10.1007/978-981-13-9431-7]

[43] Sun Y, Yang T, K, Leak R, Chen J, Zhang F. Preventive and protective roles of dietary Nrf2 activators against central nervous system diseases. CNS & Neurological Disorders-Drug Targets 2017; 16(13): 326-8.
[http://dx.doi.org/10.2174/1871527316666170102120211]

[44] Johnson DA, Johnson JA. Nrf2—a therapeutic target for the treatment of neurodegenerative diseases. Free Radic Biol Med 2015; 88(Pt B): 253-67.
[http://dx.doi.org/10.1016/j.freeradbiomed.2015.07.147] [PMID: 26281945]

[45] Ahmed SMU, Luo L, Namani A, Wang XJ, Tang X. Nrf2 signaling pathway: Pivotal roles in inflammation. Biochim Biophys Acta Mol Basis Dis 2017; 1863(2): 585-97.
[http://dx.doi.org/10.1016/j.bbadis.2016.11.005] [PMID: 27825853]

[46] Cuadrado A, Manda G, Hassan A, *et al.* Transcription factor Nrf2 as a therapeutic target for chronic

diseases: a systems medicine approach. Pharmacol Rev 2018; 70(2): 348-83.
[http://dx.doi.org/10.1124/pr.117.014753] [PMID: 29507103]

[47]   Brandes MS, Gray NE. Nrf2 as a therapeutic target in neurodegenerative diseases. ASN Neuro 2020; 12.
[http://dx.doi.org/10.1177/1759091419899782] [PMID: 31964153]

[48]   Hilliard A, Mendonca P, Russell TD, Soliman KFA. The Protective Effects of Flavonoids in Cataract Formation through the Activation of Nrf2 and the Inhibition of MMP-9. Nutrients 2020; 12(12): 3651.
[http://dx.doi.org/10.3390/nu12123651] [PMID: 33261005]

[49]   Chapple SJ, Siow RCM, Mann GE. Crosstalk between Nrf2 and the proteasome: Therapeutic potential of Nrf2 inducers in vascular disease and aging. Int J Biochem Cell Biol 2012; 44(8): 1315-20.
[http://dx.doi.org/10.1016/j.biocel.2012.04.021] [PMID: 22575091]

[50]   Vriend J, Reiter RJ. The Keap1-Nrf2-antioxidant response element pathway: A review of its regulation by melatonin and the proteasome. Mol Cell Endocrinol 2015; 401: 213-20.
[http://dx.doi.org/10.1016/j.mce.2014.12.013] [PMID: 25528518]

[51]   Murakami S, Motohashi H. Roles of Nrf2 in cell proliferation and differentiation. Free Radic Biol Med 2015; 88(Pt B): 168-78.
[http://dx.doi.org/10.1016/j.freeradbiomed.2015.06.030] [PMID: 26119783]

[52]   Hayes JD, Ashford MLJ. Nrf2 orchestrates fuel partitioning for cell proliferation. Cell Metab 2012; 16(2): 139-41.
[http://dx.doi.org/10.1016/j.cmet.2012.07.009] [PMID: 22883227]

[53]   Fan Z, Wirth A, Chen D, *et al.* Nrf2-Keap1 pathway promotes cell proliferation and diminishes ferroptosis. Oncogenesis 2017; 6(8): e371-e.
[http://dx.doi.org/10.1038/oncsis.2017.65]

[54]   Wu S, Lu H, Bai Y. Nrf2 in cancers: A double-edged sword. Cancer Med 2019; 8(5): 2252-67.
[http://dx.doi.org/10.1002/cam4.2101] [PMID: 30929309]

[55]   Janssen-Heininger YMW, Mossman BT, Heintz NH, *et al.* Redox-based regulation of signal transduction: Principles, pitfalls, and promises. Free Radic Biol Med 2008; 45(1): 1-17.
[http://dx.doi.org/10.1016/j.freeradbiomed.2008.03.011] [PMID: 18423411]

[56]   Ma Q. Role of Nrf2 in oxidative stress and toxicity. Annu Rev Pharmacol Toxicol 2013; 53(1): 401-26.
[http://dx.doi.org/10.1146/annurev-pharmtox-011112-140320] [PMID: 23294312]

[57]   Lu MC, Ji JA, Jiang ZY, You QD. The Keap1–Nrf2–ARE pathway as a potential preventive and therapeutic target: an update. Med Res Rev 2016; 36(5): 924-63.
[http://dx.doi.org/10.1002/med.21396] [PMID: 27192495]

[58]   Copple IM, Dinkova-Kostova AT, Kensler TW, Liby KT, Wigley WC. Nrf2 as an emerging therapeutic target. Hindawi 2017.
[http://dx.doi.org/10.1155/2017/8165458]

[59]   Wang YY, Chen J, Liu XM, Zhao R, Zhe H. Nrf2-mediated metabolic reprogramming in cancer. Oxidative medicine and cellular longevity 2018.
[http://dx.doi.org/10.1155/2018/9304091]

[60]   Singh S, Rai S, Birla H, Eds., *et al.* Chlorogenic acid protects against MPTP induced neurotoxicity in parkinsonian mice model *via* its anti-apoptotic activity. Journal of Neurochemistry. Hoboken 07030-5774, NJ USA: Wiley 111 River St 2019.

[61]   Rai SN, Birla H, Singh SS, *et al.* Pathophysiology of the Disease Causing Physical Disability. Biomedical Engineering and its Applications in Healthcare. Springer 2019; pp. 573-95.

[62]   Rai SN, Singh BK, Rathore AS, *et al.* Quality control in huntington's disease: a therapeutic target. Neurotox Res 2019; 36(3): 612-26.

[http://dx.doi.org/10.1007/s12640-019-00087-x] [PMID: 31297710]

[63] Rai SN, Dilnashin H, Birla H, *et al.* The role of PI3K/Akt and ERK in neurodegenerative disorders. Neurotox Res 2019; 35(3): 775-95.
[http://dx.doi.org/10.1007/s12640-019-0003-y] [PMID: 30707354]

[64] Moi P, Chan K, Asunis I, Cao A, Kan YW. Isolation of NF-E2-related factor 2 (Nrf2), a NF-E2-like basic leucine zipper transcriptional activator that binds to the tandem NF-E2/AP1 repeat of the beta-globin locus control region. Proc Natl Acad Sci USA 1994; 91(21): 9926-30.
[http://dx.doi.org/10.1073/pnas.91.21.9926] [PMID: 7937919]

[65] Nguyen T, Yang CS, Pickett CB. The pathways and molecular mechanisms regulating Nrf2 activation in response to chemical stress. Free Radic Biol Med 2004; 37(4): 433-41.
[http://dx.doi.org/10.1016/j.freeradbiomed.2004.04.033] [PMID: 15256215]

[66] Dai X, Yan X, Wintergerst KA, Cai L, Keller BB, Tan Y. Nrf2: redox and metabolic regulator of stem cell state and function. Trends Mol Med 2020; 26(2): 185-200.
[http://dx.doi.org/10.1016/j.molmed.2019.09.007] [PMID: 31679988]

[67] Vargas MR, Johnson JA. The Nrf2–ARE cytoprotective pathway in astrocytes. Expert Rev Mol Med 2009; 11: e17.
[http://dx.doi.org/10.1017/S1462399409001094] [PMID: 19490732]

[68] Jakel RJ, Townsend JA, Kraft AD, Johnson JA. Nrf2-mediated protection against 6-hydroxydopamine. Brain Res 2007; 1144: 192-201.
[http://dx.doi.org/10.1016/j.brainres.2007.01.131] [PMID: 17336276]

[69] Chen PC, Vargas MR, Pani AK, *et al.* Nrf2-mediated neuroprotection in the MPTP mouse model of Parkinson's disease: Critical role for the astrocyte. Proc Natl Acad Sci USA 2009; 106(8): 2933-8.
[http://dx.doi.org/10.1073/pnas.0813361106] [PMID: 19196989]

[70] Sandberg M, Patil J, D'Angelo B, Weber SG, Mallard C. Nrf2-regulation in brain health and disease: Implication of cerebral inflammation. Neuropharmacology 2014; 79: 298-306.
[http://dx.doi.org/10.1016/j.neuropharm.2013.11.004] [PMID: 24262633]

[71] Dinkova-Kostova AT, Abramov AY. The emerging role of Nrf2 in mitochondrial function. Free Radic Biol Med 2015; 88(Pt B): 179-88.
[http://dx.doi.org/10.1016/j.freeradbiomed.2015.04.036] [PMID: 25975984]

[72] Buendia I, Michalska P, Navarro E, Gameiro I, Egea J, León R. Nrf2–ARE pathway: An emerging target against oxidative stress and neuroinflammation in neurodegenerative diseases. Pharmacol Ther 2016; 157: 84-104.
[http://dx.doi.org/10.1016/j.pharmthera.2015.11.003] [PMID: 26617217]

[73] Hayashi G, Jasoliya M, Sahdeo S, *et al.* Dimethyl fumarate mediates Nrf2-dependent mitochondrial biogenesis in mice and humans. Hum Mol Genet 2017; 26(15): 2864-73.
[http://dx.doi.org/10.1093/hmg/ddx167] [PMID: 28460056]

[74] Sivandzade F, Prasad S, Bhalerao A, Cucullo L. Nrf2 and NF-κB interplay in cerebrovascular and neurodegenerative disorders: Molecular mechanisms and possible therapeutic approaches. Redox Biol 2019; 21: 101059.
[http://dx.doi.org/10.1016/j.redox.2018.11.017] [PMID: 30576920]

[75] Vomund S, Schäfer A, Parnham M, Brüne B, von Knethen A. Nrf2, the master regulator of anti-oxidative responses. Int J Mol Sci 2017; 18(12): 2772.
[http://dx.doi.org/10.3390/ijms18122772] [PMID: 29261130]

[76] Zahra W, Rai SN, Birla H, *et al.* Neuroprotection of rotenone-induced Parkinsonism by ursolic acid in PD mouse model. CNS & Neurological Disorders-Drug Targets 2020; 19(7): 527-40.
[http://dx.doi.org/10.2174/1871527319666200812224457]

[77] Rai SN, Zahra W, Singh SS, *et al.* Anti-inflammatory activity of ursolic acid in MPTP-induced parkinsonian mouse model. Neurotox Res 2019; 36(3): 452-62.

[http://dx.doi.org/10.1007/s12640-019-00038-6] [PMID: 31016688]

[78]   Singh SS, Rai SN, Birla H, *et al.* Neuroprotective effect of chlorogenic acid on mitochondrial dysfunction-mediated apoptotic death of DA neurons in a Parkinsonian mouse model. Oxid Med Cell Longev 2020; 2020: 1-14.
[http://dx.doi.org/10.1155/2020/6571484] [PMID: 32566093]

[79]   Zahra W, Rai SN, Birla H, *et al.* Economic Importance of Medicinal Plants in Asian Countries. Bioeconomy for Sustainable Development. Springer 2020; pp. 359-77.
[http://dx.doi.org/10.1007/978-981-13-9431-7_19]

[80]   Ranganathan VK, Siemionow V, Liu JZ, Sahgal V, Yue GH. From mental power to muscle power—gaining strength by using the mind. Neuropsychologia 2004; 42(7): 944-56.
[http://dx.doi.org/10.1016/j.neuropsychologia.2003.11.018] [PMID: 14998709]

[81]   Manini TM, Hong SL, Clark BC. Aging and muscle. Curr Opin Clin Nutr Metab Care 2013; 16(1): 21-6.
[http://dx.doi.org/10.1097/MCO.0b013e32835b5880] [PMID: 23222705]

[82]   Martinet W, De Meyer GRY, Herman AG, Kockx MM. Reactive oxygen species induce RNA damage in human atherosclerosis. Eur J Clin Invest 2004; 34(5): 323-7.
[http://dx.doi.org/10.1111/j.1365-2362.2004.01343.x] [PMID: 15147328]

[83]   Vana L, Kanaan NM, Hakala K, Weintraub ST, Binder LI. Peroxynitrite-induced nitrative and oxidative modifications alter tau filament formation. Biochemistry 2011; 50(7): 1203-12.
[http://dx.doi.org/10.1021/bi101735m] [PMID: 21210655]

[84]   Weingarten MD, Lockwood AH, Hwo SY, Kirschner MW. A protein factor essential for microtubule assembly. Proc Natl Acad Sci USA 1975; 72(5): 1858-62.
[http://dx.doi.org/10.1073/pnas.72.5.1858] [PMID: 1057175]

[85]   Gilgun-Sherki Y, Melamed E, Offen D. Oxidative stress induced-neurodegenerative diseases: the need for antioxidants that penetrate the blood brain barrier. Neuropharmacology 2001; 40(8): 959-75.
[http://dx.doi.org/10.1016/S0028-3908(01)00019-3] [PMID: 11406187]

[86]   Uttara B, Singh A, Zamboni P, Mahajan R. Oxidative stress and neurodegenerative diseases: a review of upstream and downstream antioxidant therapeutic options. Curr Neuropharmacol 2009; 7(1): 65-74.
[http://dx.doi.org/10.2174/157015909787602823] [PMID: 19721819]

[87]   Souza BWS, Cerqueira MA, Bourbon AI, *et al.* Chemical characterization and antioxidant activity of sulfated polysaccharide from the red seaweed *Gracilaria birdiae*. Food Hydrocoll 2012; 27(2): 287-92.
[http://dx.doi.org/10.1016/j.foodhyd.2011.10.005]

[88]   Chiu SP, Wu MJ, Chen PY, *et al.* Neurotrophic action of 5-hydroxylated polymethoxyflavones: 5-demethylnobiletin and gardenin A stimulate neuritogenesis in PC12 cells. J Agric Food Chem 2013; 61(39): 9453-63.
[http://dx.doi.org/10.1021/jf4024678] [PMID: 24003765]

[89]   Maitra U, Harding T, Liang Q, Ciesla L. GardeninA confers neuroprotection against environmental toxin in a Drosophila model of Parkinson's disease. Commun Biol 2021; 4(1): 162.
[http://dx.doi.org/10.1038/s42003-021-01685-2] [PMID: 33547411]

[90]   Birla H, Keswani C, Singh SS, *et al.* Unraveling the Neuroprotective Effect of *Tinospora cordifolia* in Parkinsonian Mouse Model Through Proteomics Approach. ACS Chem Neurosci 2021.12, 22, 4319–35..
[http://dx.doi.org/10.1021/acschemneuro.1c00481]

[91]   Keswani C, Dilnashin H, Birla H, Singh SP. Unravelling efficient applications of agriculturally important microorganisms for alle*via*tion of induced inter-cellular oxidative stress in crops. Acta Agric Slov 2019; 114(1): 121-30.
[http://dx.doi.org/10.14720/aas.2019.114.1.14]

[92]   Birla H, Keswani C, Rai SN, *et al.* Neuroprotective effects of *Withania somnifera* in BPA induced-cognitive dysfunction and oxidative stress in mice. Behav Brain Funct 2019; 15(1): 9.
[http://dx.doi.org/10.1186/s12993-019-0160-4] [PMID: 31064381]

[93]   Niccoli T, Partridge L. Ageing as a risk factor for disease. Curr Biol 2012; 22(17): R741-52.
[http://dx.doi.org/10.1016/j.cub.2012.07.024] [PMID: 22975005]

[94]   Chen WW, Zhang X, Huang WJ. Role of neuroinflammation in neurodegenerative diseases (Review). Mol Med Rep 2016; 13(4): 3391-6.
[http://dx.doi.org/10.3892/mmr.2016.4948] [PMID: 26935478]

[95]   Organization WH. World Health Organization 2010.

[96]   Cuadrado A. Nrf2 in neurodegenerative diseases. Curr Opin Toxicol 2016; 1: 46-53.
[http://dx.doi.org/10.1016/j.cotox.2016.09.004]

[97]   Bruns DR, Drake JC, Biela LM, Peelor FF, Miller BF, Hamilton KL. Nrf2 signaling and the slowed aging phenotype: evidence from long-lived models. Oxid Med Cell Longev 2015 2015:732596
[http://dx.doi.org/10.1155/2015/732596]

[98]   Nguyen T, Nioi P, Pickett CB. The Nrf2-antioxidant response element signaling pathway and its activation by oxidative stress. J Biol Chem 2009; 284(20): 13291-5.
[http://dx.doi.org/10.1074/jbc.R900010200] [PMID: 19182219]

[99]   Tebay LE, Robertson H, Durant ST, *et al.* Mechanisms of activation of the transcription factor Nrf2 by redox stressors, nutrient cues, and energy status and the pathways through which it attenuates degenerative disease. Free Radic Biol Med 2015; 88(Pt B): 108-46.
[http://dx.doi.org/10.1016/j.freeradbiomed.2015.06.021] [PMID: 26122708]

[100]   Osama A, Zhang J, Yao J, Yao X, Fang J. Nrf2: a dark horse in Alzheimer's disease treatment. Ageing Res Rev 2020; 64: 101206.
[http://dx.doi.org/10.1016/j.arr.2020.101206] [PMID: 33144124]

[101]   Jannat S, Balupuri A, Ali MY, *et al.* Inhibition of β-site amyloid precursor protein cleaving enzyme 1 and cholinesterases by pterosins *via* a specific structure–activity relationship with a strong BBB permeability. Exp Mol Med 2019; 51(2): 1-18.
[http://dx.doi.org/10.1038/s12276-019-0205-7] [PMID: 30755593]

[102]   Park J, Wetzel I, Marriott I, *et al.* A 3D human triculture system modeling neurodegeneration and neuroinflammation in Alzheimer's disease. Nat Neurosci 2018; 21(7): 941-51.
[http://dx.doi.org/10.1038/s41593-018-0175-4] [PMID: 29950669]

[103]   Lu Z, Harris TB, Shiroma EJ, Leung J, Kwok T. Patterns of physical activity and sedentary behavior for older adults with Alzheimer's disease, mild cognitive impairment, and cognitively normal in Hong Kong. J Alzheimers Dis 2018; 66(4): 1453-62.
[http://dx.doi.org/10.3233/JAD-180805] [PMID: 30412502]

[104]   Ossenkoppele R, Pijnenburg YAL, Perry DC, *et al.* The behavioural/dysexecutive variant of Alzheimer's disease: clinical, neuroimaging and pathological features. Brain 2015; 138(9): 2732-49.
[http://dx.doi.org/10.1093/brain/awv191] [PMID: 26141491]

[105]   Deibel MA, Ehmann WD, Markesbery WR. Copper, iron, and zinc imbalances in severely degenerated brain regions in Alzheimer's disease: possible relation to oxidative stress. J Neurol Sci 1996; 143(1-2): 137-42.
[http://dx.doi.org/10.1016/S0022-510X(96)00203-1] [PMID: 8981312]

[106]   Huang X, Atwood CS, Hartshorn MA, *et al.* The A β peptide of Alzheimer's disease directly produces hydrogen peroxide through metal ion reduction. Biochemistry 1999; 38(24): 7609-16.
[http://dx.doi.org/10.1021/bi990438f] [PMID: 10386999]

[107]   Wang J, Xiong S, Xie C, Markesbery WR, Lovell MA. Increased oxidative damage in nuclear and mitochondrial DNA in Alzheimer's disease. J Neurochem 2005; 93(4): 953-62.

[http://dx.doi.org/10.1111/j.1471-4159.2005.03053.x] [PMID: 15857398]

[108] Zhang J, Zhang B, Li X, Han X, Liu R, Fang J. Small molecule inhibitors of mammalian thioredoxin reductase as potential anticancer agents: An update. Med Res Rev 2019; 39(1): 5-39.
[http://dx.doi.org/10.1002/med.21507] [PMID: 29727025]

[109] Ramsey CP, Glass CA, Montgomery MB, *et al.* Expression of Nrf2 in neurodegenerative diseases. J Neuropathol Exp Neurol 2007; 66(1): 75-85.
[http://dx.doi.org/10.1097/nen.0b013e31802d6da9] [PMID: 17204939]

[110] Mota SI, Costa RO, Ferreira IL, *et al.* Oxidative stress involving changes in Nrf2 and ER stress in early stages of Alzheimer's disease. Biochim Biophys Acta Mol Basis Dis 2015; 1852(7): 1428-41.
[http://dx.doi.org/10.1016/j.bbadis.2015.03.015] [PMID: 25857617]

[111] Feng Y, Wang X. Antioxidant therapies for Alzheimer's disease. Oxidative medicine and cellular longevity 2012.
[http://dx.doi.org/10.1155/2012/472932]

[112] Grundman M, Delaney P, Delaney P. Antioxidant strategies for Alzheimer's disease. Proc Nutr Soc 2002; 61(2): 191-202.
[http://dx.doi.org/10.1079/PNS2002146] [PMID: 12133201]

[113] Behl C, Moosmann B. Antioxidant neuroprotection in Alzheimer's disease as preventive and therapeutic approach. Free Rad Biol Med 2002; 33(2):182-91.
[http://dx.doi.org/10.1016/S0891-5849(02)00883-3] [PMID: 12106814]

[114] Lee HP, Zhu X, Casadesus G, *et al.* Antioxidant approaches for the treatment of Alzheimer's disease. Expert Rev Neurother 2010; 10(7): 1201-8.
[http://dx.doi.org/10.1586/ern.10.74] [PMID: 20586698]

[115] Veurink G, Perry G, Singh SK. Role of antioxidants and a nutrient rich diet in Alzheimer's disease. Open Biol 2020; 10(6): 200084.
[http://dx.doi.org/10.1098/rsob.200084] [PMID: 32543351]

[116] Hybertson BM, Gao B, Bose SK, McCord JM. Oxidative stress in health and disease: The therapeutic potential of Nrf2 activation. Mol Aspects Med 2011; 32(4-6): 234-46.
[http://dx.doi.org/10.1016/j.mam.2011.10.006] [PMID: 22020111]

[117] Chen QM, Maltagliati AJ. Nrf2 at the heart of oxidative stress and cardiac protection. Physiol Genomics 2018; 50(2): 77-97.
[http://dx.doi.org/10.1152/physiolgenomics.00041.2017] [PMID: 29187515]

[118] Eftekharzadeh B, Maghsoudi N, Khodagholi F. Stabilization of transcription factor Nrf2 by tBHQ prevents oxidative stress-induced amyloid β formation in NT2N neurons. Biochimie 2010; 92(3): 245-53.
[http://dx.doi.org/10.1016/j.biochi.2009.12.001] [PMID: 20026169]

[119] Fu MH, Wu CW, Lee YC, Hung CY, Chen IC, Wu KLH. Nrf2 activation attenuates the early suppression of mitochondrial respiration due to the α-synuclein overexpression. Biomed J 2018; 41(3): 169-83.
[http://dx.doi.org/10.1016/j.bj.2018.02.005] [PMID: 30080657]

[120] Schmidlin CJ, Dodson MB, Madhavan L, Zhang DD. Redox regulation by Nrf2 in aging and disease. Free Radic Biol Med 2019; 134: 702-7.
[http://dx.doi.org/10.1016/j.freeradbiomed.2019.01.016] [PMID: 30654017]

[121] Dinkova-Kostova AT, Kostov RV, Kazantsev AG. The role of Nrf2 signaling in counteracting neurodegenerative diseases. FEBS J 2018; 285(19): 3576-90.
[http://dx.doi.org/10.1111/febs.14379] [PMID: 29323772]

[122] Bahn G, Park JS, Yun UJ, *et al.* Nrf2/ARE pathway negatively regulates BACE1 expression and ameliorates cognitive deficits in mouse Alzheimer's models. Proc Natl Acad Sci USA 2019; 116(25): 12516-23.

[http://dx.doi.org/10.1073/pnas.1819541116] [PMID: 31164420]

[123] Kitaoka Y, Tamura Y, Takahashi K, Takeda K, Takemasa T, Hatta H. Effects of Nrf2 deficiency on mitochondrial oxidative stress in aged skeletal muscle. Physiol Rep 2019; 7(3): e13998.
[http://dx.doi.org/10.14814/phy2.13998] [PMID: 30756520]

[124] Tang M, Ji C, Pallo S, Rahman I, Johnson GVW. Nrf2 mediates the expression of BAG3 and autophagy cargo adaptor proteins and tau clearance in an age-dependent manner. Neurobiol Aging 2018; 63: 128-39.
[http://dx.doi.org/10.1016/j.neurobiolaging.2017.12.001] [PMID: 29304346]

[125] Sotolongo K, Ghiso J, Rostagno A. Nrf2 activation through the PI3K/GSK-3 axis protects neuronal cells from Aβ-mediated oxidative and metabolic damage. Alzheimers Res Ther 2020; 12(1): 13.
[http://dx.doi.org/10.1186/s13195-019-0578-9] [PMID: 31931869]

[126] Wijesinghe P, Shankar SK, Chickabasaviah YT, *et al.* Cytoskeletal Pathologies of Age-Related Diseases between Elderly Sri Lankan (Colombo) and Indian (Bangalore) Brain Samples. Curr Alzheimer Res 2016; 13(3): 268-80.
[http://dx.doi.org/10.2174/1567205013031602171212101210] [PMID: 26906356]

[127] Wijesinghe P, Shankar SK, Yasha TC, *et al.* Vascular contributions in Alzheimer's disease-related neuropathological changes: First autopsy evidence from a South Asian aging population. J Alzheimers Dis 2016; 54(4): 1607-18.
[http://dx.doi.org/10.3233/JAD-160425] [PMID: 27589527]

[128] Deshmukh P, Unni S, Krishnappa G, Padmanabhan B. The Keap1–Nrf2 pathway: promising therapeutic target to counteract ROS-mediated damage in cancers and neurodegenerative diseases. Biophys Rev 2017; 9(1): 41-56.
[http://dx.doi.org/10.1007/s12551-016-0244-4] [PMID: 28510041]

[129] Francisqueti-Ferron FV, Ferron AJT, Garcia JL, *et al.* Silva CCVdA, Costa MR, Gregolin CS, Moreto F, Ferreira ALA, Minatel IO, Correa CR. Basic concepts on the role of nuclear factor erythroid-derived 2-like 2 (Nrf2) in age-related diseases. Int J Mol Sci 2019; 20(13): 3208.
[http://dx.doi.org/10.3390/ijms20133208] [PMID: 31261912]

[130] Silva-Palacios A, Ostolga-Chavarría M, Zazueta C, Königsberg M. Nrf2: Molecular and epigenetic regulation during aging. Ageing Res Rev 2018; 47: 31-40.
[http://dx.doi.org/10.1016/j.arr.2018.06.003] [PMID: 29913211]

[131] Hou Y, Li X, Peng S, Yao J, Bai F, Fang J. Lipoamide ameliorates oxidative stress *via* induction of Nrf2/ARE signaling pathway in PC12 cells. J Agric Food Chem 2019; 67(29): 8227-34.
[http://dx.doi.org/10.1021/acs.jafc.9b02680] [PMID: 31299148]

[132] Hou Y, Peng S, Li X, Yao J, Xu J, Fang J. Honokiol alleviates oxidative stress-induced neurotoxicity *via* activation of Nrf2. ACS Chem Neurosci 2018; 9(12): 3108-16.
[http://dx.doi.org/10.1021/acschemneuro.8b00290] [PMID: 29989791]

[133] Peng S, Hou Y, Yao J, Fang J. Activation of Nrf2 by costunolide provides neuroprotective effect in PC12 cells. Food Funct 2019; 10(7): 4143-52.
[http://dx.doi.org/10.1039/C8FO02249F] [PMID: 31241085]

[134] Peng S, Hou Y, Yao J, Fang J. Neuroprotection of mangiferin against oxidative damage *via* arousing Nrf2 signaling pathway in PC12 cells. Biofactors 2019; 45(3): 381-92.
[http://dx.doi.org/10.1002/biof.1488] [PMID: 30633833]

[135] Peng S, Zhang B, Yao J, Duan D, Fang J. Dual protection of hydroxytyrosol, an olive oil polyphenol, against oxidative damage in PC12 cells. Food Funct 2015; 6(6): 2091-100.
[http://dx.doi.org/10.1039/C5FO00097A] [PMID: 26037629]

[136] Yao J, Ge C, Duan D, *et al.* Activation of the phase II enzymes for neuroprotection by ginger active constituent 6-dehydrogingerdione in PC12 cells. J Agric Food Chem 2014; 62(24): 5507-18.
[http://dx.doi.org/10.1021/jf405553v] [PMID: 24869427]

[137] Lang AE, Espay AJ. Disease modification in Parkinson's disease: current approaches, challenges, and future considerations. Mov Disord 2018; 33(5): 660-77.
[http://dx.doi.org/10.1002/mds.27360] [PMID: 29644751]

[138] Tanner CM, Ottman R, Goldman SM, *et al.* Parkinson disease in twins: an etiologic study. JAMA 1999; 281(4): 341-6.
[http://dx.doi.org/10.1001/jama.281.4.341] [PMID: 9929087]

[139] Kouli A, Torsney KM, Kuan W-L. Parkinson's disease: etiology, neuropathology, and pathogenesis. Exon Publications 2018; pp. 3-26.

[140] Lang AE, Melamed E, Poewe W, Rascol O. Trial designs used to study neuroprotective therapy in Parkinson's disease. Mov Disord 2013; 28(1): 86-95.
[http://dx.doi.org/10.1002/mds.24997] [PMID: 22927060]

[141] Dinkova-Kostova AT, Talalay P, Sharkey J, *et al.* An exceptionally potent inducer of cytoprotective enzymes: elucidation of the structural features that determine inducer potency and reactivity with Keap1. J Biol Chem 2010; 285(44): 33747-55.
[http://dx.doi.org/10.1074/jbc.M110.163485] [PMID: 20801881]

[142] Aiken CT, Kaake RM, Wang X, Huang L. Oxidative stress-mediated regulation of proteasome complexes. Molecular & Cellular Proteomics 2011; 10(5): R110. 006924.

[143] Chen X, Guo C, Kong J. Oxidative stress in neurodegenerative diseases. Neural Regen Res 2012; 7(5): 376-85.
[PMID: 25774178]

[144] Nakabeppu Y, Tsuchimoto D, Yamaguchi H, Sakumi K. Oxidative damage in nucleic acids and Parkinson's disease. J Neurosci Res 2007; 85(5): 919-34.
[http://dx.doi.org/10.1002/jnr.21191] [PMID: 17279544]

[145] Johnson WM, Wilson-Delfosse AL, Mieyal JJ. Dysregulation of glutathione homeostasis in neurodegenerative diseases. Nutrients 2012; 4(10): 1399-440.
[http://dx.doi.org/10.3390/nu4101399] [PMID: 23201762]

[146] Dias V, Junn E, Mouradian MM. The role of oxidative stress in Parkinson's disease. J Parkinsons Dis 2013; 3(4): 461-91.
[http://dx.doi.org/10.3233/JPD-130230] [PMID: 24252804]

[147] Alfieri A, Srivastava S, Siow RCM, Modo M, Fraser PA, Mann GE. Targeting the Nrf2-Keap1 antioxidant defence pathway for neurovascular protection in stroke. J Physiol 2011; 589(17): 4125-36.
[http://dx.doi.org/10.1113/jphysiol.2011.210294] [PMID: 21646410]

[148] Petrillo S, D'Amico J, La Rosa P, Bertini ES, Piemonte F. Targeting Nrf2 for the treatment of Friedreich's ataxia: a comparison among drugs. Int J Mol Sci 2019; 20(20): 5211.
[http://dx.doi.org/10.3390/ijms20205211] [PMID: 31640150]

[149] Zhang SM, Hernán MA, Chen H, Spiegelman D, Willett WC, Ascherio A. Intakes of vitamins E and C, carotenoids, vitamin supplements, and PD risk. Neurology 2002; 59(8): 1161-9.
[http://dx.doi.org/10.1212/01.WNL.0000028688.75881.12] [PMID: 12391343]

[150] Seidl SE, Potashkin JA. The promise of neuroprotective agents in Parkinson's disease. Front Neurol 2011; 2: 68.
[http://dx.doi.org/10.3389/fneur.2011.00068] [PMID: 22125548]

[151] Wijeyekoon R, Suriyakumara V, Gamage R, *et al.* Associations Between Lifestyle Factors And Parkinson's Disease In An Urban Sri Lankan Clinic Study. Int Arch Med 2017; 10: 10.
[http://dx.doi.org/10.3823/2516] [PMID: 29057010]

[152] Coles LD, Tuite PJ, Öz G, *et al.* Repeated-dose oral N-acetylcysteine in Parkinson's disease: pharmacokinetics and effect on brain glutathione and oxidative stress. J Clin Pharmacol 2018; 58(2): 158-67.

[http://dx.doi.org/10.1002/jcph.1008] [PMID: 28940353]

[153] Taghizadeh M, Tamtaji OR, Dadgostar E, *et al.* The effects of omega-3 fatty acids and vitamin E co-supplementation on clinical and metabolic status in patients with Parkinson's disease: A randomized, double-blind, placebo-controlled trial. Neurochem Int 2017; 108: 183-9.
[http://dx.doi.org/10.1016/j.neuint.2017.03.014] [PMID: 28342967]

[154] Goswami A, Dikshit P, Mishra A, Mulherkar S, Nukina N, Jana NR. Oxidative stress promotes mutant huntingtin aggregation and mutant huntingtin-dependent cell death by mimicking proteasomal malfunction. Biochem Biophys Res Commun 2006; 342(1): 184-90.
[http://dx.doi.org/10.1016/j.bbrc.2006.01.136] [PMID: 16472774]

[155] Sorolla MA, Reverter-Branchat G, Tamarit J, Ferrer I, Ros J, Cabiscol E. Proteomic and oxidative stress analysis in human brain samples of Huntington disease. Free Radic Biol Med 2008; 45(5): 667-78.
[http://dx.doi.org/10.1016/j.freeradbiomed.2008.05.014] [PMID: 18588971]

[156] Browne SE, Bowling AC, Macgarvey U, *et al.* Oxidative damage and metabolic dysfunction in Huntington's disease: Selective vulnerability of the basal ganglia. Ann Neurol 1997; 41(5): 646-53.
[http://dx.doi.org/10.1002/ana.410410514] [PMID: 9153527]

[157] Browne SE, Beal MF. Oxidative damage in Huntington's disease pathogenesis. Antioxid Redox Signal 2006; 8(11-12): 2061-73.
[http://dx.doi.org/10.1089/ars.2006.8.2061] [PMID: 17034350]

[158] Chen CM, Wu YR, Cheng ML, *et al.* Increased oxidative damage and mitochondrial abnormalities in the peripheral blood of Huntington's disease patients. Biochem Biophys Res Commun 2007; 359(2): 335-40.
[http://dx.doi.org/10.1016/j.bbrc.2007.05.093] [PMID: 17543886]

[159] Klepac N, Relja M, Klepac R, Hećimović S, Babić T, Trkulja V. Oxidative stress parameters in plasma of Huntington's disease patients, asymptomatic Huntington's disease gene carriers and healthy subjects. J Neurol 2007; 254(12): 1676-83.
[http://dx.doi.org/10.1007/s00415-007-0611-y] [PMID: 17990062]

[160] Chang KH, Chen YC, Wu YR, Lee WF, Chen CM. Downregulation of genes involved in metabolism and oxidative stress in the peripheral leukocytes of Huntington's disease patients. PLoS One 2012; 7(9): e46492.
[http://dx.doi.org/10.1371/journal.pone.0046492] [PMID: 23029535]

[161] Browne SE. Mitochondria and Huntington's disease pathogenesis: insight from genetic and chemical models. Ann N Y Acad Sci 2008; 1147(1): 358-82.
[http://dx.doi.org/10.1196/annals.1427.018] [PMID: 19076457]

[162] Damiano M, Galvan L, Déglon N, Brouillet E. Mitochondria in Huntington's disease. Biochim Biophys Acta Mol Basis Dis 2010; 1802(1): 52-61.
[http://dx.doi.org/10.1016/j.bbadis.2009.07.012]

[163] Kim J, Moody JP, Edgerly CK, *et al.* Mitochondrial loss, dysfunction and altered dynamics in Huntington's disease. Hum Mol Genet 2010; 19(20): 3919-35.
[http://dx.doi.org/10.1093/hmg/ddq306] [PMID: 20660112]

[164] Pavese N, Gerhard A, Tai YF, *et al.* Microglial activation correlates with severity in Huntington disease: A clinical and PET study. Neurology 2006; 66(11): 1638-43.
[http://dx.doi.org/10.1212/01.wnl.0000222734.56412.17] [PMID: 16769933]

[165] Tai YF, Pavese N, Gerhard A, *et al.* Microglial activation in presymptomatic Huntington's disease gene carriers. Brain 2007; 130(7): 1759-66.
[http://dx.doi.org/10.1093/brain/awm044] [PMID: 17400599]

[166] Björkqvist M, Wild EJ, Thiele J, *et al.* A novel pathogenic pathway of immune activation detectable before clinical onset in Huntington's disease. J Exp Med 2008; 205(8): 1869-77.

[http://dx.doi.org/10.1084/jem.20080178] [PMID: 18625748]

[167] Politis M, Pavese N, Tai YF, *et al.* Microglial activation in regions related to cognitive function predicts disease onset in Huntington's disease: A multimodal imaging study. Hum Brain Mapp 2011; 32(2): 258-70.
[http://dx.doi.org/10.1002/hbm.21008] [PMID: 21229614]

[168] Prasad KN, Bondy SC. C Bondy S. Inhibition of early biochemical defects in prodromal Huntington's disease by simultaneous activation of Nrf2 and elevation of multiple micronutrients. Curr Aging Sci 2016; 9(1): 61-70.
[http://dx.doi.org/10.2174/1874609809666151124231127] [PMID: 26601664]

[169] Prasad KN. Simultaneous activation of Nrf2 and elevation of antioxidant compounds for reducing oxidative stress and chronic inflammation in human Alzheimer's disease. Mech Ageing Dev 2016; 153: 41-7.
[http://dx.doi.org/10.1016/j.mad.2016.01.002] [PMID: 26811881]

[170] Quinti L, Dayalan Naidu S, Träger U, *et al.* KEAP1-modifying small molecule reveals muted Nrf2 signaling responses in neural stem cells from Huntington's disease patients. Proc Natl Acad Sci USA 2017; 114(23): E4676-85.
[http://dx.doi.org/10.1073/pnas.1614943114] [PMID: 28533375]

[171] Chang KH, Chen WL, Wu YR, *et al.* Aqueous extract of Gardenia jasminoides targeting oxidative stress to reduce polyQ aggregation in cell models of spinocerebellar ataxia 3. Neuropharmacology 2014; 81: 166-75.
[http://dx.doi.org/10.1016/j.neuropharm.2014.01.032] [PMID: 24486383]

[172] Chen CM, Weng YT, Chen WL, *et al.* Aqueous extract of Glycyrrhiza inflata inhibits aggregation by upregulating PPARGC1A and NFE2L2–ARE pathways in cell models of spinocerebellar ataxia 3. Free Radic Biol Med 2014; 71: 339-50.
[http://dx.doi.org/10.1016/j.freeradbiomed.2014.03.023] [PMID: 24675225]

[173] Wu YL, Chang JC, Lin WY, *et al.* Treatment with caffeic acid and resveratrol alleviates oxidative stress induced neurotoxicity in cell and drosophila models of spinocerebellar ataxia type3. Sci Rep 2017; 7(1): 11641.
[http://dx.doi.org/10.1038/s41598-017-11839-0] [PMID: 28912527]

[174] Khairallah RJ, Shi G, Sbrana F, *et al.* Microtubules underlie dysfunction in duchenne muscular dystrophy. Sci Signal 2012; 5(236): ra56.
[http://dx.doi.org/10.1126/scisignal.2002829] [PMID: 22871609]

[175] Petrillo S, Pelosi L, Piemonte F, *et al.* Oxidative stress in Duchenne muscular dystrophy: focus on the Nrf2 redox pathway. Hum Mol Genet 2017; 26(14): 2781-90.
[http://dx.doi.org/10.1093/hmg/ddx173] [PMID: 28472288]

[176] Pelosi L, Forcina L, Nicoletti C, Scicchitano BM, Musarò A. Increased circulating levels of interleukin-6 induce perturbation in redox-regulated signaling cascades in muscle of dystrophic mice. Oxid Med Cell Longev 2017; 2017:1987218
[http://dx.doi.org/10.1155/2017/1987218]

[177] Canton M, Menazza S, Di Lisa F. Oxidative stress in muscular dystrophy: from generic evidence to specific sources and targets. J Muscle Res Cell Motil 2014; 35(1): 23-36.
[http://dx.doi.org/10.1007/s10974-014-9380-2] [PMID: 24619215]

[178] Prosser BL, Khairallah RJ, Ziman AP, Ward CW, Lederer WJ. X-ROS signaling in the heart and skeletal muscle: Stretch-dependent local ROS regulates $[Ca^{2+}]i$. J Mol Cell Cardiol 2013; 58: 172-81.
[http://dx.doi.org/10.1016/j.yjmcc.2012.11.011] [PMID: 23220288]

[179] Cheng AJ, Andersson DC, Lanner JT. Can't live with or without it: calcium and its role in Duchenne muscular dystrophy-induced muscle weakness. Focus on "SERCA1 overexpression minimizes skeletal muscle damage in dystrophic mouse models". Am J Physiol Cell Physiol 2015; 308(9): C697-8.
[http://dx.doi.org/10.1152/ajpcell.00056.2015] [PMID: 25740154]

[180] Hughes MC, Ramos SV, Turnbull PC, *et al.* Early myopathy in Duchenne muscular dystrophy is associated with elevated mitochondrial H_2O_2 emission during impaired oxidative phosphorylation. J Cachexia Sarcopenia Muscle 2019; 10(3): 643-61.
[http://dx.doi.org/10.1002/jcsm.12405] [PMID: 30938481]

[181] Timpani CA, Goodman CA, Stathis CG, *et al.* Adenylosuccinic acid therapy ameliorates murine Duchenne Muscular Dystrophy. Sci Rep 2020; 10(1): 1125.
[http://dx.doi.org/10.1038/s41598-020-57610-w] [PMID: 31980663]

[182] Moulin M, Ferreiro A, Eds. Muscle redox disturbances and oxidative stress as pathomechanisms and therapeutic targets in early-onset myopathies. Seminars in cell & developmental biology. Elsevier 2017.

[183] Woodman K, Coles C, Lamandé S, White J. Nutraceuticals and their potential to treat duchenne muscular dystrophy: separating the credible from the conjecture. Nutrients 2016; 8(11): 713.
[http://dx.doi.org/10.3390/nu8110713] [PMID: 27834844]

[184] Kourakis S, Timpani CA, Campelj DG, *et al.* Standard of care versus new-wave corticosteroids in the treatment of Duchenne muscular dystrophy: Can we do better? Orphanet J Rare Dis 2021; 16(1): 117.
[http://dx.doi.org/10.1186/s13023-021-01758-9] [PMID: 33663533]

[185] Gillard GO, Collette B, Anderson J, *et al.* DMF, but not other fumarates, inhibits NF-κB activity in vitro in an Nrf2-independent manner. J Neuroimmunol 2015; 283: 74-85.
[http://dx.doi.org/10.1016/j.jneuroim.2015.04.006] [PMID: 26004161]

[186] Casili G, Lanza M, Filippone A, *et al.* Dimethyl fumarate alleviates the nitroglycerin (NTG)-induced migraine in mice. J Neuroinflammation 2020; 17(1): 59.
[http://dx.doi.org/10.1186/s12974-020-01736-1] [PMID: 32066464]

[187] Geyik S, Altunısık E, Neyal AM, Taysi S. Oxidative stress and DNA damage in patients with migraine. J Headache Pain 2016; 17(1): 10.
[http://dx.doi.org/10.1186/s10194-016-0606-0] [PMID: 26883365]

[188] Tuncel D, Tolun FI, Gokce M, İmrek S, Ekerbiçer H. Oxidative stress in migraine with and without aura. Biol Trace Elem Res 2008; 126(1-3): 92-7.
[http://dx.doi.org/10.1007/s12011-008-8193-9] [PMID: 18690416]

[189] Yilmaz G, Sürer H, Inan LE, Coskun Ö, Yücel D. Increased nitrosative and oxidative stress in platelets of migraine patients. Tohoku J Exp Med 2007; 211(1): 23-30.
[http://dx.doi.org/10.1620/tjem.211.23] [PMID: 17202769]

[190] Alp R, Selek S, Alp SI, Taşkin A, Koçyiğit A. Oxidative and antioxidative balance in patients of migraine. Eur Rev Med Pharmacol Sci 2010; 14(10): 877-82.
[PMID: 21222375]

[191] Neri M, Frustaci A, Milic M, *et al.* A meta-analysis of biomarkers related to oxidative stress and nitric oxide pathway in migraine. Cephalalgia 2015; 35(10): 931-7.
[http://dx.doi.org/10.1177/0333102414564888] [PMID: 25573894]

[192] Chung CS. Drug therapy for migraine. J Korean Med Assoc 2007; 50(10): 917-23.
[http://dx.doi.org/10.5124/jkma.2007.50.10.917]

[193] Borkum J. Harnessing migraines for neural regeneration. Neural Regen Res 2018; 13(4): 609-15.
[http://dx.doi.org/10.4103/1673-5374.230275] [PMID: 29722303]

[194] Di W, Shi X, Lv H, *et al.* Activation of the nuclear factor E2-related factor 2/anitioxidant response element alleviates the nitroglycerin-induced hyperalgesia in rats. J Headache Pain 2016; 17(1): 99.
[http://dx.doi.org/10.1186/s10194-016-0694-x] [PMID: 27778243]

[195] Giniatullin R, Nistri A, Fabbretti E. Molecular mechanisms of sensitization of pain-transducing P2X3 receptors by the migraine mediators CGRP and NGF. Mol Neurobiol 2008; 37(1): 83-90.
[http://dx.doi.org/10.1007/s12035-008-8020-5] [PMID: 18459072]

[196]　Giniatullin R, Nistri A. Desensitization properties of P2X3 receptors shaping pain signaling. Front Cell Neurosci 2013; 7: 245.
[http://dx.doi.org/10.3389/fncel.2013.00245] [PMID: 24367291]

[197]　Das J, Ramani R, Suraju MO. Polyphenol compounds and PKC signaling. Biochim Biophys Acta, Gen Subj 2016; 1860(10): 2107-21.
[http://dx.doi.org/10.1016/j.bbagen.2016.06.022]

[198]　Matzinger M, Fischhuber K, Heiss EH. Activation of Nrf2 signaling by natural products-can it alleviate diabetes? Biotechnol Adv 2018; 36(6): 1738-67.
[http://dx.doi.org/10.1016/j.biotechadv.2017.12.015] [PMID: 29289692]

[199]　Lopresti AL, Smith SJ, Drummond PD. Herbal treatments for migraine: A systematic review of randomised-controlled studies. Phytother Res 2020; 34(10): 2493-517.
[http://dx.doi.org/10.1002/ptr.6701] [PMID: 32310327]

[200]　Suwanwela N, Poungvarin N, Asap . Asian Stroke Advisory Panel. Stroke burden and stroke care system in Asia. Neurol India 2016; 64(7) (Suppl.): 46.
[http://dx.doi.org/10.4103/0028-3886.178042] [PMID: 26954968]

[201]　Benjamin EJ, Virani SS, Callaway CW, *et al.* American Heart Association Council on Epidemiology and Prevention Statistics Committee and Stroke Statistics Subcommittee. Heart disease and stroke statistics—2018 update: a report from the American Heart Association. Circulation 2018; 137(12): e67-e492.
[http://dx.doi.org/10.1161/CIR.0000000000000558] [PMID: 29386200]

[202]　Prabhakaran S, Ruff I, Bernstein RA. Acute stroke intervention: a systematic review. JAMA 2015; 313(14): 1451-62.
[http://dx.doi.org/10.1001/jama.2015.3058] [PMID: 25871671]

[203]　Romano JG, Sacco RL. Progress in acute ischaemic stroke treatment and prevention. Nat Rev Neurol 2015; 11(11): 619-21.
[http://dx.doi.org/10.1038/nrneurol.2015.199] [PMID: 26481298]

[204]　Hacke W, Kaste M, Bluhmki E, *et al.* ECASS Investigators. Thrombolysis with alteplase 3 to 4.5 hours after acute ischemic stroke. N Engl J Med 2008; 359(13): 1317-29.
[http://dx.doi.org/10.1056/NEJMoa0804656] [PMID: 18815396]

[205]　Fonarow GC, Smith EE, Saver JL, *et al.* Timeliness of tissue-type plasminogen activator therapy in acute ischemic stroke: patient characteristics, hospital factors, and outcomes associated with door-t--needle times within 60 minutes. circulation 2011; 123(7): 750-8.

[206]　Sandercock P, Wardlaw JM, Lindley RI, *et al.* The benefits and harms of intravenous thrombolysis with recombinant tissue plasminogen activator within 6 h of acute ischaemic stroke (the third international stroke trial [IST-3]): a randomised controlled trial. IST-3 collaborative group. Lancet 2012; 379(9834): 2352-63.
[http://dx.doi.org/10.1016/S0140-6736(12)60768-5] [PMID: 22632908]

[207]　Emberson J, Lees KR, Lyden P, *et al.* Stroke Thrombolysis Trialists' Collaborative Group. Effect of treatment delay, age, and stroke severity on the effects of intravenous thrombolysis with alteplase for acute ischaemic stroke: a meta-analysis of individual patient data from randomised trials. Lancet 2014; 384(9958): 1929-35.
[http://dx.doi.org/10.1016/S0140-6736(14)60584-5] [PMID: 25106063]

[208]　Chang CW, Lai MC, Cheng TJ, Lau MT, Hu ML. Plasma levels of antioxidant vitamins, selenium, total sulfhydryl groups and oxidative products in ischemic-stroke patients as compared to matched controls in Taiwan. Free Radic Res 1998; 28(1): 15-24.
[http://dx.doi.org/10.3109/10715769809097872] [PMID: 9554829]

[209]　Žitňanová I, Šiarnik P, Kollár B, *et al.* Oxidative stress markers and their dynamic changes in patients after acute ischemic stroke.Oxid Med Cell Longev 2016; 2016:9761697.

[210] Lo EH, Dalkara T, Moskowitz MA. Mechanisms, challenges and opportunities in stroke. Nat Rev Neurosci 2003; 4(5): 399-414.
[http://dx.doi.org/10.1038/nrn1106] [PMID: 12728267]

[211] Moskowitz MA, Lo EH, Iadecola C. The science of stroke: mechanisms in search of treatments. Neuron 2010; 67(2): 181-98.
[http://dx.doi.org/10.1016/j.neuron.2010.07.002] [PMID: 20670828]

[212] Zhang J, Wang X, Vikash V, *et al.* ROS and ROS-mediated cellular signaling. Oxidative medicine and cellular longevity 2016.

[213] Bae YS, Oh H, Rhee SG, Yoo YD. Regulation of reactive oxygen species generation in cell signaling. Mol Cells 2011; 32(6): 491-509.
[http://dx.doi.org/10.1007/s10059-011-0276-3] [PMID: 22207195]

[214] Dang J, Brandenburg LO, Rosen C, *et al.* Nrf2 expression by neurons, astroglia, and microglia in the cerebral cortical penumbra of ischemic rats. J Mol Neurosci 2012; 46(3): 578-84.
[http://dx.doi.org/10.1007/s12031-011-9645-9] [PMID: 21932039]

[215] Guruswamy R, ElAli A. Complex roles of microglial cells in ischemic stroke pathobiology: new insights and future directions. Int J Mol Sci 2017; 18(3): 496.
[http://dx.doi.org/10.3390/ijms18030496] [PMID: 28245599]

[216] Jayaraj RL, Azimullah S, Beiram R, Jalal FY, Rosenberg GA. Neuroinflammation: friend and foe for ischemic stroke. J Neuroinflammation 2019; 16(1): 142.
[http://dx.doi.org/10.1186/s12974-019-1516-2] [PMID: 31291966]

[217] Iadecola C, Anrather J. The immunology of stroke: from mechanisms to translation. Nat Med 2011; 17(7): 796-808.
[http://dx.doi.org/10.1038/nm.2399] [PMID: 21738161]

[218] Alfieri A, Srivastava S, Siow RCM, *et al.* Sulforaphane preconditioning of the Nrf2/HO-1 defense pathway protects the cerebral vasculature against blood–brain barrier disruption and neurological deficits in stroke. Free Radic Biol Med 2013; 65: 1012-22.
[http://dx.doi.org/10.1016/j.freeradbiomed.2013.08.190] [PMID: 24017972]

[219] Gutteridge JMC, Halliwell B. Free radicals and antioxidants in the year 2000. A historical look to the future. Ann N Y Acad Sci 2000; 899(1): 136-47.
[http://dx.doi.org/10.1111/j.1749-6632.2000.tb06182.x] [PMID: 10863535]

[220] Wardyn JD, Ponsford AH, Sanderson CM. Dissecting molecular cross-talk between Nrf2 and NF-κB response pathways. Biochem Soc Trans 2015; 43(4): 621-6.
[http://dx.doi.org/10.1042/BST20150014] [PMID: 26551702]

[221] Cuadrado A, Martín-Moldes Z, Ye J, Lastres-Becker I. Transcription factors Nrf2 and NF-κB are coordinated effectors of the Rho family, GTP-binding protein RAC1 during inflammation. J Biol Chem 2014; 289(22): 15244-58.
[http://dx.doi.org/10.1074/jbc.M113.540633] [PMID: 24759106]

[222] Liu L, Locascio LM, Doré S. Critical role of Nrf2 in experimental ischemic stroke. Front Pharmacol 2019; 10: 153.
[http://dx.doi.org/10.3389/fphar.2019.00153] [PMID: 30890934]

[223] Liu L, Vollmer MK, Fernandez VM, Dweik Y, Kim H, Doré S. Korean red ginseng pretreatment protects against long-term sensorimotor deficits after ischemic stroke likely through Nrf2. Front Cell Neurosci 2018; 12: 74.
[http://dx.doi.org/10.3389/fncel.2018.00074] [PMID: 29628876]

[224] Leonardo CC, Mendes M, Ahmad AS, Doré S. Efficacy of prophylactic flavan-3-ol in permanent focal ischemia in 12-mo-old mice. Am J Physiol Heart Circ Physiol 2015; 308(6): H583-91.
[http://dx.doi.org/10.1152/ajpheart.00239.2014] [PMID: 25576625]

[225] Leonardo CC, Agrawal M, Singh N, Moore JR, Biswal S, Doré S. Oral administration of the flavanol (−)-epicatechin bolsters endogenous protection against focal ischemia through the Nrf2 cytoprotective pathway. Eur J Neurosci 2013; 38(11): 3659-68.
[http://dx.doi.org/10.1111/ejn.12362] [PMID: 24112193]

[226] Wang B, Cao W, Biswal S, Doré S. Carbon monoxide-activated Nrf2 pathway leads to protection against permanent focal cerebral ischemia. Stroke 2011; 42(9): 2605-10.
[http://dx.doi.org/10.1161/STROKEAHA.110.607101] [PMID: 21852618]

[227] Shih AY, Li P, Murphy TH. A small-molecule-inducible Nrf2-mediated antioxidant response provides effective prophylaxis against cerebral ischemia *in vivo*. J Neurosci 2005; 25(44): 10321-35.
[http://dx.doi.org/10.1523/JNEUROSCI.4014-05.2005] [PMID: 16267240]

[228] Clausen BH, Lundberg L, Yli-Karjanmaa M, *et al*. Fumarate decreases edema volume and improves functional outcome after experimental stroke. Exp Neurol 2017; 295: 144-54.
[http://dx.doi.org/10.1016/j.expneurol.2017.06.011] [PMID: 28602832]

[229] Zhao Y, Fu B, Zhang X, *et al*. Paeonol pretreatment attenuates cerebral ischemic injury *via* upregulating expression of pAkt, Nrf2, HO-1 and ameliorating BBB permeability in mice. Brain Res Bull 2014; 109: 61-7.
[http://dx.doi.org/10.1016/j.brainresbull.2014.09.008] [PMID: 25286445]

[230] Zhang J, Fu B, Zhang X, *et al*. Bicyclol upregulates transcription factor Nrf2, HO-1 expression and protects rat brains against focal ischemia. Brain Res Bull 2014; 100: 38-43.
[http://dx.doi.org/10.1016/j.brainresbull.2013.11.001] [PMID: 24252362]

[231] Meng H, Guo J, Wang H, Yan P, Niu X, Zhang J. Erythropoietin activates Keap1–Nrf2/ARE pathway in rat brain after ischemia. Int J Neurosci 2014; 124(5): 362-8.
[http://dx.doi.org/10.3109/00207454.2013.848439] [PMID: 24063261]

[232] Zhang L, Zhang X, Zhang C, *et al*. Nobiletin promotes antioxidant and anti-inflammatory responses and elicits protection against ischemic stroke *in vivo*. Brain Res 2016; 1636: 130-41.
[http://dx.doi.org/10.1016/j.brainres.2016.02.013] [PMID: 26874072]

[233] Chang CY, Kuan YH, Li JR, *et al*. Docosahexaenoic acid reduces cellular inflammatory response following permanent focal cerebral ischemia in rats. J Nutr Biochem 2013; 24(12): 2127-37.
[http://dx.doi.org/10.1016/j.jnutbio.2013.08.004] [PMID: 24139673]

[234] Wang M, Wang K, Gao X, Zhao K, Chen H, Xu M. Anti-inflammatory effects of isoalantolactone on LPS-stimulated BV2 microglia cells through activating GSK-3β-Nrf2 signaling pathway. Int Immunopharmacol 2018; 65: 323-7.
[http://dx.doi.org/10.1016/j.intimp.2018.10.008] [PMID: 30343259]

[235] Chen L, Wang L, Zhang X, *et al*. The protection by Octreotide against experimental ischemic stroke: Up-regulated transcription factor Nrf2, HO-1 and down-regulated NF-κB expression. Brain Res 2012; 1475: 80-7.
[http://dx.doi.org/10.1016/j.brainres.2012.07.052] [PMID: 22885292]

[236] Chang CY, Kao TK, Chen WY, *et al*. Tetramethylpyrazine inhibits neutrophil activation following permanent cerebral ischemia in rats. Biochem Biophys Res Commun 2015; 463(3): 421-7.
[http://dx.doi.org/10.1016/j.bbrc.2015.05.088] [PMID: 26043690]

[237] Kao TK, Chang CY, Ou YC, *et al*. Tetramethylpyrazine reduces cellular inflammatory response following permanent focal cerebral ischemia in rats. Exp Neurol 2013; 247: 188-201.
[http://dx.doi.org/10.1016/j.expneurol.2013.04.010] [PMID: 23644042]

[238] Chen M, Dai LH, Fei A, Pan SM, Wang HR. Isoquercetin activates the ERK1/2-Nrf2 pathway and protects against cerebral ischemia-reperfusion injury *in vivo* and *in vitro*. Exp Ther Med 2017; 13(4): 1353-9.
[http://dx.doi.org/10.3892/etm.2017.4093] [PMID: 28413477]

[239] Sun X, Zuo H, Liu C, Yang Y. Overexpression of miR-200a protects cardiomyocytes against hypoxia-

induced apoptosis by modulating the kelch-like ECH-associated protein 1-nuclear factor erythroid 2-related factor 2 signaling axis. Int J Mol Med 2016; 38(4): 1303-11.
[http://dx.doi.org/10.3892/ijmm.2016.2719] [PMID: 27573160]

[240]   Kou X, Kirberger M, Yang Y, Chen N. Natural products for cancer prevention associated with Nrf2–ARE pathway. Food Sci Hum Wellness 2013; 2(1): 22-8.
[http://dx.doi.org/10.1016/j.fshw.2013.01.001]

[241]   Zhu J, Wang H, Chen F, *et al.* An overview of chemical inhibitors of the Nrf2-ARE signaling pathway and their potential applications in cancer therapy. Free Radic Biol Med 2016; 99: 544-56.
[http://dx.doi.org/10.1016/j.freeradbiomed.2016.09.010] [PMID: 27634172]

[242]   Mallouk N, Jacquemond V, Allard B. Elevated subsarcolemmal Ca $^{2+}$ in *mdx* mouse skeletal muscle fibers detected with Ca $^{2+}$ -activated K $^+$ channels. Proc Natl Acad Sci USA 2000; 97(9): 4950-5.
[http://dx.doi.org/10.1073/pnas.97.9.4950] [PMID: 10781103]

[243]   Tsurumi F, Baba S, Yoshinaga D, *et al.* The intracellular Ca $^{2+}$ concentration is elevated in cardiomyocytes differentiated from hiPSCs derived from a Duchenne muscular dystrophy patient. PLoS One 2019; 14(3): e0213768.
[http://dx.doi.org/10.1371/journal.pone.0213768] [PMID: 30875388]

[244]   Zaichick SV, McGrath KM, Caraveo G. The role of Ca $^{2+}$ signaling in Parkinson's disease. Dis Model Mech 2017; 10(5): 519-35.
[http://dx.doi.org/10.1242/dmm.028738] [PMID: 28468938]

[245]   Marambaud P, Dreses-Werringloer U, Vingtdeux V. Calcium signaling in neurodegeneration. Mol Neurodegener 2009; 4(1): 20.
[http://dx.doi.org/10.1186/1750-1326-4-20] [PMID: 19419557]

[246]   Bezprozvanny I, Hiesinger P. The synaptic maintenance problem: membrane recycling, Ca $^{2+}$ homeostasis and late onset degeneration. Mol Neurodegener 2013; 8(1): 23.
[http://dx.doi.org/10.1186/1750-1326-8-23] [PMID: 23829673]

[247]   Pal R, Palmieri M, Loehr JA, *et al.* Src-dependent impairment of autophagy by oxidative stress in a mouse model of Duchenne muscular dystrophy. Nat Commun 2014; 5(1): 4425.
[http://dx.doi.org/10.1038/ncomms5425] [PMID: 25028121]

[248]   Duchen MR. Mitochondria and calcium: from cell signalling to cell death. J Physiol 2000; 529(1): 57-68.
[http://dx.doi.org/10.1111/j.1469-7793.2000.00057.x] [PMID: 11080251]

[249]   Goonasekera SA, Lam CK, Millay DP, *et al.* Mitigation of muscular dystrophy in mice by SERCA overexpression in skeletal muscle. J Clin Invest 2011; 121(3): 1044-52.
[http://dx.doi.org/10.1172/JCI43844] [PMID: 21285509]

[250]   Granatiero V, Konrad C, Bredvik K, Manfredi G, Kawamata H. Nrf2 signaling links ER oxidative protein folding and calcium homeostasis in health and disease. Life Sci Alliance 2019; 2(5): e201900563.
[http://dx.doi.org/10.26508/lsa.201900563] [PMID: 31658977]

[251]   Morciano G, Marchi S, Morganti C, *et al.* Role of mitochondria-associated ER membranes in calcium regulation in cancer-specific settings. Neoplasia 2018; 20(5): 510-23.
[http://dx.doi.org/10.1016/j.neo.2018.03.005] [PMID: 29626751]

[252]   Bai X, Chen Y, Hou X, Huang M, Jin J. Emerging role of Nrf2 in chemoresistance by regulating drug-metabolizing enzymes and efflux transporters. Drug Metab Rev 2016; 48(4): 541-67.
[http://dx.doi.org/10.1080/03602532.2016.1197239] [PMID: 27320238]

[253]   Nitahara-Kasahara Y, Takeda S, Okada T. Inflammatory predisposition predicts disease phenotypes in muscular dystrophy. Inflamm Regen 2016; 36(1): 14.
[http://dx.doi.org/10.1186/s41232-016-0019-0]

[254]   Giunta B, Fernandez F, Nikolic WV, *et al.* Inflammaging as a prodrome to Alzheimer's disease. J

Neuroinflammation 2008; 5(1): 51.
[http://dx.doi.org/10.1186/1742-2094-5-51] [PMID: 19014446]

[255] Hoozemans JJM, Veerhuis R, Rozemuller JM, Eikelenboom P. Neuroinflammation and regeneration in the early stages of Alzheimer's disease pathology. Int J Dev Neurosci 2006; 24(2-3): 157-65.
[http://dx.doi.org/10.1016/j.ijdevneu.2005.11.001] [PMID: 16384684]

[256] Schuitemaker A, Dik MG, Veerhuis R, *et al.* Inflammatory markers in AD and MCI patients with different biomarker profiles. Neurobiol Aging 2009; 30(11): 1885-9.
[http://dx.doi.org/10.1016/j.neurobiolaging.2008.01.014] [PMID: 18378357]

[257] Choi T-M, Chiu C-H, Chan H-K. Risk management of logistics systems. Elsevier 2016.
[http://dx.doi.org/10.1016/j.tre.2016.03.007]

[258] Sun CC, Li SJ, Yang CL, *et al.* Sulforaphane attenuates muscle inflammation in dystrophin-deficient mdx mice *via* NF-E2-related factor 2 (Nrf2)-mediated inhibition of NF-κB signaling pathway. J Biol Chem 2015; 290(29): 17784-95.
[http://dx.doi.org/10.1074/jbc.M115.655019] [PMID: 26013831]

[259] Kobayashi E, Suzuki T, Yamamoto M. Roles Nrf2 plays in myeloid cells and related disorders. Oxidative medicine and cellular longevity.Oxid Med Cell Longev 2013; 2013:529219.
[http://dx.doi.org/10.1155/2013/529219]

[260] Wakabayashi N, Slocum SL, Skoko JJ, Shin S, Kensler TW. When Nrf2 talks, who's listening? Antioxid Redox Signal 2010; 13(11): 1649-63.
[http://dx.doi.org/10.1089/ars.2010.3216] [PMID: 20367496]

[261] Seldon MP, Silva G, Pejanovic N, *et al.* Heme oxygenase-1 inhibits the expression of adhesion molecules associated with endothelial cell activation *via* inhibition of NF-kappaB RelA phosphorylation at serine 276. J Immunol 2007; 179(11): 7840-51.
[http://dx.doi.org/10.4049/jimmunol.179.11.7840] [PMID: 18025230]

[262] Wang CH, Chou PC, Chung FT, Lin HC, Huang KH, Kuo HP. Heat shock protein70 is implicated in modulating NF-κB activation in alveolar macrophages of patients with active pulmonary tuberculosis. Sci Rep 2017; 7(1): 1214.
[http://dx.doi.org/10.1038/s41598-017-01405-z] [PMID: 28127051]

[263] Pietraszek-Gremplewicz K, Kozakowska M, Bronisz-Budzynska I, *et al.* Heme oxygenase-1 influences satellite cells and progression of Duchenne muscular dystrophy in mice. Antioxid Redox Signal 2018; 29(2): 128-48.
[http://dx.doi.org/10.1089/ars.2017.7435] [PMID: 29669436]

[264] Holmström KM, Baird L, Zhang Y, *et al.* Nrf2 impacts cellular bioenergetics by controlling substrate availability for mitochondrial respiration. Biol Open 2013; 2(8): 761-70.
[http://dx.doi.org/10.1242/bio.20134853] [PMID: 23951401]

[265] Ludtmann MHR, Angelova PR, Zhang Y, Abramov AY, Dinkova-Kostova AT. Nrf2 affects the efficiency of mitochondrial fatty acid oxidation. Biochem J 2014; 457(3): 415-24.
[http://dx.doi.org/10.1042/BJ20130863] [PMID: 24206218]

[266] Kovac S, Angelova PR, Holmström KM, Zhang Y, Dinkova-Kostova AT, Abramov AY. Nrf2 regulates ROS production by mitochondria and NADPH oxidase. Biochim Biophys Acta, Gen Subj 2015; 1850(4): 794-801.
[http://dx.doi.org/10.1016/j.bbagen.2014.11.021]

[267] Murata H, Takamatsu H, Liu S, Kataoka K, Huh N, Sakaguchi M. Nrf2 regulates PINK1 expression under oxidative stress conditions. PLoS One 2015; 10(11): e0142438.
[http://dx.doi.org/10.1371/journal.pone.0142438] [PMID: 26555609]

[268] Kwon J, Han E, Bui CB, *et al.* Assurance of mitochondrial integrity and mammalian longevity by the p62–Keap1–Nrf2–Nqo1 cascade. EMBO Rep 2012; 13(2): 150-6.
[http://dx.doi.org/10.1038/embor.2011.246] [PMID: 22222206]

[269]   Soto C, Pritzkow S. Protein misfolding, aggregation, and conformational strains in neurodegenerative diseases. Nat Neurosci 2018; 21(10): 1332-40.
[http://dx.doi.org/10.1038/s41593-018-0235-9] [PMID: 30250260]

[270]   Schieber M, Chandel NS. ROS function in redox signaling and oxidative stress. Curr Biol 2014; 24(10): R453-62.
[http://dx.doi.org/10.1016/j.cub.2014.03.034] [PMID: 24845678]

[271]   Dodson M, Redmann M, Rajasekaran NS, Darley-Usmar V, Zhang J. KEAP1–Nrf2 signalling and autophagy in protection against oxidative and reductive proteotoxicity. Biochem J 2015; 469(3): 347-55.
[http://dx.doi.org/10.1042/BJ20150568] [PMID: 26205490]

[272]   White E, Karp C, Strohecker AM, Guo Y, Mathew R. Role of autophagy in suppression of inflammation and cancer. Curr Opin Cell Biol 2010; 22(2): 212-7.
[http://dx.doi.org/10.1016/j.ceb.2009.12.008] [PMID: 20056400]

[273]   Kansanen E, Jyrkkänen HK, Levonen AL. Activation of stress signaling pathways by electrophilic oxidized and nitrated lipids. Free Radic Biol Med 2012; 52(6): 973-82.
[http://dx.doi.org/10.1016/j.freeradbiomed.2011.11.038] [PMID: 22198184]

[274]   Al-Sawaf O, Fragoulis A, Rosen C, et al. Nrf2 augments skeletal muscle regeneration after ischaemia-reperfusion injury. J Pathol 2014; 234(4): 538-47.
[http://dx.doi.org/10.1002/path.4418] [PMID: 25111334]

[275]   Sala D, Cunningham TJ, Stec MJ, et al. The Stat3-Fam3a axis promotes muscle stem cell myogenic lineage progression by inducing mitochondrial respiration. Nat Commun 2019; 10(1): 1796.
[http://dx.doi.org/10.1038/s41467-019-09746-1] [PMID: 30996264]

[276]   Yamaguchi M, Murakami S, Yoneda T, et al. Evidence of Notch-Hesr-Nrf2 axis in muscle stem cells, but absence of Nrf2 has no effect on their quiescent and undifferentiated state. PLoS One 2015; 10(9): e0138517.
[http://dx.doi.org/10.1371/journal.pone.0138517] [PMID: 26418810]

[277]   Cerletti M, Jurga S, Witczak CA, et al. Highly efficient, functional engraftment of skeletal muscle stem cells in dystrophic muscles. Cell 2008; 134(1): 37-47.
[http://dx.doi.org/10.1016/j.cell.2008.05.049] [PMID: 18614009]

[278]   Montarras D, Morgan J, Collins C, et al. Direct isolation of satellite cells for skeletal muscle regeneration. Science 2005; 309(5743): 2064-7.
[http://dx.doi.org/10.1126/science.1114758] [PMID: 16141372]

[279]   Qu-Petersen Z, Deasy B, Jankowski R, et al. Identification of a novel population of muscle stem cells in mice. J Cell Biol 2002; 157(5): 851-64.
[http://dx.doi.org/10.1083/jcb.200108150] [PMID: 12021255]

[280]   Chen D, Zhou Y, Lyons KE, Pahwa R, Reddy MB. Green tea consumption reduces oxidative stress in Parkinson's disease patients. J Behav Brain Sci 2015; 5(6): 194-202.
[http://dx.doi.org/10.4236/jbbs.2015.56020]

[281]   Coimbra S, Castro E, Rocha-Pereira P, Rebelo I, Rocha S, Santos-Silva A. The effect of green tea in oxidative stress. Clin Nutr 2006; 25(5): 790-6.
[http://dx.doi.org/10.1016/j.clnu.2006.01.022] [PMID: 16698148]

[282]   Zareie A, Sahebkar A, Khorvash F, Bagheriya M, Hasanzadeh A, Askari G. Effect of cinnamon on migraine attacks and inflammatory markers: A randomized double-blind placebo-controlled trial. Phytother Res 2020; 34(11): 2945-52.
[http://dx.doi.org/10.1002/ptr.6721] [PMID: 32638445]

[283]   Nelson MD, Rosenberry R, Barresi R, et al. Sodium nitrate alleviates functional muscle ischaemia in patients with Becker muscular dystrophy. J Physiol 2015; 593(23): 5183-200.
[http://dx.doi.org/10.1113/JP271252] [PMID: 26437761]

[284] Kalia V. Effect of cinnamon and honey on on-time and off-time in parkinson's disease: a case report. Journal of the Gujarat Research Society 2019; 21(10s): 650-4.

[285] Hishikawa N, Takahashi Y, Amakusa Y, *et al.* Effects of turmeric on Alzheimer's disease with behavioral and psychological symptoms of dementia. Ayu 2012; 33(4): 499-504.
[http://dx.doi.org/10.4103/0974-8520.110524] [PMID: 23723666]

[286] de la Rubia Ortí JE, García-Pardo MP, Drehmer E, *et al.* Improvement of main cognitive functions in patients with alzheimer's disease after treatment with coconut oil enriched mediterranean diet: a pilot study. J Alzheimers Dis 2018; 65(2): 577-87.
[http://dx.doi.org/10.3233/JAD-180184] [PMID: 30056419]

[287] Xu SS, Gao ZX, Weng Z, *et al.* Efficacy of tablet huperzine-A on memory, cognition, and behavior in Alzheimer's disease. 1995; 16(5): 391-995.

[288] Kanowski S, Herrmann W, Stephan K, Wierich W, Hörr R. Proof of efficacy of the ginkgo biloba special extract EGb 761 in outpatients suffering from mild to moderate primary degenerative dementia of the Alzheimer type or multi-infarct dementia. Pharmacopsychiatry 1996; 29(2): 47-56.
[http://dx.doi.org/10.1055/s-2007-979544] [PMID: 8741021]

[289] Singh H, Raghav S, Dalal PK, Srivastava JS, Asthana OP. Randomized controlled trial of standardized Bacopa monniera extract in age-associated memory impairment. Indian J Psychiatry 2006; 48(4): 238-42.
[http://dx.doi.org/10.4103/0019-5545.31555] [PMID: 20703343]

[290] Chan DKY, Woo J, Ho SC, *et al.* Genetic and environmental risk factors for Parkinson's disease in a Chinese population. J Neurol Neurosurg Psychiatry 1998; 65(5): 781-4.
[http://dx.doi.org/10.1136/jnnp.65.5.781] [PMID: 9810958]

[291] Checkoway H, Powers K, Smith-Weller T, Franklin GM, Longstreth WT Jr, Swanson PD. Parkinson's disease risks associated with cigarette smoking, alcohol consumption, and caffeine intake. Am J Epidemiol 2002; 155(8): 732-8.
[http://dx.doi.org/10.1093/aje/155.8.732] [PMID: 11943691]

[292] Hu G, Bidel S, Jousilahti P, Antikainen R, Tuomilehto J. Coffee and tea consumption and the risk of Parkinson's disease. Mov Disord 2007; 22(15): 2242-8.
[http://dx.doi.org/10.1002/mds.21706] [PMID: 17712848]

[293] Kandinov B, Giladi N, Korczyn AD. Smoking and tea consumption delay onset of Parkinson's disease. Parkinsonism Relat Disord 2009; 15(1): 41-6.
[http://dx.doi.org/10.1016/j.parkreldis.2008.02.011] [PMID: 18434232]

[294] Fadaeinasab M, Basiri A, Kia Y, Karimian H, Ali HM, Murugaiyah V. New indole alkaloids from the bark of Rauvolfia reflexa and their cholinesterase inhibitory activity. Cell Physiol Biochem 2015; 37(5): 1997-2011.
[http://dx.doi.org/10.1159/000438560] [PMID: 26584298]

[295] Zhan G, Miao R, Zhang F, *et al.* Monoterpene indole alkaloids with diverse skeletons from the stems of Rauvolfia vomitoria and their acetylcholinesterase inhibitory activities. Phytochemistry 2020; 177: 112450.
[http://dx.doi.org/10.1016/j.phytochem.2020.112450] [PMID: 32580106]

[296] Fadaeinasab M, Hadi A, Kia Y, Basiri A, Murugaiyah V. Cholinesterase enzymes inhibitors from the leaves of Rauvolfia reflexa and their molecular docking study. Molecules 2013; 18(4): 3779-88.
[http://dx.doi.org/10.3390/molecules18043779] [PMID: 23529036]

[297] Kashyap P, Kalaiselvan V, Kumar R, Kumar S. Ajmalicine and reserpine: indole alkaloids as multi-target directed ligands towards factors implicated in Alzheimer's disease. Molecules 2020; 25(7): 1609.
[http://dx.doi.org/10.3390/molecules25071609] [PMID: 32244635]

[298] Rahman H, Shaik HA, Madhavi P, Eswaraiah MC. A review: pharmacognostics and pharmacological

profiles of Nardastachys jatamansi DC. Elixir pharmacy 2011; : 5017-20.

[299] Saroya AS, Singh J. Neuropharmacology of nardostachys jatamansi dc. pharmacotherapeutic potential of natural products in neurological disorders. Springer 2018; pp. 167-74.
[http://dx.doi.org/10.1007/978-981-13-0289-3_17]

[300] Ahmad M, Yousuf S, Khan MB, *et al.* Attenuation by Nardostachys jatamansi of 6-hydroxydopamin--induced parkinsonism in rats: behavioral, neurochemical, and immunohistochemical studies. Pharmacol Biochem Behav 2006; 83(1): 150-60.
[http://dx.doi.org/10.1016/j.pbb.2006.01.005] [PMID: 16500697]

[301] Bose B, Tripathy D, Chatterjee A, Tandon P, Kumaria S. Secondary metabolite profiling, cytotoxicity, anti-inflammatory potential and in vitro inhibitory activities of Nardostachys jatamansi on key enzymes linked to hyperglycemia, hypertension and cognitive disorders. Phytomedicine 2019; 55: 58-69.
[http://dx.doi.org/10.1016/j.phymed.2018.08.010] [PMID: 30668444]

[302] Joshi H, Parle M. Nardostachys jatamansi improves learning and memory in mice. J Med Food 2006; 9(1): 113-8.
[http://dx.doi.org/10.1089/jmf.2006.9.113] [PMID: 16579738]

[303] Godkar PB, Gordon RK, Ravindran A, Doctor BP. *Celastrus paniculatus* seed water soluble extracts protect against glutamate toxicity in neuronal cultures from rat forebrain. J Ethnopharmacol 2004; 93(2-3): 213-9.
[http://dx.doi.org/10.1016/j.jep.2004.03.051] [PMID: 15234755]

[304] Nalini K, Karanth KS, Rao A, Aroor AR. Effects of *Celastrus paniculatus* on passive avoidance performance and biogenic amine turnover in albino rats. J Ethnopharmacol 1995; 47(2): 101-8.
[http://dx.doi.org/10.1016/0378-8741(95)01264-E] [PMID: 7500635]

[305] Bhanumathy M, Harish MS, Shivaprasad HN, Sushma G. Nootropic activity of *Celastrus paniculatus* seed. Pharm Biol 2010; 48(3): 324-7.
[http://dx.doi.org/10.3109/13880200903127391] [PMID: 20645820]

[306] Orhan IE. *Centella asiatica* (L.) Urban: from traditional medicine to modern medicine with neuroprotective potential. Evidence-based complementary and alternative medicine 2012.

[307] Farhana KM, Malueka RG, Wibowo S, Gofir A. Effectiveness of gotu kola extract 750 mg and 1000 mg compared with folic acid 3 mg in improving vascular cognitive impairment after stroke. > Evid Based Complement Alternat Med 2016; 2016:2795915
[http://dx.doi.org/10.1155/2016/2795915]

[308] Tiwari S, Singh S, Patwardhan K, Gehlot S, Gambhir I. Effect of *Centella asiatica* on mild cognitive impairment (MCI) and other common age-related clinical problems. Dig J Nanomater Biostruct 2008; 3(4): 215-20.

[309] Thu NTK, Hai NT, Tung BT. *In vitro* antioxidant and acetylcholinesterase inhibitory activities of fractions from *Centella asiatica* (Linn.) extract. Curr Bioact Compd 2018; 14(1): 86-91.
[http://dx.doi.org/10.2174/1573407213666161129124609]

[310] Kumar MHV, Gupta YK. Antioxidant property of *Celastrus paniculatus* Willd.: a possible mechanism in enhancing cognition. Phytomedicine 2002; 9(4): 302-11.
[http://dx.doi.org/10.1078/0944-7113-00136] [PMID: 12120811]

[311] Ganesan K, Gani SB. Ethnomedical and Pharmacological Potentials of Plumbago zeylanica L-A.Amer J Phytomed Clin Therapeutics 2013.

[312] Uplanchiwar V, Mk G, Gautam RK. Bioactivity-guided isolation of memory-enhancing compound from chloroform extract of roots of *plumbago zeylanica* linn. Asian J Pharm Clin Res 2018; 11(7): 497-500.
[http://dx.doi.org/10.22159/ajpcr.2018.v11i7.27028]

[313] Thompson SV, Winham DM, Hutchins AM. Bean and rice meals reduce postprandial glycemic

response in adults with type 2 diabetes: a cross-over study. Nutr J 2012; 11(1): 23.
[http://dx.doi.org/10.1186/1475-2891-11-23] [PMID: 22494488]

[314] Srinath S. Memory enhancing medicinal herbs. Journal of Pharmaceutical Sciences and Research 2014; 6(10): 331.

[315] Ahirwar S, Tembhre M. Assessment of Acetylcholinestrase Inhibiton by *Bacopa Monneiri* and Acephate in Hippocampus of Chick Brain for Impediment of Alzheimer's Disease. Pharm Pharmacol Int J 2016; 4(5): 00088.

[316] Mokhtarian A, Esfandiari E, Ghanadian M, Rashidi B, Vatankhah A. The effects of *Acorus calamus* L. in preventing memory loss, anxiety, and oxidative stress on lipopolysaccharide-induced neuroinflammation rat models. Int J Prev Med 2018; 9(1): 85.
[http://dx.doi.org/10.4103/ijpvm.IJPVM_75_18] [PMID: 30450168]

[317] Mukherjee P, Kumar V, Mal M, Houghton P. *In vitro* acetylcholinesterase inhibitory activity of the essential oil from *Acorus calamus* and its main constituents. Planta Med 2007; 73(3): 283-5.
[http://dx.doi.org/10.1055/s-2007-967114] [PMID: 17286241]

[318] Mukherjee PK, Kumar V, Mal M, Houghton PJ. *Acorus calamus.*: Scientific validation of Ayurvedic tradition from natural resources. Pharm Biol 2007; 45(8): 651-66.
[http://dx.doi.org/10.1080/13880200701538724]

[319] Chaudhary AK, Solanki R, Singh V, Singh UK. Inhibitory effect of *Capparis zeylanica* Linn. on acetylcholinesterase activity and attenuation of scopolamine-induced amnesia. CELLMED 2012; 2(2): 19.1-6.

[320] Yadav MK, Singh SK, Singh M, *et al.* Neuroprotective activity of *evolvulus alsinoides* & *centella asiatica* ethanolic extracts in scopolamine-induced amnesia in swiss albino mice. Open Access Maced J Med Sci 2019; 7(7): 1059-66.
[http://dx.doi.org/10.3889/oamjms.2019.247] [PMID: 31049081]

[321] Mathew M, Subramanian S. *In vitro* screening for anti-cholinesterase and antioxidant activity of methanolic extracts of ayurvedic medicinal plants used for cognitive disorders. PLoS One 2014; 9(1): e86804.
[http://dx.doi.org/10.1371/journal.pone.0086804] [PMID: 24466247]

[322] Mehla J, Pahuja M, Dethe SM, Agarwal A, Gupta YK. Amelioration of intracerebroventricular streptozotocin induced cognitive impairment by *Evolvulus alsinoides* in rats: *In vitro* and*in vivo*evidence. Neurochem Int 2012; 61(7): 1052-64.
[http://dx.doi.org/10.1016/j.neuint.2012.07.022] [PMID: 22892278]

[323] Solanki R, Chaudhary AK, Singh R. Effect of leaf extract of *Capparis zeylanica* Linn. on spatial learning and memory in rats. J Nat Med 2012; 66(4): 600-7.
[http://dx.doi.org/10.1007/s11418-012-0626-2] [PMID: 22261859]

[324] Sethiya NK, Nahata A, Dixit VK, Mishra SH. Cognition boosting effect of *Canscora decussata* (a South Indian Shankhpushpi). Eur J Integr Med 2012; 4(1): e113-21.
[http://dx.doi.org/10.1016/j.eujim.2011.11.003]

[325] Gaikwad N, Bhadoria PS, Mitra A. Root cultures of *Canscora decussata* as a potential source of acetylcholinesterase inhibitors. Planta Medica 81(16): PW_135.2015;
[http://dx.doi.org/10.1055/s-0035-1565759]

[326] Ranasinghe P, Pigera S, Premakumara GAS, Galappaththy P, Constantine GR, Katulanda P. Medicinal properties of 'true' cinnamon (*Cinnamomum zeylanicum*): a systematic review. BMC Complement Altern Med 2013; 13(1): 275.
[http://dx.doi.org/10.1186/1472-6882-13-275] [PMID: 24148965]

[327] Qais FA, Khan MS, Althubiani AS, Al-Ghamdi SB, Ahmad I. Understanding biochemical and molecular mechanism of complications of glycation and its management by herbal medicine. New Look to Phytomedicine. Elsevier 2019; pp. 331-66.

[328] Choi YH. trans-Cinnamaldehyde Prevents Oxidative Stress-Induced Apoptosis in V79-4 Chinese Hamster Lung Fibroblasts through the Nrf2-Mediated HO-1 Activation. Biol Pharm Bull 2020; 43(11): 1707-14.
[http://dx.doi.org/10.1248/bpb.b20-00407] [PMID: 33132316]

[329] Abou El-ezz D, Maher A, Sallam N, El-brairy A, Kenawy S. Trans-cinnamaldehyde modulates hippocampal Nrf2 factor and inhibits amyloid beta aggregation in LPS-induced neuroinflammation mouse model. Neurochem Res 2018; 43(12): 2333-42.
[http://dx.doi.org/10.1007/s11064-018-2656-y] [PMID: 30302613]

[330] Ismail H, Wijekoon N, Gonawala L, *et al.* Tapping into the potential of cinnamon as a therapeutic agent in neurological disorders and metabolic syndrome. Cinnamon. Springer 2020; pp. 273-305.
[http://dx.doi.org/10.1007/978-3-030-54426-3_11]

[331] Fakhri S, Pesce M, Patruno A, *et al.* Attenuation of Nrf2/Keap1/ARE in Alzheimer's disease by plant secondary metabolites: A mechanistic review. Molecules 2020; 25(21): 4926.
[http://dx.doi.org/10.3390/molecules25214926] [PMID: 33114450]

[332] Liao BC, Hsieh CW, Liu YC, Tzeng TT, Sun YW, Wung BS. Cinnamaldehyde inhibits the tumor necrosis factor-α-induced expression of cell adhesion molecules in endothelial cells by suppressing NF-κB activation: Effects upon IκB and Nrf2. Toxicol Appl Pharmacol 2008; 229(2): 161-71.
[http://dx.doi.org/10.1016/j.taap.2008.01.021] [PMID: 18304597]

[333] Wang F, Pu C, Zhou P, *et al.* Cinnamaldehyde prevents endothelial dysfunction induced by high glucose by activating Nrf2. Cell Physiol Biochem 2015; 36(1): 315-24.
[http://dx.doi.org/10.1159/000374074] [PMID: 25967970]

[334] Wondrak GT, Cabello CM, Villeneuve NF, *et al.* Cinnamoyl-based Nrf2-activators targeting human skin cell photo-oxidative stress. Free Radic Biol Med 2008; 45(4): 385-95.
[http://dx.doi.org/10.1016/j.freeradbiomed.2008.04.023] [PMID: 18482591]

[335] Bhakkiyalakshmi E, Sireesh D, Rajaguru P, Paulmurugan R, Ramkumar KM. The emerging role of redox-sensitive Nrf2–Keap1 pathway in diabetes. Pharmacol Res 2015; 91: 104-14.
[http://dx.doi.org/10.1016/j.phrs.2014.10.004] [PMID: 25447793]

[336] Yokozawa T, Kim HY, Kim HJ, *et al.* Amla (*Emblica officinalis* Gaertn.) attenuates age-related renal dysfunction by oxidative stress. J Agric Food Chem 2007; 55(19): 7744-52.
[http://dx.doi.org/10.1021/jf072105s] [PMID: 17715896]

[337] Yamamoto H, Morino K, Mengistu L, *et al.* Amla enhances mitochondrial spare respiratory capacity by increasing mitochondrial biogenesis and antioxidant systems in a murine skeletal muscle cell line. Oxid Med Cell Longev 2016; 2016:1735841.
[http://dx.doi.org/10.1155/2016/1735841]

[338] Lesmana R, Sinha RA, Singh BK, *et al.* Thyroid hormone stimulation of autophagy is essential for mitochondrial biogenesis and activity in skeletal muscle. Endocrinology 2016; 157(1): 23-38.
[http://dx.doi.org/10.1210/en.2015-1632] [PMID: 26562261]

[339] Ding Y, Zhang B, Zhou K, *et al.* Dietary ellagic acid improves oxidant-induced endothelial dysfunction and atherosclerosis: Role of Nrf2 activation. Int J Cardiol 2014; 175(3): 508-14.
[http://dx.doi.org/10.1016/j.ijcard.2014.06.045] [PMID: 25017906]

[340] Husain I, Akhtar M, Madaan T, *et al.* Tannins enriched fraction of *Emblica officinalis* fruits alleviates high-salt and cholesterol diet-induced cognitive impairment in rats *via* Nrf2–ARE pathway. Front Pharmacol 2018; 9: 23.
[http://dx.doi.org/10.3389/fphar.2018.00023] [PMID: 29441016]

[341] Ding Y, Ren D, Xu H, *et al.* Antioxidant and pro-angiogenic effects of corilagin in rat cerebral ischemia *via* Nrf2 activation. Oncotarget 2017; 8(70): 114816-28.
[http://dx.doi.org/10.18632/oncotarget.22023] [PMID: 29383122]

[342] Leung HW, Foo G, Banumurthy G, *et al.* The effect of *Bacopa monnieri* on gene expression levels in

SH-SY5Y human neuroblastoma cells. PLoS One 2017; 12(8): e0182984.
[http://dx.doi.org/10.1371/journal.pone.0182984] [PMID: 28832626]

[343] Wu J, Li Q, Wang X, *et al.* Neuroprotection by curcumin in ischemic brain injury involves the Akt/Nrf2 pathway. PLoS One 2013; 8(3): e59843.
[http://dx.doi.org/10.1371/journal.pone.0059843] [PMID: 23555802]

[344] Lee DS, Ko W, Kim DC, Kim YC, Jeong GS. Cudarflavone B provides neuroprotection against glutamate-induced mouse hippocampal HT22 cell damage through the Nrf2 and PI3K/Akt signaling pathways. Molecules 2014; 19(8): 10818-31.
[http://dx.doi.org/10.3390/molecules190810818] [PMID: 25061726]

[345] Kim WS, Kim YE, Cho EJ, *et al.* Neuroprotective effect of *Annona muricata* -derived polysaccharides in neuronal HT22 cell damage induced by hydrogen peroxide. Biosci Biotechnol Biochem 2020; 84(5): 1001-12.
[http://dx.doi.org/10.1080/09168451.2020.1715201] [PMID: 31960754]

[346] Ola-Davies OE, Oyagbemi AA, Omobowale TO, Akande I, Ashafa A. Ameliorative effects of *Annona muricata* Linn. (Annonaceae) against potassium dichromate-induced hypertension *in vivo* : involvement of Kim-1/p38 MAPK/Nrf2 signaling. J Basic Clin Physiol Pharmacol 2019; 30(4): 20180172.
[http://dx.doi.org/10.1515/jbcpp-2018-0172] [PMID: 31050655]

[347] Yasurin P, Sriariyanun M, Phusantisampan T. the bioavailability activity of *Centella asiatica*. Applied Science and Engineering Progress 2016; 9(1): 1-9.

[348] Hanapi NA, Arshad ASM, Abdullah JM, Muhammad TST, Yusof SR. Blood-brain barrier permeability of asiaticoside, madecassoside and asiatic acid in porcine brain endothelial cell model. J Pharm Sci 2020.
[PMID: 32949562]

[349] Matthews DG, Caruso M, Murchison CF, *et al.* *Centella asiatica* improves memory and promotes antioxidative signaling in 5XFAD mice. Antioxidants 2019; 8(12): 630.
[http://dx.doi.org/10.3390/antiox8120630] [PMID: 31817977]

[350] Qi Z, Ci X, Huang J, *et al.* Asiatic acid enhances Nrf2 signaling to protect HepG2 cells from oxidative damage through Akt and ERK activation. Biomed Pharmacother 2017; 88: 252-9.
[http://dx.doi.org/10.1016/j.biopha.2017.01.067] [PMID: 28110191]

[351] Higdon JV, Frei B. Tea catechins and polyphenols: health effects, metabolism, and antioxidant functions. Crit Rev Food Sci Nutr 2003; 43(1):89-143.
[http://dx.doi.org/10.1080/10408690390826464]

[352] Mandel SA, Avramovich-Tirosh Y, Reznichenko L, *et al.* Multifunctional activities of green tea catechins in neuroprotection. Modulation of cell survival genes, iron-dependent oxidative stress and PKC signaling pathway. Neurosignals 2005; 14(1-2): 46-60.
[http://dx.doi.org/10.1159/000085385] [PMID: 15956814]

[353] Mandel SA, Amit T, Weinreb O, Reznichenko L, Youdim MBH. Simultaneous manipulation of multiple brain targets by green tea catechins: a potential neuroprotective strategy for Alzheimer and Parkinson diseases. CNS Neurosci Ther 2008; 14(4): 352-65.
[http://dx.doi.org/10.1111/j.1755-5949.2008.00060.x] [PMID: 19040558]

[354] Han J, Wang M, Jing X, Shi H, Ren M, Lou H. (-)-Epigallocatechin gallate protects against cerebral ischemia-induced oxidative stress *via* Nrf2/ARE signaling. Neurochem Res 2014; 39(7): 1292-9.
[http://dx.doi.org/10.1007/s11064-014-1311-5] [PMID: 24792731]

[355] Romeo L, Intrieri M, D'Agata V, *et al.* The major green tea polyphenol,(-)-epigallocatechin-3-gallate, induces heme oxygenase in rat neurons and acts as an effective neuroprotective agent against oxidative stress. Journal of the American College of Nutrition 2009; 28(sup4): 492S-9S.

[356] Arafa MH, Atteia HH. Protective role of epigallocatechin gallate in a rat model of cisplatin-induced

cerebral inflammation and oxidative damage: Impact of modulating NF-κB and Nrf2. Neurotox Res 2020; 37(2): 380-96.
[http://dx.doi.org/10.1007/s12640-019-00095-x] [PMID: 31410684]

[357] Shanmugam T, Abdulla S, Yakulasamy V, Selvaraj M, Mathan R. A mechanism underlying the neurotoxicity induced by sodium fluoride and its reversal by epigallocatechin gallate in the rat hippocampus: Involvement of Nrf2/Keap-1 signaling pathway. J Basic Appl Zool 2018; 79(1): 1-19.

[358] Pervin M, Unno K, Nakagawa A, *et al.* Blood brain barrier permeability of (−)-epigallocatechin gallate, its proliferation-enhancing activity of human neuroblastoma SH-SY5Y cells, and its preventive effect on age-related cognitive dysfunction in mice. Biochem Biophys Rep 2017; 9: 180-6.
[http://dx.doi.org/10.1016/j.bbrep.2016.12.012] [PMID: 28956003]

[359] Lee SH, Nam HJ, Kang HJ, Kwon HW, Lim YC. Epigallocatechin-3-gallate attenuates head and neck cancer stem cell traits through suppression of Notch pathway. Eur J Cancer 2013; 49(15): 3210-8.
[http://dx.doi.org/10.1016/j.ejca.2013.06.025] [PMID: 23876835]

[360] Chen D, Tavana O, Chu B, *et al.* Nrf2 is a major target of ARF in p53-independent tumor suppression. Molecular cell 2017; 8(1): 224-32.
[http://dx.doi.org/10.1016/j.molcel.2017.09.009]

[361] Ortiz-López L, Márquez-Valadez B, Gómez-Sánchez A, *et al.* Green tea compound epigallo-catechi--3-gallate (EGCG) increases neuronal survival in adult hippocampal neurogenesis*in vivo*and in vitro. Neuroscience 2016; 322: 208-20.
[http://dx.doi.org/10.1016/j.neuroscience.2016.02.040] [PMID: 26917271]

[362] Lin CL, Chen TF, Chiu MJ, Way TD, Lin JK. Epigallocatechin gallate (EGCG) suppresses β-amyloi--induced neurotoxicity through inhibiting c-Abl/FE65 nuclear translocation and GSK3β activation. Neurobiol Aging 2009; 30(1): 81-92.
[http://dx.doi.org/10.1016/j.neurobiolaging.2007.05.012] [PMID: 17590240]

[363] Kohda K, Goda H, Itoh K, Samejima K, Fukuuchi T. Aged garlic extract reduces ROS production and cell death induced by 6-hydroxydopamine through activation of the Nrf2-ARE pathway in SH-SY5Y cells. Pharmacol Pharm 2013; 04(01): 31-40.

[364] Chung LY. The antioxidant properties of garlic compounds: allyl cysteine, alliin, allicin, and allyl disulfide. J Med Food 2006; 9(2): 205-13.
[http://dx.doi.org/10.1089/jmf.2006.9.205] [PMID: 16822206]

[365] Chen S, Chen W, Shen X, *et al.* Analysis of the genetic diversity of garlic (Allium sativum L.) by simple sequence repeat and inter simple sequence repeat analysis and agro-morphological traits. Biochem Syst Ecol 2014; 55: 260-7.
[http://dx.doi.org/10.1016/j.bse.2014.03.021]

[366] Gao X, Xue Z, Ma Q, *et al.* Antioxidant and antihypertensive effects of garlic protein and its hydrolysates and the related mechanism. J Food Biochem 2020; 44(2): e13126.
[http://dx.doi.org/10.1111/jfbc.13126] [PMID: 31877235]

[367] Mohd Sahardi NFN, Makpol S. Ginger (zingiber officinale roscoe) in the prevention of ageing and degenerative diseases: Review of current evidence. Evidence-Based Complementary and Alternative Medicine 2019.

[368] Nile SH, Park SW. Chromatographic analysis, antioxidant, anti-inflammatory, and xanthine oxidase inhibitory activities of ginger extracts and its reference compounds. Ind Crops Prod 2015; 70: 238-44.
[http://dx.doi.org/10.1016/j.indcrop.2015.03.033]

[369] Hussein U, Hassan N, Elhalwagy M, *et al.* Ginger and propolis exert neuroprotective effects against monosodium glutamate-induced neurotoxicity in rats. Molecules 2017; 22(11): 1928.
[http://dx.doi.org/10.3390/molecules22111928] [PMID: 29117134]

[370] Tanaka K, Arita M, Sakurai H, Ono N, Tezuka Y. Analysis of chemical properties of edible and medicinal ginger by metabolomics approach. BioMed Research International 2015.

[http://dx.doi.org/10.1155/2015/671058]

[371] Seow SLS, Hong SL, Lee GS, Malek SNA, Sabaratnam V. 6-shogaol, a neuroactive compound of ginger (jahe gajah) induced neuritogenic activity *via* NGF responsive pathways in PC-12 cells. BMC Complement Altern Med 2017; 17(1): 334.
[http://dx.doi.org/10.1186/s12906-017-1837-6] [PMID: 28646880]

[372] Lee C, Park GH, Kim CY, Jang JH. [6]-Gingerol attenuates β-amyloid-induced oxidative cell death *via* fortifying cellular antioxidant defense system. Food Chem Toxicol 2011; 49(6): 1261-9.
[http://dx.doi.org/10.1016/j.fct.2011.03.005] [PMID: 21396424]

[373] Yerer MB, Tiryaki MK, Demirpolat E. GSK-3beta inhibitory effects of 6-gingerol and 6-shogaol help to the recovery of SHSY-5Y cells after amyloid beta1–42 oligomer or aggregate toxicity. Journal of Cellular Biotechnology 2017; 2(2): 145-57.
[http://dx.doi.org/10.3233/JCB-15035]

[374] Wang L, Cai X, Shi M, *et al.* Identification and optimization of piperine analogues as neuroprotective agents for the treatment of Parkinson's disease *via* the activation of Nrf2/keap1 pathway. Eur J Med Chem 2020; 199: 112385.
[http://dx.doi.org/10.1016/j.ejmech.2020.112385] [PMID: 32402936]

[375] Takooree H, Aumeeruddy MZ, Rengasamy KR, *et al.* A systematic review on black pepper (Piper nigrum L.): From folk uses to pharmacological applications. Critical reviews in food science and nutrition 59(sup1): S210-43.2019.

[376] Roshanbakhsh H, Elahdadi Salmani M, Dehghan S, Nazari A, Javan M, Pourabdolhossein F. Piperine ameliorated memory impairment and myelin damage in lysolecethin induced hippocampal demyelination. Life Sci 2020; 253: 117671.
[http://dx.doi.org/10.1016/j.lfs.2020.117671] [PMID: 32335165]

[377] Niture SK, Kaspar JW, Shen J, Jaiswal AK. Nrf2 signaling and cell survival. Toxicol Appl Pharmacol 2010; 244(1): 37-42.
[http://dx.doi.org/10.1016/j.taap.2009.06.009] [PMID: 19538984]

[378] Kitamura H, Motohashi H. Nrf2 addiction in cancer cells. Cancer Sci 2018; 109(4): 900-11.
[http://dx.doi.org/10.1111/cas.13537] [PMID: 29450944]

[379] Panieri E, Saso L. Potential applications of Nrf2 inhibitors in cancer therapy. Oxidative medicine and cellular longevity 2019.
[http://dx.doi.org/10.1155/2019/8592348]

[380] Zang H, Mathew RO, Cui T. The dark side of Nrf2 in the heart. Front Physiol 2020; 11: 722.
[http://dx.doi.org/10.3389/fphys.2020.00722] [PMID: 32733266]

[381] Tao S, Rojo de la Vega M, Chapman E, Ooi A, Zhang DD. The effects of Nrf2 modulation on the initiation and progression of chemically and genetically induced lung cancer. Mol Carcinog 2018; 57(2): 182-92.
[http://dx.doi.org/10.1002/mc.22745] [PMID: 28976703]

[382] Wang Y, Miao Y, Mir AZ, *et al.* Inhibition of beta-amyloid-induced neurotoxicity by pinocembrin through Nrf2/HO-1 pathway in SH-SY5Y cells. J Neurol Sci 2016; 368: 223-30.
[http://dx.doi.org/10.1016/j.jns.2016.07.010] [PMID: 27538638]

[383] DeNicola GM, Karreth FA, Humpton TJ, *et al.* Oncogene-induced Nrf2 transcription promotes ROS detoxification and tumorigenesis. Nature 2011; 475(7354): 106-9.
[http://dx.doi.org/10.1038/nature10189] [PMID: 21734707]

[384] Mitsuishi Y, Motohashi H, Yamamoto M. The Keap1–Nrf2 system in cancers: stress response and anabolic metabolism. Front Oncol 2012; 2: 200.
[http://dx.doi.org/10.3389/fonc.2012.00200] [PMID: 23272301]

[385] McCarthy N. Tumorigenesis: oncogene detox programme. Nat Rev Cancer 2011; 11(9): 622-3.
[PMID: 21779002]

[386] Oh ET, Kim J, Kim JM, *et al.* NQO1 inhibits proteasome-mediated degradation of HIF-1α. Nat Commun 2016; 7(1): 13593.
[http://dx.doi.org/10.1038/ncomms13593] [PMID: 31911652]

[387] Niture SK, Jaiswal AK. Nrf2-induced antiapoptotic Bcl-xL protein enhances cell survival and drug resistance. Free Radic Biol Med 2013; 57: 119-31.
[http://dx.doi.org/10.1016/j.freeradbiomed.2012.12.014] [PMID: 23275004]

[388] Kensler TW, Wakabayashi N, Biswal S. Cell survival responses to environmental stresses *via* the Keap1-Nrf2-ARE pathway. Annu Rev Pharmacol Toxicol 2007; 47(1): 89-116.
[http://dx.doi.org/10.1146/annurev.pharmtox.46.120604.141046] [PMID: 16968214]

[389] Rojo de la Vega M, Chapman E, Zhang DD. Nrf2 and the hallmarks of cancer. Cancer Cell 2018; 34(1): 21-43.
[http://dx.doi.org/10.1016/j.ccell.2018.03.022] [PMID: 29731393]

[390] Panieri E, Buha A, Telkoparan-Akillilar P, *et al.* Potential applications of Nrf2 modulators in cancer therapy. Antioxidants 2020; 9(3): 193.
[http://dx.doi.org/10.3390/antiox9030193] [PMID: 32106613]

[391] Qin JJ, Cheng XD, Zhang J, Zhang WD. Dual roles and therapeutic potential of Keap1-Nrf2 pathway in pancreatic cancer: a systematic review. Cell Commun Signal 2019; 17(1): 121.
[http://dx.doi.org/10.1186/s12964-019-0435-2] [PMID: 31511020]

[392] Zhang L, Wang H, Fan Y, *et al.* Fucoxanthin provides neuroprotection in models of traumatic brain injury *via* the Nrf2-ARE and Nrf2-autophagy pathways. Sci Rep 2017; 7(1): 46763.
[http://dx.doi.org/10.1038/srep46763] [PMID: 28429775]

[393] Shin D, Kim EH, Lee J, Roh JL. Nrf2 inhibition reverses resistance to GPX4 inhibitor-induced ferroptosis in head and neck cancer. Free Radic Biol Med 2018; 129: 454-62.
[http://dx.doi.org/10.1016/j.freeradbiomed.2018.10.426] [PMID: 30339884]

[394] Roh JL, Jang H, Kim EH, Shin D. Targeting of the glutathione, thioredoxin, and Nrf2 antioxidant systems in head and neck cancer. Antioxid Redox Signal 2017; 27(2): 106-14.
[http://dx.doi.org/10.1089/ars.2016.6841] [PMID: 27733046]

[395] Tang W, Jiang Y-F, Ponnusamy M, Diallo M. Role of Nrf2 in chronic liver disease. World J Gastroenterol 2014; 20(36): 13079-87.
[http://dx.doi.org/10.3748/wjg.v20.i36.13079] [PMID: 25278702]

[396] Vartanian S, Ma TP, Lee J, *et al.* Application of mass spectrometry profiling to establish brusatol as an inhibitor of global protein synthesis. Mol Cell Proteomics 2016; 15(4): 1220-31.
[http://dx.doi.org/10.1074/mcp.M115.055509] [PMID: 26711467]

[397] Sun J, Hu H, Ren X, Simpkins JW. Tert-butylhydroquinone compromises survival in murine experimental stroke. Neurotoxicol Teratol 2016; 54: 15-21.
[http://dx.doi.org/10.1016/j.ntt.2016.01.004] [PMID: 26827673]

[398] Harder B, Tian W, La Clair JJ, *et al.* Brusatol overcomes chemoresistance through inhibition of protein translation. Mol Carcinog 2017; 56(5): 1493-500.
[http://dx.doi.org/10.1002/mc.22609] [PMID: 28019675]

[399] Lin R, Yi S, Gong L, *et al.* Inhibition of TGF-β signaling with halofuginone can enhance the antitumor effect of irradiation in Lewis lung cancer. OncoTargets Ther 2015; 8: 3549-59.
[http://dx.doi.org/10.2147/OTT.S92518] [PMID: 26664138]

[400] Xia X, Wang L, Zhang X, *et al.* Halofuginone-induced autophagy suppresses the migration and invasion of MCF-7 cells *via* regulation of STMN1 and p53. J Cell Biochem 2018; 119(5): 4009-20.
[http://dx.doi.org/10.1002/jcb.26559] [PMID: 29231257]

[401] Xia X, Wang X, Zhang S, *et al.* miR-31 shuttled by halofuginone-induced exosomes suppresses MFC-7 cell proliferation by modulating the HDAC2/cell cycle signaling axis. J Cell Physiol 2019; 234(10):

18970-84.
[http://dx.doi.org/10.1002/jcp.28537] [PMID: 30916359]

[402]   Elahi-Gedwillo KY, Carlson M, Zettervall J, Provenzano PP. Antifibrotic therapy disrupts stromal barriers and modulates the immune landscape in pancreatic ductal adenocarcinoma. Cancer Res 2019; 79(2): 372-86.
[http://dx.doi.org/10.1158/0008-5472.CAN-18-1334] [PMID: 30401713]

[403]   Tsuchida K, Tsujita T, Hayashi M, *et al.* Halofuginone enhances the chemo-sensitivity of cancer cells by suppressing Nrf2 accumulation. Free Radic Biol Med 2017; 103: 236-47.
[http://dx.doi.org/10.1016/j.freeradbiomed.2016.12.041] [PMID: 28039084]

[404]   Davatgaran-Taghipour Y, Masoomzadeh S, Farzaei MH, *et al.* Polyphenol nanoformulations for cancer therapy: experimental evidence and clinical perspective. Int J Nanomedicine 2017; 12: 2689-702.
[http://dx.doi.org/10.2147/IJN.S131973] [PMID: 28435252]

[405]   Li X, Huang Q, Ong CN, Yang XF, Shen HM. Chrysin sensitizes tumor necrosis factor-α-induced apoptosis in human tumor cells *via* suppression of nuclear factor-kappaB. Cancer Lett 2010; 293(1): 109-16.
[http://dx.doi.org/10.1016/j.canlet.2010.01.002] [PMID: 20133051]

[406]   Wang J, Wang H, Sun K, *et al.* Chrysin suppresses proliferation, migration, and invasion in glioblastoma cell lines *via* mediating the ERK/Nrf2 signaling pathway. Drug Des Devel Ther 2018; 12: 721-33.
[http://dx.doi.org/10.2147/DDDT.S160020] [PMID: 29662304]

[407]   Wang S, Zhong Z, Wan J, *et al.* Oridonin induces apoptosis, inhibits migration and invasion on highly-metastatic human breast cancer cells. Am J Chin Med 2013; 41(1): 177-96.
[http://dx.doi.org/10.1142/S0192415X13500134] [PMID: 23336515]

[408]   Ren CM, Li Y, Chen QZ, *et al.* Oridonin inhibits the proliferation of human colon cancer cells by upregulating BMP7 to activate p38 MAPK. Oncol Rep 2016; 35(5): 2691-8.
[http://dx.doi.org/10.3892/or.2016.4654] [PMID: 26986967]

[409]   Li F, Yi S, Wen L, *et al.* Li F-f. Oridonin induces NPM mutant protein translocation and apoptosis in NPM1c+ acute myeloid leukemia cells in vitro. Acta Pharmacol Sin 2014; 35(6): 806-13.
[http://dx.doi.org/10.1038/aps.2014.25] [PMID: 24902788]

[410]   Abdel-Hafeez EH, Ahmad AK, Kamal AM, Abdellatif MZM, Abdelgelil NH. *in vivo* antiprotozoan effects of garlic (*Allium sativum*) and ginger (*Zingiber officinale*) extracts on experimentally infected mice with Blastocystis spp. Parasitol Res 2015; 114(9): 3439-44.
[http://dx.doi.org/10.1007/s00436-015-4569-x] [PMID: 26085068]

[411]   Inbaraj JJ, Chignell CF. Cytotoxic action of juglone and plumbagin: a mechanistic study using HaCaT keratinocytes. Chem Res Toxicol 2004; 17(1): 55-62.
[http://dx.doi.org/10.1021/tx034132s] [PMID: 14727919]

[412]   Kapur A, Beres T, Rathi K, *et al.* Oxidative stress *via* inhibition of the mitochondrial electron transport and Nrf-2-mediated anti-oxidative response regulate the cytotoxic activity of plumbagin. Sci Rep 2018; 8(1): 1073.
[http://dx.doi.org/10.1038/s41598-018-19261-w] [PMID: 29348410]

[413]   Pan S-T, Qin Y, Zhou Z-W, *et al.* Plumbagin induces G2/M arrest, apoptosis, and autophagy *via* p38 MAPK- and PI3K/Akt/mTOR-mediated pathways in human tongue squamous cell carcinoma cells. Drug Des Devel Ther 2015; 9: 1601-26.
[PMID: 25834400]

[414]   La Rosa P, Petrillo S, Bertini ES, Piemonte F. Oxidative stress in DNA repeat expansion disorders: A focus on Nrf2 signaling involvement. Biomolecules 2020; 10(5): 702.
[http://dx.doi.org/10.3390/biom10050702] [PMID: 32369911]

[415] Cuadrado A, Rojo AI, Wells G, *et al.* Therapeutic targeting of the Nrf2 and KEAP1 partnership in chronic diseases. Nat Rev Drug Discov 2019; 18(4): 295-317.
[http://dx.doi.org/10.1038/s41573-018-0008-x] [PMID: 30610225]

[416] Wijekoon N, Gonawala L, Wijesinghe P, Steinbusch HWM, Mohan C, de Silva KRD. A biobank in Sri Lanka that links East and West. Lancet Neurol 2020; 19(12): 972.
[http://dx.doi.org/10.1016/S1474-4422(20)30405-1] [PMID: 33212058]

CHAPTER 5

Phytochemicals from Indian Medicinal Herbs in the Treatment of Neurodegenerative Disorders

Himanshu Verma[1], **Naveen Shivavedi**[2] and **Prasanta Kumar Nayak**[1,*]

¹ Department of Pharmaceutical Engineering and Technology, Indian Institute of Technology, Banaras Hindu University, Varanasi, 221005 (U.P.), India

² Shri Ram Group of Institutions, Faculty of Pharmacy, Jabalpur-482002 (M.P.), India

Abstract: Neurodegenerative disorders such as Alzheimer's disease, Parkinson's disease, Huntington's disease, and Amyotrophic lateral sclerosis are the major cause of disability and mortality. These disorders are appearing in the current era due to aging and stress-full lifestyles. For the treatments of these disorders, several conventional drugs are available but due to higher cost and dangerous adverse effects. Therefore, scientists are focusing more on medicinal herbs containing phytochemicals because these medicinal herbs are more effective, low cost, and show less harmful side effects to cure neurodegenerative disorders. Indian medicinal herbs are the most effective medicines and indigenous to India. Since ancient times, medicinal herbs have been used for treating neurodegenerative disorders. Indian medicinal herbs containing phytochemicals possess beneficial therapeutic effects for the treatment of neurodegenerative disorders, majorly having various compounds such as alkaloids, sesquiterpenes, triterpenoids, polyphenols, flavonoids, saponins, and essential oils which show anti-inflammatory and anti-oxidative properties. In this chapter, we highlighted and discussed the importance of some Indian medicinal herbs, such as *Bacopa monnieri* (Brahmi), *Centella asiatica*, *Curcuma longa* (turmeric), *Allium sativum* (garlic), *Terminalia chebula* (haritaki), *Celastrus paniculatus* (Jyotishmati), *Glycyrrhiza glabra* (Licorice), and *Acorus calamus* (Vacha) containing phytochemicals with their mechanism of action on neurodegenerative disorders.

Keywords: Alzheimer's disease, Flavonoids, Huntington's disease, Parkinson's disease, Phytochemicals, Polyphenols.

INTRODUCTION

Neurodegenerative disorders such as Alzheimer's disease (AD), Parkinson's disease (PD), Huntington's disease (HD), and Amyotrophic lateral sclerosis

* **Corresponding author Prasanta Kumar Nayak:** Department of Pharmaceutical Engineering and Technology, Indian Institute of Technology, Banaras Hindu University, Varanasi, 221005 (U.P.), India; E-mail: pknayak.phe@iitbhu.ac.in

Surya Pratap Singh, Hagera Dilnashin, Hareram Birla & Chetan Keswani (Eds.)

(ALS) occurred due to degeneration of neurons or neuronal damage. Neuroprotection is the strategies and mechanisms used against neuronal damage to treat neurodegenerative disorders [1]. Degeneration of neuronal cells and protein aggregation are the major factors involved in neuropathological and brain aging [1 - 3]. Neurodegenerative disorders are the main cause of morbidity and mortality with cognitive impairment in elderly people [4]. Etiologically, aging is the primary risk factor for neurodegeneration [5, 6]. Growing populations day by day and average life span increase the prevalence and incidences of neurodegenerative diseases [4]. Epidemiologically, these diseases are the second leading cause of death worldwide among elderly people by the 2040s, and the global aging population may rise by 2050 to 2 billion people [7 - 13].

AD is the first and most common type of dementia characterized by the accumulation of amyloid and hyper-phosphorylated tau protein in the brain, which is marked by progressive memory loss in elderly people [14]. PD is another common neurodegenerative disorder (movement disorder), and the etiology of PD is unclear, but several genetic and environmental causes have been identified [15]. HD is a common genetic disorder of autosomal dominant inheritance. In HD, degeneration of medium spiny neurons due to trinucleotide repeat expansion (CAG), causes continuous involuntary motor movements [16]. Amyotrophic lateral sclerosis is an adult-onset neurodegenerative disease characterized by the accumulation of ubiquitinated protein that occurs due to the loss of motor neurons in the central nervous system, leading to muscle atrophy and respiratory failure [17, 18].

However, several categories of synthetics drugs are available for the management of neurodegenerative disorders, such as cholinesterase inhibitors, N-methyl-D-aspartic acid receptor antagonists, dopamine agonists, catechol-o-methy-ltran-sferase inhibitors, anticholinergic drugs, dopamine decarboxylase inhibitors, monoamine oxidase inhibitors, tetrabenazine, edaravone, riluzole, *etc.* All these conventional drugs have therapeutic benefits but contain some unwanted dangerous side effects, such as psychosis, depression, low blood pressure, dry mouth, drowsiness, anxiety, difficulty with balance, *etc..*, that may harm the patients [19]. Therefore, treatment with Indian medicinal herbs got more significant as it may have potential anti-oxidative and anti-inflammatory effects, which can be safer than conventional drugs. These phytochemicals are well-accepted treatments that can modulate neuronal function and protective mechanisms against several neurodegenerative disorders [20 - 25].

Since ancient times, medicinal herbs have been used in India to treat neurodegenerative disorders. Here, we are discussing some novel studies and mechanisms of Indian medicinal herbs such as *Bacopa monnieri, Centella asiatica*, *Curcuma longa*, *Allium sativum*, *Terminalia chebula*, *Celastrus paniculatus*, *Glycyrrhiza glabra*, and *Acorus calamus* that may treat neurodegenerative disorders without any harmful effects (Fig. **1**).

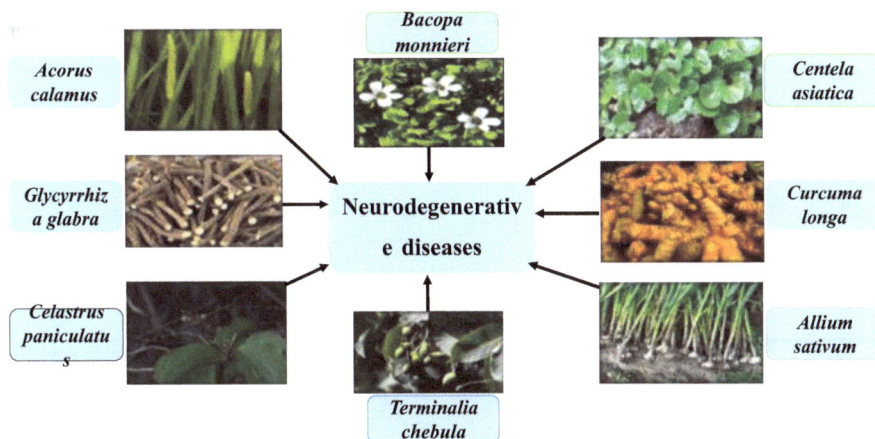

Fig. (1). Indian medicinal herbs used in the treatment of neurodegenerative disorders.

B. MONNIERI

B. monnieri (Brahmi, family: *Scrophulariaceae*) is a phytochemical found throughout the Indian subcontinents, as a most traditional herb in 'Ayurvedic Materia Medica' and used against mental disorders such as anti-anxiety, anti-epileptic, memory enhancer, tranquilizer, anti-oxidant and anti-inflammatory agent [26 - 31].

Phytoconstituents of *B. monnieri*

Triterpenoid saponins are the major constituents of *B. monnieri* called jujubacogenin, psudojubacogenin, and bacosides glycosides moieties [32]. There are several classes of saponins identified from I to XIII, and bacosides are the well-known constituents for pharmacological action [33]. Bacosides A and B, and D-mannitol play an important role in neuroprotection [34] (Table **1**).

Neuroprotective Activity of *B. monnieri*

In a clinical study, *B. monnieri* standardized extract (300 mg; orally) twice a day was used for 6 months, resulting in improved cognitive function in AD patients [35]. Numerous researches suggested that bacosides (*B. monnieri* components) work against oxidative stress and cognitive deterioration with different mechanisms of action and improve memory and the ability to learn in rodents [36 - 40]. More studies stated that "Brahmi" reduces reactive oxygen species (ROS), neuroinflammation, aggregation inhibition of amyloid-β, and better cognitive and learning behavior which states that inhibition of tau-mediated toxicity. Brahmi can be used in the treatment of AD [41].

Table 1. Phytochemicals and their mechanism of action of Indian medicinal herbs in the treatment of neurodegenerative disorders.

Scientific Name	Phytochemicals and Main Constituents	Mechanism of Action	References
B. monnieri (Brahmi, family Scrophulariaceae)	Bacoside-A and B, bacosaponins, betulinic acid	Inhibition of amyloid-β, reduction of ROS and neuroinflammation	[41]
	Bacosides, bacopasides, bacosaponins	Prevent the breakdown of MPTP to MPP⁺, decreased expression of inducible nitric oxide synthetase (iNOS)	[43]
C. asiatica (Indian Penny Wort; family: Apiaceae)	Aqueous ethanolic Extract	Increases the level of protein phosphatase 2 and mRNA expressions Bcl2 while decreasing glycogen synthase kinase-3β	[53]
	Pentacyclic triterpene (Asiatic acid)	Decreased phosphorylation of MAPK/P38 proteins (JNK and ERK), increased phosphorylation of PI3K, Akt, GSK-3β, and mTOR receptor	[57]
C. longa (Turmeric, Family: Zingiberaceae)	Ethanolic extract	Decreased expressions of miRNA-146a and Aβ, and proinflammatory cytokines	[82]
	Polyphenol (curcumin)	Anti-acetylcholinesterase, anti-inflammatory, anti-oxidant, inhibit α-synuclein, adenosine A2a receptor, angiotensin-II, increased dopamine, 5-HT, and norepinephrine	[84]
A. sativum (Garlic; family: Alliaceae)	Aged garlic extract	Anti-oxidative, anti-inflammatory, and modulation of GABAergic neurons	[100]
	Garlic extract	Anti-oxidative, anti-inflammatory, inhibition of mitochondrial dysfunction and apoptosis	[102]
T. chebula (Haritaki, family: Combretaceae)	Ellagic acid (phenolic)	Decreased amyloid-β, reactive oxygen species, and calcium ion reflex/anti-oxidative decreased amyloid-β plaques, pro-inflammatory markers, anti-acetylcholinesterase	[114, 116]
	Phenolic (ellagic acid)	Anti-oxidative, improved MAO-B, Nrf2, heme oxygenase-1, prevented the loss of tyrosine hydroxylase enzyme	[119]
C. paniculatus (Jyotishmati or black oil plant, family: Celastraceae)	Oleic, palmitic, linoleic, and stearic acid	Anticholinesterase	[121]
	Methanolic extract	Inhibits the aggregation of α-synuclein (heterologously expressed human)	[128]

(Table 1) cont.....

Scientific Name	Phytochemicals and Main Constituents	Mechanism of Action	References
G. glabra (Liquorice or sweet wood or mulaithi, family: Fabaceae)	Glycyrrhizic acid	Anticholinesterase, anti-oxidative (increased SOD and catalase)	[135]
	G. glabra extract	Inhibition of MEK-ERK-½ hyperphosphorylation, prevention of mitochondrial stress, and apoptosis	[143]
A. calamus (Vacha, family: Araceae)	Phenols, tannins, alkaloids, and flavonoids	Acetylcholine esterase inhibitor	[160]
	β-asarone (phenylpropanoid)	Increased tyrosine hydroxylase positive cells, decreased expressions of MALAT1 and α-synucleins	[159]

One of the recent studies showed that pre-treatment with *B. monnieri* exhibited a neuroprotective effect by limiting the brain inflammation in the rat model [42]. Moreover, in an *in-vivo/in-silico* study, animals were treated with *B. monnieri* (40 mg/kg/body weight) orally in a 1-methyl-4-phenyl-1,2,3,6-tetrahydropyridine model of PD significantly recover dopamine level, glutathione level, lipid peroxide, and behavioral parameters in mice [43]. Furthermore, researchers reported that *B. monnieri* ethanolic extract (180 mg/kg; orally) for 20 days of administration shows modulation of the cholinergic system and reduces the symptoms of PD induced by the rotenone model in rats [44]. In nematodes, a study shows that *B. monnieri* reduces alpha-synuclein aggregation, restores lipid contents, and prevents dopamine neurodegeneration; thereby, *B. monnieri* work against PD induced by 6-hydroxy dopamine (6-OHDA) [45].

In primary cortical cultured of neurons, glutamate-induced neurotoxicity and β-amyloid protein inhibited by "Brahmi" shows a neuroprotective effect because it protects neurons from β-amyloid accumulation by suppressing cellular acetylcholinesterase activity, promotes cell survival, and inhibits lipid peroxidation [46]. Moreover, in female Wistar rats, "Brahmi" (10 and 40 mg/kg/body weight) was used for 10 days to evaluate its anti-oxidant activity for the protection of peripheral and central neuronal systems resulting in a reduction of oxidative stress, increased tyrosine hydroxylase, and nerve growth factors [47].

C. ASIATICA

C. asiatica (Indian Penny Wort; family: Apiaceae member of the Umbelliferae) has been used as a traditional medicinal herb found in swampy areas of India and Asia for over 2000 years [48]. Ethanolic extract and aqueous extract of *C. asiatica* show the medicinal function and biological activities [48].

Phytoconstituents of *C. asiatica*

C. asiatica contains triterpenoids (asiatic acid and asiaticoside), flavonoids, alkaloids, and essential oil are the major active components of the ethanolic extract [49, 50]. It is used as a scavenger, reduces Fe^{+3} and possesses excellent anti-oxidant activity in the brain [37, 51] (Table **1**).

Neuroprotective Activity of *C. asiatica*

The researcher stated that feeding with ethanolic extract of *C. asiatica* (300 mg/kg/body weight) for 60 consecutive days improved oxidative status and reduced lipid peroxidation, causing delaying of the aging process in the rat brain [51]. *C. asiatica* contains anti-oxidative, anti-inflammatory, neuron regeneration ability, inhibition of acetylcholine esterase, and accumulation of plaques. All these multifunctional properties are responsible for making it capable of neuroprotection involved in neurodegeneration disorders [50]. Moreover, this ethanolic extract is also used in neurodegenerative disorders, such as AD, with performing several memory tasks, such as the passive avoidance test and the Morris water maze test in rats [52]. Moreover, Chiroma *et al.*, stated that *C. asiatica* alleviates D-galactose induced/aluminum chloride-induced AD *via* inhibition of hyperphosphorylated tau (P-tau) bio-synthetic protein, increased protein phosphatase-2 (PPA2), decreased glycogen synthase kinase-3 β (GSK-3β) in rats [53]. Matthews *et al.* reported that *C. asiatica* water extract improves cognitive functions in AD (Tg2576 and wild-type mice model) *via* anti-oxidative action [54]. Moreover, triterpene asiatic acid (*C. asiatica*) contains neuroprotective activity and mitigates aluminum chloride (100 mg/kg/bodyweight for 40 days) induced AD by multiple pharmacological actions [55].

Furthermore, extract of *C. asiatica* (10, 30, and 100 mg/kg; for 20 consecutive days) used in rotenone (2.5 mg/kg; *i.p.*) induces PD in rats. In this study, *C. asiatica* (30 mg/kg) increased the number and intensity of dopaminergic neurons in the striatum, substantia nigra, and decreased malondialdehyde and increased catalase levels with protecting against mitochondrial complex I inhibition, showing anti-parkinsonism effect [56]. Nataraj *et al.* reported that Asiatic acid (pentacyclic triterpene) from *C. asiatica* (100 mg/kg/body weight) for 5 weeks significantly reduces 1-methyl 4-phenyl 1,2,3, 6-tetrahydropyridine hydrochloride/probenecid (MPTP/p) induced PD by improving motor abnormality, dopamine, expression of neurotrophic factor, and tyrosine kinase receptors in mice [57]. Moreover, the researcher used a transgenic *Drosophila* model to induce PD and evaluate leaf extract activity (*C. asiatica*) [58]. This study showed that leaf extract (0.25, 0.50, and 0.1μL/mL with diet) significantly increased glutathione content and glutathione-S-transferase activity, reduced oxidative stress in the brain, and significantly delayed the loss of climbing ability and activity pattern of the transgenic *Drosophila* model [58].

Furthermore, in an *in-vitro* study, the researcher used 3-nitropropionic acid (3-NPA) to induce oxidative stress to evaluate the effectiveness of *C. asiatica* in brain mitochondria [59]. This 3-NPA model increases levels of malondialdehyde, hydroperoxide, and reactive oxygen species, indicating oxidative stress. *C. asiatica* treatment reversed the concentration of oxidative stress parameters, such as malondialdehyde, hydroperoxide, and ROS, and defense against mitochondria from different parts of the brain. Finally, this study suggests that *C. asiatica* involve in neuroprotection by its major anti-oxidative property [59]. In a similar study, the researcher administered the 3-NPA model for induction of Huntington's disease and evaluated the prophylactic activity of *C. asiatica* in juvenile mice. They found that the prophylactic action of *C. asiatica* by a significant reduction of malondialdehyde and ROS in the cytosol, and mitochondria of the striatum exhibited anti-oxidative properties [60].

C. LONGA

C. longa (Turmeric, Family: *Zingiberaceae*) is a popular natural drug extensively found in tropical areas of Asia [61]. It is used in various diseases such as dyslipidemia, liver, stomach, and neurodegenerative diseases such as Alzheimer's, Parkinson's, Huntington's, *etc*. [62 - 66].

Phytoconstituents of *C. longa*

The main polyphenolic constituents of turmeric are known as curcumin which is yellow-colored and can be isolated from the rhizome of the plant [67]. This constituents are composed of three parts curcumin-I, curcumin-II, and curcumin-III [68]. Curcumin (8%) part found in the dehydrated root part of the plant [69]. Volatile oils and diferuloylmethane are the other main active constituents of turmeric [70]. Curcumin is a constituent of the *Curcuma longa* plant, which is insoluble in water while soluble in organic solvents (ethanol) [71] (Table **1**).

Neuroprotective Activity of *C. longa*

Aluminum is one of the factors leading to amyloid aggregation, and impaired iron metabolism causes accumulation of aluminum in substantia nigra and oxidative damage [72, 73]. Chronically using aluminum leads to increasing proinflammatory cytokines observed in the cortex, hippocampus, and corpus callosum, causing neuronal damage involved in the pathogenesis of several neurodegenerative disorders [74 - 76]. Recently, a researcher used a turmeric extract essential oil combination (25 mg/kg and 50 mg/kg) to evaluate the neuroprotective effect in Swiss albino mice. In this study, aluminum chloride (40 mg/kg) was used as a model for neurotoxicity and used turmeric extract essential oil combination, which reversed the impaired spatial learning and memory, decreased glutathione, acetylcholinesterase, and catalase, increased lipid peroxidation in mice [77].

The recent finding indicated that curcumin is involved in AD pathophysiology, by the inhibition of deposition and oligomerization of Aβ and tau phosphorylation in the brain of AD animals with behavioral improvement [78]. In the *in-vitro* model (primary neuronal cortical culture) of AD, the combined effect of curcumin and vitamin-D was evaluated [79]. This combination reduces lipid peroxidation products by augmentation of anti-oxidative enzymes (superoxide dismutase, glutathione, and catalase) and upregulation of neurotrophic growth factors [79]. This study stated that this combination could be a promising therapy for the management of AD [79]. Moreover, the researcher stated that curcumin contains highly anti-inflammatory and anti-oxidative properties in the cortex and hippocampus, which improve cognitive function in mice models of AD [80]. Mir-146a is a microRNA (miRNA) involved in the pathophysiology of AD by its neuroinflammation and aging process, and expression was observed [81]. The researcher measured mir-146a as a marker of AD and used curcumin which significantly reduces neuroinflammatory mir-146a, and increases phagocytosis and clearance of amyloid-β in mice [82].

Systemic experimental literature reported that curcumin shows an anti-parkinsonism effect by reducing neuronal apoptosis, anti-inflammatory, and anti-oxidant action in toxin base animal models, which indicated that curcumin has neuroprotection activity for human PD patients [83]. Moreover, curcumin was used in rotenone induce PD animal model, which suggested that curcumin (80 mg/kg/day; orally administered) antagonizes adenosine A2a receptor gene expression and inhibits acetylcholine esterase, alpha-synuclein, malondialdehyde, C-reactive protein, caspase-3, interleukin-6, and DNA fragmentation, while significantly increasing norepinephrine, serotonin, dopamine, glutathione, and superoxide dismutase in mice [84].

A. SATIVUM

A. sativum (Garlic, family: Alliaceae) is used as a valuable spice and a well-known remedy for several diseases and physiological disorders. It was cultivated throughout the world and originated in central Asia [85]. It contains several pharmacological activities, such as neuroprotective activity, brain ischemia, Alzheimer's, Parkinson's, Huntington's, and Amyotrophic lateral sclerosis [86 -

88].

Phytoconstituents of *A. sativum*

Sulphur compounds such as allicins, ajoene, and sulfides are the major constituents of the garlic plant [89]. S-allyl-cysteine is an organosulphur compound that possesses anti-apoptotic and anti-oxidant properties, while S-allyl mercapto cysteine shows different pharmacological activity [90, 91] (Table **1**).

Neuroprotective Activity of *A. sativum*

Garlic extract reported various biological activity and pharmacological effects like anti-inflammatory effects [87, 92]. Similarly, the researcher investigated that garlic extract protects against Aβ-induced neuroinflammation and cognitive dysfunction [93]. In this study, rats were orally administered garlic extract at different doses (125, 250, and 500 mg/kg; body weight) for 56 days. After that, Aβ was used as a model for induction of neuroinflammation and cognitive dysfunction [93]. They concluded that garlic extract (250 and 500 mg/kg) significantly improves cognitive dysfunction with the reduction of microglia, and IL-1β (inflammatory mediators) shows a neuroprotective effect in rats [93].

Furthermore, literature reported that garlic extract (40 mg/g; body weight) exhibits an anti-amyloidogenic effect in mice models of AD [94]. Dietary aged extract (2%), S-allyl cysteine, and diallyl-disulfide (20 mg/kg) decreased plaques and inflammation in cerebral, Aβ species, and conformational alteration in tau protein [95]. Reactive oxygen species and lipid peroxidation are the major factors promoting neuronal death [96, 97]. Whereas, S-allyl cysteine is the major product of garlic extract that protects against Aβ-induced neurotoxicity in the brain [98, 99]. Garlic extract prevents the dysfunction of cognitive and learning memory. The *in-vitro* and *in-vivo* studies suggested the anti-oxidant, anti-inflammatory, and modulation of neurotransmitters in brain regions of AD [100].

Moreover, garlic extract containing S-allyl cysteine shows a higher anti-oxidative property. Rojas *et al.* reported that S-allyl cysteine shows a neuroprotective effect against oxidative stress induced by 1-methyl-4-phenylpyridinium (MPP$^+$) in mice [101]. In this study, S-allyl cysteine was administered (125 mg/kg; *i.p.*) daily for 17 days. Then, MPP$^+$ was used for the induction of oxidative stress in the striatum of the brain. Results state that S-allyl cysteine significantly reversed the reduced dopamine level, locomotor activity, and oxidative stress induced by MPP$^+$ in mice and exhibited a neuroprotective effect due to its high anti-oxidant activity [101]. Furthermore, recently researchers reported that garlic extract protects against 6-OHDA-induced PD in rats. In this study, Bigham *et al.* investigated that garlic extract can protect the cell from inflammation, oxidative stress, apoptosis, and mitochondrial dysfunction [102]. Therefore, they concluded that garlic extract protects dopaminergic neurons and decreases movements and behavioral dysfunctions [102].

In recent years studies indicated that H_2S exhibited neuroprotection activity in PD [103]. *A. sativum* contains a number of sulfur compounds that release hydrogen disulfide. Some researchers stated that H_2S shows neuroprotective effects in PD [104 - 107].

T. CHEBULA

T. chebula (Haritaki, family: Combretaceae) occurs in India and other countries. This plant is used for long diarrhea, as anti-tussive and leucorrhoea, headache, mental abnormality, loss of memory, and epilepsy [108]. It also contains neuroprotective, anti-inflammatory, and anti-oxidant properties [109].

Phytoconstituents of *T. chebula*

Haritaki contains major active phytoconstituents such as chebulic acid, ellagic acid, oleanane-type triterpenoids, and chebulagic acid [110 - 112]. Hydrolyzable tannins (chebulic acid, gallic acid, chebulanin, corilagin, chebulagic, ellagic acid, and chebulinic acid) are also found in aqueous fruit extract [112, 113] (Table **1**).

Neuroprotective Activity of *T. chebula*

Neuroprotective activity with their mechanism is mainly due to anti-oxidative and anti-inflammatory effects. Researchers reported that cell toxicity induced by β-amyloid for induction of AD. In this study, water and methanol extract of *T. chebula* and ellagic acid showed neuroprotection *via* inhibition of reactive oxygen species or oxidative stress [114]. Moreover, *T. chebula* improves the activity of learning and memory impairments using ethanol-induced cognitive impairment, and the Morris water maze test was used for the evaluation of learning and memory dysfunction in rats. This study concluded that extract of *T. chebula* significantly exhibited a protective effect against oxidative stress and neurodegenerative disorders in rats [115]. Sporadic AD is the neuronal loss of age-related dementia and marked cognitive impairment. Ellagic acid is the phenolic constituents using 50 mg/kg per oral for 30 days exhibited a reduction of streptozocin induced sporadic Alzheimer's disease with biochemical abnormalities in rats *via* reduction of amyloid β, anti-oxidative and anti-inflammatory effect [116].

Moreover, the study reported that ellagic acid work against PD induced by 6-

OHDA, *via* its anti-oxidant activity. In this study, ellagic acid (50 mg/kg/mL) was administered to significantly improve motor impairment, decreased malonaldehyde while increased superoxide dismutase and glutathione peroxidase activity. The results of this study showed that ellagic acid can be used in PD because it increases cerebral anti-oxidant activity in rats [117]. Farbood *et al.*, reported the anti-inflammatory activity of ellagic acid and stated that it can improve PD by reduction of motor impairment in the medial forebrain bundle *via* reducing neuroinflammatory cytokines (TNF-α and IL-6) and decreased free radicals in the rat brain [118]. Moreover, ellagic acid protects from PD *via* an anti-oxidative mechanism (reduced malonaldehyde and reactive oxygen species), amelioration of apoptosis, improvement in monoamine oxidase-B, prevented loss of tyrosine hydroxylase within substantia nigra part of the brain in rats [119].

C. PANICULATUS

C. paniculatus (Jyotishmati or black oil plant, Family: *Celastraceae*) is a well-known Indian medicinal plant [120]. In the traditional Ayurvedic system of medicines, this plant has been used for 1000 years for the treatment of several diseases, such as memory enhancer, nervine tonic, anti-depressant, AD, and other neurodegenerative disorders [121].

Phytoconstituents of *C. paniculatus*

Alkaloids (celastrin and paniculatin), tannins, terpenoids, sesquiterpene polyesters, and fixed oil are the major components of this plant and show several pharmacological activities such as anti-inflammatory, anti-convulsant, anti-epileptic, and nootropic action [122 - 124] (Table **1**).

Neuroprotective Activity of *C. paniculatus*

C. paniculatus is a well-known folk medicine for the enhancement of memory and improving attention. Generally, seeds of *C. paniculatus* play an important role in neuroprotective activity because seeds contain major active constituents, which may protect brain function [121]. At different doses (5-15 drop seed oil or 1 gm seed powder), these seeds are used as a memory booster and treat memory disorders and AD *via* inhibition of the cholinesterase enzyme in the brain [121].

C. paniculatus contain anti-oxidative activity, which is the possible mechanism for improvement in cognitive functions [125]. The methanolic extract (100, 200, and 400 mg/kg) of *C. paniculatus* exhibited nootropic or memory-enhancing activity in the rats [126]. In another study, *C. paniculatus* seed oil was used to treat dementia, which exhibited a memory-enhancing effect in mice. In this study, scopolamine (3 mg/kg; *i.p.*) was used for induction of memory impairment which was reversed by seed oil (200 mg/kg/day) evaluated by using an elevated plus maze test (spatial memory) and passive avoidance test (fear memory) in mice [127].

Moreover, the PD model (Caenorhabditis elegance BZ555 and NL5901 strains) is induced by 1-methyl-4-phenylpyridinium iodide and accumulation of α-synuclein protein. In this study, *C. paniculatus* shows neuroprotective and mitigation of protein aggregation effect [128]. Furthermore, ethanolic extract of *C. paniculatus* (100 and 200 mg/kg) and aqueous extract (36 mg/kg) was used in Huntington's disease induced by 3-nitropropionic acid in the rats. This study showed that ethanolic extract and aqueous extract significantly improve behavioral tests and oxidative parameters in rats [129].

G. GLABRA

G. glabra (Liquorice or sweet wood or mulaithi, family: Fabaceae) is found in the part of Asia and other continents [130]. It contains several pharmacological activities, such as anti-viral, anti-inflammatory, anti-diabetic, and neuroprotective activity [131].

Phytoconstituents of *G. glabra*

It contains major bioactive molecules such as glycyrrhizin, glycyrrhizic acid, isoliquiritigenin, liquiritigenin, licochalcone-A, α-terpineol, licoriphenone, licoaryl coumarin, furfuraldehyde, and several volatile components. All these constituents are reported to have several pharmacological effects such as anti-oxidative, anti-inflammatory, anti-diabetic, neuroprotective, *etc.* [130] (Table **1**).

Neuroprotective Activity of *G. glabra*

Glycyrrhizic acid (triterpenoid saponin) is one of the major active constituents which contain anti-inflammatory, anti-microbial, anti-oxidant, and anti-aging activities [132, 133]. High mobility group box-1 is a ubiquitous protein, which acts as proinflammatory cytokines. This protein is inhibited by glycyrrhizic acid and shows neuroprotective properties [132, 133]. Sathyamoorthy *et al.* reported that glycyrrhizic acid protects the brain by inhibiting reactive oxygen species and oxidative stress [134]. This property of glycyrrhizic acid occurs due to restoring mitochondrial complex I and IV, enzymatic anti-oxidant activity, and showing neuroprotective action in rats [134].

Moreover, *G. glabra* contains glycyrrhizic acid to protect against cognitive impairment in mice. The researcher uses scopolamine (1 mg/kg) for induction of cognitive impairment in mice. Whereas, glycyrrhizic acid (10 and 20 mg/kg) was used for 21 days, and the Y maze and passive avoidance test were tested for measurement of cognitive functions in mice. This study showed that glycyrrhizic acid significantly ameliorates acetylcholine esterase, superoxide dismutase, and catalase in scopolamine-induced cognitive dysfunction in mice [135]. Furthermore, the study reported that glycyrrhizin improves isoflurane-induced cognitive deficits in neonatal rats *via* the alleviation of neuroinflammation (TNF-α and IL-1β), hippocampal apoptosis, and restoration of protein synthesis. These results stated that glycyrrhizin is a potential treatment against neurotoxicity and cognitive deficits [136]. Dhingra *et al.* reported that *G. glabra* (75, 150, and 300 mg/kg) was used for seven successive days increased memory in mice, which stated that 150 mg/kg was more effective, so it can be used as a memory enhancer and could be helpful in the treatment of AD [137]. In another study, glabridin isolated from *G. glabra* was effective for the treatment of AD by the inhibition of cholinesterase activity in mice [138].

In PD, several factors are involved in dopaminergic neurodegeneration, such as apoptosis and hyperphosphorylation [139]. The researcher reported that *G. glabra* (Yashtimadhu) can be used against PD induced by the rotenone cellular model. By this study, they stated that "Yashtimadhu" prevents the development of PD *via* preventing apoptosis and mitochondrial oxidative stress [140]. In a randomized clinical study, the researcher selected some patients and used licorice or placebo syrup 5 mL (136 mg of licorice extract, 12.14 mg of glycyrrhizic acid, and 136 µg of polyphenol) orally for 6 months daily in twice form. They used a unified Parkinson's rating scale to measure PD symptoms and found that patients' syrup use improved symptoms without any side effects [141]. Furthermore, methanolic extract of *G. glabra* is the best adjuvant for the treatment of PD. *G. glabra* (30 and 100 mg/kg, *i.p.*) was significantly effective against haloperidol-induced catalepsy in mice [142]. A recent study showed "Yashtimadhu choorna" prepared from dried roots of *G. glabra* (licorice). This "Yashtimadhu" can be used as a memory enhancer and contain a neuroprotective effect [143]. The researcher uses "Yashtimadhu" as a therapeutic strategy against PD *via* inhibition of mitogen-activated protein kinase/extracellular regulated kinase hyperactivation, mitochondrial stress, and apoptosis in rotenone-induced cellular and molecular aberrations [143 - 146].

A. CALAMUS

A. calamus (Vacha, Family: Araceae) is a known plant in the Indian medicines ayurvedic system [147]. This plant contains rhizome, essential oil, and several biological activities, such as allelopathic, anti-cellular, and immunosuppressive [147, 148].

Phytoconstituents of *A. calamus*

It contains several major active constituents such as volatile oils α and β-asarones, sesquiterpenes, phenylpropanoids, monoterpenes, saponins, coumarins, flavones, lignans, and xanthone glycosides [147]. It contains several pharmacological activities, such as anti-convulsant, acetylcholinesterase inhibitory, anti-oxidative, memory enhancing, anti-inflammatory, cytoprotective, and neuroprotective activity [149] (Table **1**).

Neuroprotective Activity of *A. calamus*

The chemical compounds such as β-asarone (82.42%), calarene (2.41%), euasarone (1.92%), and 2-methoxy-3-allyl phenol (1.91%) are isolated from *Acorus calamus*. These chemical compounds show several biological activities (anti-inflammatory, anti-oxidant, anti-microbial, and cytotoxicity activities) [150]. Furthermore, rhizome extract of *A. calamus* exhibited a neuromodulatory effect on stressed rats. In this study, rats were orally treated with A. calamus extract for 21 days against restrained stress. This study concluded that rhizome extract prevents restrain stress-induced cognitive dysfunction and exhibited modulatory effect in Na^+ - K^+ ATPase and anti-oxidants activity in rats [151]. Similarly, in another study, *A. calamus* (hydroalcoholic root extract) shows a protective effect against memory loss, oxidative stress, and anxiety [152].

Moreover, AD is one of the major neurodegenerative disorders that occur due to aging, decreased levels of acetylcholine by enzyme acetylcholinesterase, and lifestyle changes [151 - 154]. Those molecules that can inhibit this enzyme may protect and ameliorate the symptoms of AD [151, 152]. Out of several medicinal herbs, *A. calamus* is also one of the herbs that are used in memory loss and exhibited neuroprotective activity [151, 152].

Indian traditional plant *A. calamus* and its constituents α-asarone contain higher anti-oxidant and anti-inflammatory activities [149]. Mikami *et al.,* investigated the *in-vitro* effect of *A. calamus* and α-asarone extract on endoplasmic reticulum and oxidative stress-induced hippocampal HT22 cells death by tunicamycin and L- glutamate [155]. As result, both *A. calamus* and α-asarone reduced ROS (oxidative stress) and phosphorylation of protein kinase RNA-like kinase (PERK) endoplasmic reticulum kinase. This study suggested that both *A. calamus* and α-asarone inhibit endoplasmic reticulum and oxidative stress by reduction of PERK and ROS inhibition, protecting the hippocampal cell damage [155]. It concluded that asarone candidates can be useful in neurodegenerative disorders, AD [155].

In Parkinsonism rats, *A. calamus* containing asarone plays an important role in maintaining dopaminergic activity [156]. Researchers reported that β-asarone has the capability to inhibit the autophagy process and contribute to the treatment of 6-OHDA-induced damage in rats [156]. This study investigated beclin-1, light chain 3B, and P62 expression, which are autophagy-related proteins. As a result, β-asarone decreased beclin-1 and light chain 3B while increased nucleoporin 62 (P62) expressions. All data suggested that β-asarone used against 6-OHDA induced damage in rats [156]. Another study reported that α-asarone contains a protective effect against MPTP-induced PD in the mice model. In this study, α-asarone inhibits MPTP induction PD *via* inhibition of inflammatory response and NF-kB activation in microglial cells and protects dopaminergic neurons with the attenuation of behavioral impairments (Y-maze and pole test) in MPTP-induced PD in mice [157]. Inositol-requiring enzyme 1(IRE1), X- box protein 1 (XBP1), glucose-related protein 78, and homologous binding protein, and α-synuclein expression induced by 6-OHDA and MPTP are some important pathways that are involved in the PD and protect using the administration of β-asarone in rodents [158, 159].

OTHER IMPORTANT INDIAN MEDICINAL HERBS FOR THE TREATMENT OF NEURODEGENERATIVE DISORDERS

The active component of *Crocus sativus*, crocin, contains a major anti-oxidative property that can be used for the treatment of neurodegenerative disorder either by reducing oxidative stress or inflammation in rats [161]. The extract of *Crocus sativus* possesses inhibitory activity and prevents acetylcholine breakdown showing a therapeutic strategy against AD [162]. Other Indian medicinal herbs such as *Coriandrum sativum* [163] and *Ocimum sanctum* [164] also have the property to treat neurodegenerative disorders.

CONCLUSION

Environmental, aging, and lifestyle factors endorse the health of the nervous system by causing stress, memory loss, and neurodegeneration. Today's phytochemicals are available in the form of herbs, spices, and dietary supplements that contain infinite sources of constituents for improving the health of patients. Several phytochemicals recently reported that these molecules can exert a protective effect against neurodegenerative disorders. In this chapter, the information collected is based on Indian medicinal herbs containing phytochemicals that showed therapeutic effects in preclinical, cell culture models, and clinical treatment in neurodegenerative disorders. Pharmacologically, several Indian medicinal herbs, phytochemicals, and herbal extracts target particular mechanisms. For instance, anti-Alzheimer's drugs inhibited acetylcholine esterase enzyme, anti-Parkinson's drugs increased dopaminergic neurons, *etc.*. however, several medicinal herbs containing phytochemicals possess anti-inflammatory, anti-oxidant, and neuroprotective action. Hence, these natural plants and their phytochemicals provide a new source of effective and beneficial neurodegenerative drugs.

CONSENT FOR PUBLICATION

Not applicable.

CONFLICT OF INTEREST

The author declares no conflict of interest, financial or otherwise.

ACKNOWLEDGMENTS

The authors thank the Central Library, Banaras Hindu University, Varanasi, India, for providing the facilities required to access relevant papers.

REFERENCES

[1]   Onyango I, Bennett J, Stokin G. Regulation of neuronal bioenergetics as a therapeutic strategy in neurodegenerative diseases. Neural Regen Res 2021; 16(8): 1467-82.
[http://dx.doi.org/10.4103/1673-5374.303007] [PMID: 33433460]

[2]   Giri M, Bhalke R, Prakash KV, Kasture S. Evaluation Of *Camellia sinensis*, *Withania somnifera* and their Combination for Anti-oxidant and Antiparkinsonian Effect. J Pharma Sci Res 2020; 12(8): 1093-9.

[3]   Trancikova A, Ramonet D, Moore DJ. Genetic mouse models of neurodegenerative diseases. Prog Mol Biol Transl Sci 2011; 100: 419-82.
[http://dx.doi.org/10.1016/B978-0-12-384878-9.00012-1] [PMID: 21377633]

[4]   Erkkinen MG, Kim MO, Geschwind MD. Clinical neurology and epidemiology of the major neurodegenerative diseases. Cold Spring Harb Perspect Biol 2018; 10(4): a033118.
[http://dx.doi.org/10.1101/cshperspect.a033118] [PMID: 28716886]

[5]   Hou Y, Dan X, Babbar M, *et al.* Ageing as a risk factor for neurodegenerative disease. Nat Rev Neurol 2019; 15(10): 565-81.
[http://dx.doi.org/10.1038/s41582-019-0244-7] [PMID: 31501588]

[6]   Mattson MP, Arumugam TV. Hallmarks of brain aging: adaptive and pathological modification by metabolic states. Cell Metab 2018; 27(6): 1176-99.
[http://dx.doi.org/10.1016/j.cmet.2018.05.011] [PMID: 29874566]

[7]   World Health Organization. Global strategy and action plan on ageing and health. 2017.

[8]   Rudnicka E, Napierała P, Podfigurna A, Męczekalski B, Smolarczyk R, Grymowicz M. The World Health Organization (WHO) approach to healthy ageing. Maturitas 2020; 139: 6-11.
[http://dx.doi.org/10.1016/j.maturitas.2020.05.018] [PMID: 32747042]

[9]   Ansari JA, Siraj A, Inamdar NN. Pharmacotherapeutic approaches of Parkinson's disease. Int J Pharmacol 2010; 6(5): 584-90.
[http://dx.doi.org/10.3923/ijp.2010.584.590]

[10]   Rai SN, Birla H, Singh SS, *et al.* Biomedical engineering and its applications in healthcare pathophysiology of the disease causing physical disability. biomedical engineering and its applications in healthcare. Springer 2019; pp. 573-95.

[11]   Rai SN, Dilnashin H, Birla H, *et al.* The role of PI3K/Akt and ERK in neurodegenerative disorders. Neurotox Res 2019; 35(3): 775-95.
        [http://dx.doi.org/10.1007/s12640-019-0003-y] [PMID: 30707354]

[12]   Rai SN, Singh BK, Rathore AS, *et al.* Quality control in huntington's disease: a therapeutic target. Neurotox Res 2019; 36(3): 612-26.
        [http://dx.doi.org/10.1007/s12640-019-00087-x] [PMID: 31297710]

[13]   Singh SS, Rai SN, Birla H, *et al.* Techniques Related to Disease Diagnosis and Therapeutics. Application of Biomedical Engineering in Neuroscience. Springer 2019; pp. 437-56.
        [http://dx.doi.org/10.1007/978-981-13-7142-4_22]

[14]   Muralidar S, Ambi SV, Sekaran S, Thirumalai D, Palaniappan B. Role of tau protein in Alzheimer's disease: The prime pathological player. Int J Biol Macromol 2020; 163: 1599-617.
        [http://dx.doi.org/10.1016/j.ijbiomac.2020.07.327] [PMID: 32784025]

[15]   Balestrino R, Schapira AHV. Parkinson disease. Eur J Neurol 2020; 27(1): 27-42.
        [http://dx.doi.org/10.1111/ene.14108] [PMID: 31631455]

[16]   Cuturic M. Huntington's Disease. Mind and Brain. Springer 2020; pp. 81-108.

[17]   Vicencio E, Beltrán S, Labrador L, Manque P, Nassif M, Woehlbier U. Implications of selective autophagy dysfunction for ALS pathology. Cells 2020; 9(2): 381.
        [http://dx.doi.org/10.3390/cells9020381] [PMID: 32046060]

[18]   Sharkey LM, Sandoval-Pistorius SS, Moore SJ, *et al.* Modeling UBQLN2-mediated neurodegenerative disease in mice: Shared and divergent properties of wild type and mutant UBQLN2 in phase separation, subcellular localization, altered proteostasis pathways, and selective cytotoxicity. Neurobiol Dis 2020; 143: 105016.
        [http://dx.doi.org/10.1016/j.nbd.2020.105016] [PMID: 32653673]

[19]   Hosamani R. The efficacy of *Bacopa monnieri* extract in modulating Parkinson's disease. Genetics, Neurology, Behavior, and Diet in Parkinson's Disease. Elsevier 2020; pp. 609-24.
        [http://dx.doi.org/10.1016/B978-0-12-815950-7.00039-4]

[20]   Birla H, Keswani C, Rai SN, *et al.* Neuroprotective effects of *Withania somnifera* in BPA induced-cognitive dysfunction and oxidative stress in mice. Behav Brain Funct 2019; 15(1): 9.
        [http://dx.doi.org/10.1186/s12993-019-0160-4] [PMID: 31064381]

[21]   Birla H, Keswani C, Singh SS, *et al.* Unraveling the Neuroprotective Effect of *Tinospora cordifolia* in Parkinsonian Mouse Model Through Proteomics Approach. 2021.
        [http://dx.doi.org/10.1021/acschemneuro.1c00481]

[22]   Rai SN, Zahra W, Singh SS, *et al.* Anti-inflammatory activity of ursolic acid in MPTP-induced parkinsonian mouse model. Neurotox Res 2019; 36(3): 452-62.
        [http://dx.doi.org/10.1007/s12640-019-00038-6] [PMID: 31016688]

[23]   Zahra W, Rai SN, Birla H, *et al.* The global economic impact of neurodegenerative diseases: Opportunities and challenges. Bioeconomy for Sustainable Development 2020; pp. 333-45.

[24]   Zahra W, Rai SN, Birla H, *et al.* Economic Importance of Medicinal Plants in Asian Countries. Bioeconomy for Sustainable Development. Springer 2020; pp. 359-77.
        [http://dx.doi.org/10.1007/978-981-13-9431-7_19]

[25]   Zahra W, Rai SN, Birla H, *et al.* Neuroprotection of rotenone-induced Parkinsonism by ursolic acid in PD mouse model. CNS & Neurological Disorders-Drug Targets (Formerly Current Drug Targets-CNS & Neurological Disorders) 2020; 14: 527-40.
        [http://dx.doi.org/10.2174/1871527319666200812224457]

[26]   Sarkar S, Jha S. Effects associated with insertion of rol genes on morphogenic potential in explants derived from transgenic *Bacopa monnieri* (L.). Wettst, 2021.
        [http://dx.doi.org/10.1007/s11240-021-02092-5]

[27] Vishwakarma RK, Kumari U, Khan BM. Memory booster plant *Bacopa monniera* (Brahmi): Biotechnology and molecular aspects of bacoside biosynthesis. Medicinal Plants-Recent Advances in Research and Development. Springer 2016; pp. 167-89.

[28] Jeyasri R, Muthuramalingam P, Suba V, Ramesh M, Chen JT. *Bacopa monnieri* and their bioactive compounds inferred multi-target treatment strategy for neurological diseases: a cheminformatics and system pharmacology approach. Biomolecules 2020; 10(4): 536.
[http://dx.doi.org/10.3390/biom10040536] [PMID: 32252235]

[29] Chopra RN, Nayar SL, Chopra IC. Glossary of Indian medicinal plants. Council of Scientific & Industrial Research New Delhi 1956.

[30] Singh AK, Solanki S, Prasad D. Antioxidant determination and thin layer chromatography of extract *Withania somnifera, Terminalia arjuna, Bacopa monnieri, Ranunculus sceleratus* and *Acalypha indica*. Eur J Mol Clin Med 2021; 7(11): 4394-408.

[31] Nemetchek MD, Stierle AA, Stierle DB, Lurie DI. The Ayurvedic plant *Bacopa monnieri* inhibits inflammatory pathways in the brain. J Ethnopharmacol 2017; 197: 92-100.
[http://dx.doi.org/10.1016/j.jep.2016.07.073] [PMID: 27473605]

[32] Ganzera M, Gampenrieder J, Pawar RS, Khan IA, Stuppner H. Separation of the major triterpenoid saponins in *Bacopa monnieri* by high-performance liquid chromatography. Anal Chim Acta 2004; 516(1-2): 149-54.
[http://dx.doi.org/10.1016/j.aca.2004.04.002]

[33] Rauf K, Subhan F, Al-Othman AM, Khan I, Zarrelli A, Shah MR. Preclinical profile of bacopasides from *Bacopa monnieri* (BM) as an emerging class of therapeutics for management of chronic pains. Curr Med Chem 2013; 20(8): 1028-37.
[PMID: 23210787]

[34] Kumar GP, Anilakumar KR, Naveen S. Phytochemicals having neuroprotective properties from dietary sources and medicinal herbs. Pharmacogn J 2015; 7(1): 01-17.
[http://dx.doi.org/10.5530/pj.2015.1.1]

[35] Goswami S, Kumar N, Thawani V, Tiwari M, Thawani M. Effect of *Bacopa monnieri* on cognitive functions in Alzheimer's disease patients. International Journal of Collaborative Research on Internal Medicine & Public Health 2011; 3(4): 0.

[36] Saraf MK, Prabhakar S, Khanduja KL, Anand A. *Bacopa monniera* attenuates scopolamine-induced impairment of spatial memory in mice. Evidence-Based Complementary and Alternative Medicine 2011.

[37] Kulkarni O, Mukherjee S, Bhandare R, *et al.* Evaluation of comparative free-radical quenching potential of Brahmi (*Bacopa monnieri*) and Mandookparni (*Centella asiatica*). Ayu 2011; 32(2): 258-64.
[http://dx.doi.org/10.4103/0974-8520.92549] [PMID: 22408313]

[38] Rajan KE, Preethi J, Singh HK. Molecular and functional characterization of *Bacopa monniera*: a retrospective review. Evidence-Based Complementary and Alternative Medicine 2015.

[39] Keswani C, Dilnashin H, Birla H, Singh SP. Unravelling efficient applications of agriculturally important microorganisms for alleviation of induced inter-cellular oxidative stress in crops. Acta Agric Slov 2019; 114(1): 121-30.
[http://dx.doi.org/10.14720/aas.2019.114.1.14]

[40] Keswani C, Dilnashin H, Birla H, Singh S. Re-addressing the commercialization and regulatory hurdles for biopesticides in India. Rhizosphere 2019; 11(100155): 10.1016.

[41] Dubey T, Chinnathambi S. Brahmi (*Bacopa monnieri*): An ayurvedic herb against the Alzheimer's disease. Arch Biochem Biophys 2019; 676: 108153.
[http://dx.doi.org/10.1016/j.abb.2019.108153] [PMID: 31622587]

[42] Singh B, Pandey S, Rumman M, Mahdi AA. Neuroprotective effects of *Bacopa monnieri* in Parkinson's disease model. Metab Brain Dis 2020; 35(3): 517-25.
[http://dx.doi.org/10.1007/s11011-019-00526-w] [PMID: 31834548]

[43] Singh B, Pandey S, Rumman M, *et al.* Neuroprotective and Neurorescue Mode of Action of *Bacopa monnieri* (L.) Wettst in 1-Methyl-4-phenyl-1,2,3,6-tetrahydropyridine-Induced Parkinson's Disease: An *In Silico* and *in vivo* Study. Front Pharmacol 2021; 12: 616413.
[http://dx.doi.org/10.3389/fphar.2021.616413] [PMID: 33796021]

[44] Swathi G, Bhuvaneswar C, Rajendra W. Alterations of cholinergic neurotransmission in rotenone induced parkinson's disease: protective role of *Bacopa monnieri*. Int J Pharm Biol Sci 2013; 3: 286-92.

[45] Jadiya P, Khan A, Sammi SR, Kaur S, Mir SS, Nazir A. Anti-Parkinsonian effects of *Bacopa monnieri*: Insights from transgenic and pharmacological Caenorhabditis elegans models of Parkinson's disease. Biochem Biophys Res Commun 2011; 413(4): 605-10.
[http://dx.doi.org/10.1016/j.bbrc.2011.09.010] [PMID: 21925152]

[46] Limpeanchob N, Jaipan S, Rattanakaruna S, Phrompittayarat W, Ingkaninan K. Neuroprotective effect of *Bacopa monnieri* on beta-amyloid-induced cell death in primary cortical culture. J Ethnopharmacol 2008; 120(1): 112-7.
[http://dx.doi.org/10.1016/j.jep.2008.07.039] [PMID: 18755259]

[47] Priyanka HP, Bala P, Ankisettipalle S, ThyagaRajan S. *Bacopa monnieri* and L-deprenyl differentially enhance the activities of antioxidant enzymes and the expression of tyrosine hydroxylase and nerve growth factor *via* ERK 1/2 and NF-κB pathways in the spleen of female wistar rats. Neurochem Res 2013; 38(1): 141-52.
[http://dx.doi.org/10.1007/s11064-012-0902-2] [PMID: 23076629]

[48] Lakshmi Pravallika P, Krishna Mohan G, Venkateswara Rao K, Shanker K. Biosynthesis, characterization and acute oral toxicity studies of synthesized iron oxide nanoparticles using ethanolic extract of *Centella asiatica* plant. Mater Lett 2019; 236: 256-9.
[http://dx.doi.org/10.1016/j.matlet.2018.10.037]

[49] James J, Dubery I. Pentacyclic triterpenoids from the medicinal herb, *Centella asiatica* (L.) Urban. Molecules 2009; 14(10): 3922-41.
[http://dx.doi.org/10.3390/molecules14103922] [PMID: 19924039]

[50] Sabaragamuwa R, Perera CO, Fedrizzi B. *Centella asiatica* (Gotu kola) as a neuroprotectant and its potential role in healthy ageing. Trends Food Sci Technol 2018; 79: 88-97.
[http://dx.doi.org/10.1016/j.tifs.2018.07.024]

[51] Subathra M, Shila S, Devi MA, Panneerselvam C. Emerging role of *Centella asiatica* in improving age-related neurological antioxidant status. Exp Gerontol 2005; 40(8-9): 707-15.
[http://dx.doi.org/10.1016/j.exger.2005.06.001] [PMID: 16026958]

[52] Veerendra Kumar MH, Gupta YK. Effect of different extracts of *Centella asiatica* on cognition and markers of oxidative stress in rats. J Ethnopharmacol 2002; 79(2): 253-60.
[http://dx.doi.org/10.1016/S0378-8741(01)00394-4] [PMID: 11801389]

[53] Chiroma SM, Baharuldin MTH, Mat Taib CN, *et al.* *Centella asiatica* protects d-galactose/AlCl3 mediated Alzheimer's disease-like rats *via* PP2A/GSK-3β signaling pathway in their Hippocampus. Int J Mol Sci 2019; 20(8): 1871.
[http://dx.doi.org/10.3390/ijms20081871] [PMID: 31014012]

[54] Matthews DG, Caruso M, Murchison CF, *et al.* *Centella asiatica* improves memory and promotes antioxidative signaling in 5XFAD mice. Antioxidants 2019; 8(12): 630.
[http://dx.doi.org/10.3390/antiox8120630] [PMID: 31817977]

[55] Ahmad Rather M, Justin Thenmozhi A, Manivasagam T, Dhivya Bharathi M, Essa MM, Guillemin GJ. Neuroprotective role of Asiatic acid in aluminium chloride induced rat model of Alzheimer's disease. Front Biosci (Schol Ed) 2018; 10(2): 262-75.

[PMID: 28930532]

[56] Teerapattarakan N, Benya-aphikul H, Tansawat R, Wanakhachornkrai O, Tantisira MH, Rodsiri R. Neuroprotective effect of a standardized extract of *Centella asiatica* ECa233 in rotenone-induced parkinsonism rats. Phytomedicine 2018; 44: 65-73.
[http://dx.doi.org/10.1016/j.phymed.2018.04.028] [PMID: 29895494]

[57] Nataraj J, Manivasagam T, Justin Thenmozhi A, Essa MM. Neurotrophic effect of asiatic acid, a triterpene of *Centella asiatica* against chronic 1-methyl 4-phenyl 1, 2, 3, 6-tetrahydropyridine hydrochloride/probenecid mouse model of Parkinson's disease: The role of MAPK, PI3K-Akt-GSK3β and mTOR signalling pathways. Neurochem Res 2017; 42(5): 1354-65.
[http://dx.doi.org/10.1007/s11064-017-2183-2] [PMID: 28181071]

[58] Siddique YH, Naz F, Jyoti S, *et al.* Effect of *Centella asiatica* leaf extract on the dietary supplementation in transgenic Drosophila model of Parkinson's disease. Parkinson's Disease 2014.

[59] Shinomol GK, Muralidhara . Effect of *Centella asiatica* leaf powder on oxidative markers in brain regions of prepubertal mice *in vivo* and its *in vitro* efficacy to ameliorate 3-NPA-induced oxidative stress in mitochondria. Phytomedicine 2008; 15(11): 971-84.
[http://dx.doi.org/10.1016/j.phymed.2008.04.010] [PMID: 18539017]

[60] Shinomol GK, Ravikumar H, Muralidhara . Muralidhara. Prophylaxis with *Centella asiatica* confers protection to prepubertal mice against 3-nitropropionic-acid-induced oxidative stress in brain. Phytother Res 2010; 24(6): 885-92.
[http://dx.doi.org/10.1002/ptr.3042] [PMID: 19943239]

[61] Gupta SC, Sung B, Kim JH, Prasad S, Li S, Aggarwal BB. Multitargeting by turmeric, the golden spice: From kitchen to clinic. Mol Nutr Food Res 2013; 57(9): 1510-28.
[http://dx.doi.org/10.1002/mnfr.201100741] [PMID: 22887802]

[62] Delgado-Vargas F, Paredes-Lopez O. Natural colorants for food and nutraceutical uses. CRC press 2002.
[http://dx.doi.org/10.1201/9781420031713]

[63] Tayyem RF, Heath DD, Al-Delaimy WK, Rock CL. Curcumin content of turmeric and curry powders. Nutr Cancer 2006; 55(2): 126-31.
[http://dx.doi.org/10.1207/s15327914nc5502_2] [PMID: 17044766]

[64] Bagheri H, Ghasemi F, Barreto GE, Rafiee R, Sathyapalan T, Sahebkar A. Effects of curcumin on mitochondria in neurodegenerative diseases. Biofactors 2020; 46(1): 5-20.
[http://dx.doi.org/10.1002/biof.1566] [PMID: 31580521]

[65] Monroy A, Lithgow GJ, Alavez S. Curcumin and neurodegenerative diseases. Biofactors 2013; 39(1): 122-32.
[http://dx.doi.org/10.1002/biof.1063] [PMID: 23303664]

[66] Shanmugam M, Rane G, Kanchi M, *et al.* The multifaceted role of curcumin in cancer prevention and treatment. Molecules 2015; 20(2): 2728-69.
[http://dx.doi.org/10.3390/molecules20022728] [PMID: 25665066]

[67] Ireson CR, Jones DJ, Orr S, *et al.* Metabolism of the cancer chemopreventive agent curcumin in human and rat intestine. Cancer Epidemiol Biomarkers Prev 2002; 11(1): 105-11.
[PMID: 11815407]

[68] Phan TT, See P, Lee ST, Chan SY. Protective effects of curcumin against oxidative damage on skin cells *in vitro*: its implication for wound healing. J Trauma 2001; 51(5): 927-31.
[http://dx.doi.org/10.1097/00005373-200111000-00017] [PMID: 11706342]

[69] Ruby AJ, Kuttan G, Dinesh Babu K, Rajasekharan KN, Kuttan R. Anti-tumour and antioxidant activity of natural curcuminoids. Cancer Lett 1995; 94(1): 79-83.
[http://dx.doi.org/10.1016/0304-3835(95)03827-J] [PMID: 7621448]

[70] Nurrulhidayah A, Rafi M, Lukitaningsih E, Widodo H, Rohman A, Windarsih A. Review on *in vitro*

anti-oxidant activities of *Curcuma* species commonly used as herbal components in Indonesia. Food Res 2020; 4(2): 286-93.

[71]   Aggarwal BB, Kumar A, Bharti AC. Anticancer potential of curcumin: preclinical and clinical studies. Anticancer research 2003; 23(1/A): 363-98.

[72]   Hirsch EC, Brandel JP, Galle P, Javoy-Agid F, Agid Y. Iron and aluminum increase in the substantia nigra of patients with Parkinson's disease: an X-ray microanalysis. J Neurochem 1991; 56(2): 446-51.
        [http://dx.doi.org/10.1111/j.1471-4159.1991.tb08170.x] [PMID: 1988548]

[73]   Exley C. Aluminium and Alzheimer's Disease: The science that describes the link. Elsevier 2001.

[74]   Platt B, Fiddler G, Riedel G, Henderson Z. Aluminium toxicity in the rat brain: histochemical and immunocytochemical evidence. Brain Res Bull 2001; 55(2): 257-67.
        [http://dx.doi.org/10.1016/S0361-9230(01)00511-1] [PMID: 11470325]

[75]   Jangra A, Kasbe P, Pandey SN, *et al.* Hesperidin and silibinin ameliorate aluminum-induced neurotoxicity: modulation of anti-oxidants and inflammatory cytokines level in mice hippocampus. Biol Trace Elem Res 2015; 168(2): 462-71.
        [http://dx.doi.org/10.1007/s12011-015-0375-7] [PMID: 26018497]

[76]   Inan-Eroglu E, Ayaz A. Is aluminum exposure a risk factor for neurological disorders? Journal of research in medical sciences: The official journal of Isfahan University of Medical Sciences 2018; 33.

[77]   Banji D, Banji OJ, Srinivas K. Neuroprotective Effect of Turmeric Extract in Combination with Its Essential Oil and Enhanced Brain Bioavailability in an Animal Model. Bio Med Research International 2021.
        [http://dx.doi.org/10.1155/2021/6645720]

[78]   Mukhopadhyay CD, Ruidas B, Chaudhury S. Role of curcumin in treatment of Alzheimer disease. Int J Neurorehabilitation 2017; 4(274): 2376-0281.1000274.
        [http://dx.doi.org/10.4172/2376-0281.1000274]

[79]   Alamro AA, Alsulami EA, Almutlaq M, Alghamedi A, Alokail M, Haq SH. Therapeutic potential of vitamin d and curcumin in an *in vitro* model of alzheimer disease. J Cent Nerv Syst Dis 2020; 12.
        [http://dx.doi.org/10.1177/1179573520924311] [PMID: 32528227]

[80]   Lin L, Li C, Zhang D, Yuan M, Chen C, Li M. Synergic effects of berberine and curcumin on improving cognitive function in an Alzheimer's disease mouse model. Neurochem Res 2020; 45(5): 1130-41.
        [http://dx.doi.org/10.1007/s11064-020-02992-6] [PMID: 32080784]

[81]   Ansari A, Maffioletti E, Milanesi E, *et al.* PharmaCog Consortium. miR-146a and miR-181a are involved in the progression of mild cognitive impairment to Alzheimer's disease. Neurobiol Aging 2019; 82: 102-9.
        [http://dx.doi.org/10.1016/j.neurobiolaging.2019.06.005] [PMID: 31437718]

[82]   Gong J, Sun D. Study on the mechanism of curcumin to reduce the inflammatory response of temporal lobe in Alzheimer's disease by regulating miR-146a. Minerva Med 2020.
        [PMID: 32207596]

[83]   Wang XS, Zhang ZR, Zhang MM, Sun MX, Wang WW, Xie CL. Neuroprotective properties of curcumin in toxin-base animal models of Parkinson's disease: a systematic experiment literatures review. BMC Complement Altern Med 2017; 17(1): 412.
        [http://dx.doi.org/10.1186/s12906-017-1922-x] [PMID: 28818104]

[84]   Motawi TK, Sadik NAH, Hamed MA, Ali SA, Khalil WKB, Ahmed YR. Potential therapeutic effects of antagonizing adenosine A_{2A} receptor, curcumin and niacin in rotenone-induced Parkinson's disease mice model. Mol Cell Biochem 2020; 465(1-2): 89-102.
        [http://dx.doi.org/10.1007/s11010-019-03670-0] [PMID: 31820278]

[85]   Londhe V. Role of garlic (*Allium sativum*) in various diseases: An overview. angiogenesis 2011.

[86]   Kosuge Y. Neuroprotective mechanisms of *S*-allyl-L-cysteine in neurological disease. Exp Ther Med 2020; 19(2): 1565-9.
[PMID: 32010340]

[87]   El-Saber Batiha G, Magdy Beshbishy A, G Wasef L, *et al.* Chemical Constituents and Pharmacological Activities of Garlic (*Allium sativum* L.): A Review. Nutrients 2020; 12(3): 872.
[http://dx.doi.org/10.3390/nu12030872] [PMID: 32213941]

[88]   Rahman K. Historical perspective on garlic and cardiovascular disease. J Nutr 2001; 131(3): 977S-9S.
[http://dx.doi.org/10.1093/jn/131.3.977S] [PMID: 11238800]

[89]   Al-Snafi AE. Pharmacological effects of Allium species grown in Iraq. An overview International Journal of Pharmaceutical and health care Research 2013; 1(4): 132-47.

[90]   Souza GA, Ebaid GX, Seiva FR, *et al.* N-acetylcysteine an Allium plant compound improves high-sucrose diet-induced obesity and related effects. Evidence-Based Complementary and Alternative Medicine 2011.

[91]   Liu Y, Yan J, Han X, Hu W. Garlic-derived compound S-allylmercaptocysteine (SAMC) is active against anaplastic thyroid cancer cell line 8305C (HPACC). Technol Health Care 2015; 23(s1) (Suppl. 1): S89-93.
[http://dx.doi.org/10.3233/thc-150936] [PMID: 26410334]

[92]   Nile SH, Park SW. Chromatographic analysis, antioxidant, anti-inflammatory, and xanthine oxidase inhibitory activities of ginger extracts and its reference compounds. Ind Crops Prod 2015; 70: 238-44.
[http://dx.doi.org/10.1016/j.indcrop.2015.03.033]

[93]   Nillert N, Pannangrong W, Welbat J, Chaijaroonkhanarak W, Sripanidkulchai K, Sripanidkulchai B. Neuroprotective effects of aged garlic extract on cognitive dysfunction and neuroinflammation induced by β-amyloid in rats. Nutrients 2017; 9(1): 24.
[http://dx.doi.org/10.3390/nu9010024] [PMID: 28054940]

[94]   Chauhan NB. Anti-amyloidogenic effect of *Allium sativum* in Alzheimer's transgenic model Tg2576. J Herb Pharmacother 2003; 3(1): 95-107.
[http://dx.doi.org/10.1080/J157v03n01_05] [PMID: 15277073]

[95]   Chauhan NB. Effect of aged garlic extract on APP processing and tau phosphorylation in Alzheimer's transgenic model Tg2576. J Ethnopharmacol 2006; 108(3): 385-94.
[http://dx.doi.org/10.1016/j.jep.2006.05.030] [PMID: 16842945]

[96]   Cassarino DS, Bennett JP Jr. An evaluation of the role of mitochondria in neurodegenerative diseases: mitochondrial mutations and oxidative pathology, protective nuclear responses, and cell death in neurodegeneration. Brain Res Brain Res Rev 1999; 29(1): 1-25.
[http://dx.doi.org/10.1016/S0165-0173(98)00046-0] [PMID: 9974149]

[97]   Ishige K, Chen Q, Sagara Y, Schubert D. The activation of dopamine D4 receptors inhibits oxidative stress-induced nerve cell death. J Neurosci 2001; 21(16): 6069-76.
[http://dx.doi.org/10.1523/JNEUROSCI.21-16-06069.2001] [PMID: 11487630]

[98]   Miranda S, Opazo C, Larrondo LF, *et al.* The role of oxidative stress in the toxicity induced by amyloid β-peptide in Alzheimer's disease. Prog Neurobiol 2000; 62(6): 633-48.
[http://dx.doi.org/10.1016/S0301-0082(00)00015-0] [PMID: 10880853]

[99]   Ito Y, Ito M, Takagi N, Saito H, Ishige K. Neurotoxicity induced by amyloid β-peptide and ibotenic acid in organotypic hippocampal cultures: protection by S-allyl-l-cysteine, a garlic compound. Brain Res 2003; 985(1): 98-107.
[http://dx.doi.org/10.1016/S0006-8993(03)03173-1] [PMID: 12957372]

[100]   Sripanidkulchai B. Benefits of aged garlic extract on Alzheimer's disease: Possible mechanisms of action. Exp Ther Med 2020; 19(2): 1560-4.
[PMID: 32010339]

[101] Rojas P, Serrano-García N, Medina-Campos ON, Pedraza-Chaverri J, Maldonado PD, Ruiz-Sánchez E. S-Allylcysteine, a garlic compound, protects against oxidative stress in 1-methyl-4-phenylpyridinium-induced parkinsonism in mice. J Nutr Biochem 2011; 22(10): 937-44.
[http://dx.doi.org/10.1016/j.jnutbio.2010.08.005] [PMID: 21190833]

[102] Bigham M, Mohammadipour A, Hosseini M, Malvandi AM, Ebrahimzadeh-Bideskan A. Neuroprotective effects of garlic extract on dopaminergic neurons of substantia nigra in a rat model of Parkinson's disease: motor and non-motor outcomes. Metab Brain Dis 2021; 36(5): 927-37.
[http://dx.doi.org/10.1007/s11011-021-00705-8] [PMID: 33656625]

[103] Cao X, Cao L, Ding L, Bian JS. A new hope for a devastating disease: hydrogen sulfide in Parkinson's disease. Mol Neurobiol 2018; 55(5): 3789-99.
[PMID: 28536975]

[104] Mostafa DK, El Azhary NM, Nasra RA. The hydrogen sulfide releasing compounds ATB-346 and diallyl trisulfide attenuate streptozotocin-induced cognitive impairment, neuroinflammation, and oxidative stress in rats: involvement of asymmetric dimethylarginine. Can J Physiol Pharmacol 2016; 94(7): 699-708.
[http://dx.doi.org/10.1139/cjpp-2015-0316] [PMID: 27088818]

[105] Rao PSS, Midde N, Miller D, Chauhan S, Kumar A, Kumar S. M Midde N, D Miller D, Chauhan S, Kumar A, Kumar S. Diallyl sulfide: potential use in novel therapeutic interventions in alcohol, drugs, and disease mediated cellular toxicity by targeting cytochrome P450 2E1. Curr Drug Metab 2015; 16(6): 486-503.
[http://dx.doi.org/10.2174/1389200216666150812123554] [PMID: 26264202]

[106] Liu H, Mao P, Wang J, Wang T, Xie CH. Allicin protects PC12 cells against 6-OHDA-induced oxidative stress and mitochondrial dysfunction *via* regulating mitochondrial dynamics. Cell Physiol Biochem 2015; 36(3): 966-79.
[http://dx.doi.org/10.1159/000430271] [PMID: 26087780]

[107] Mathew B, Biju R. Neuroprotective effects of garlic a review. Libyan J Med 2008; 3(1): 23-33.
[PMID: 21499478]

[108] Akbar S. *Terminalia chebula* Retz.(*Combretaceae*). Handbook of 200 medicinal plants. Springer 2020; pp. 1779-93.
[http://dx.doi.org/10.1007/978-3-030-16807-0_184]

[109] Nigam M, Mishra AP, Adhikari-Devkota A, *et al.* Fruits of *Terminalia chebula* Retz.: A review on traditional uses, bioactive chemical constituents and pharmacological activities. Phytother Res 2020; 34(10): 2518-33.
[http://dx.doi.org/10.1002/ptr.6702] [PMID: 32307775]

[110] Wang W, Ali Z, Li XC, Shen Y, Khan I. Triterpenoids from two *Terminalia* species. Planta Med 2010; 76(15): 1751-4.
[http://dx.doi.org/10.1055/s-0030-1249809] [PMID: 20383817]

[111] Bajpai M, Pande A, Tewari SK, Prakash D. Phenolic contents and antioxidant activity of some food and medicinal plants. Int J Food Sci Nutr 2005; 56(4): 287-91.
[http://dx.doi.org/10.1080/09637480500146606] [PMID: 16096138]

[112] Han Q, Song J, Qiao C, Wong L, Xu H. Preparative isolation of hydrolysable tannins chebulagic acid and chebulinic acid from *Terminalia chebula* by high-speed counter-current chromatography. J Sep Sci 2006; 29(11): 1653-7.
[http://dx.doi.org/10.1002/jssc.200600089] [PMID: 16922284]

[113] Juang LJ, Sheu SJ. Chemical identification of the sources of commercial fructus chebulae. Phytochem Anal 2005; 16(4): 246-51.
[http://dx.doi.org/10.1002/pca.823] [PMID: 16042149]

[114] Shen YC, Juan CW, Lin CS, Chen CC, Chang CL. Neuroprotective effect of *Terminalia chebula*

extracts and ellagic acid in pc12 cells. Afr J Tradit Complement Altern Med 2017; 14(4): 22-30.
[http://dx.doi.org/10.21010/ajtcam.v14i4.3] [PMID: 28638863]

[115] Lakshmi K, Karishma S, Sekhar NC, Babu NA, Kumar BN. *Terminalia chebula* Retz improve memory and learning in Alzheimer's Model:(Experimental Study in Rat). Research. J Pharm Technol 2018; 11(11): 4888-91.

[116] Jha AB, Panchal SS, Shah A. Ellagic acid: Insights into its neuroprotective and cognitive enhancement effects in sporadic Alzheimer's disease. Pharmacol Biochem Behav 2018; 175: 33-46.
[http://dx.doi.org/10.1016/j.pbb.2018.08.007] [PMID: 30171934]

[117] Sarkaki A, Farbood Y, Dolatshahi M, Mansouri SMT, Khodadadi A. Neuroprotective effects of ellagic acid in a rat model of Parkinson's disease. Acta Med Iran 2016; 54(8): 494-502.
[PMID: 27701719]

[118] Farbood Y, Sarkaki A, Dolatshahi M, Taqhi Mansouri SM, Khodadadi A. Ellagic acid protects the brain against 6-hydroxydopamine induced neuroinflammation in a rat model of Parkinson's disease. Basic Clin Neurosci 2015; 6(2): 83-9.
[PMID: 27307952]

[119] Baluchnejadmojarad T, Rabiee N, Zabihnejad S, Roghani M. Ellagic acid exerts protective effect in intrastriatal 6-hydroxydopamine rat model of Parkinson's disease: Possible involvement of ERβ/Nrf2/HO-1 signaling. Brain Res 2017; 1662: 23-30.
[http://dx.doi.org/10.1016/j.brainres.2017.02.021] [PMID: 28238669]

[120] Kalam MA, Khanday S, Salim S, Nida K, Ahmad Amalkangi. (*Celastrus paniculatus* Wild.): Neuropharmacological properties in perspective of Unani medicine and pharmacological studies. Review 2018.

[121] Maurya H, Arya RK, Belwal T, Rana M, Kumar A. *Celastrus paniculatus*. Naturally Occurring Chemicals Against Alzheimer's Disease. Elsevier 2021; pp. 425-35.
[http://dx.doi.org/10.1016/B978-0-12-819212-2.00036-0]

[122] Avinash DK, NandaWaman S. Phytochemical constituents of leaves of *Celastrus paniculatus* wild: Endangered medicinal plant. Inter J Pharmacog Phytochem Res 2014; 6: 792-4.

[123] Bhanumathy M, Chandrasekar S, Chandur U, Somasundaram T. Phyto-pharmacology of *Celastrus paniculatus*: an Overview. Int J Pharm Sci Drug Res 2010; 2(3): 176-81.

[124] Shashank D, Rajendra S, Mistry A. An overview of phytoconstituents and pharmacological activities of *Celastrus paniculatus* willd. J Pharm Res 2018; 16(4): 307-13.

[125] Kumar MHV, Gupta YK. Antioxidant property of *Celastrus paniculatus* Willd.: a possible mechanism in enhancing cognition. Phytomedicine 2002; 9(4): 302-11.
[http://dx.doi.org/10.1078/0944-7113-00136] [PMID: 12120811]

[126] Jakka AL. A study on nootropic activity of Celastrus paniculata willd whole plant methanolic extract in rats. Asian J Pharm Clin Res 2016; 9: 336-41.

[127] Jadhav KS, Marathe PA, Rege NN, Raut SB, Parekar RR. Effect of Jyotiṣmatī seed oil on spatial and fear memory using scopolamine induced amnesia in mice. Anc Sci Life 2015; 34(3): 130-3.
[http://dx.doi.org/10.4103/0257-7941.157149] [PMID: 26120226]

[128] Anjaneyulu J, R V, Godbole A. Differential effect of Ayurvedic nootropics on *C. elegans* models of Parkinson's disease. J Ayurveda Integr Med 2020; 11(4): 440-7.
[http://dx.doi.org/10.1016/j.jaim.2020.07.006] [PMID: 32978047]

[129] Malik J, Karan M, Dogra R. Ameliorating effect of *Celastrus paniculatus* standardized extract and its fractions on 3-nitropropionic acid induced neuronal damage in rats: possible antioxidant mechanism. Pharm Biol 2017; 55(1): 980-90.
[http://dx.doi.org/10.1080/13880209.2017.1285945] [PMID: 28164735]

[130] El-Saber Batiha G, Magdy Beshbishy A, El-Mleeh A, Abdel-Daim MM, Prasad Devkota H.

Traditional uses, bioactive chemical constituents, and pharmacological and toxicological activities of *Glycyrrhiza glabra* L.(*Fabaceae*). Biomolecules 2020; 10(3): E352.
[http://dx.doi.org/10.3390/biom10030352] [PMID: 32106571]

[131] Sharma V, Katiyar A, Agrawal R. Glycyrrhiza glabra: chemistry and pharmacological activity. Sweeteners 2018; p. 87.

[132] Ohnishi M, Katsuki H, Fukutomi C, *et al.* HMGB1 inhibitor glycyrrhizin attenuates intracerebral hemorrhage-induced injury in rats. Neuropharmacology 2011; 61(5-6): 975-80.
[http://dx.doi.org/10.1016/j.neuropharm.2011.06.026] [PMID: 21752338]

[133] Paudel YN, Angelopoulou E, Semple B, Piperi C, Othman I, Shaikh MF. Potential neuroprotective effect of the HMGB1 inhibitor Glycyrrhizin in neurological disorders. ACS Chem Neurosci 2020; 11(4): 485-500.
[http://dx.doi.org/10.1021/acschemneuro.9b00640] [PMID: 31972087]

[134] Sathyamoorthy Y, Kaliappan K, Nambi P, Radhakrishnan R. Glycyrrhizic acid renders robust neuroprotection in rodent model of vascular dementia by controlling oxidative stress and curtailing cytochrome-c release. Nutr Neurosci 2020; 23(12): 955-70.
[http://dx.doi.org/10.1080/1028415X.2019.1580935] [PMID: 30794076]

[135] Ban JY, Park HK, Kim SK. Effect of glycyrrhizic acid on scopolamine-induced cognitive impairment in mice. Int Neurourol J 2020; 24 (Suppl. 1): S48-55.
[http://dx.doi.org/10.5213/inj.2040154.077] [PMID: 32482057]

[136] Wang W, Chen X, Zhang J, *et al.* Glycyrrhizin attenuates isoflurane-induced cognitive deficits in neonatal rats *via* its anti-inflammatory activity. Neuroscience 2016; 316: 328-36.
[http://dx.doi.org/10.1016/j.neuroscience.2015.11.001] [PMID: 26550949]

[137] Dhingra D, Parle M, Kulkarni SK. Memory enhancing activity of *Glycyrrhiza glabra* in mice. J Ethnopharmacol 2004; 91(2-3): 361-5.
[http://dx.doi.org/10.1016/j.jep.2004.01.016] [PMID: 15120462]

[138] Cui YM, Ao MZ, Li W, Yu LJ. Effect of glabridin from *Glycyrrhiza glabra* on learning and memory in mice. Planta Med 2008; 74(4): 377-80.
[http://dx.doi.org/10.1055/s-2008-1034319] [PMID: 18484526]

[139] Lev N, Melamed E, Offen D. Apoptosis and Parkinson's disease. Prog Neuropsychopharmacol Biol Psychiatry 2003; 27(2): 245-50.
[http://dx.doi.org/10.1016/S0278-5846(03)00019-8] [PMID: 12657363]

[140] Karthikkeyan G, Najar MA, Pervaje R, Pervaje SK, Modi PK, Prasad TSK. Identification of Molecular Network Associated with Neuroprotective Effects of Yashtimadhu (*Glycyrrhiza glabra* L.) by Quantitative Proteomics of Rotenone-Induced Parkinson's Disease Model. ACS Omega 2020; 5(41): 26611-25.
[http://dx.doi.org/10.1021/acsomega.0c03420] [PMID: 33110989]

[141] Petramfar P, Hajari F, Yousefi G, Azadi S, Hamedi A. Efficacy of oral administration of licorice as an adjunct therapy on improving the symptoms of patients with Parkinson's disease, A randomized double blinded clinical trial. J Ethnopharmacol 2020; 247: 112226.
[http://dx.doi.org/10.1016/j.jep.2019.112226] [PMID: 31574343]

[142] Kasture SB, Barhate SA, Mohan M. *Glycyrrhiza glabra* as an adjuvant in treatment of Parkinsonism and depression. Planta Med 2008; 74(9): PA310.
[http://dx.doi.org/10.1055/s-0028-1084308]

[143] Karthikkeyan G, Pervaje R, Pervaje SK, Prasad TSK, Modi PK. Prevention of MEK-ERK-1/2 hyper-activation underlines the neuroprotective effect of *Glycyrrhiza glabra* L. (Yashtimadhu) against rotenone-induced cellular and molecular aberrations. J Ethnopharmacol 2021; 274: 114025.
[http://dx.doi.org/10.1016/j.jep.2021.114025] [PMID: 33775804]

[144] Rathore AS, Birla H, Singh SS, *et al.* Epigenetic Modulation in Parkinson's Disease and Potential

Treatment Therapies. Neurochem Res 2021; 46(7): 1618-26.
[http://dx.doi.org/10.1007/s11064-021-03334-w] [PMID: 33900517]

[145] Singh S, Rai S, Birla H, Eds., *et al.* Chlorogenic acid protects against MPTP induced neurotoxicity in parkinsonian mice model *via* its anti-apoptotic activity. J Neurochem. Hoboken 07030-5774, NJ USA: Wiley 111 River St 2019.

[146] Singh SS, Rai SN, Birla H, *et al.* Neuroprotective effect of chlorogenic acid on mitochondrial dysfunction-mediated apoptotic death of DA neurons in a Parkinsonian mouse model. Oxid Med Cell Longev 2020; 2020: 1-14.
[http://dx.doi.org/10.1155/2020/6571484] [PMID: 32566093]

[147] Devi SA, Ganjewala D. Antimicrobial activity of *Acorus calamus* (L.) rhizome and leaf extract. Acta Biol Szeged 2009; 53(1): 45-9.

[148] Abu Bakar MF, Mohamed M, Rahmat A, Fry J. Phytochemicals and antioxidant activity of different parts of bambangan (*Mangifera pajang*) and tarap (*Artocarpus odoratissimus*). Food Chem 2009; 113(2): 479-83.
[http://dx.doi.org/10.1016/j.foodchem.2008.07.081]

[149] Umamaheshwari N, Rekha A. Sweet flag: (*Acarus calamus*) - An incredible medicinal herb. J Pharmacogn Phytochem 2018; 7(6): 15-22.

[150] Loying R, Gogoi R, Sarma N, *et al.* Chemical compositions, in-vitro anti-oxidant, anti-microbial, anti-inflammatory and cytotoxic activities of essential oil of *Acorus calamus* L. rhizome from North-East India. J Essent Oil-Bear Plants 2019; 22(5): 1299-312.
[http://dx.doi.org/10.1080/0972060X.2019.1696236]

[151] Reddy S, Rao G, Shetty B, Hn G. Effects of *acorus calamus* rhizome extract on the neuromodulatory system in restraint stress male rats. Turk Neurosurg 2015; 25(3): 425-31.
[PMID: 26037183]

[152] Mokhtarian A, Esfandiari E, Ghanadian M, Rashidi B, Vatankhah A. The effects of *Acorus calamus* L. in preventing memory loss, anxiety, and oxidative stress on lipopolysaccharide-induced neuroinflammation rat models. Int J Prev Med 2018; 9(1): 85.
[http://dx.doi.org/10.4103/ijpvm.IJPVM_75_18] [PMID: 30450168]

[153] Keswani C. Bioeconomy for Sustainable Development. Springer 2020.
[http://dx.doi.org/10.1007/978-981-13-9431-7]

[154] Keswani C. Agri-based Bioeconomy: Reintegrating Trans-disciplinary Research and Sustainable Development Goals. CRC Press 2021.
[http://dx.doi.org/10.1201/9781003033394]

[155] Mikami M, Takuya O, Yoshino Y, *et al. Acorus calamus* extract and its component α-asarone attenuate murine hippocampal neuronal cell death induced by L -glutamate and tunicamycin. Biosci Biotechnol Biochem 2021; 85(3): 493-501.
[http://dx.doi.org/10.1093/bbb/zbaa071] [PMID: 33589895]

[156] Huang LP, Deng MZ, He YP, Fang YQ. β-asarone and levodopa co-administration protects against 6-hydroxydopamine-induced damage in parkinsonian rat mesencephalon by regulating autophagy: down-expression Beclin-1 and light chain 3B and up-expression P62. Clin Exp Pharmacol Physiol 2015; 42(3): 269-77.
[http://dx.doi.org/10.1111/1440-1681.12344] [PMID: 25424835]

[157] Kim BW, Koppula S, Kumar H, *et al.* α-Asarone attenuates microglia-mediated neuroinflammation by inhibiting NF kappa B activation and mitigates MPTP-induced behavioral deficits in a mouse model of Parkinson's disease. Neuropharmacology 2015; 97: 46-57.
[http://dx.doi.org/10.1016/j.neuropharm.2015.04.037] [PMID: 25983275]

[158] Ning B, Deng M, Zhang Q, Wang N, Fang Y. β-Asarone inhibits IRE1/XBP1 endoplasmic reticulum stress pathway in 6-OHDA-induced parkinsonian rats. Neurochem Res 2016; 41(8): 2097-101.

[http://dx.doi.org/10.1007/s11064-016-1922-0] [PMID: 27097550]

[159] Zhang QS, Wang ZH, Zhang JL, Duan YL, Li GF, Zheng DL. Beta-asarone protects against MPTP-induced Parkinson's disease *via* regulating long non-coding RNA MALAT1 and inhibiting α-synuclein protein expression. Biomed Pharmacother 2016; 83: 153-9.
[http://dx.doi.org/10.1016/j.biopha.2016.06.017] [PMID: 27470562]

[160] Adarlo LET, Andal MAM, Magpayo FLM, Reyes JMM, Alejandro DCB. In *Vitro* Acetyl cholinesterase Inhibition of *Acorus calamus* (Lubigan) Rhizome Fractions for Alzheimer's Disease.

[161] Khalili M, Hamzeh F. Effects of active constituents of *Crocus sativus* L., crocin on streptozocin-induced model of sporadic Alzheimer's disease in male rats. Iran Biomed J 2010; 14(1-2): 59-65.
[PMID: 20683499]

[162] Geromichalos GD, Lamari FN, Papandreou MA, *et al.* Saffron as a source of novel acetylcholinesterase inhibitors: molecular docking and *in vitro* enzymatic studies. J Agric Food Chem 2012; 60(24): 6131-8.
[http://dx.doi.org/10.1021/jf300589c] [PMID: 22655699]

[163] Mani V, Parle M. Memory-enhancing activity of *Coriandrum sativum* in rats. Pharmacologyonline 2009; 2: 827-39.

[164] Raditya MN, Bagus AMM, Kustiati U, Wihadmadyatami H, Kusindarta DL. Data of the expression of serotonin in alzheimer's disease (AD) rat model under treatment of ethanolic extract *ocimum sanctum* linn. Data Brief 2020; 30: 105654.
[http://dx.doi.org/10.1016/j.dib.2020.105654] [PMID: 32395598]

CHAPTER 6

Neuroprotective Alkaloids: Neuromodulatory Action on Neurotransmitter Pathway

Pratibha Thakur[1,*]

[1] *Department of Bioscience, Endocrinology Unit, Barkatullah University, Bhopal- 462026 (M.P.), India*

Abstract: Equilibrium in excitatory and inhibitory neurotransmitter signal transmission is necessary for the proper functioning of the brain, and alteration can stimulate the negative feedback mechanism that causes various neuropathogenesis. Disturbances like oxidative stress and alteration in the metabolism of neurotransmitters like γ-aminobutyric acid (GABA), acetylcholine (Ach), serotonin, dopamine, and glutamate, are important factors for the progression of neurodegenerative disorder (NDDs). Plant alkaloids have the potential to modulate the neurotransmitter signal transmission in the central nervous system and can provide a better alternative to the synthetic molecule. In the present chapter, we summarize the potential efficacy of plant alkaloids *via* functioning as anti-oxidant, monoamine oxidase (MAO) inhibitor, glutamate receptors-N-methyl-D-aspartate (NMDA) antagonist, acetylcholinesterase (AcHE) inhibitor and shows potential therapeutic effects against NDDs.

Keywords: Alkaloids, Central nervous system, Neurodegenerative disorder, Neurotransmitter.

INTRODUCTION

Different conditions affecting the nervous system, and nerve cells due to degeneration in the structure and functioning of the nervous system, are described under the superordinate phrase "neurodegenerative diseases" (NDDs). Studies from different clinical and experimental investigations showed that the alteration in physical and chemical properties of protein results in aggregation of these proteins and consequently degeneration in the structure and function of neurons [1 - 7]. The main symptoms of the NDDs are problems with movement (ataxia) or mental functioning (dementia), or both, causing morbidity and fatality. The most common neuropsychiatric and neurological disorders are schizophrenia, anxiety, depression, Alzheimer's disease (AD), Huntington's disease (HD), Parkinson's

* **Corresponding author Pratibha Thakur:** Department of Bioscience, Endocrinology Unit, Barkatullah University, Bhopal- 462026 (M.P.), India; E-mail: pratibha000136@gmail.com

disease (PD), Amyotrophic lateral sclerosis (ALS), spinocerebellar ataxia (SCA), spinal muscular atrophy (SMA) and seizure disorder [8]. The available treatment for these diseases gives only symptomatic relief to the patient, therefore, there is a need to explore actual treatment. Since prehistoric times, herbal medicine has been used in traditional systems by different cultures throughout the world. As per the world health organization (WHO) recommendation, any plant which contains a bioactive component with medicinal properties can be used directly or indirectly to cure the disease as well as drug synthesis and design [9]. The traditional system of herbal medicine is still being used for the treatment of many diseases, especially in the rural area, and is in high demand due to various factors like the high cost of modern medicine, inadequate supply of drugs, rise in population, and side effects of synthetic drugs. 50% of modern medicines are derived from plants, and approximately 391,000 species of plants are present on earth, but only limited have been highlighted with medicinal properties [10]. In the past decades, researchers have focused on the continuous failure of synthetic drugs in various clinical trials [11 - 16]. A medicinal plant contains different chemical compositions, including alkaloids, phenolics, flavonoids, terpenoids, steroids, saponins, and glycosides with a broad range of biological activities like anti-oxidative, anti-carcinogenic, anti-bacterial, anti-thrombotic, anti-inflammatory, and regulate blood pressure, blood cholesterol, and blood sugar concentration [17 - 19]. The multiple components of herbal medicines and multiple targeting natures of NDDs suggest that herbal medicines may achieve an effective clinical outcome by dealing with the complex mechanism of NDDs. Among many functions, bioactive plant compound shows positive effects on the central nervous system by neuromodulatory action on some neurotransmitter [20 - 25]. Studies from the clinical and non-clinical investigation showed that some NDDs, and mood affective disorders like AD, and PD are caused by an alteration in glutamate, γ-aminobutyric acid (GABA), or acetylcholine (Ach) [20, 21, 26, 27]. Along with this, Ach is also responsible for the cholinergic signaling in the central nervous system (CNS), as well as associated with β-amyloid (Aβ) plaque distribution in the brain [28]. There are a number of bioactive compounds of plants with neuroprotective properties, and alkaloids are one of them with antidepressant properties by dopaminergic agonists and inhibition of the acetylcholinesterase (AChE), monoamine oxidase (MAO), and glutamate toxicity [8, 20, 29].

SOURCE STRUCTURE AND CLASSIFICATION OF ALKALOIDS

Alkaloids are one of the important groups of phytoconstituents containing carbon, hydrogen, nitrogen, and oxygen and naturally occur in plants [20]. The nitrogen present in the alkaloid molecule ring system causes the alkalinity of these compounds and is classified into different classes like indoles, quinolines, isoquinolines, pyridines, pyrrolidines, pyrrolizidines, steroids, tropanes, and terpenoids. Alkaloids are also classified on the basis of the family of plant species in which they occur, like opium alkaloids present in the opium poppy (*Papaver somniferum*) [30]. In pure form, alkaloids are colorless, odorless, and crystalline solid, and to date, more than 3000 alkaloids have been explored in over different 4000 plant species. Furthermore, the study showed that several families of plants like Solanaceae, Ranunculaceae, Papaveraceae, and Amaryllidaceae are rich in different types of alkaloids [31].

Alkaloids show various pharmacological potential in modern medicine, such as anti-hyperglycemic, analgesic, anticancer, antibacterial, and antiarrhythmic, but are only specifically used in modern medicine [32]. Along with this, some alkaloids like cocaine, caffeine, and nicotine show stimulant effect in CNS, and psilocin exhibits a psychotropic effect. Alkaloids show different neuroprotective properties against NDDs through inhibition of AChE enzyme kinetics [33], the elevation of inhibitory neurotransmitters, *i.e.*, GABA [33], and much more, as described in Table **1**.

Table 1. Different classes of alkaloids and effective in neurodegenerative disorders.

Alkaloid	Class	Source	Mechanism	Disease	Refs.
Aporphine alkaloids	Nantenine	*Nandina domestica*	Inhibit the Ca^{2+} influx AChE Inhibitor	Epilepsy AD	[34, 35]
Isoquinoline alkaloids	Galantamine	*Galanthus nivalis* *Leucojum aestivum* *Galanthus woronovii*	AChE Inhibitor, allosteric modulation of nicotinic Ach receptor	PD	[36]
	Berberine	*Berberis aristata* *Berberis aquifolium* *Hydrastis canadensis* *Coptis chinensis*	AChE inhibitor, NMDA inhibitor, up-regulation of autophagic function	Epilepsy HD, PD, AD	[37]
	Salsoline	*Salsola oppositefolia*	AChE inhibitor	AD	[38]
	Morphine	*Papaver somniferum*	Anti-oxidant, increase GABA	AD	[31, 39]
	Montanine	*Hippeastrum vittatum*	AChE inhibitor	AD, Epilepsy	[40]
Indole Alkaloids	Geissospermine	*Geissospermum vellosii*	AChE inhibitor	AD	[41 - 44]

(Table 1) cont.....

Alkaloid	Class	Source	Mechanism	Disease	Refs.
Piperidine alkaloids	Piperine	*Piper nigrum* *Piper longum*	MAO inhibitor, Anti-oxidant, AcHE inhibitor	PD, AD Epilepsy	[45 - 47]
	Lobeline	*Lobelia inflate*	Nicotinic agonist, MAO-B inhibitor	AD, PD	[48, 49]
Pyrroloindole alkaloids	Physostigmine	*Physostigma venosum*	AcHE inhibitor	AD, PD	[50 - 53]
Pyrindine alkaloids	Nicotine	*Nicotiana tobacum*	Anti-amyloid Nicotinic agonist	AD, PD	[54, 55]
	Arecoline	*Areca catechunut*	Muscarinic receptor agonist	AD Schizophrenia	[56, 57]
Indole β-carboline	Harmine	*Peganum harmala*	AcHE inhibitor	PD, AD	[58, 59]
Methylxanthine derivatives	Caffeine	*Coffea arabica*	Inhibits Aβ aggregation	PD, AD	[60, 61]
Vinca alkaloids	Vinpocetine	*Vinca minor*	Anti-inflammatory	Hypoxia & Ischemia	[62, 63]
Lycopodium alkaloids	Huperzine A	*Huperzia serrata*	Anti-oxidant, AcHE inhibitor, Inhibits NMDA & glutamate toxicity	AD	[64, 65]

NEUROTRANSMITTERS

Neurotransmitters are chemical messengers synthesized from an amino acid and transmit the signals between the neurons, and neuromuscular junctions [66, 67]. Acetylcholine is synthesized from serine, γ-amino butyric acid from glutamate, dopamine from L-tyrosine/L-phenylalanine, and serotonin from L-tryptophan [68, 69]. These are the main neurotransmitters, and their alteration is an important factor in the pathogenesis of NDDs, but alkaloids have shown the potential to treat NDDs by the modulation of neurotransmitters in different clinical, and preclinical studies.

Cholinergic Signaling and Alkaloids

Cholinergic neurons, *i.e.*, Acetylcholine (Ach) producing neurons, play an important role in the pathogenesis of NDDs, especially Parkinson's disease (PD). Acetylcholine is also known as an anti-Alzheimer's agent, which may be due to its neuroprotective effect against the toxicity of β-amyloid protein (Aβ) [68]. The pathological hallmark of NDDs includes extracellular plaques of Aβ, and cholinergic neuronal degeneration in the brain [70]. Furthermore, the alteration in cholinergic signal results in cognitive, and behavioral symptoms in AD. Therefore, the cholinergic system is the main therapeutic target for the treatment of either by inhibition of acetylcholinesterase enzyme (AcHE) or by an agonist of the receptors [70, 71]. The mechanism of action of inhibition of AcHE is based on the inhibition of the degradation of Ach neurotransmitter and to improve dysfunction of cholinergic neuronal, and associated cognitive and behavioral functions [72].

Alkaloids Acetylcholinesterase Inhibitor

It has been documented that some alkaloids showed AcHE inhibitory activity which may be due to the presence of positively charged nitrogen part of alkaloids, and restore the Ach level in the hippocampus and cortical area of the brain as cholinergic deficiency has been noticed in these areas in AD [73]. Apart from this, the AcHE enzyme has two active sites, *i.e.*, the catalytic site and a peripheral anionic site (PAS) [74, 75]. The catalytic site binds with the substrate Ach neurotransmitter resulting in its degradation, and evidence showed that AcHE facilitates the formation of amyloid fibrils by the amino acids present around the PAS [76, 77], and some alkaloid prevents Aβ toxicity and restore acetylcholine *via* its dual inhibitory activity [70, 77]. This effect was reported for nantenine-aporphine alkaloid isolated from *Nandina domestica*, a berberine-isoquinoline alkaloid obtained from several plants, *i.e.*, *Berberis aristata, Berberis aquifolium, Hydrastis Canadensis* and *Coptis chinensis*, and crosses the blood-brain barrier (BBB), which will be important for designing potential anti-AD drugs [35, 78]. A similar inhibitory action on AcHE was observed using geissospermine-indole alkaloid extracted from the bark of Brazilian *Geissospermum vellosii* [59] and piperine-piperidine alkaloid isolated from *Piper nigrum, Piper longum* and prevents neuronal toxicity *via* the inhibition of Aβ peptides in the hippocampus, ameliorates cognition and decreases oxidative stress [79].

Apart from this, huperzine A is also a potent inhibitor of AcHE binding with the active site of the cholinesterase enzyme [80, 81] and prevents mitochondrial damage and oxidative stress [82, 83]. Furthermore, similar inhibitory activity was also shown by other alkaloids like physostigmine (*Physostigma venosum*) [84], and harmine (*Peganum harmala)* [85].

Galantamine is an alkaloid extracted from the flower, and bulb of *Narcissus tazetta, Galanthus nivalis, Leucojum aestivum, Galanthus woronovii* [36]. It crosses BBB, affects the cholinergic system in the brain, and was approved in 2000 as an anti-Alzheimer drug in Asia, Europe, and United States [86 - 88]. Inhibitory action of galantamine is due to binding with the catalytic site of AcHE [89] and restoring the deficiency of Ach [90]. Along with this, AcHE inhibiting activity of galantamine has also been identified modulator of nicotinic acetylcholine receptor (nAchR) [87]. The stimulation of nAchRs showed a significant increase in Ca^{2+} and noradrenaline results improve cognitive brain functioning [91]. A study reported that female rat hippocampal cells treated with montanine-isoquinoline alkaloid found in *Hippeastrum* vittatum plant and salsoline-isoquinoline alkaloid isolated from *Salsola oppositefolia* showed significant inhibition of AcHE in a dose-dependent manner [92, 93]. Pagliosa *et al.* [92], reported that montanine decreased the activity of AcHE at higher concentrations than galantamine. Further, *in vivo* investigations on these alkaloids regarding structural activity relationship, interaction with AcHE, and cognition are necessary.

Glutamatergic Signaling and Alkaloid

Glutamatergic neurotransmission in CNS is responsible for memory, learning, and plasticity; therefore, it is involved in the establishment of long-term potentiation (LTP), which gets affected in AD patients. In AD, aggregation of Aβ peptides induces oxidative stress and consequently deregulates glutamatergic neurotransmission, ultimately causing failure in memory, learning, and cognition in AD patients [94]. Glutamate is the excitatory neurotransmitter in the nervous system, and the disturbances in the metabolism and excessive release of this excitatory neurotransmitter results in epilepsy, AD, PD, and affective disorder. Glutamate activates the receptors of excitatory glutamate; therefore, the compound, which blocks receptors or inhibits glutamate secretion, could be neuroprotective when used in the therapy of neurodegenerative disorders. It has been confirmed that elevation in glutamate level and overstimulation of glutamate receptors, *i.e.*, NMDA results in the initiation of free radical formation and causes cell death and neuronal degeneration due to oxidative stress [95]. Thus, anti-oxidant for the inhibition of NMDA and glutamate toxicity will be a powerful therapeutic approach for the treatment of a neurodegenerative disorder. It has been reported that plant alkaloid huperzine A and berberine shows inhibitory effects for NMDA and glutamate toxicity [96, 97].

It has been reported that *in vitro* and *in vivo* studies huperzine A which ameliorates the pathogenesis of AD *via* its neuroprotective property; it prevents mitochondrial damage by blocking the aggregation of Aβ peptides [81, 82]. But, a number of indications from clinical and basic research propose that Aβ causes an increase in the level of glutamate in extra-synaptic space, consequently overstimulation in NMDA receptors, and finally results in synaptic loss as well as cell death [95, 98]. Huperzine A also inhibits the level of glutamate *via* the action of the non-competitive antagonist of the NMDA receptor and prevents neuronal cell death [96]. Along with this, berberine also protects neurons from hydrogen peroxide-induced apoptosis *via* its anti-oxidant property [99] and inhibiting NMDA receptors [100].

Gabaergic Signaling and Alkaloid

GABA is the principal inhibitory neurotransmitter in the mammalian brain. It is reported that $GABA_A$ receptors are major inhibitory receptors in the brain [101, 102], and the drugs which boost chloride ion influx through $GABA_A$ receptor channels are used for the treatment of epilepsy, AD, PD, schizophrenia, anxiety, and mood disorder [103 - 108]. Benzodiazepine drugs are commonly used for the modulation of GABA-ergic neurotransmission but show many side effects like addiction, cognitive decline, and impairment in long-term memory [109]. Therefore, there is a high medical need for a $GABA_A$ receptors modulator with a lack of side effects.

In this context, a researcher reported some alkaloids, *i.e.*, piperine [110], montanine [111], and morphine [31], modulate $GABA_A$ receptors and showed anxiolytic action with little sedation and can be used in the synthesis of modified $GABA_A$ receptors. Morphine results in the elevation of GABA levels in the synaptic region of the brain by binding with the μ-opioid receptor (MOR) [31] and protects from oxidative stress-induced neurotoxicity [112].

Alkaloids as Monoamine Inhibitors

Alterations in the dopaminergic and serotonergic systems are the main cause of depression, and most of the anti-depressant drugs are inhibitors of monoamine oxidase (MAO). MAOs are the enzyme responsible for the oxidative deamination of monoamines. The activation of the MAO-B enzyme results in the deamination of dopamine, and the loss of dopaminergic neurons is the hallmark of PD. Therefore, MAO-B inhibitors are clinically used to inhibit MAO-B and elevate the dopamine level [113]. The previous study shows that alkaloids have the potential to inhibit MAO-A and MAO-B enzyme activity. *In vivo* study piperidine alkaloids-piperine and lobeline extracted from *Piper nigrum, Piper longum,* and *Lobelia inflate,* which showed the antidepressant property in mice brain model of PD *via* inhibiting both MAO-A and MAO-B [114]. These results suggest that monoamine oxidase enzyme inhibition *via* piperidine alkaloids can increase the level of monoamines, *i.e.*, dopamine, serotonin, and noradrenaline, in patientssuffering from depression and side effects.

CONCLUSION

There are a number of drugs available in markets that have been used for the treatment of NDDs, but they do not have the potential to inhibit the progression of the disease instead of side effects. Many alkaloids show inhibitory, anti-oxidant, and anti-apoptosis *via* modulating neurotransmitter signal transmission. In this chapter, we have summarized only the selective mechanism of neuroprotection evoked by plant alkaloids (Fig. **1**). Alkaloids show neuroprotective properties, but further studies are required on their toxicity effect. It has been reported that natural alkaloids are more effective and safe for therapeutic application in NDDs. But, only limited implementation in clinical application, and there is a requirement to further explore & design a clinical trial for such compound.

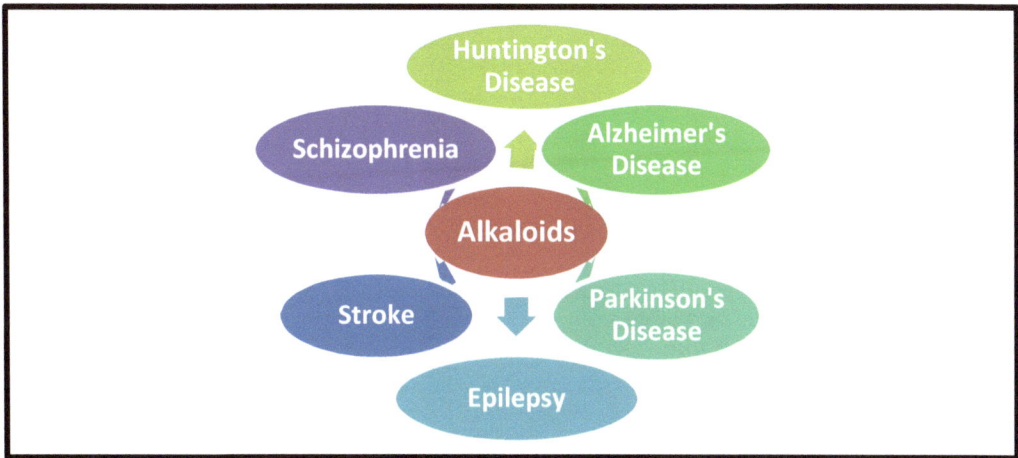

Fig. (1). Alkaloids neuroprotection in various neurodegenerative disorders.

CONSENT FOR PUBLICATION

Not applicable.

CONFLICT OF INTEREST

The author declares no conflict of interest, financial or otherwise.

ACKNOWLEDGEMENTS

Declared none.

REFERENCES

[1]   Kovacs GG. Molecular pathology of neurodegenerative diseases: principles and practice. J Clin Pathol 2019; 72(11): 725-35.
[http://dx.doi.org/10.1136/jclinpath-2019-205952] [PMID: 31395625]

[2]   Singh S, Rai S, Birla H, Eds., *et al.* Chlorogenic acid protects against MPTP induced neurotoxicity in parkinsonian mice model *via* its anti-apoptotic activity. J Neurochem. Hoboken 07030-5774, NJ USA: Wiley 111 River St 2019.

[3]   Rai SN, Birla H, Singh SS, *et al.* Pathophysiology of the Disease Causing Physical Disability.

Biomedical Engineering and its Applications in Healthcare. Springer 2019; pp. 573-95.

[4]   Rai SN, Singh BK, Rathore AS, *et al.* Quality control in huntington's disease: a therapeutic target. Neurotox Res 2019; 36(3): 612-26.
[http://dx.doi.org/10.1007/s12640-019-00087-x] [PMID: 31297710]

[5]   Rai SN, Dilnashin H, Birla H, *et al.* The role of PI3K/Akt and ERK in neurodegenerative disorders. Neurotox Res 2019; 35(3): 775-95.
[http://dx.doi.org/10.1007/s12640-019-0003-y] [PMID: 30707354]

[6]   Zahra W, Rai SN, Birla H, *et al.* Neuroprotection of rotenone-induced Parkinsonism by ursolic acid in PD mouse model. CNS & Neurological Disorders-Drug Targets 2020; 14: 527-40.
[http://dx.doi.org/10.2174/1871527319666200812224457]

[7]   Rai SN, Zahra W, Singh SS, *et al.* Anti-inflammatory activity of ursolic acid in MPTP-induced parkinsonian mouse model. Neurotox Res 2019; 36(3): 452-62.
[http://dx.doi.org/10.1007/s12640-019-00038-6] [PMID: 31016688]

[8]   Hussain G, Shahzad A, Anwar H, Mahmood Baig S, Shabbir A. De Aaguilar J-lG. Neurological disorder burden in faisalabad, punjab-pakistan: data from the major tertiary carecenters of the city. Pakistan Journal of Neurological Sciences 2017; 12(3): 3-10.

[9]   Mawoza T, Nhachi C, Magwali T. Prevalence of traditional medicine use during pregnancy, at labour and for postpartum care in a rural area in Zimbabwe. Clin Mother Child Health 2019; 16(2): 321.
[PMID: 31341518]

[10]   Sonter LJ, Ali SH, Watson JE. Mining and biodiversity: key issues and research needs in conservation science. Proceedings of the Royal Society B. 285(1892): 20181926.
[http://dx.doi.org/10.1098/rspb.2018.1926]

[11]   Mehta D, Jackson R, Paul G, Shi J, Sabbagh M. Why do trials for Alzheimer's disease drugs keep failing? A discontinued drug perspective for 2010-2015. Expert Opin Investig Drugs 2017; 26(6): 735-9.
[http://dx.doi.org/10.1080/13543784.2017.1323868] [PMID: 28460541]

[12]   Singh SS, Rai SN, Birla H, *et al.* Neuroprotective effect of chlorogenic acid on mitochondrial dysfunction-mediated apoptotic death of DA neurons in a Parkinsonian mouse model. Oxid Med Cell Longev 2020; 2020: 1-14.
[http://dx.doi.org/10.1155/2020/6571484] [PMID: 32566093]

[13]   Zahra W, Rai SN, Birla H, *et al.* Economic Importance of Medicinal Plants in Asian Countries Bioeconomy for Sustainable Development. Springer 2020; pp. 359-77.
[http://dx.doi.org/10.1007/978-981-13-9431-7_19]

[14]   Birla H, Keswani C, Singh SS, *et al.* Unraveling the neuroprotective effect of *tinospora cordifolia* in parkinsonian mouse model through proteomics approach. ACS Chem Neurosci 2021, 12(22): 4319–35.
[http://dx.doi.org/10.1021/acschemneuro.1c00481]

[15]   Keswani C, Dilnashin H, Birla H, Singh SP. Unravelling efficient applications of agriculturally important microorganisms for alleviation of induced inter-cellular oxidative stress in crops. Acta Agric Slov 2019; 114(1): 121-30.
[http://dx.doi.org/10.14720/aas.2019.114.1.14]

[16]   Birla H, Keswani C, Rai SN, *et al.* Neuroprotective effects of *Withania somnifera* in BPA induced-cognitive dysfunction and oxidative stress in mice. Behav Brain Funct 2019; 15(1): 9.
[http://dx.doi.org/10.1186/s12993-019-0160-4] [PMID: 31064381]

[17]   Niaz K, Shah MA, Khan F, Saleem U, Vargas C, Panichayupakaranant P. Bioavailability and safety of phytonutrients. Phytonutrients in Food. Elsevier 2020; pp. 117-36.
[http://dx.doi.org/10.1016/B978-0-12-815354-3.00003-4]

[18]   Melini F, Melini V, Luziatelli F, Ficca AG, Ruzzi M. Health-promoting components in fermented

foods: An up-to-date systematic review. Nutrients 2019; 11(5): 1189.
[http://dx.doi.org/10.3390/nu11051189] [PMID: 31137859]

[19]   Keswani C. Bioeconomy for Sustainable Development. Springer 2020.
[http://dx.doi.org/10.1007/978-981-13-9431-7]

[20]   Renaud J, Martinoli MG. Considerations for the use of polyphenols as therapies in neurodegenerative diseases. Int J Mol Sci 2019; 20(8): 1883.
[http://dx.doi.org/10.3390/ijms20081883] [PMID: 30995776]

[21]   Gonçalves S, Mansinhos I, Romano A. Neuroprotective compounds from plant sources and their modes of action: an update. Plant-derived Bioactives. Springer 2020; pp. 417-40.
[http://dx.doi.org/10.1007/978-981-15-2361-8_19]

[22]   Keswani C, Dilnashin H, Birla H, Singh S. Re-addressing the commercialization and regulatory hurdles for biopesticides in India. Rhizosphere 2019; 11(100155): 10.1016.

[23]   Rathore AS, Birla H, Singh SS, *et al.* Epigenetic modulation in parkinson's disease and potential treatment therapies. Neurochem Res 2021; 46(7): 1618-26.
[http://dx.doi.org/10.1007/s11064-021-03334-w] [PMID: 33900517]

[24]   Singh SS, Rai SN, Birla H, *et al.* Techniques related to disease diagnosis and therapeutics. application of biomedical engineering in neuroscience. Springer 2019; pp. 437-56.
[http://dx.doi.org/10.1007/978-981-13-7142-4_22]

[25]   Zahra W, Rai SN, Birla H, *et al.* The global economic impact of neurodegenerative diseases: Opportunities and challenges. Bioeconomy for Sustainable Development 2020; pp. 333-45.

[26]   Dey A, Mukherjee A. Plant-derived alkaloids: a promising window for neuroprotective drug discovery. Discovery and Development of Neuroprotective Agents from Natural Products. Elsevier 2018; pp. 237-320.
[http://dx.doi.org/10.1016/B978-0-12-809593-5.00006-9]

[27]   Dhivya PS, Selvamani P, Latha S, Mani V, Azahan NSM. *In vitro* evaluation of acetylcholinesterase inhibitory and neuroprotective activity in commiphora species: a comparative study. Pharmacogn J 2020; 12(6): 1223-31.
[http://dx.doi.org/10.5530/pj.2020.12.171]

[28]   John SK, Chandrapragasam V. *In vitro* anti-oxidant activity of *Lactobacillus plantarum* against hydrogen peroxide-induced neuronal damage on PC12 cells. Journal of Applied Biology & Biotechnology Vol 2020; 8(05): 84-7.

[29]   dos Santos RG, Hallak JEC. Effects of the natural β-carboline alkaloid harmine, a main constituent of ayahuasca, in memory and in the hippocampus: A systematic literature review of preclinical studies. J Psychoactive Drugs 2017; 49(1): 1-10.
[http://dx.doi.org/10.1080/02791072.2016.1260189] [PMID: 27918874]

[30]   Živić T. Encyclopædia Britannica Online: mrežno izdanje pouzdanoga priručnika (2012.–2020.). Studia lexicographica: časopis za leksikografiju i enciklopedistiku 2020;14(27):109-23 2020; 14(27): 109-23.

[31]   Cushnie TPT, Cushnie B, Lamb AJ. Alkaloids: An overview of their antibacterial, antibiotic-enhancing and antivirulence activities. Int J Antimicrob Agents 2014; 44(5): 377-86.
[http://dx.doi.org/10.1016/j.ijantimicag.2014.06.001] [PMID: 25130096]

[32]   Ng YP, Or TCT, Ip NY. Plant alkaloids as drug leads for Alzheimer's disease. Neurochem Int 2015; 89: 260-70.
[http://dx.doi.org/10.1016/j.neuint.2015.07.018] [PMID: 26220901]

[33]   Burr GL. The Encyclopaedia Britannica: a dictionary of arts, sciences, literature and general information. JSTOR 1911.

[34]   Ribeiro RA, Leite JR. Nantenine alkaloid presents anticonvulsant effect on two classical animal

models. Phytomedicine 2003; 10(6-7): 563-8.
[http://dx.doi.org/10.1078/094471103322331557] [PMID: 13678244]

[35] Pecic S, McAnuff MA, Harding WW. Nantenine as an acetylcholinesterase inhibitor: SAR, enzyme kinetics and molecular modeling investigations. J Enzyme Inhib Med Chem 2011; 26(1): 46-55.
[http://dx.doi.org/10.3109/14756361003671078] [PMID: 20583856]

[36] Heinrich M, Lee Teoh H. Galanthamine from snowdrop—the development of a modern drug against Alzheimer's disease from local Caucasian knowledge. J Ethnopharmacol 2004; 92(2-3): 147-62.
[http://dx.doi.org/10.1016/j.jep.2004.02.012] [PMID: 15137996]

[37] Jiang W, Li S, Li X. Therapeutic potential of berberine against neurodegenerative diseases. Sci China Life Sci 2015; 58(6): 564-9.
[http://dx.doi.org/10.1007/s11427-015-4829-0] [PMID: 25749423]

[38] Williams P, Sorribas A, Howes MJR. Natural products as a source of Alzheimer's drug leads. Nat Prod Rep 2011; 28(1): 48-77.
[http://dx.doi.org/10.1039/C0NP00027B] [PMID: 21072430]

[39] Almeida MB, Costa-Malaquias A, Nascimento JLM, Oliveira KR, Herculano AM, Crespo-López ME. Therapeutic concentration of morphine reduces oxidative stress in glioma cell line. Braz J Med Biol Res 2014; 47(5): 398-402.
[http://dx.doi.org/10.1590/1414-431X20143697] [PMID: 24728211]

[40] Ghafari S, Golalipour MJ. Prenatal morphine exposure reduces pyramidal neurons in CA1, CA2 and CA3 subfields of mice hippocampus. Iran J Basic Med Sci 2014; 17(3): 155-61.
[PMID: 24847417]

[41] Sarbishegi M, Mahmoudzadeh-sagheb H, Heidari Z, Baharvand F. The protective effect of celecoxib on CA1 hippocampal neurons and oxidative stress in a rat model of parkinson's disease. Acta Med Iran 2019; 94-102.
[http://dx.doi.org/10.18502/acta.v57i2.1763]

[42] Panda SS, Jhanji N. Natural products as potential anti-Alzheimer agents. Curr Med Chem 2020; 27(35): 5887-917.
[http://dx.doi.org/10.2174/0929867326666190618113613] [PMID: 31215372]

[43] Mohammadzadeh N, Mehri S, Hosseinzadeh H. *Berberis vulgaris* and its constituent berberine as antidotes and protective agents against natural or chemical toxicities. Iran J Basic Med Sci 2017; 20(5): 538-51.
[PMID: 28656089]

[44] Huang M, Jiang X, Liang Y, Liu Q, Chen S, Guo Y. Berberine improves cognitive impairment by promoting autophagic clearance and inhibiting production of β-amyloid in APP/tau/PS1 mouse model of Alzheimer's disease. Exp Gerontol 2017; 91: 25-33.
[http://dx.doi.org/10.1016/j.exger.2017.02.004] [PMID: 28223223]

[45] Srivastav S, Anand BG, Fatima M, *et al.* Piperine-Coated Gold Nanoparticles Alle*via*te Paraquat-Induced Neurotoxicity in *Drosophila melanogaster*. ACS Chem Neurosci 2020; 11(22): 3772-85.
[http://dx.doi.org/10.1021/acschemneuro.0c00366] [PMID: 33125229]

[46] Hussain G, Rasul A, Anwar H, *et al.* Role of plant derived alkaloids and their mechanism in neurodegenerative disorders. Int J Biol Sci 2018; 14(3): 341-57.
[http://dx.doi.org/10.7150/ijbs.23247] [PMID: 29559851]

[47] Chaurasiya ND, Midiwo J, Pandey P, *et al.* Selective Interactions of *O*-Methylated Flavonoid Natural Products with Human Monoamine Oxidase-A and -B. Molecules 2020; 25(22): 5358.
[http://dx.doi.org/10.3390/molecules25225358] [PMID: 33212830]

[48] Engelbrecht I, Petzer JP, Petzer A. Evaluation of selected natural compounds as dual inhibitors of catechol-O-methyltransferase and monoamine oxidase. Central Nervous System Agents in Medicinal Chemistry 2019; 19(2): 133-45.

[http://dx.doi.org/10.2174/1871524919666190619090852]

[49]   Zheng Q, Fang L, Huang X, Wang Y, Zhang S. Investigation of the mechanisms of neuroprotection mediated by Lobelia species via computational network pharmacology and molecular modeling 2020.
[http://dx.doi.org/10.21203/rs.3.rs-61537/v1]

[50]   Sanabria-Castro A, Alvarado-Echeverría I, Monge-Bonilla C. Molecular pathogenesis of Alzheimer's disease: an update. Ann Neurosci 2017; 24(1): 46-54.
[http://dx.doi.org/10.1159/000464422] [PMID: 28588356]

[51]   Manchishi SM. M Manchishi S. recent advances in antiepileptic herbal medicine. Curr Neuropharmacol 2018; 16(1): 79-83.
[PMID: 28521703]

[52]   Araújo JQ, Lima JA, Pinto AC, de Alencastro RB, Albuquerque MG. Docking of the alkaloid geissospermine into acetylcholinesterase: a natural scaffold targeting the treatment of Alzheimer's disease. J Mol Model 2011; 17(6): 1401-12.
[http://dx.doi.org/10.1007/s00894-010-0841-2] [PMID: 20844909]

[53]   Kumar A, Singh A, Ekavali . A review on Alzheimer's disease pathophysiology and its management: an update. Pharmacol Rep 2015; 67(2): 195-203.
[http://dx.doi.org/10.1016/j.pharep.2014.09.004] [PMID: 25712639]

[54]   White HK, Levin ED. Chronic transdermal nicotine patch treatment effects on cognitive performance in age-associated memory impairment. Psychopharmacology (Berl) 2004; 171(4): 465-71.
[http://dx.doi.org/10.1007/s00213-003-1614-8] [PMID: 14534771]

[55]   Ma C, Liu Y, Neumann S, Gao X. Nicotine from cigarette smoking and diet and Parkinson disease: a review. Transl Neurodegener 2017; 6(1): 18.
[http://dx.doi.org/10.1186/s40035-017-0090-8] [PMID: 28680589]

[56]   Woo T-UW. Neurobiology of schizophrenia onset. The neurobiology of childhood 2013; 267-95.
[http://dx.doi.org/10.1007/978-3-662-45758-0_243]

[57]   Houghton PJ, Howes MJ. Natural products and derivatives affecting neurotransmission relevant to Alzheimer's and Parkinson's disease. Neurosignals 2005; 14(1-2): 6-22.
[http://dx.doi.org/10.1159/000085382] [PMID: 15956811]

[58]   Yalcin D, Bayraktar O. Inhibition of catechol-O-methyltransferase (COMT) by some plant-derived alkaloids and phenolics. J Mol Catal, B Enzym 2010; 64(3-4): 162-6.
[http://dx.doi.org/10.1016/j.molcatb.2009.04.014]

[59]   Choudhury B, Saytode P, Shah V. Neurodegenrative disorders: Past, present and future. Int J Appl Pharm Biotechnol 2014; 5(2): 14-28.

[60]   Arendash GW, Mori T, Cao C, *et al.* Caffeine reverses cognitive impairment and decreases brain amyloid-β levels in aged Alzheimer's disease mice. J Alzheimers Dis 2009; 17(3): 661-80.
[http://dx.doi.org/10.3233/JAD-2009-1087] [PMID: 19581722]

[61]   Hernán MA, Takkouche B, Caamaño-Isorna F, Gestal-Otero JJ. A meta-analysis of coffee drinking, cigarette smoking, and the risk of Parkinson's disease. Ann Neurol 2002; 52(3): 276-84.
[http://dx.doi.org/10.1002/ana.10277] [PMID: 12205639]

[62]   Wang H, Zhang K, Zhao L, Tang J, Gao L, Wei Z. Anti-inflammatory effects of vinpocetine on the functional expression of nuclear factor-kappa B and tumor necrosis factor-alpha in a rat model of cerebral ischemia–reperfusion injury. Neurosci Lett 2014; 566: 247-51.
[http://dx.doi.org/10.1016/j.neulet.2014.02.045] [PMID: 24598438]

[63]   Rivera-Oliver M, Díaz-Ríos M. Using caffeine and other adenosine receptor antagonists and agonists as therapeutic tools against neurodegenerative diseases: A review. Life Sci 2014; 101(1-2): 1-9.
[http://dx.doi.org/10.1016/j.lfs.2014.01.083] [PMID: 24530739]

[64]   Zhang Z, Wang X, Chen Q, Shu L, Wang J, Shan G. Clinical efficacy and safety of huperzine Alpha in

treatment of mild to moderate Alzheimer disease, a placebo-controlled, double-blind, randomized trial. Zhonghua Yi Xue Za Zhi 2002; 82(14): 941-4.
[PMID: 12181083]

[65] Liu J, Zhang HY, Tang XC, Wang B, He XC, Bai DL. Effects of synthetic (-)-huperzine A on cholinesterase activities and mouse water maze performance. Chung Kuo Yao Li Hsueh Pao 1998; 19(5): 413-6.
[PMID: 10375798]

[66] Snyder SH, Innis RB. Peptide Neurotransmitters. Annu Rev Biochem 1979; 48(1): 755-82.
[http://dx.doi.org/10.1146/annurev.bi.48.070179.003543] [PMID: 38738]

[67] Waxham MN. Neuro transmitter receptorsFrom Molecules to Networks. Elsevier 2014; pp. 285-321.
[http://dx.doi.org/10.1016/B978-0-12-397179-1.00010-5]

[68] Grimaldi M, Marino SD, Florenzano F, *et al.* β-Amyloid-acetylcholine molecular interaction: new role of cholinergic mediators in anti-Alzheimer therapy? Future Med Chem 2016; 8(11): 1179-89.
[http://dx.doi.org/10.4155/fmc-2016-0006] [PMID: 27402297]

[69] Sapolsky R. Biology and Human Behavior: The Neurological Origins of Individuality. 2nd ed., The Teaching Company Limited Partnership 2005.

[70] Holzgrabe U, Kapková P, Alptüzün V, Scheiber J, Kugelmann E. Targeting acetylcholinesterase to treat neurodegeneration. Expert Opin Ther Targets 2007; 11(2): 161-79.
[http://dx.doi.org/10.1517/14728222.11.2.161] [PMID: 17227232]

[71] Parri HR, Hernandez CM, Dineley KT. Research update: Alpha7 nicotinic acetylcholine receptor mechanisms in Alzheimer's disease. Biochem Pharmacol 2011; 82(8): 931-42.
[http://dx.doi.org/10.1016/j.bcp.2011.06.039] [PMID: 21763291]

[72] Howes M. Alkaloids and drug discovery for neurodegenerative diseases. Natural products Phytochemistry, botany and metabolism of alkaloids, phenolics and terpenes 2013; 1331-65.
[http://dx.doi.org/10.1007/978-3-642-22144-6_43]

[73] Girdhar S, Girdhar A, Verma SK, Lather V, Pandita D. Plant derived alkaloids in major neurodegenerative diseases: from animal models to clinical trials. Journal of Ayurvedic and Herbal Medicine 2015; 1(3): 91-100.
[http://dx.doi.org/10.31254/jahm.2015.1307]

[74] Bolognesi M, Minarini A, Rosini M, Tumiatti V, Melchiorre C. From dual binding site acetylcholinesterase inhibitors to multi-target-directed ligands (MTDLs): a step forward in the treatment of Alzheimer's disease. Mini Rev Med Chem 2008; 8(10): 960-7.
[http://dx.doi.org/10.2174/138955708785740652] [PMID: 18782050]

[75] Cavalli A, Bottegoni G, Raco C, De Vivo M, Recanatini M. A computational study of the binding of propidium to the peripheral anionic site of human acetylcholinesterase. J Med Chem 2004; 47(16): 3991-9.
[http://dx.doi.org/10.1021/jm040787u] [PMID: 15267237]

[76] Inestrosa NC, Sagal JP, Colombres M. Acetylcholinesterase interaction with Alzheimer amyloid β. Alzheimer's Disease 2005; pp. 299-317.

[77] De Ferrari GV, Canales MA, Shin I, Weiner LM, Silman I, Inestrosa NC. A structural motif of acetylcholinesterase that promotes amyloid β-peptide fibril formation. Biochemistry 2001; 40(35): 10447-57.
[http://dx.doi.org/10.1021/bi0101392] [PMID: 11523986]

[78] Huang L, Shi A, He F, Li X. Synthesis, biological evaluation, and molecular modeling of berberine derivatives as potent acetylcholinesterase inhibitors. Bioorg Med Chem 2010; 18(3): 1244-51.
[http://dx.doi.org/10.1016/j.bmc.2009.12.035] [PMID: 20056426]

[79] Mishra A, Punia JK, Bladen C, Zamponi GW, Goel RK. Anticonvulsant mechanisms of piperine, a piperidine alkaloid. Channels (Austin) 2015; 9(5): 317-23.

[http://dx.doi.org/10.1080/19336950.2015.1092836] [PMID: 26542628]

[80]   Wong DM, Greenblatt HM, Dvir H, *et al.* Acetylcholinesterase complexed with bivalent ligands related to huperzine a: experimental evidence for species-dependent protein-ligand complementarity. J Am Chem Soc 2003; 125(2): 363-73.
[http://dx.doi.org/10.1021/ja021111w] [PMID: 12517147]

[81]   Raves ML, Harel M, Pang YP, Silman I, Kozikowski AP, Sussman JL. Structure of acetylcholinesterase complexed with the nootropic alkaloid, (–)-huperzine A. Nat Struct Mol Biol 1997; 4(1): 57-63.
[http://dx.doi.org/10.1038/nsb0197-57] [PMID: 8989325]

[82]   Francis PT, Nordberg A, Arnold SE. A preclinical view of cholinesterase inhibitors in neuroprotection: do they provide more than symptomatic benefits in Alzheimer's disease? Trends Pharmacol Sci 2005; 26(2): 104-11.
[http://dx.doi.org/10.1016/j.tips.2004.12.010] [PMID: 15681028]

[83]   Howes MJR, Houghton PJ. Plants used in Chinese and Indian traditional medicine for improvement of memory and cognitive function. Pharmacol Biochem Behav 2003; 75(3): 513-27.
[http://dx.doi.org/10.1016/S0091-3057(03)00128-X] [PMID: 12895669]

[84]   Orhan G, Orhan I, Subutay-Oztekin N, Ak F, Sener B. Contemporary anticholinesterase pharmaceuticals of natural origin and their synthetic analogues for the treatment of Alzheimer's disease. Recent Patents CNS Drug Discov 2009; 4(1): 43-51.
[http://dx.doi.org/10.2174/157488909787002582] [PMID: 19149713]

[85]   Klein-Junior L, Santos Passos C, Moraes A, *et al.* Indole alkaloids and semisynthetic indole derivatives as multifunctional scaffolds aiming the inhibition of enzymes related to neurodegenerative diseases--a focus on *Psychotria* L. Genus. Curr Top Med Chem 2014; 14(8): 1056-75.
[http://dx.doi.org/10.2174/1568026614666140324142409] [PMID: 24660679]

[86]   Parys W. Development of Reminyl (R)(galantamine), a novel acetylcholinesterase inhibitor, for the treatment of Alzheimer's disease. Alzheimers Rep 1998; 1: S19-20.

[87]   Farlow MR. Pharmacokinetic profiles of current therapiesfor Alzheimer's disease: implications for switching to galantamine. Clin Ther 2001; 23 (Suppl. A): A13-24.
[http://dx.doi.org/10.1016/S0149-2918(01)80164-8] [PMID: 11396867]

[88]   Marco-Contelles J, do Carmo Carreiras M, Rodríguez C, Villarroya M, García AG. Synthesis and pharmacology of galantamine. Chem Rev 2006; 106(1): 116-33.
[http://dx.doi.org/10.1021/cr040415t] [PMID: 16402773]

[89]   Doytchinova I, Atanasova M, Stavrakov G, Philipova I, Zheleva-Dimitrova D. Galantamine Derivatives as Acetylcholinesterase Inhibitors: Docking, Design, Synthesis, and Inhibitory Activity Computational Modeling of Drugs Against Alzheimer's Disease. Springer 2018; pp. 163-76.

[90]   Dall'Acqua S. Plant-derived acetylcholinesterase inhibitory alkaloids for the treatment of Alzheimer's disease. Botanics 2013; 3: 19-28.
[http://dx.doi.org/10.2147/BTAT.S17297]

[91]   Wang D, Noda Y, Zhou Y, *et al.* The allosteric potentiation of nicotinic acetylcholine receptors by galantamine ameliorates the cognitive dysfunction in beta amyloid25-35 i.c.v.-injected mice: involvement of dopaminergic systems. Neuropsychopharmacology 2007; 32(6): 1261-71.
[http://dx.doi.org/10.1038/sj.npp.1301256] [PMID: 17133263]

[92]   Pagliosa LB, Monteiro SC, Silva KB, *et al.* Effect of isoquinoline alkaloids from two *Hippeastrum* species on *in vitro* acetylcholinesterase activity. Phytomedicine 2010; 17(8-9): 698-701.
[http://dx.doi.org/10.1016/j.phymed.2009.10.003] [PMID: 19969445]

[93]   Tundis R, Menichini F, Conforti F, *et al.* A potential role of alkaloid extracts from *Salsola* species (Chenopodiaceae) in the treatment of Alzheimer's disease. J Enzyme Inhib Med Chem 2009; 24(3): 818-24.

[http://dx.doi.org/10.1080/14756360802399662] [PMID: 18720188]

[94]   Butterfield DA, Pocernich CB. The glutamatergic system and Alzheimer's disease: therapeutic implications. CNS Drugs 2003; 17(9): 641-52.
[http://dx.doi.org/10.2165/00023210-200317090-00004] [PMID: 12828500]

[95]   Bonfoco E, Krainc D, Ankarcrona M, Nicotera P, Lipton SA. Apoptosis and necrosis: two distinct events induced, respectively, by mild and intense insults with N-methyl-D-aspartate or nitric oxide/superoxide in cortical cell cultures. Proc Natl Acad Sci USA 1995; 92(16): 7162-6.
[http://dx.doi.org/10.1073/pnas.92.16.7162] [PMID: 7638161]

[96]   Zhang JM, Hu GY. Huperzine A, a nootropic alkaloid, inhibits N-methyl-D-aspartate-induced current in rat dissociated hippocampal neurons. Neuroscience 2001; 105(3): 663-9.
[http://dx.doi.org/10.1016/S0306-4522(01)00206-8] [PMID: 11516831]

[97]   Popik P, Layer RT, Fossom LH, *et al.* NMDA antagonist properties of the putative antiaddictive drug, ibogaine. J Pharmacol Exp Ther 1995; 275(2): 753-60.
[PMID: 7473163]

[98]   Anggono V, Tsai L-H, Götz J. Glutamate receptors in Alzheimer's Disease: mechanisms and therapies. Hindawi 2016.

[99]   Zhu X, Guo X, Mao G, *et al.* Hepatoprotection of berberine against hydrogen peroxide-induced apoptosis by upregulation of Sirtuin 1. Phytother Res 2013; 27(3): 417-21.
[http://dx.doi.org/10.1002/ptr.4728] [PMID: 22628222]

[100] Cui HS, Matsumoto K, Murakami Y, Hori H, Zhao Q, Obi R. Berberine exerts neuroprotective actions against *in vitro* ischemia-induced neuronal cell damage in organotypic hippocampal slice cultures: involvement of B-cell lymphoma 2 phosphorylation suppression. Biol Pharm Bull 2009; 32(1): 79-85.
[http://dx.doi.org/10.1248/bpb.32.79] [PMID: 19122285]

[101] Macdonald RL, Olsen RW. GABAA receptor channels. Annu Rev Neurosci 1994; 17(1): 569-602.
[http://dx.doi.org/10.1146/annurev.ne.17.030194.003033] [PMID: 7516126]

[102] Sieghart W. Structure and pharmacology of γ-aminobutyric acidA receptor subtypes. Pharmacol Rev 1995; 47(2): 181-234.
[PMID: 7568326]

[103] Thakur P, Shrivastava R, Shrivastava VK. Effects of exogenous oxytocin and atosiban antagonist on GABA in different region of brain. IBRO Rep 2019; 6: 185-9.
[http://dx.doi.org/10.1016/j.ibror.2019.04.001] [PMID: 31211283]

[104] Möhler H. GABAA receptors in central nervous system disease: anxiety, epilepsy, and insomnia. J Recept Signal Transduct Res 2006; 26(5-6): 731-40.
[http://dx.doi.org/10.1080/10799890600920035] [PMID: 17118808]

[105] Macdonald RL, Kang JQ, Gallagher MJ. Mutations in GABA $_A$ receptor subunits associated with genetic epilepsies. J Physiol 2010; 588(11): 1861-9.
[http://dx.doi.org/10.1113/jphysiol.2010.186999] [PMID: 20308251]

[106] Engin E, Liu J, Rudolph U. α2-containing GABAA receptors: A target for the development of novel treatment strategies for CNS disorders. Pharmacol Ther 2012; 136(2): 142-52.
[http://dx.doi.org/10.1016/j.pharmthera.2012.08.006] [PMID: 22921455]

[107] Rudolph U, Knoflach F. Beyond classical benzodiazepines: novel therapeutic potential of GABAA receptor subtypes. Nat Rev Drug Discov 2011; 10(9): 685-97.
[http://dx.doi.org/10.1038/nrd3502] [PMID: 21799515]

[108] Letizia Trincavelli M, Da Pozzo E, Daniele S, Martini C. The GABAA-BZR complex as target for the development of anxiolytic drugs. Curr Top Med Chem 2012; 12(4): 254-69.
[http://dx.doi.org/10.2174/1568026799078787] [PMID: 22204488]

[109] Uzun S, Kozumplik O, Jakovljević M, Sedić B. Side effects of treatment with benzodiazepines.

Psychiatr Danub 2010; 22(1): 90-3.
[PMID: 20305598]

[110] Schöffmann A, Wimmer L, Goldmann D, *et al.* Efficient modulation of γ-aminobutyric acid type A receptors by piperine derivatives. J Med Chem 2014; 57(13): 5602-19.
[http://dx.doi.org/10.1021/jm5002277] [PMID: 24905252]

[111] Mojarad TB, Roghani M. The anticonvulsant and anti-oxidant effects of berberine in kainate-induced temporal lobe epilepsy in rats. Basic Clin Neurosci 2014; 5(2): 124-30.
[PMID: 25337370]

[112] Cui J, Wang Y, Dong Q, *et al.* Morphine protects against intracellular amyloid toxicity by inducing estradiol release and upregulation of Hsp70. J Neurosci 2011; 31(45): 16227-40.
[http://dx.doi.org/10.1523/JNEUROSCI.3915-11.2011] [PMID: 22072674]

[113] Youdim MBH, Bakhle YS. Monoamine oxidase: isoforms and inhibitors in Parkinson's disease and depressive illness. Br J Pharmacol 2006; 147(S1) (Suppl. 1): S287-96.
[http://dx.doi.org/10.1038/sj.bjp.0706464] [PMID: 16402116]

[114] Lee SA, Hong SS, Han XH, *et al.* Piperine from the fruits of *Piper longum* with inhibitory effect on monoamine oxidase and antidepressant-like activity. Chem Pharm Bull (Tokyo) 2005; 53(7): 832-5.
[http://dx.doi.org/10.1248/cpb.53.832] [PMID: 15997146]

CHAPTER 7

South Indian Medicinal Herb: An Extensive Comparison of the Neuroprotective Activity

Pratistha Singh[1,*], **Ashutosh Kumar**[2,*] and **Anil Kumar Singh**[1]

[1] *Department of Dravyguna, Faculty of Ayurveda, Institute of Medical Sciences, Banaras Hindu University, Varanasi-221005 (U.P.), India*

[2] *Department of Pharmacology, Faculty of Medicine, Institute of Medical Sciences, Banaras Hindu University, Varanasi-221005 (U.P.), India*

Abstract: Medicinal Plants have secondary metabolites containing various phytoconstituents. Traditionally, medicinal plants are used in several diseases like cancer, diabetes, neurodegenerative disorder, *etc.* Flavonoids, Tannin, Phenols, Phenylpropanoids, Isoprenoids, and alkaloids are present in several medicinal plants, which play a very important role to promote health benefits and defensiveness for other disorders. Neurological disorders are prone to the elderly and difficult to treat. Several medicinal plants have been recognized as beneficial in neurological disorders. Various types of plant extract and formulations are present in ancient texts, which are effective in such disorders and should be explored scientifically to mitigate neurodegenerative disorders. In this chapter, we will focus on South Indian medicinal plants which are effective in neurological disorders or have neuroprotective properties.

Keywords: Anti-oxidant, Medicinal plants, Neuroprotective activity, Secondary metabolites, South India.

INTRODUCTION

Chronic neurodegenerative disorders such as Parkinson's disease (PD), and Alzheimer's disease (AD), occur due to unable to defend the central nervous system against any type of neural injury. Neuroinflammation has been concerned with the pathogenesis of several neurodegenerative diseases such as AD, PD, and multiple sclerosis (MS) [1]. Herbal medicine has precious resources in mitigating and prophylaxis several CNS disorders and helps improve health. Increasing irregularity in normal life leads to several disorders in the human body. In allopa-

* Corresponding authors Pratistha Singh & Ashutosh Kumar: Department of Dravyguna, Faculty of Ayurveda, Institute of Medical Sciences, Banaras Hindu University, Varanasi-221005 (U.P.), India & Department of Pharmacology, Faculty of Medicine, Institute of Medical Sciences, Banaras Hindu University, Varanasi221005 (U.P.), India; E-mails: psingh30.bhu@gmail.com & ashusingh1612@gmail.com

Surya Pratap Singh, Hagera Dilnashin, Hareram Birla & Chetan Keswani (Eds.)

ths, several medicines and surgery methods are present which are effective but do not cure permanently. Herbal products contain complex mixtures or formulations of bioactive compounds such phytochemicals, phenylpropanoids, isoprenoids and alkaloids, and saponin, which are responsible for biological activity [2]. Medicinal plant extract has become the most common supplement to prevent several neural disorders. The standardized extract of several medicinal plants is effective in the local area; it should be explored on a global level. Developing countries depend on traditional medicine, such as plant products and formulations for primary health, as estimated by WHO [3]. India is full of biodiversity, and 12 major biodiversity regions are present in the Southern part of India and blessed with a huge number of medicinal plants, including two major biodiversity zone, Western Ghat and Eastern Ghat. It is reported that approximately 2000 medical species are present in Western Ghat. The majority of plant species are limited to the southern isthmus [4]. In the present study, we described medicinal plants and their phytoconstituents as neuroprotective medicine (Fig. **1**). We briefly discussed neurodegenerative diseases, AD and PD in particular, with emphasis on the preventive strategies represented by herbal medicine [5 - 10]. We provide an ethnobiological approach, focusing on medicinal herbs used by different traditional medicines and their neuroprotective components.

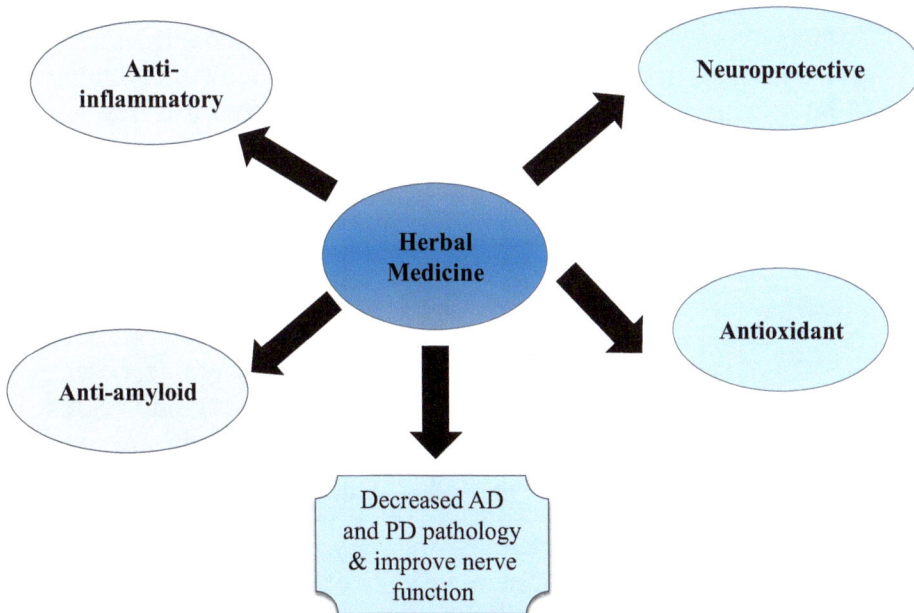

Fig. (1).   Effects of plant secondary metabolites present in herbal medicine; Anti-inflammatory, neuroprotective, anti-amyloid, and anti-oxidant activities. It is effective in the inhibition of the formation of amyloid plaques in neurological disorders, inhibition of reactive oxygen species, and prevent inflammatory.

NEURODEGENERATIVE DISEASE

Neurodegeneration is a process that leads to damage of neurons and also loss of the function and structure of neurons. This result leads to impaired cognition and neurological disorder leading to PD, AD, dementia, epilepsy, and cerebral ischemia.

AD is an accumulation of beta-amyloid plaques between nerve cells (Neurons) present in the brain. It is a common form of dementia in adults and is an unalterable degeneration of the brain that causes an interruption in memory and other neural function. It causes many other troubles such as confusion, visual complication, agitation, poor judgment, and hallucination and may lead to neuron death. Genetic and environmental factors are also responsible for the disease, such as diet, smoking, brain injury, diabetes, and other medical conditions [11].

PD was first described by James Parkinson. It is the second most common neurodegenerative disease. Young children and people mostly over 50-60 years are most affected [12]. PD is characterized by the loss of 50-70% of dopaminergic neurons in the substantia nigra (SN), which results in a fall in dopamine levels in the brain. PD causes several abnormalities in the body: slow movements (Bradykinesia) and muscle rigidity [13 - 16]. Several other abnormalities are seen in PD: cramped handwriting, expressionlessness, difficulty swallowing, and mitochondrial dysfunction. Genetic and Reactive oxygen species generation causes such types of neurodegenerative diseases [17 - 21].

MEDICINAL PLANTS

Avicennia marina forssk. Vierh

A. marina, commonly known as grey mangrove or white mangrove, belongs to the Acanthaceae family. It is found in Kerala and Tamil Nadu region in South India. The plant is a rich source of phytocompounds such as alkaloids, aromatic lipids, phenylethanoid glycosides (PGs), and other effective compounds. It has pharmacological activities such as anti-microbial activity [22]. Marinoid J was obtained from fruits of *A. marina* that significantly improve cognitive deficits in vascular dementia (VD) rats model, regulate a set of proteins that affect oxidative stress and apoptosis, and decrease oxidative stress, and apoptosis of hippocampal CA1 neurons. Marinoid J shows a novel opening treatment of VD [23].

Azadirachta indica A. Juss

A. indica is commonly known as Neem in India. It is a traditional medicine used as a tonic in immune potentiator, anti-inflammatory, and anti-microbial agents [24]. It is commonly found in the Tamil Nadu region of south India. It has several phytoconstituents as its leaves contain quercetin, catechin, carotenes, and vitamin C. It is reported that treatment of *A. indica* significantly reduced Parkinson's disease; it induces catalase, glutathione- peroxidase, and decreases ROS. *A. indica* significantly decreased the PD-induced rotational behavior in rats. The same result was found in another study; PD-induced catalase, glutathione-peroxidase, iNOS activity, and iNOS protein expression were significantly suppressed by treatment with *A. indica*. It has been confirmed that it shows neuroprotective, anti-oxidant, and anti-apoptotic effects on Parkinson's disease [25]. Leave extract of *A. indica* used in neuroprotection against Partial Sciatic nerve Ligation (PSNL) induced neuropathic pain *via* inhibition of oxidative –nitrosative stress. It also helps in the release of proinflammatory cytokines and apoptosis to improve Motor nerve conduction velocity [26].

Aloe vera (L.) Burm. f.

Aloe Vera is a succulent plant. It is an evergreen perennial plant, commonly found in south India, and belongs to *Asphodelaceae* (Liliaceae) family. It is found in some parts of Tamil Nadu. The leaf extract of *Aloevera* is used in the treatment of wound healing, anti-fungal, anti-diabetic, immunomodulator, and gastroprotective properties [27]. Major phytoconstituents present in Aloe Vera are Anthraquinones, aloe-emodin, aloe-resin, aloeninma [28]. Aloin present in aloe Vera helps to reduce ROS generation in the intracellular regions. The calcium ion generation is decreased by aloin which is responsible for depolarization and death of neurons [29].

Asparagus racemosa Willd

A. racemosa, known as Shatavari, belongs to the Asparagaceae family. It is commonly found in the Himalayas belt region and predominately present in the southern part of India. Root, stem, and fruits are used for medical purposes. In Ayurveda, it has entitled as a queen of Herb. It has been reported that its constituent's arsasapogenin has neuroprotective properties in the rodent AD models. It is a steroidal saponin, as a targeted ligand that helps in the treatment of Alzheimer's disease. The aqueous root extract of Shatavari helps to inhibit an enzyme responsible progression of Alzheimer's disease, such as Acetylcholinesterase and MAO-B and it also showed possible anti-amyloidogenic properties in *in-vitro* studies [30]. Racemosol and Rhamnose present in the extract of *A. racemosa* has neuroprotective properties against PD [31]. Methanolic extract of Shatavari has anti-oxidant effects and enhanced neuronal activity in the hippocampus and striatum [32].

Baccopa monnieri (L.) Pennell

B. monnieri, commonly known as Jal Brahmi, belongs to the Scrophulariaceae family. It is a perennial, creeping herb found in wetlands of the southern and eastern parts of India. It has been used in several health complications since the ancient era [33]. There are several phytoconstituents present in *B. monnieri,* mainly saponins, terpenoids, and alkaloids. The presence of Nicotin and herpestine has been reported in *B. monnieri.* It has several pharmacological activities: anticonvulsant, anti-inflammatory, immunostimulatory, anti-oxidant, and hepatoprotective. Bacoside A3, bacopasaponin X, bacopasaponin C and bacopaside I and II are present in ethanolicextract of *B. monnieri*. It helps in the improvement of cognitive abilities and is neuroprotective in Alzheimer's model [34]. It has been demonstrated that extract of *B. monieri* has protective effects against rotenone-induced PD in PC-12 cell lines [35]. Its extract also has the ability to decrease lipoxygenase action [36]. *B. monnieri* as a formulation with ferula narthex Drude, *Gardenia gummifers* L. *Elettaria cardamomum* L., and cow ghee showed significant neuroprotective activity [37].

Centella asiatica (L.) Urban

C. asiatica, commonly known as "Brahmi", "Gotu kola", belongs to the Apiaceae family. It is an herbaceous, perennial medicinal plant. It is found in Karnataka, South India. Asiaticosides, Asiatic acid, madecassoside and madasiatic acid are the main chemical constituents, and also contains centelloside brahminoside, brahmoside, isothankuniside, and thankuniside [38, 39]. In the Ayurvedic system, the leave of *C. asiatica* has been used as a memory enhancer, rejuvenating effects, improving brain function and preventing cognitive deficits [40]. It has several pharmacological activities, such as cardioprotective, anti-diabetic, anti-bacterial, anti-inflammatory, anti-oxidant, anti-depressant, and immunostimulant [38]. *In vitro* studies found that *C. asiatica* is associated with increased mitochondrial activity, increasing anti-oxidant activity, and inhibiting the pro-inflammatory enzyme, phospholipase A2. A recent study reported that caffeoylquinic acid is found in *C. asiatica*. A group of active compounds found in *C. asiatica* has the potential of enhancing Nrf2, an anti-oxidant response pathway [41]. 11-ox--asiaticoside B is a triterpenoid saponin found in methanolic extract of *C. asiatica,* displayed the best neuroprotective effects, reduced cell apoptosis, increased the mRNA expression of anti-oxidant enzymes, and activated phosphatidylinositol 3-kinase/Akt pathway [42].

Curcuma longa L.

C. longa Linn, commonly known as turmeric, belongs to the Zingiberaceae family. It is obtained from the rhizome of the plant. It is found in most of the areas of Tamil Nadu, Orissa, Karnataka, and Kerala. In Ayurveda, several times, it has been used in different medical conditions [43]. Curcumin, demethoxycurcumin, and bisdemethoxy curcmin are the main chemical constituents, and other constituents are α, β- turmerone, artumerone, curlone, curcumol and zingibereneetc, present in *C. longa* [44]. Several pharmacological properties are reported in *C. longa,* such as immunostimulant, anti-diabetic, cardioprotective, anti-bacterial, anti-inflammatory, anti-oxidant, anti-depressant, hypotensive, anti-microbial, and anti-rheumatic [45]. Curcumin was isolated from the rhizome of *C. longa*, can chelate with metal ions, and have anti-oxidant properties. It was investigated that the protective effects of complexes of curcumin with Cu II or Zn II possess significant neuroprotective effects on hydrogen peroxide-induced injury and inhibit cell apoptosis *via* down regulating the nuclear factor NF-kB pathway and upregulating the Bcl-2 pathway [46]. A study reported that curcumin reduced TNF α, MCP-1, IL- 1β, IL-6, TLR4 expression, and neuronal and apoptotic cell death [47]. Ethanolic extract of turmeric (200mg/kg) prohibited oxidative stress and increased SOD, CAT, and GPx enzyme activities [48].

Desmodium gangedicum (L.) DC

D. gedicum, commonly known as Salvan or Salpani, belongs to the Leguminosae family, distributed in Andhra Pradesh, Tamil Nadu, Kerala, and Odisha. It is a perennial shrub. There are several phytoconstituents reported in *D. gangedicum,* such as phospholipid, sterol, flavones, pterocarpanoids (gangetin and desmodin) and alkaloids (tryptamines and phenylethylamines) [49]. It shows pharmacological activities as immunomodulatory, anti-oxidant, anti-inflammatory, anti-nociceptive, cardioprotective, anti-ulcer, and hepatoprotective. [50]. *D. gangedicum* has pharmacological properties that indicate the potential for the management of AD. 100 and 200 mg/kg aqueous extract of *D. gangedicum* was administered to improve memory in mice because of AchE inhibitory activity [51].

Evolvulus alsinoides Linn.

E. alsinoides, commonly known as Vishnu Krantha, belongs to the Convolvulaceae family, and is a perennial herb found in the Tamil Nadu region of India. In Ayurveda, it is also known as Shankhpushpi, traditionally used as a memory enhancer [52]. Octadecanoic acid, n-hexadecanoic acid, piperine, squalene, ethyl oleate, and cholesterol are the chemical constituents of the plant [53]. It has anti-oxidant, and immunomodulatory properties [54]. Hydroalcoholic extract of *E. alsinoides* reported anti-inflammatory and other enzymes inhibitory activity such as cholinesterase, prolylendopeptidase, glycogen synthase kinase-3-β and enzymes inhibitory activity; all these enzymes are involved in AD pathology condition [55]. Another study showed that methanol and water extract of *E. alsinoides* is reported to help treat neurodegenerative disorders like managing AD [56].

Foeniculum vulgare Mill

F. vulgare, commonly known as fennel, belongs to Umbelliferae (Apiaceae) family. It is an upright branching perennial herb found in Kerala, and Tamil Nadu regions in South India. It has several pharmacological properties such as memory-enhancing, antimicrobial, antiviral, anti-inflammatory, anti-nociceptive, anti-pyretic, anti-spasmodic, hypoglycemic, and hypolipidemic. Its phytocomponds are quercetin-3-glucuronide, isoquercitrin, quercetin-3-arabinoside, kaemp-fero--3-glucuronide, kaempferol-3-arabinoside and isorhamnetin [57]. *F. vulgare* and their phytocompounds have several pharmacological activities such as antimicrobial, anti-inflammatory, anti-thirsutism, anti-colitic, anti-mutagenic, anti-nociceptive, anti-stress, anti-thrombotic, anti-tumor, cytotoxicity, diuretic, estrogenic properties, hypoglycemic, hypolipidemic, memory-enhancing properties, *etc.* [58]. Ethanolic extract of *F. vulgare* seed (200 mg/kg/day) decreases neuronal toxicity, attenuating the expression level of Amyloid precursor protein isoform and oxidative stress [59]. Another study reported that *F. vulgare* has therapeutic potential that increases functional improvement of peripheral nerve injury and reduces oxidative stress [60]. Anethole (1-methoxy -4-propenylbenzene) present in *F. vulgare*, has been reported to reduce mechanical allodynia and hyperalgesia in neuropathic pain and protect against nerve damage [61].

Ficus religiosa Linn.

F. religiosa is, commonly known as peepal, belongs to the Moraceae family. It is a large perennial tree, found throughout India and Kerala in south India, enriched with this medicinal plant. *F. religiosa* contains Phyosterol, flavonoids, tannins, Kaempeferol, quercetin, and myricetin [62]. In Ayurveda, the bark of *F. religiosa* is used in the treatment of ulcers, skin disease, gonorrhea, and diabetes [63]. A study reported that methanolic extract of leaf of *F. religiosa* (200mg/kg) has neuroprotective potential [64]. Petroleum ether extract of *F. religiosa* leaves a significantly enhanced motor performance and decreases oxidative damage [65]. In a study, a flavonoid-rich fraction of *F. religiosa* and phenytoin combination reduced AChE activity and increased CAT levels [66].

Garcinia indica Choisy

G. indica choisy, known as kokum, brindon, or bhirand, belongs to the Guttiferae family. It is found in the tropical humid evergreen rain forest of the Western Ghats of south India and north India. Garcinol is the important phytoconstituents of *G. indica* [67], efficiently reinstates the balance between glutamate neurotransmitters and γ aminobutyric acid (GABA). It also saves neural precursor cells and their rapid growth and enhances memory. It acts as an inhibitor of histone acetyltransferase, and in this way, it protects against rapid neurodegeneration complications [68, 69]. A recent study reported that it represses MPP + induced cell death [70]. Garcinol helps to avoid the production of toxic dopamine metabolites, such as homocysteine, 3-o-methyldopa, 3-methoxytyramine, and 3,4 dihydroxyphenylacetaldehyde [71].

Hippophae rhamnoides L.

H. rhamnoides, commonly known as Seabuckthorn, belongs to the *Elaeagnaceae* family. It is a thorny nitrogen-fixing deciduous shrub found in South India. Major phytocompounds of *H. rhamnoides* are riboflavin, folic acid, carotenoids, phytosterol, organic acid, polyunsaturated fatty acid, essential amino acid, and Vitamin A, C, E [72]. Anti-oxidant, anti-atherogenic, anti-stress, hepatoprotective, immunomodulatory, radioprotective, cardioprotective, anti-carcinogenic, immunomodulatory, anti-viral, and anti-bacterial are the major known pharmacological properties of the plant [73]. Extracting *H. rhamnoides* has potential free radical scavenging activity and regulates lipid peroxidation activity, leading to neuroprotective activity [74]. A polyhedral formulation of *B. monnieri*, *H. rhamnoides*, and *Dioscorea bulbifera* has a protective effect against neural disorders such as AD [74]. Flavonolignans are present in fruits of *H. rhamnoide*, and show neuroprotective and immunosuppressive activities [75].

Moringa oligofera Lam.

M. oleifera Lam., commonly known as drumstick tree, horseradish tree, and ben oil tree, belongs to the Moringaceae family. It is a perennial deciduous tropical tree, cultivated in India and occurs mainly in southern states (Tamil Nadu, Karnataka, Kerala, and Andhra Pradesh) of India. It has several phytocompounds such as flavonoids, isothiocyanates. It possesses anti-diabetic activity, and is beneficial in neurodysfunctional disease, neuroprotective, hypoglycemic, and anti-inflammatory activities [76]. Methanolic extract of *M. oleifera* leaves possesses anti-oxidant and neuroprotective activities [77]. Several previous studies mentioned that *M. oleifera* significantly showed positive effects on neural disorders [78]. *M. oleifera* seed extract has neuroprotective effects; it prevents brain damage, promotes hippocampal neurogenesis, and improves cholinergic function [79].

Morinda pubescens Sm

It is commonly known as Manjanathi Maram, and belongs to the *Rubiaceae* family. It is a medicinal plant of southern India; its leaves are mainly used for treatment. It has several pharmacological activities, such as anti-oxidant and cytotoxic effects [62]. It has been reported in a survey and documentation of medicinal plants in 2013 in Uthapuram Madurai district. It is used in the treatment of nerve problems [4].

Pedalium murex Linn

P. murex Linn commonly known as Gokhru, belongs to the Pedaliaceae family. It is a shrub found in the southern part and Deccan region of India, Known as Aalsomotha-malvi-gokharu in Malayalam, Ananerinnil in Tamil. Several phytoconstituents are present in *P. murex,* such as diosgenin and vanillin, quercetin, ursolic acid, caffeic acid, and amino acid, (Glycine, Histamine, tyrosine, threonine, aspartic acid). Several pharmacological activities are present in this plant, such as nephroprotective, hypolipidemic, aphrodisiac, anti-oxidant, anti-microbial, and insecticidal [80]. In a study, it has been reported that ethanol extract of *P. Murex* Linn shows neuroprotective activity. It shows potential beneficial effects on (Lipopolysaccharides) LPS-induced brain damage that indicates the presence of anti-oxidant in *P. Murex* leaves [81].

Punica granatum L.

P. granatum, commonly known as pomegranate, belongs to the Lythraceae family. It is a fruit-bearing deciduous shrub. It is commonly found in Karnataka, Kerala, and all districts of Tamil Nadu as well as in North India. It has several phytoconstituents such as rutin, catechinellagic acid, tannic acid, pedunculagin, anthocyanins, and polyphenols [82]. Several pharmaceutical properties are anti-inflammatory, anti-angiogenic, anti-cancerous, anti-mutagenic, hepatoprotective, anti-diabetic, anti-bacterial, and effective in cardiovascular diseases [82]. Peel extract of pomegranate is a rich source of phytocompounds and anti-oxidant properties that have the potential to delay the progression of dementia associated with AD. It reduces the accumulation of senile plaques and reduces lipid peroxidation and inflammatory cytokine TNF-α [83]. Punicalagin (PG) is a phytocompound in *P. granatum*. It has been reported that PG decreases neuronal damage by sodium-potassium adenosine triphosphate activity, downregulating the malondialdehyde, and decreasing the mitochondrial-generated reactive oxygen species [84].

Phyllanthus amarus Schumah & Thonn

P. amarus, commonly known as Bhumi amla, belongs to the Euphorbiaceae family. It is an upright herb and shrub found in Hotspots in South India [85]. *P.amarus* contains various phytocompounds such as volatile oil, sterol, flavonoids, tannins, terpenes and phenolics [80]. Major compounds of the plant are isonirtetralin, phyltetralin, hypophyllanthin, ellagic acid, corilagin and geraniin andniranthin. It is used in several pharmacological properties, such as anti-amnesic, anti-lipidemic, anti-hyperglycemic, hepatoprotective, anti-viral, anti-fungal, anti-cancer, anti-inflammatory, and immunomodulatory [80]. Ethanol extract of *P. amarus* shows protective effects on neural complications; It decreases TNF-α, IL-1β, NO level, integrin expression, and iNOS in the brain [86]. In a recent study, it has been found that alkaloid, present in the leaves of *Andrographis paniculata* and *P. amarus*, shows therapeutic effects on neurodegenerative disease [87].

Portulaca oleracea L

P. oleracea (L.) is commonly well-known as Pasali keerai portula. It is found in Uthapuram Madurai district in Tamil Nadu (a state of South India), and belongs to Portulacaceae. *P. oleracea* has various biological activities such as anti-oxidant anti-microbial, hepatoprotective, and neuroprotective. It has various phycompounds present in plant parts, such as alkaloids, flavonoids, fatty acids, minerals, and vitamins [88]. It has been reported that leaves are used in nerve weakness [4].

Sesbania grandiflora L.

S. grandiflora, commonly known as Agast or Agathi, belongs to the legume family. It is a small, loosely legume plant found in South India. Leaves contain several phytocompounds, such as amino acids, minerals, riboflavin, nicotinic acid, and Vitamin A, C [89]. *S. grandiflora* has pharmacological properties such as hepatoprotective, anticonvulsive, anxiolytic, rheumatism, gout, anti-leprosy, anti-inflammatory, treatment of bronchitis, smallpox, fever, and headache. *S. grandiflora* has high anti-oxidant properties. Ethanolic extract of *S. grandiflora* seeds has been investigated that enhance memory and decrease the activity of Acetylcholine Esterase activity (AchE) and Malondialdehyde (MDA) in the brain [90].

Terminalia chebula Retz.

T. chebula belongs to the Combretaceae family. Phytocompounds of *T. chebula* are gallic acid, ellagic acid, tannic acid, chebulic acid, corilagin, mannitol, ascorbic acid, and other compounds like Vitamin C [91]. It has several pharmacological activities such as cardiotonic, diuretic, laxative, Cancer, cardiovascular disease, paralysis, urinary tract infection, arthritis, epilepsy, gastroenteritis, urinary tract infection, and wound infection [92]. It exhibits neuroprotective activities and may be a possible candidate for the treatment of neurodegenerative disease. It reduces H_2O_2- induced toxicity toward PC 12 cells [93]. There are neuroprotective and anti-oxidant activities found in *T. chebula*, which are beneficial for the treatment of AD [94].

CONCLUSION

We discussed many neuroprotective plants that are effective in treating various neurological diseases. Phytoconstituents of the plants show many pharmacological properties such as anti-oxidant, anti- β amyloid, anti-ACHE, increased Dopamine level in the brain, anti-depressant, anti-epileptic, cognition enhancer, *etc.* Further, there is a need for isolation and standardization of phytocompounds to treat neurological diseases and improve life.

CONSENT FOR PUBLICATION

Not applicable.

CONFLICT OF INTEREST

The author declares no conflict of interest, financial or otherwise.

ACKNOWLEDGMENTS

The authors gratefully acknowledge the Department of Biotechnology, Government of India, New Delhi, for providing fellowship. They would also like to thank the Department of Biochemistry, Faculty of Science, Banaras Hindu University.

REFERENCES

[1]   Stephenson J, Nutma E, van der Valk P, Amor S. Inflammation in CNS neurodegenerative diseases. Immunology 2018; 154(2): 204-19.
[http://dx.doi.org/10.1111/imm.12922] [PMID: 29513402]

[2]   Atanasov AG, Waltenberger B, Pferschy-Wenzig EM, *et al.* Discovery and resupply of pharmacologically active plant-derived natural products: A review. Biotechnol Adv 2015; 33(8): 1582-614.
[http://dx.doi.org/10.1016/j.biotechadv.2015.08.001] [PMID: 26281720]

[3]   Vines G. Herbal harvests with a future: towards sustainable sources for medicinal plants: Plantlife International 2004.

[4]   Sivasankari B, Pitchaimani S, Anandharaj M. A study on traditional medicinal plants of Uthapuram, Madurai District, Tamilnadu, South India. Asian Pac J Trop Biomed 2013; 3(12): 975-9.
[http://dx.doi.org/10.1016/S2221-1691(13)60188-4] [PMID: 24093789]

[5]   Rai SN, Zahra W, Singh SS, *et al.* Anti-inflammatory activity of ursolic acid in MPTP-induced parkinsonian mouse model. Neurotox Res 2019; 36(3): 452-62.
[http://dx.doi.org/10.1007/s12640-019-00038-6] [PMID: 31016688]

[6]   Singh SS, Rai SN, Birla H, *et al.* Neuroprotective effect of chlorogenic acid on mitochondrial dysfunction-mediated apoptotic death of DA neurons in a Parkinsonian mouse model. Oxid Med Cell Longev 2020; 2020: 1-14.
[http://dx.doi.org/10.1155/2020/6571484] [PMID: 32566093]

[7]   Zahra W, Rai SN, Birla H, *et al.* Economic Importance of Medicinal Plants in Asian Countries. Bioeconomy for Sustainable Development. Springer 2020; pp. 359-77.
[http://dx.doi.org/10.1007/978-981-13-9431-7_19]

[8]   Birla H, Keswani C, Singh SS, *et al.* Unraveling the Neuroprotective Effect of Tinospora cordifolia in Parkinsonian Mouse Model Through Proteomics Approach 2021.

[9]   Keswani C, Dilnashin H, Birla H, Singh SP. Unravelling efficient applications of agriculturally important microorganisms for alleviation of induced inter-cellular oxidative stress in crops. Acta Agric Slov 2019; 114(1): 121-30.
[http://dx.doi.org/10.14720/aas.2019.114.1.14]

[10]   Birla H, Keswani C, Rai SN, *et al.* Neuroprotective effects of *Withania somnifera* in BPA induced-cognitive dysfunction and oxidative stress in mice. Behav Brain Funct 2019; 15(1): 9.
[http://dx.doi.org/10.1186/s12993-019-0160-4] [PMID: 31064381]

[11] Tublin JM, Adelstein JM, del Monte F, Combs CK, Wold LE. Getting to the heart of Alzheimer disease. Circ Res 2019; 124(1): 142-9.
[http://dx.doi.org/10.1161/CIRCRESAHA.118.313563] [PMID: 30605407]

[12] Chen J, Zhang C, Wu Y, Zhang D. Association between hypertension and the risk of Parkinson's disease: a meta-analysis of analytical studies. Neuroepidemiology 2019; 52(3-4): 181-92.
[http://dx.doi.org/10.1159/000496977] [PMID: 30726850]

[13] Rai SN, Birla H, Singh SS, *et al.* Pathophysiology of the Disease Causing Physical Disability. Biomedical Engineering and its Applications in Healthcare. Springer 2019; pp. 573-95.

[14] Rai SN, Singh BK, Rathore AS, *et al.* Quality control in huntington's disease: a therapeutic target. Neurotox Res 2019; 36(3): 612-26.
[http://dx.doi.org/10.1007/s12640-019-00087-x] [PMID: 31297710]

[15] Rai SN, Dilnashin H, Birla H, *et al.* The role of PI3K/Akt and ERK in neurodegenerative disorders. Neurotox Res 2019; 35(3): 775-95.
[http://dx.doi.org/10.1007/s12640-019-0003-y] [PMID: 30707354]

[16] Zahra W, Rai SN, Birla H, *et al.* Neuroprotection of rotenone-induced Parkinsonism by ursolic acid in PD mouse model. CNS & Neurological Disorders-Drug Targets 2020; (14): 527-40.
[http://dx.doi.org/10.2174/1871527319666200812224457]

[17] Rathore AS, Birla H, Singh SS, *et al.* Epigenetic modulation in parkinson's disease and potential treatment therapies. Neurochem Res 2021; 46(7): 1618-26.
[http://dx.doi.org/10.1007/s11064-021-03334-w] [PMID: 33900517]

[18] Keswani C, Dilnashin H, Birla H, Singh S. Re-addressing the commercialization and regulatory hurdles for biopesticides in India 2019; 11(100155): 10.1016.

[19] Singh SS, Rai SN, Birla H, *et al.* Techniques Related to Disease Diagnosis and Therapeutics. Application of Biomedical Engineering in Neuroscience. Springer 2019; pp. 437-56.
[http://dx.doi.org/10.1007/978-981-13-7142-4_22]

[20] Zahra W, Rai SN, Birla H, *et al.* The global economic impact of neurodegenerative diseases: Opportunities and challenges. Bioeconomy for Sustainable Development 2020; pp. 333-45.

[21] Singh S, Rai S, Birla H, Eds., *et al.* Chlorogenic acid protects against MPTP induced neurotoxicity in parkinsonian mice model via its anti-apoptotic activity. 2019.

[22] Karthi S, Vinothkumar M, Karthic U, *et al.* Biological effects of *Avicennia marina* (Forssk.) vierh. extracts on physiological, biochemical, and antimicrobial activities against three challenging mosquito vectors and microbial pathogens. Environ Sci Pollut Res Int 2020; 27(13): 15174-87.
[http://dx.doi.org/10.1007/s11356-020-08055-1] [PMID: 32072409]

[23] Yi X, Li J, Tang Z, *et al.* Marinoid J, a phenylglycoside from *Avicennia marina* fruit, ameliorates cognitive impairment in rat vascular dementia: a quantitative iTRAQ proteomic study. Pharm Biol 2020; 58(1): 1220-9.
[http://dx.doi.org/10.1080/13880209.2020.1837187] [PMID: 33280468]

[24] Dkhil MA, Al-Quraishy S, Abdel Moneim AE, Delic D. Protective effect of *Azadirachta indica* extract against Eimeria papillata-induced coccidiosis. Parasitol Res 2013; 112(1): 101-6.
[http://dx.doi.org/10.1007/s00436-012-3109-1] [PMID: 22972359]

[25] Xiang X, Wu L, Mao L, Liu Y. Anti-oxidative and anti-apoptotic neuroprotective effects of *Azadirachta indica* in Parkinson-induced functional damage. Mol Med Rep 2018; 17(6): 7959-65.
[PMID: 29620282]

[26] Kandhare AD, Mukherjee AA, Bodhankar SL. Neuroprotective effect of *Azadirachta indica* standardized extract in partial sciatic nerve injury in rats: Evidence from anti-inflammatory, antioxidant and anti-apoptotic studies. EXCLI J 2017; 16: 546-65.
[PMID: 28694757]

[27]   Rath M, Bhattacharya A, Rath K, Santra S, Ghosh G, Nanda BB. A comprehensive study of the neuropharmacological profile of methanol leaf extract of *aloe vera* and identification of associated neuroprotective compounds through gas chromatography-mass spectrometry analysis. Indian J Pharm Sci 2020; 82(6): 996-1005.

[28]   Speranza G, Gramatica P, Dadá G, Manitto P. Aloeresin c, a bitter c,o-diglucoside from cape aloe. Phytochemistry 1985; 24(7): 1571-3.
[http://dx.doi.org/10.1016/S0031-9422(00)81068-7]

[29]   Chang R, Zhou R, Qi X, *et al.* Protective effects of aloin on oxygen and glucose deprivation-induced injury in PC12 cells. Brain Res Bull 2016; 121: 75-83.
[http://dx.doi.org/10.1016/j.brainresbull.2016.01.001] [PMID: 26772628]

[30]   Kashyap P, Muthusamy K, Niranjan M, Trikha S, Kumar S. Sarsasapogenin: A steroidal saponin from Asparagus racemosus as multi target directed ligand in Alzheimer's disease. Steroids 2020; 153: 108529.
[http://dx.doi.org/10.1016/j.steroids.2019.108529] [PMID: 31672628]

[31]   Bhaskar K. Ethnobotany and conservation status of saponin rich plants of gangetic plain having both medicinal and Cleansing properties. Plant Arch 2018; 18(1): 81-97.

[32]   Singh R, Geetanjali . *Asparagus racemosus* : a review on its phytochemical and therapeutic potential. Nat Prod Res 2016; 30(17): 1896-908.
[http://dx.doi.org/10.1080/14786419.2015.1092148] [PMID: 26463825]

[33]   Aguiar S, Borowski T. Neuropharmacological review of the nootropic herb *Bacopa monnieri*. Rejuvenation Res 2013; 16(4): 313-26.
[http://dx.doi.org/10.1089/rej.2013.1431] [PMID: 23772955]

[34]   Dhanasekaran M, Tharakan B, Holcomb LA, Hitt AR, Young KA, Manyam BV. Neuroprotective mechanisms of ayurvedic antidementia botanical *Bacopa monniera*. Phytother Res 2007; 21(10): 965-9.
[http://dx.doi.org/10.1002/ptr.2195] [PMID: 17604373]

[35]   Swathi G, Ramaiah CV, Rajendra W. Protective role of *Bacopa monnieri* against Rotenone- induced Parkinson's disease in PC 12 cell lines. Int J Phytomed 2017; 9(2): 219-22.
[http://dx.doi.org/10.5138/09750185.2008]

[36]   Abdul Manap AS, Vijayabalan S, Madhavan P, *et al. Bacopa monnieri*, a neuroprotective lead in Alzheimer Disease: a review on its properties, mechanisms of action, and preclinical and clinical studies. Drug Target Insights 2019; 13
[http://dx.doi.org/10.1177/1177392819866412] [PMID: 31391778]

[37]   Achliya GS, Wadodkar SG, Dorle AK. Evaluation of sedative and anticonvulsant activities of Unmadnashak Ghrita. J Ethnopharmacol 2004; 94(1): 77-83.
[http://dx.doi.org/10.1016/j.jep.2004.04.020] [PMID: 15261966]

[38]   Gohil K, Patel J, Gajjar A. Pharmacological review on *Centella asiatica*: A potential herbal cure-all. Indian J Pharm Sci 2010; 72(5): 546-56.
[http://dx.doi.org/10.4103/0250-474X.78519] [PMID: 21694984]

[39]   Belwal T, Andola HC, Atanassova MS, *et al.* Gotu Kola (*Centella asiatica*). Nonvitamin and nonmineral nutritional supplements: Elsevier 2019; 265-75.

[40]   Mohandas Rao KG, Muddanna Rao S, Gurumadhva Rao S. *Centella asiatica* (L.) leaf extract treatment during the growth spurt period enhances hippocampal CA3 neuronal dendritic arborization in rats. Evid Based Complement Alternat Med 2006; 3(3): 349-57.
[http://dx.doi.org/10.1093/ecam/nel024] [PMID: 16951719]

[41]   Gray NE, Alcazar Magana A, Lak P, *et al. Centella asiatica*: phytochemistry and mechanisms of neuroprotection and cognitive enhancement. Phytochem Rev 2018; 17(1): 161-94.
[http://dx.doi.org/10.1007/s11101-017-9528-y] [PMID: 31736679]

[42]   Wu ZW, Li WB, Zhou J, *et al.* Oleanane- and ursane-type triterpene saponins from *centella asiatica* exhibit neuroprotective effects. J Agric Food Chem 2020; 68(26): 6977-86.
[http://dx.doi.org/10.1021/acs.jafc.0c01476] [PMID: 32502339]

[43]   Majeed M, Badmaev V, Murray F. Turmeric and the healing curcuminoids: McGraw Hill Professional 1999.

[44]   Perrone D, Ardito F, Giannatempo G, *et al.* Biological and therapeutic activities, and anticancer properties of curcumin. Exp Ther Med 2015; 10(5): 1615-23.
[http://dx.doi.org/10.3892/etm.2015.2749] [PMID: 26640527]

[45]   Sharifi-Rad J, Rayess YE, Rizk AA, *et al.* Turmeric and its major compound curcumin on health: bioactive effects and safety profiles for food, pharmaceutical, biotechnological and medicinal applications 2020.
[http://dx.doi.org/10.3389/fphar.2020.01021]

[46]   Yan FS, Sun JL, Xie WH, Shen L, Ji HF. Neuroprotective effects and mechanisms of curcumin–Cu (II) and–Zn (II) complexes systems and their pharmacological implications. Nutrients 2017; 10(1): 28.
[http://dx.doi.org/10.3390/nu10010028]

[47]   Zhu H, Bian C, Yuan J, *et al.* Curcumin attenuates acute inflammatory injury by inhibiting the TLR4/MyD88/NF-κB signaling pathway in experimental traumatic brain injury. J Neuroinflammation 2014; 11(1): 59.
[http://dx.doi.org/10.1186/1742-2094-11-59] [PMID: 24669820]

[48]   Yuliani S, Mustofa , Partadiredja G. The neuroprotective effects of an ethanolic turmeric (*Curcuma longa* L.) extract against trimethyltin-induced oxidative stress in rats. Nutr Neurosci 2019; 22(11): 797-804.
[http://dx.doi.org/10.1080/1028415X.2018.1447267] [PMID: 29513140]

[49]   Mishra PK, Singh N, Ahmad G, Dube A, Maurya R. Glycolipids and other constituents from *Desmodium gangeticum* with antileishmanial and immunomodulatory activities. Bioorg Med Chem Lett 2005; 15(20): 4543-6.
[http://dx.doi.org/10.1016/j.bmcl.2005.07.020] [PMID: 16099649]

[50]   Rastogi S, Pandey MM, Rawat AKS. An ethnomedicinal, phytochemical and pharmacological profile of *Desmodium gangeticum* (L.) DC. and Desmodium adscendens (Sw.) DC. J Ethnopharmacol 2011; 136(2): 283-96.
[http://dx.doi.org/10.1016/j.jep.2011.04.031] [PMID: 21530632]

[51]   Joshi H, Parle M. Antiamnesic effects of *Desmodium gangeticum* in mice. Yakugaku Zasshi 2006; 126(9): 795-804.
[http://dx.doi.org/10.1248/yakushi.126.795] [PMID: 16946593]

[52]   Chatterjee A, Pakrashi SC. Treatise on Indian medicinal plants: Publications & Information Directorate 1991.

[53]   Gomathi D, Kalaiselvi M, Ravikumar G, Devaki K, Uma C. GC-MS analysis of bioactive compounds from the whole plant ethanolic extract of *Evolvulus alsinoides* (L.) L. J Food Sci Technol 2015; 52(2): 1212-7.
[http://dx.doi.org/10.1007/s13197-013-1105-9] [PMID: 25694742]

[54]   Ganju L, Karan D, Chanda S, Srivastava KK, Sawhney RC, Selvamurthy W. Immunomodulatory effects of agents of plant origin. Biomed Pharmacother 2003; 57(7): 296-300.
[http://dx.doi.org/10.1016/S0753-3322(03)00095-7] [PMID: 14499177]

[55]   Mehla J, Pahuja M, Dethe SM, Agarwal A, Gupta YK. Amelioration of intracerebroventricular streptozotocin induced cognitive impairment by *Evolvulus alsinoides* in rats: *In vitro* and *in vivo* evidence. Neurochem Int 2012; 61(7): 1052-64.
[http://dx.doi.org/10.1016/j.neuint.2012.07.022] [PMID: 22892278]

[56]   Patel SS, Raghuwanshi R, Masood M, Acharya A, Jain SK. Medicinal plants with acetylcholinesterase

inhibitory activity. Rev Neurosci 2018; 29(5): 491-529.
[http://dx.doi.org/10.1515/revneuro-2017-0054] [PMID: 29303784]

[57]   Kunzemann J, Herrmann K. Isolation and identification of flavon(ol)-O-glycosides in caraway (*Carum carvi* L.), fennel (*Foeniculum vulgare* Mill.), anise (*Pimpinella anisum* L.), and coriander (*Coriandrum sativum* L.), and of flavon-C-glycosides in anise. Z Lebensm Unters Forsch 1977; 164(3): 194-200.
[http://dx.doi.org/10.1007/BF01263030] [PMID: 910554]

[58]   Badgujar SB, Patel VV, Bandivdekar AH. *Foeniculum vulgare* Mill: a review of its botany, phytochemistry, pharmacology, contemporary application, and toxicology. BioMed research international 2014.

[59]   Bhatti S, Ali Shah SA, Ahmed T, Zahid S. Neuroprotective effects of *Foeniculum vulgare* seeds extract on lead-induced neurotoxicity in mice brain. Drug Chem Toxicol 2018; 41(4): 399-407.
[http://dx.doi.org/10.1080/01480545.2018.1459669] [PMID: 29742941]

[60]   Imran A, Xiao L, Ahmad W, *et al. Foeniculum vulgare* (Fennel) promotes functional recovery and ameliorates oxidative stress following a lesion to the sciatic nerve in mouse model. J Food Biochem 2019; 43(9): e12983.
[http://dx.doi.org/10.1111/jfbc.12983] [PMID: 31489666]

[61]   Wang B, Zhang G, Yang M, *et al.* Neuroprotective effect of anethole against neuropathic pain induced by chronic constriction injury of the sciatic nerve in mice. Neurochem Res 2018; 43(12): 2404-22.
[http://dx.doi.org/10.1007/s11064-018-2668-7] [PMID: 30367337]

[62]   Sultana B, Anwar F. Flavonols (kaempferol, quercetin, myricetin) contents of selected fruits, vegetables and medicinal plants. Food Chem 2008; 108(3): 879-84.
[http://dx.doi.org/10.1016/j.foodchem.2007.11.053] [PMID: 26065748]

[63]   Khare CP. Indian medicinal plants: an illustrated dictionary. Springer Science & Business Media 2008.

[64]   Veerendra Kumar MH, Gupta YK. Effect of *Centella asiatica* on cognition and oxidative stress in an intracerebroventricular streptozotocin model of Alzheimer's disease in rats. Clin Exp Pharmacol Physiol 2003; 30(5-6): 336-42.
[http://dx.doi.org/10.1046/j.1440-1681.2003.03842.x] [PMID: 12859423]

[65]   Bhangale JO, Acharya NS, Acharya SR. Protective effect of *Ficus religiosa* (L.) against 3-nitropropionic acid induced Huntington disease. Orient Pharm Exp Med 2016; 16(3): 165-74.
[http://dx.doi.org/10.1007/s13596-016-0237-7]

[66]   Singh P, Singh D, Goel RK. *Ficus religiosa* L. figs — A potential herbal adjuvant to phenytoin for improved management of epilepsy and associated behavioral comorbidities. Epilepsy Behav 2014; 41: 171-8.
[http://dx.doi.org/10.1016/j.yebeh.2014.10.002] [PMID: 25461211]

[67]   Nayak CA, Rastogi NK, Raghavarao KSMS. Bioactive constituents present in *Garcinia indica* Choisy and its potential food applications: A review. Int J Food Prop 2010; 13(3): 441-53.
[http://dx.doi.org/10.1080/10942910802626754]

[68]   Balasubramanyam K, Altaf M, Varier RA, *et al.* Polyisoprenylated benzophenone, garcinol, a natural histone acetyltransferase inhibitor, represses chromatin transcription and alters global gene expression. J Biol Chem 2004; 279(32): 33716-26.
[http://dx.doi.org/10.1074/jbc.M402839200] [PMID: 15155757]

[69]   Hegarty S, O'Keeffe GW, Sullivan AM. The Epigenome as a therapeutic target for Parkinson's disease. Neural Regen Res 2016; 11(11): 1735-8.
[http://dx.doi.org/10.4103/1673-5374.194803] [PMID: 28123403]

[70]   Park G, Tan J, Garcia G, Kang Y, Salvesen G, Zhang Z. Regulation of histone acetylation by autophagy in Parkinson disease. J Biol Chem 2016; 291(7): 3531-40.
[http://dx.doi.org/10.1074/jbc.M115.675488] [PMID: 26699403]

[71]   Deb S, Phukan BC, Mazumder MK, *et al.* Garcinol, a multifaceted sword for the treatment of Parkinson's disease. Neurochem Int 2019; 128: 50-7.
[http://dx.doi.org/10.1016/j.neuint.2019.04.004] [PMID: 30986504]

[72]   Beveridge T, Li TSC, Oomah BD, Smith A. Sea buckthorn products: manufacture and composition. J Agric Food Chem 1999; 47(9): 3480-8.
[http://dx.doi.org/10.1021/jf981331m] [PMID: 10552673]

[73]   Krejcarová J, Straková E, Suchý P, Herzig I, Karásková K. Sea buckthorn (*Hippophae rhamnoides* L.) as a potential source of nutraceutics and its therapeutic possibilities - a review. Acta Vet Brno 2015; 84(3): 257-68.
[http://dx.doi.org/10.2754/avb201584030257]

[74]   Shivapriya S, Ilango K, Dubey GP. Evaluation of antioxidant and neuroprotective effect of *Hippophae rhamnoides* (L.) on oxidative stress induced cytotoxicity in human neural cell line IMR32. Saudi J Biol Sci 2015; 22(5): 645-50.
[http://dx.doi.org/10.1016/j.sjbs.2015.04.011] [PMID: 26288571]

[75]   Ma QG, Wei RR, Shang DL, Sang ZP, Dong JH. Structurally Diverse Flavonolignans with Immunosuppressive and Neuroprotective Activities from the Fruits of *Hippophae rhamnoides* L. J Agric Food Chem 2020; 68(24): 6564-75.
[http://dx.doi.org/10.1021/acs.jafc.0c01432] [PMID: 32437606]

[76]   Kou X, Li B, Olayanju J, Drake J, Chen N. Nutraceutical or pharmacological potential of *Moringa oleifera* Lam. Nutrients 2018; 10(3): 343.
[http://dx.doi.org/10.3390/nu10030343] [PMID: 29534518]

[77]   Idoga ES, Ambali SF, Ayo JO, Mohammed A. Assessment of antioxidant and neuroprotective activities of methanol extract of *Moringa oleifera* Lam. leaves in subchronic chlorpyrifos-intoxicated rats. Comp Clin Pathol 2018; 27(4): 917-25.
[http://dx.doi.org/10.1007/s00580-018-2682-9]

[78]   Omotoso GO, Gbadamosi IT, Afolabi TT, Abdulwahab AB, Akinlolu AA. Ameliorative effects of *Moringa* on cuprizone-induced memory decline in rat model of multiple sclerosis. Anat Cell Biol 2018; 51(2): 119-27.
[http://dx.doi.org/10.5115/acb.2018.51.2.119] [PMID: 29984057]

[79]   Zeng K, Li Y, Yang W, *et al. Moringa oleifera* seed extract protects against brain damage in both the acute and delayed stages of ischemic stroke. Exp Gerontol 2019; 122: 99-108.
[http://dx.doi.org/10.1016/j.exger.2019.04.014] [PMID: 31039389]

[80]   Patel DK, Laloo D, Kumar R, Hemalatha S. *Pedalium murex* Linn.: An overview of its phytopharmacological aspects. Asian Pac J Trop Med 2011; 4(9): 748-55.
[http://dx.doi.org/10.1016/S1995-7645(11)60186-7] [PMID: 21967701]

[81]   Gomathi S, Sundaram RS, Annapandian VM, Vijayabaskaran M. Neuroprotective effect of *pedalium murex* linn. Leaf against lipopolysaccharide induced behavioural disorders in rats. Pharmacogn J 2017; 9(6): 957-62.
[http://dx.doi.org/10.5530/pj.2017.6.150]

[82]   Puneeth HR, Chandra SSP. A review on potential therapeutic properties of Pomegranate (*Punica granatum* L.). Plant Sci Today 2020; 7(1): 9-16.
[http://dx.doi.org/10.14719/pst.2020.7.1.619]

[83]   Yaidikar L, Byna B, Thakur SR. Neuroprotective effect of punicalagin against cerebral ischemia reperfusion-induced oxidative brain injury in rats. J Stroke Cerebrovasc Dis 2014; 23(10): 2869-78.
[http://dx.doi.org/10.1016/j.jstrokecerebrovasdis.2014.07.020] [PMID: 25282190]

[84]   Morzelle MC, Salgado JM, Telles M, *et al.* Neuroprotective effects of pomegranate peel extract after chronic infusion with amyloid-β peptide in mice. PLoS One 2016; 11(11): e0166123.
[http://dx.doi.org/10.1371/journal.pone.0166123] [PMID: 27829013]

[85] Meena J, Sharma R, Rolania R. A review on phytochemical and pharmacological properties of *Phyllanthus amarus*Schum. and Thonn. Int J Pharm Sci Res 2018; 9(4): 1377-86.

[86] Alagan A, Jantan I, Kumolosasi E, Ogawa S, Abdullah MA, Azmi N. Protective effects of *Phyllanthus amarus* against lipopolysaccharide-induced neuroinflammation and cognitive impairment in rats. Front Pharmacol 2019; 10: 632.
[http://dx.doi.org/10.3389/fphar.2019.00632] [PMID: 31231221]

[87] Adedayo BC, Ogunsuyi OB, Akinniyi ST, Oboh G. Effect of *Andrographis paniculata* and *Phyllanthus amarus* leaf extracts on selected biochemical indices in *Drosophila melanogaster* model of neurotoxicity. Drug Chem Toxicol 2020; 1-10.
[PMID: 31899970]

[88] Petropoulos S, Karkanis A, Martins N, Ferreira ICFR. Phytochemical composition and bioactive compounds of common purslane (*Portulaca oleracea* L.) as affected by crop management practices. Trends Food Sci Technol 2016; 55: 1-10.
[http://dx.doi.org/10.1016/j.tifs.2016.06.010]

[89] Ramesh T, Mahesh R, Sureka C, Begum VH. Cardioprotective effects of Sesbania grandiflora in cigarette smoke-exposed rats. J Cardiovasc Pharmacol 2008; 52(4): 338-43.
[http://dx.doi.org/10.1097/FJC.0b013e3181888383] [PMID: 18791462]

[90] Semwal BC, Verma M, Murti Y, Yadav HN. Neuroprotective activity of *Sesbania grandifolara* seeds extract against celecoxib induced amnesia in mice. Pharmacogn J 2018; 10(4): 747-52.
[http://dx.doi.org/10.5530/pj.2018.4.125]

[91] Chattopadhyay R, Bhattacharyya S. PHCOG REV.: Plant Review *Terminalia chebula*: An update. Pharmacogn Rev 2007; 1(1): 151-6.

[92] Rathinamoorthy R, Thilagavathi G. *Terminalia chebula*-review on pharmacological and biochemical studies. Int J Pharm Tech Res 2014; 6(1): 97-116.

[93] Chang CL, Lin CS. Phytochemical composition, anti-oxidant activity, and neuroprotective effect of *Terminalia chebula* Retzius extracts. Evidence-Based Complementary and Alternative Medicine 2012.

[94] Sadeghnia HR, Jamshidi R, Afshari AR, Mollazadeh H, Forouzanfar F, Rakhshandeh H. *Terminalia chebula* attenuates quinolinate-induced oxidative PC12 and OLN-93 cell death. Mult Scler Relat Disord 2017; 14: 60-7.
[http://dx.doi.org/10.1016/j.msard.2017.03.012] [PMID: 28619434]

CHAPTER 8

Therapeutic Anti-Parkinson's Role of *Bacopa monnieri* and Reconsideration of Underlying Mechanisms

Vartika Gupta[1] and **Sukala Prasad[1,*]**

[1] *Biochemistry & Molecular Biology Laboratory, Department of Zoology, Brain Research Centre, Banaras Hindu University, Varanasi-221005 (U.P.), India*

Abstract: Neurodegeneration leads to several life-threatening brain disorders such as Parkinson's disease, Alzheimer's disease, and many more. Such kinds of diseases have a great impact on normal life patterning and may cause other severe symptoms, which are sometimes incurable. PD is the second most common disease characterized by the symptoms like Bradykinesia, resting tremor, postural instability, and some motor symptoms involving cognitive impairment and sleep disturbance. Memory plays a major role in sustaining the life of an individual. The development of an advanced molecular technique for treating PD increases day by day, but the complications in these techniques also cannot be ignored, so scientists move towards ayurvedic herbs to treat such kinds of disorders. *Bacopa monnieri* is an ayurvedic medicinal creeping plant used since ancient times to treat several kinds of diseases, including brain diseases. It has many components which are useful in neuroprotection and ameliorating PD. The core aim of the present chapter is to summarize and discuss how *B. monnieri* plays a therapeutic role in PD

Keywords: Alpha-synuclein, Antioxidant, *B. monneiri*, Nootropic herb, Oxidative stress, Parkinson's disease.

INTRODUCTION

The brain is the most important and complex organ of the body, which serves to control and coordinate the mental and physical activity of humans and other vertebrates. It consists of millions of neuronal cells, and each neuronal cell is connected to itself *via* a synapse. Synapse acts as a junction between two nerve cells, passing the impulse by diffusion of neurotransmitters [1, 2]. These neurons act in coordination with each other to acquire new information and store them for

* **Corresponding author Sukala Prasad:** Biochemistry & Molecular Biology Laboratory, Department of Zoology, Brain Research Centre, Banaras Hindu University, Varanasi-221005 (U.P.), India; E-mail: s.sprasadbhu@gmail.com

Surya Pratap Singh, Hagera Dilnashin, Hareram Birla & Chetan Keswani (Eds.)

future use, and this ability of the brain is known as learning and memory. Conversely, learning is the process of acquisition of new information or experiences, and storing the learned information for later use is termed as memory, both of which are complex and major functions of the brain [3]. The molecular mechanism of learning and memory is governed by synaptic plasticity, which is the ability of neurons to strengthen and weaken in response to an increase and decrease in the given signals [4]. In short, the brain is the master controller of the body and a very complex organ that learns and forms memory with the help of neurons which can be retrieved for later use.

However, sometimes, the brain also loses its ability to do all these functions due to disturbance in their neurophysiological process which leads to several kinds of neurodegenerative disorders such as Alzheimer's disease [AD], Parkinson's disease [PD], Huntington's disease [HD] and undergo other neuropathological conditions like brain injury, aging, metabolic disorders, and neuropsychiatric problems. AD and PD are the first and second most common neurogenerative diseases, respectively. The key difference lies in their onset period, associated key protein, memory, cognition, personality, more prominent movement, *etc.* [5]. PD is an age-related neurodegenerative disorder characterized by motor impairment involving rigidity, bradykinesia, rest tremor, and postural instability, along with non-motor complications, such as autonomic dysfunctions, cognitive neuropsychiatric changes, and sleep disturbances [6, 7]. The pathological hallmark underlying PD comprises the loss of the dopaminergic (DAergic) neurons in the substantia nigra pars compacta (SNpc) region and the aggregation of intracytoplasmic proteins known as Lewy bodies [8]. Treatment for PD has been progressed at different stages such developments at surgery, chemical drugs, therapies, *etc.*. have been observed. Currently, no cure is available for PD, however, these therapies and medications address some of the symptoms and improve the quality of life for patients. In the recent past, complementary and alternative therapies with herbal or ayurvedic compounds or products have shown their potential as a drug and improved the lives of patients with PD [9, 10]. As a result, many researchers are currently focusing on herbs of ayurvedic medicine to cure or reverse the symptoms of PD. A wide variety of ayurvedic herbs like "Brahmi", "Ashwagandha", "Shankhpushpi", *etc.*, and their solutions, compounds, and extracts have shown very high potential as nootropic herbs to improve neurodegenerative conditions and serve as the potential therapy for neurological disorders.

THE LINK BETWEEN NEURODEGENERATION AND AYURVEDIC HERB

Ayurveda has a great emphasis on treatment and encourages the maintenance of health by paying proximate attention to a balanced lifestyle. Medical science deals with the ideas of screening, understanding, and medicinal attributes of naturally occurring plants or plant products and their role in the treatment of various diseases [11]. According to the Ayurveda, the living body is controlled by the three energies "Vata", "Pitta", and "Kapha" if any of these get impaired, which leads to the development of several kinds of diseases [12, 13]. The imbalance in the "Vata" leads to neurological disorders symptomized as memory loss, impaired locomotory control, anxiety, poor blood circulation, *etc*. [14]. Ayurvedic plants play a considerable role in the treatment of neurodegenerative diseases. Neurodegenerative diseases are the result of the gradual loss of the neurons in the brain, which affects many body activities such as balance, movement, talking, cognition, breathing, *etc*. [15]. These can be caused due to genetic as well as environmental factors and sometimes influenced by medical conditions like a tumor, stroke, alcoholism, *etc*.. Neurodegeneration can range from mild to chronic to life-threatening, which depends on the type of disease. There is various type of neurodegenerative disorders/disease, and some of which are:

- Alzheimer's disease
- Parkinson's disease
- Huntington's disease
- Spinal muscular atrophy
- Amyotrophic lateral sclerosis
- Friedreich's ataxia

Treatment for these diseases/disorders has been observed in the developing stage, like surgery, chemical drugs, therapies, *etc*. [16]. Currently, no cure is available for PD, however, these therapies and medications address some of the symptoms and improve the quality of life for patients. In the recent past, complementary and alternative therapies with herbal or ayurvedic compounds or products have shown their potential as a drug in animal models and improved the lives of patients with PD [9, 10]. As a result, many researchers are currently focusing on herbs of ayurvedic medicine to cure or reverse the symptoms of PD. It has been remarkably noticed in the past few years by modern sciences and epidemiological as well as experimental approaches indicating the benefits of naturally occurring plants and plant products, of Ayurveda. A wide variety of ayurvedic medicinal herbs and their extract have been used against neurodegeneration like *B. monneiri* (Bramhi), *Withania somnifera* (Ashwagandha), *Convolvulus pluricaulis*

(Shankhpushpi), *Rauwolfia sepentina* (Sarpgandha) and *Nardostachys jatamansi* (Jatamansi) [17] (Table **1**). These have shown very high potential as nootropic herbs to improve neurodegenerative conditions and serve as the potential therapy for neurological disorders.

Table 1. otential effect of ayurvedic herbs on neurological disorder.

S. No.	Name of Ayurvedic Herb	Botanical Name	Biologically Active Compounds	Function	Ref.
1.	Ashwagandha	*W. somnifera*	Withanine, Withananine, Somniferine, Sominone	Reduce neuroinflammation, memory deficit, depression	[18]
2.	Awla	*Emblica officinalis*	Pyrogallol	Memory improvement	[19]
3.	Brahmi	*B. monnieri*	Bacoside A, Betulininc Acid, Bacoposide	Enhancement in memory and cognition	[20]
4.	Bringraj	*Eclipta alba*	Wedelolactone	Antioxidant and learning improvement	[21]
5.	Clove	*Syzygium aromaticum*	Euginol	Anti-depressant	[22]
6.	Giloy	*Tinospora cordifolia*	Tinocordioside, Cordiosides	Anti-depressant	[23]
7.	Jatamansi	*N. jatamansi*	Sesquiterpenoids, Valeriananoids	Memory deficit, insomnia (sleep disorder)	[24]
8.	Kesar	*Crocus sativus*	Crocins	Anti-parkinsonian and antioxidant	[25]
9.	Neem	*Azadirchta indica*	Limonoids	Cognitive improvement	[26]
10.	Pepper	*Piper nigrum*	Piperine	Neurodegeneration protection and memory impairment	[27]
11.	Shankhpushpi	*C. pluricaulis*	Shankhapushpine, Convolamine, Convoline,	Memory and learning improvement, reduction of tau- mediate toxicity	[28]
12.	Shatavar	*Asparagus racemosus*	Shatavarin IV	Anti-parkinsonian and antioxidant	[29]
13.	Tulsi	*Ocimum santum*	Eugenol	Inhibition of acetyl-choline	[30]
14.	Turmeric	*Curcuma longa*	Curcumin	Reduce neuroinflammation, memory deficit, depression, neurodegeneration	[31]

PD

PD is the second most common progressive neurodegenerative disease, also referred to as shaking palsy, characterized by loss of DAergic neurons in the SNpc [31] and accumulation of Lewy bodies in surviving neurons or simply Parkinson's is a neurodegenerative disease, and it was first medically described by James Parkinson in 1917 [32]. It is a long-term degenerative disorder that involves the degeneration or death of neurons. This leads to the development of motor and non-motor symptoms, which include tremors, muscle rigidity, slowness of movement (bradykinesia), cognitive dysfunction and subtle language problems.

PREVALENCE OF PD

The prevalence of PD varies, affecting around 7 to 10 million people [33, 34]. It is remarkably common throughout the world, and the estimated number of cases per 100,000 individuals is 8-18, in a year. Cases of PD doubled from 1990 to 2015 [35], which may be due to the increasing number of older people, longer disease duration, increased reporting of cases, changes in the environmental conditions, and food preferences. It mostly impacts the people of the age group 40-60 and older people above 60 [36], who are at the greatest risk of developing PD. It can develop at any stage of life, from young to older age, with a mean onset of age 60 years. The chance, *i.e.*, rate of developing PD varies with age group, was 3-4% before the age of 40, 5-10% in 20-50 age group, 1% over 60, and 4% above 80 years [34, 37, 38]. More than 90% of cases of PD are sporadic, while mutations induce PD in a small proportion [39].

SYMPTOMS OF PD

The major factor involved in PD generation is the loss of DAergic neurons and aggregation of Alpha-Synuclein (α-syn) [7]. DAergic neurons are present in the SNpc region of the brain, which degenerates as time progresses. This leads to a low level of dopamine in the basal ganglia, which majorly affects the movement. Many environmental and genetic factors will lead to their degeneration. This degeneration is slowly emerged and spotted *via* symptoms, and as the disease worsens, non-motor symptoms become more common. The presence of α-syn containing intracellular aggregation leads to the most common and recognizable symptoms of PD, primarily including movement-related problems like bradykinesia, resting tremor, slowness of movement, postural instability, rigidity, and difficulty with walking, further cognitive and behavioral problems may also occur [40 - 44]. Emotional, sensory and sleep problems are some other symptoms of PD, which may lead to depression and anxiety in one-third of patients [45]. In the advanced stage of PD, dementia becomes more common, which includes loss of memory, language, problem-solving, and other thinking abilities that are severe enough to interfere with daily life [46]. Neuroinflammation, generation of ROS, cognitive impairment, and neuropsychiatric symptoms have also been seen in PD patients [47]. The cause of PD is not fully understood yet, but the combination of environmental and genetic factors is likely involved. Researchers worldwide look to determine the exact cause of PD and, at the same time, find better ways to treat these conditions with natural/ayurvedic herbs [44, 48 - 54].

Motor Symptoms

Bradykinesia: Over time, PD patients move slowly due to motor disturbance in the planning of the initiation of the motion making the simple task difficult and time-consuming. In this condition, steps become shorter, and affected people experience struggling in walking.

Tremor: This is related to shaking, which generally begins with the limb, mainly in hand and fingers. As the disease progresses, it affects the whole arm and its voluntary movement.

Postural instability: In this condition, posture becomes stooped, leading to impaired balance and repeated falls. The number of falls is related to the severity of PD.

Rigidity: Rigidity is stiffness and resistance to limb movement caused by increased muscle tone, an excessive and continuous contraction of muscles. Rigidity may be associated with joint pain, such pain being a frequent initial manifestation of the disease. Rigidity is often asymmetrical in the early onset of PD, and it tends to affect the neck and shoulder muscles before the muscles of the face and extremities. With the progression of the disease, rigidity typically affects the whole body and reduces the ability to move [51, 55 - 57].

Non-Motor Symptoms

Along with the motor symptoms, PD is also characterized by non-motor manifestations such as cognitive impairment, sleep disturbance, autonomic disturbance, and other health issues like Dementia, depression, psychosis, anxiety, apathy, hallucinations, delusions, *etc*.

Cognition disturbances: As the severity of the disease increases, the memory fades and dementia-like symptoms start appearing. The most common complication found in PD is the execution, which includes problem-solving capacity, planning, abstract thinking, cognition flexibility, working memory, impaired recall or memory acquisition, perception, *etc..*, leading to overall cognitive decline [43, 57, 58].

RISK FACTORS: ENVIRONMENTAL AND GENETIC FACTORS

The epidemiology of PD suggests that exposure to air pollutants, pesticides, dietary contaminants, and environmental toxins is involved in PD pathogenesis. Microorganisms such as viruses may enter the human body *via* the nose and/or mouth, and may initiate PD pathogenesis at the olfactory bulb or the gut enteric nerves; over time, the pathogenesis may spread to the brain *via* the olfactory and/or the vagus nerve, and eventually lead to DAergic neuron deaths in the SNpc [49, 51, 55]. The majority of environmental toxins lead to mitochondrial dysfunction resulting in oxidative stress and proteinaceous aggregation like 1-methyl-4-phenyl-1,2,3,6-tetrahydropyridine (MPTP) and rotenone. Cigarette smoking, and alcohols also show their adverse effect on PD [50, 52].

Several genetic factors are involved as the causative agent for familial as well as sporadic PD (Table 2). In genome-wide association studies (GWAS), single nucleotide polymorphisms (SNP) of several genes, including the SNCA gene that codes for α-syn, were found to be associated with an increased risk for PD. These genes give a better idea at the molecular level, which aids to develop successful therapies for treating PD. Some such genes are SNCA, LRRK2, VPS35, CHCHD2, BF4G1, SNCA, MAPT, LRRK2, HLA DRB5, BST1, GAK, ACMSD, STK39, MCCC1/LAMP3, SYT11, CCDC62/HIP1R, Parkin, PINK1, DJ1, ATP13A2, PLA2G6, FBXO7, DNAJC6, RAB39B, *etc..* which involved in synaptic transmission, lysosomal and endosomal pathways, mitochondrial functions and vesicular trafficking [59].

Table 2. Genes responsible for both the familial and sporadic forms.

α-syn (SNCA) (Park 1 and 4)	Point mutations in an autosomal dominant pattern. Duplications. Triplications and post-translational modifications cause the protein product to change into fibrillar form. It constitutes the major component of the Lewy body. Expression level changes are also seen in sporadic cases
Parkin (Park 2)	Autosomal recessive causes juvenile parkinsonism but not all cases contain Lewy body
PARK 3 (not known)	Autosomal dominant
Ubiquitin C-terminal hydrolase like- I (**UCHL-1**) (PARK 5)	The missense mutation, Autosomal dominant, Role is uncertain

(Table 2) cont.....

PTEN-induced putative kinase **(PINK1)** (PARK 6)	A second most common form of juvenile parkinsonism. A heterozygous mutation of PINK is also seen in sporadic cases. Causes Lewy body pathology.
DJ-1 (PARK 7)	A rare form of autosomal recessive parkinsonism. It is localized in mitochondria and modulates to oxidative stress
Leucine-rich repeat kinase 2 **(LRRK 2** or Dardarin) (PARK 8)	Most common familial autosomal dominant. Lewy body pathology, nigral degeneration, progressive supranuclear palsy-like tau aggregation seen in LRRK2 mutation
ATP 13 A2 (PARK 9)	Autosomal recessive phenotypes like Parkinson's with spasticity and dementia
PARK 10, 11 & 12	Unknown function, Autosomal Dominants
OMI/HtrA2 (PARK 13)	Its function is a mitochondrial serine protease
Phospholipase A2 (PLA2G6) (PARK 14)	An autosomal recessive, missense mutation
F-box protein 7 FBXO7 (PARK 15)	Missense mutations, and truncations cause parkinsonism, Autosomal recessive

HALLMARK OF PD: A -SYN

PD is histopathologically defined by the presence of Lewy Bodies (LB) and Lewy neurites. LB are discovered by Frederic Heinrich Lewy in 1912, and are the large protein aggregates of α-syn and considered a hallmark of the PD pathogenesis [7]. α-syn aggregation increase with disease progression. In the initial stage of PD, the site of aggregation is the central nervous system (CNS), the dorsal motor nucleus of the brainstem, and the olfactory bulb. After disease progression, these aggregates will appear in the pontine tegmentum, followed by the amygdala and SNpc. At the terminal stage of the disease, these eventually will reach the temporal cortex and neocortex. Along with aggregation in the CNS, α-syn also forms aggregates in the peripheral nervous system (PNS), and it is found in the spinal cord, sympathetic ganglia, vagus, sciatic nerves, and gastrointestinal system [60]. In short, α-syn is present throughout the PD spatially, and temporally stereotypic patterns and its localization can be used deliberately to understand the symptoms and mechanism of PD. Its presence in CNS is the causal factor for the motor as well as non-motor symptoms, conversely, PNS may be the potential cause of the non-motor symptoms [61]. α-syn is present at the end of pre-synaptic neurons and is the defining component of LBs. Its impairment will lead to the spectrum of the disease called synucleinopathy, which is a key inducer and progressor of the PD. It is the causal factor of two types of PD: familial PD, and sporadic PD [62]. It is generally present and functional in the native monomeric soluble unfolded stage, but in PD it forms aggregates, which are the main component of LBs. These aggregate forms, also called α-syn toxicity or synuclein pathology, causes oxidative stress and neuronal degradation [63]. This toxicity and widespread distribution of the α-syn suggested that it may spread from cell to cell in a prion-like manner [64]. These aggregates are formed due to alteration in α-syn encoding gene SNCA gene, which is present on the long arm of chromosome 4, through Missense mutation, promotor alteration, polymorphisms or multiplications, and phosphorylation [65]. Various missense mutations have been identified in the SNCA gene, which leads to the formation of aggregation of α-syn: G209A, A30P, E46K, H50Q, G51D, A53E, A18T, and A29S [66]. These missense mutations produce impaired α-syn by increasing the aggregation kinetics, which causes to disrupt the membrane binding [67]. Mutation in the promoter region of the SNCA gene has been identified to increase the risk factor of PD.

PATHOPHYSIOLOGY OF PD

The primary neuropathology of PD is problems related to movement, which is a major and first appeared symptom. This movement-related problem is largely induced due to degeneration of the DAergic neurons, which are subcortical nuclei present in the region of the basal ganglia called the substantia nigra (SN) [7]. DAergic neuron is a key producer of dopamine, and their neurodegeneration in PD causes to alter or complete loss of dopamine [68]. This degeneration, also called toxicity, may be induced by genetic or environmental factors that may occur due to protein misfolding, defective proteolysis, and mitochondrial dysfunctions to enhance the production of the reactive oxygen species (ROS) [68]. Dopamine act in paracrine fashion in the areas of basal ganglia, which contain different regions: striatum (or caudate/putamen), SN, subthalamic nucleus (STN), thalamus, pedunculopontine nucleus, and globus pallidus with external and internal segments (GPe and GPi) [69]. Basal ganglia are the centre for muscle movements, and they will subconsciously control and coordinate the muscle tone from the learned movement pattern. The pathogenesis of PD has three major themes: protein aggregation, mitochondrial, and proteasomal dysfunction (Fig. **1**). Inflammation mainly associated with microglia activation is also seen in other neurodegenerative diseases [70]. Apart from the DA system, the other system affected are noradrenergic (locus coeruleus), serotonergic (raphe) and cholinergic (nucleus basalis of Meynert, the dorsal motor nucleus of Vagus), neurotransmitter, as well as cerebral cortex (in cingulate and entorhinal cortices), olfactory lobe and autonomic nervous system resulting in the non-motor system [71, 72]. PD, progresses in six neuropathological stages known as Braak stages according to the development of inclusion bodies Lewy neurites (LN) within the cellular process and as granular aggregation known as Lewy bodies (LB) (Table **3**) [73].

Table 3. Braak stages of PD.

Stages	Affected Regions	Symptoms
Stage 1	Brain stem and olfactory system mainly dorsal motor and anterior olfactory nucleus	Pre-symptomatic
Stage 2	Locus ceruleus in the pontine tegmentum	Pre-symptomatic
Stage 3	SNpc	Motor symptoms
Stage 4	Meso cortex, amygdala (transition zone and neocortex and allocortex)	Motor symptoms
Stage 5	The neocortex, temporal, parietal, frontal lobe	Cognitive symptoms
Stage 6	Neocortex and limbic system	Cognitive symptoms

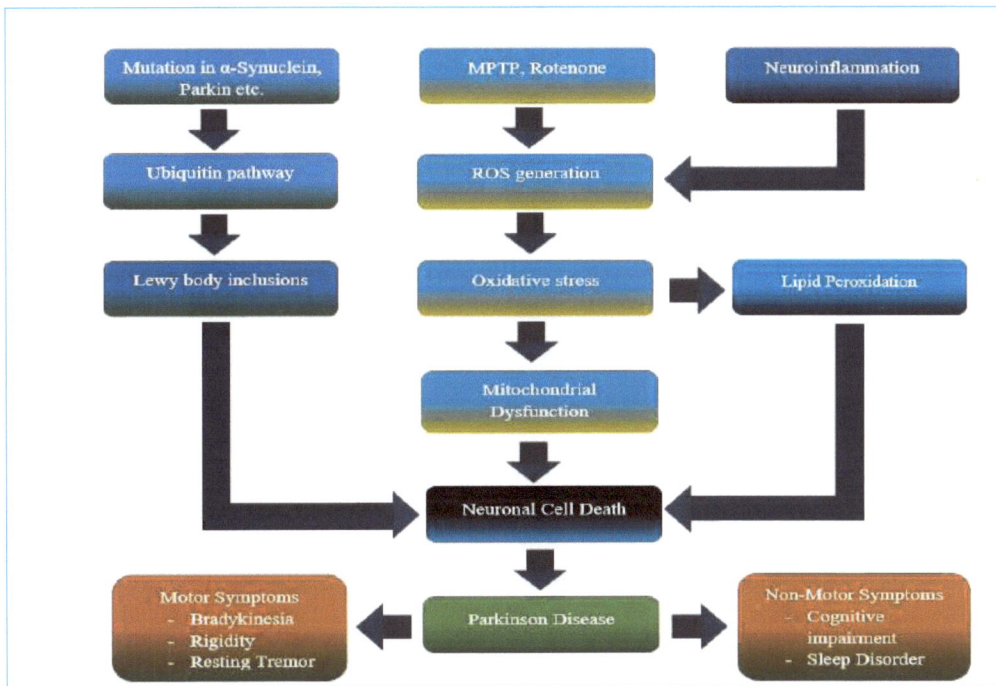

Fig. (1). Pathophysiology of PD: Pathophysiology of PD – Death of neurons is the basic cause for the pathophysiology of PD, which mostly occurs due to three reasons (left to right). 1) Mutations in Genes like α-syn will lead to the formation of Lewy bodies *via* ubiquitin pathways which is the hallmark feature of PD. 2) Oxidative stress induced by compounds like MPTP or rotenone will lead to a change the mitochondrial dysfunction and 3) Neuroinflammation.

B. MONNIERI AND ITS HISTORICAL PERSPECTIVE

B. monnieri is a traditional Ayurvedic medicine known for centuries. It is used for memory enhancing, antipyretic, sedative, analgesic, anti-inflammatory, and antiepileptic agents [74]. *B. monnieri* L., has various vernacular names (common names) such as "Brahmi" or water hyssop or Thyme-leaved Gratiola. It is described in Ayurveda, as a brain tonic. It is commonly known as "Brahmi", which is derived from the Indian god for "Bramha", the mythical "creator" in the Hindu pantheon [75]. The brain is a creative centre of the body. It is a traditional ayurvedic herb classified under the "Medhya Rasayana" since ancient times and described as a memory enhancer promoting intellect and managing mental health such as poor cognition and concentrations, in "Charka Samhita" (6th century A.D.) [76]. It has been used by the Ayurvedic medical practitioners of India for almost 3000 years and is known to alle*via*te diseases that impair intellect, memory, and knowledge. It is considered a nootropic drug because it enhances memory and performs work like a neuromodulator [77]. Brahmi is believed to be an aphrodisiac, in certain parts of India. In Sri Lanka, it is known as "Loonooweella" and is used for fevers. In the Philippines, it is used as a diuretic [74].

Geographical Distribution, Plant Description, and Classification

It is a small, creeping, and annual succulent herb with numerous branches and small fleshy, oblong leaves. Stems bear leaves and flowers, which form roots at the nodes. Flowers are blue or white with purple veins, and the fruit is a capsule with numerous seeds. Flowers and fruits appear in the summer, and the stem and the leaves of the plant are used [78]. It is dispersed throughout the subtropical areas of countries like India, China, Nepal, Shri Lanka, *etc*. It is found throughout the Indian subcontinent in wet, damp and marshy areas. It grows abundantly in marshes and wetlands of warmer regions and is recognized as weeds in rice fields [79]. It grows in wet and sandy areas and near streams in tropical regions. It is distributed widely throughout the world in the warmer parts. It belongs to the family Scrophulariaceae under the class Amognoliopsida of division Magnoliophyta in the kingdom Plantae. The genus *B. monnieri* includes over 100 species of aquatic herbs [80].

Classification [plants.usda.gov]

Kingdom: Plantae – Plants

Subkingdom: Tracheobionta – Vascular plants

Super-division: Spermatophyta – Seed plants

Division: Magnoliophyta – Flowering plants

Class: Magnoliopsida – Dicotyledons

Subclass: Asteridae

Order: Scrophulariales

Family: Scrophulariaceae – Figwort family

Genus: *Bacopa* Aubl. – waterhyssop

Species: *monnieri* (L.) Pennell – herb of grace

B. *monnieri* and its Biologically Active Components

In the indigenous system of medicine viewing the importance of this plant, systematic chemical examinations of the plant and its parts have been carried out by several groups of researchers. The phytochemical analysis of *B. monnieri* plant, plant extract, and isolated bacosides (the major active principles) have shown the presence of several bioactive components, such as triterpenoids saponins, alkaloids, glycoside, and alcohols [81]. Triterpenoid saponins of dammarane types known as bacosides are the main nootropic constituents of *B. monnieri* [82]. They contain glycone units such as jujubogenin or pseudo-jujubogenin moieties, which differ only in the position of the side chain of olefinic in aglycone and nature glycosidic chain sugar units [83]. These bacosides form includes bacosides A1-A3 and B bacopasaponins A–G, and bacopasides I–XI [83]. Recently, some novel saponins have been identified called bacopasides I–XII [81]. Along with triterpenoids saponins, many different compounds have been identified from *B. monnieri* and its different extracts like alkalosis, (brahmin, nicotine, and herpestine), saponins (monnierin, hersaponin), sterol (β-sitosterol, stigma-sterol), d-mannitol, acid A, apigenin, monnierasides I-III, cucurbitacins (Bacobitacin A–D and cucurbitacin E), plantainoside B, betulinic acid, phenylethanoid glycosides, flavonoids and stigmastanol [Aguiar, S., & Borowski, T. (2013)]. Bacoside A, [3-(α-L-arabinopyronsyl)-O-β-D-glucopyronaside, 20-dihydraoxy-16-keto-dammar-24-ene], remained one of the most studied constituents of *B. monnieri*, which is a blend of bacoside A3, bacopacide II, bacopasaponin C, and a jujubogenin isomer of bacosaponin C (Table **4**) [84]. A compound extracted by the chemical and physical-based polar fraction [85 - 90] and their structure elucidated through NMR [91, 92].

Role of B. *monnieri* as Nootropic Drug

B. monnieri has been used to promote memory and intellect, psychoneurological disorders, and rejuvenator. In the last four decades, it has increased research interaction due to its memory-enhancing activities, improving cognitive function. Many reviews have been published on *B. monnieri* about memory-enhancing activities, improving cognitive function, and some clinical trials [93 - 95]. It has been shown, in rats, to improve motor learning capabilities [96], and improve acquisition, retention of memory and consolidation [97], cognitive function and mental retention capacity [96 - 101], antidementia properties [100], the tranquilizing effect [102, 103], smooth-muscle relaxation and showed antispasmodic activity [103], prevented oxidative stress or anti-oxidant [104 - 106], acquisition or learning in mice [107], sedative and hypnotic potentiating [108]. *B. monnieri* has reduced aluminum-induced toxicity through reversal or reduction of toxicity [106, 109] by prevention of oxidative stress [109], which shows its high potential as a neuroprotective drug. Extracted or purified compounds of *B. monnieri* are used to study these effects. *B. monnieri* Ethanolic extract induced a neuroprotective role [11], inhibited protein oxidation, lipofuscin accumulation, and lipid peroxidation [11] and reversed oxidative stress [104 - 106, 109]. *B. monnieri* showed comparable activity to some of the well-established drugs α-deprenyl (a monoamine oxidase-B inhibitor and neuroprotectant used in PD) [104, 110]. These effects of *B. monnieri* can be compiled in some mechanisms; acquisition or learning may be due to an increase in acetylcholine levels [107]; anti-oxidant activity through the restoration of endogenous antioxidant enzymes [106], superoxide dismutase (SOD), catalase (CAT), and glutathione peroxidase (GPx) activities [104], and increased the activity of SOD and CAT [111]. It also has shown an elevated level of cerebral glutamic acid, gamma-aminobutyric acid (GABA) [112, 113], anticholinesterase activity [100], inhibited protein oxidation, lipofuscin accumulation, and lipid peroxidation [110], accumulation of lipid and protein damage [106, 109], increase protein kinase and protein and serotonin (5-HT) levels and lower the norepinephrine level [97, 114].

Table 4. The bioactive component of brahmi extract.

S. No.	Bioactive component	IUPAC Name	Chemical Formula	Category
1	**Bacoside A2**	2-[2-[3,4-Dihydroxy-5- (hydroxymethyl)oxolan--yl]oxy-1-[3,4- dihydroxy-5-[[16-hydr-xy-2,6,6,10,16- pentamethyl-17-(2-methylpr-p-1-enyl)-19,21dioxahexacyclo[18.2.1.01,14.02,11.05,10.015,20]tricosan-7-yl]oxy]oxolan-2-yl]ethoxy]oxane-3,4,5-triol	$C_{46}H_{74}O_{17}$	Triterpenoids, saponins
2	**Bacoside A**	[3-(α-L-arabinopyronsyl)-O-β-D- glucopyronaside, 20-dihydraoxy-16-keto- dammar-24-ene]	$C_{40}H_{64}O_{12}$	Triterpenoids, saponins
3	**Bacoside A3**	3-β-[O-β-D-glucopyronosyl (1-3)-O-[α-L-arabinofuranosy (1-2)]-O-β-D-glucopyranosyl)oxy]	$C_{47}H_{76}O_{18}$	Triterpenoids, saponins

(Table 4) cont.....

S. No.	Bioactive component	IUPAC Name	Chemical Formula	Category
4	Pseudojujubogenin	3-O-[α-1-arabinofuranosyl (1-2) β-d-glucopyranosyl]	$C_{46}H_{74}O_{17}$	Glycoside
5	Nicotine	(S)-3-[1-Methylpyrrolidin-2-yl]pyridine	$C_{10}H_{14}N_2$	Alkaloid
6	Betuinic acid	(3β)-3-hydroxy-lup-20(29)-en-28-oic acid	$C_{30}H_{48}O_3$	Triterpenoids
7	Bacopasapon in G	3-O-[α-1-arabinofuranosyl-1(1-2)]-α-L- arabino-pyrosyl jujubogenin	$C_{46}H_{74}O_{17}$	Saponins
8	Cucurbitacin E	[(E,6R)-6-[8S,9R,10R,13R,14S,16R,17R)-2,16-dihydroxy-4,4,9,13,14,pentamethyl- 3,11-dioxo-8,10,12,15,16,17-hexahydro-7H-cyclopenta[a]phenantren-17-yl]-6-hydroxy- 2-methyl-5-oxohept-3-en-2-yl] acetate	$C_{32}H_{44}O_8$	Triterpene
9	Luteolin-7-rutinoside	2-(3,4-dihydroxyphenyl)-5-hydroxy-7-[(2S,4S,5S)-3,4,5-trihydraoxy-6-[[2R,4S,5R)-3,4,5 -trihydroxy-6-methyloxan-2-yl]oxymethyl]oxan-2-yl]oxychromen-4-one	$C_{27}H_{30}O_{15}$	Triterpenoids
10	Monnieraside III	([(2R,3R,4S,5S,6R)-2-[2-(3,4-Dihydroxyphenyl)ethoxy]-4,5-dihydroxy-6-(hydroxymethyl)oxan-3-yl] 4- hydroxybenzoate)	$C_{21}H_{24}O_{10}$	Triterpenoids

MECHANISTIC UNDERSTANDING OF *B. MONNEIRI* IN THE LIGHT OF PD: PHARMACOLOGICAL EFFECTS

Anti-Inflammatory and Analgesic Effects

Recent studies reveal that inflammation plays a crucial role in the progression of PD. The other hallmark of PD is also represented by chronic neuroinflammation. The release of pro-inflammatory cytokines by the activation of microglia leads to destructive effects and also enhance the apoptosis of neuronal cell, which result in poor condition of PD [75]. Microglia activation produces pro-inflammatory enzymes, such as COX1, COX2, iNOS, and pro-inflammatory cytokines like TNF-, IL-6, and IL1β and radicals such as nitric oxide and superoxide anion, which leads to the neural cell damaging and results in PD progression [115]. Pieces of evidence suggest that oxidative stress greatly impacts neuroinflammation and intracellular protein aggregation due to the production of ROS [115]. Various drugs are used to treat the problem related to inflammation and oxidative stress, which are further used for treating PD as an anti-parkinsonian drug [116 - 118]. Therefore, the suppression or reduction of overexpressed microglia may serve as a potential therapeutic strategy to prevent the further progression of PD. On the treatment with *B. monneiri*, there is a significant decrease in the level of pro-inflammatory cytokines, including interleukin-6 (IL-6) and macrophage inflammatory proteins-1-beta (MIP1β) [119], which indicates the role of *B. monneiri* as an anti-inflammatory herb.

Antioxidative Effect

ROS are the oxygen-derived free radicals, which in accumulation, lead to the damage of cellular machinery resulting in diseases such as inflammation, cancer, and neurodegeneration [120]. The generation of oxidative stress leads to the gradual loss of neurons, protein aggregation, membrane disruption, and oxidization of enzymes [121, 122]. There are antioxidative enzymes such as SOD, CAT, GPx, and Glutathione (GSH), which reduce the ROS, in turn preventing the damaging of cells. Many types of research have evidenced antioxidant properties, and it is thought to know as *B. monneiri* reduces the ROS level by upregulating various anti-oxidant enzymes (SOD, GSH, *etc.*.) [115, 123]. Furthermore, "Brahmi" also has the ability to quench the H_2O_2-mediated oxidative stress *in vitro* as well as *in vivo* [124]. Nrf2 and NF-κB are the transcription factor that regulates the antioxidant machinery of cells. "Brahmi" was found to increase Nrf2 and NF-κB expression in okadaic acid-treated Wistar rats [125]. *B. monneiri* shows the free radical scavenging property in their aqueous and ethanolic extract [126]. Pre-treatment of *B. monneiri* increases the antioxidant enzymatic activity suggesting the anti-neurotoxic effect of rotenone.

B. monnieri Reduced α-Syn Protein Aggregation

Inhibition of α-syn aggregation is an emerging strategy for attenuation of PD. Numerous ayurvedic extracts, such as *B. monneiri* have been reported for their potency in inhibiting the α-syn mediated destruction and toxicity [81, 127]. As described earlier, the association of dopamine and α-syn in maintaining the DAergic neuron cellular homeostasis plays a major role in the pathology of PD. α-syn gene (SNCA gene) stands first as a target of mutation, overexpression, and post-translational modification and by alternative splicing, a mechanism which leads to the formation of Lewy bodies and loss of dopamine. Thus α-syn is considered the main target for PD treatment [7]. Recent studies advocated the defense property of *B. monneiri* against the PD. *B. monneiri* treatment was found to reduce α-syn -induced degeneration in the cell [81, 127]. A study on rotenone-induced PD shows the increased aggregation of α-syn however, pre-treatment with *B. monneiri* decreases the level of α-syn compared to rotenone-injected PD rats.

B. monnieri **Enhances Cognition**

α-syn aggregation and selective degeneration of DAergic neurons lead to cognition decline. α-syn is a hallmark or marker protein for the validation of PD.

Human cognition can be divided into four categories based on their function: reception/ acquisition, learning/memory, thinking/ reasoning, and expression/ action, where memory is the central aspect of all these cognitive functions. It is the learning, storage, and retrieval of information, which divides the memory into two types: primary or short-term memory and secondary or long-term memory. The process of learning process starts when sensory signals are transcribed in the cortex, which is then transmitted to the hippocampus, where new memories are formed. If the signal is strong and repeated, a long-term memory is established, which is then wired and back to the cortex for storage [9, 11, 13, 54]. This memory will be stored as a new memory in neurons and synapses of the hippocampus region of the brain, without affecting the previous one. These neurons communicate with synapses and form several synaptic connections with other neurons to form complex structures. These structures are responsible for memory formation and brain functions. The frequent use of these synapses makes them stronger to form long-term memory and non-frequent synapse weaken over time, based on synaptic pruning. This strengthening and weakening of synapses over time is central to learning and memory and is termed as synaptic plasticity. The frequent use or repeated stimulation builds up a strong connection over time and establishes long-term potentiation (LTP), which will lead to long-term memory, whereas the weakening of synapse over time is termed as long-term depression (LTD), which is the basis of short-term memory. These LTPs are thought to be the cellular basis of memory formation and are best studied at glutamatergic neuronal connections. These glutamatergic connections use glutamate as a key molecule which exhibits an important role in memory function by the multiple receptor proteins [43, 56 - 58]. Glutamatergic neuron stimulation will release glutamate from the presynaptic knob of the neuron or exon into the synaptic cleft. This released glutamate will bind to the N-methyl-D-aspartate receptors (NMDAR), which are the nascent receptors situated on the postsynaptic membrane. NMDAR is located very early in the postsynaptic membrane and induces mature receptor alpha-amino-3-hydroxy-5-methyl-4-isoxazole propionic acid receptors (AMPAR). This induction and transition to mature AMPAR mediated by the nascent NMDAR is called synapse stabilization. This synapse stabilization is mediated *via* LTP and leads to long-term memory [85 - 89, 91 - 95]. These LTPs are the basis and key mechanism for learning and memory in the hippocampus. On the other hand, if the signal from afferent stimulation is weak, *i.e.*, non-frequent, then NMDAR will not be able to induce the AMPAR, and this will lead to the LTD, *i.e.*, short-term memory. In a nutshell, NMDARs will induce signal-dependent strengthening of synapse *via* LTP and weakening *via* LTD, through insertion and removal of the AMPAR from the postsynaptic membrane. LTP and LTD are key for this change in a conduit of the synaptic strength, which not just strengthens or weakens synaptic connections (short-term plasticity), but also will trigger the addition or loss of synapses (long-term plasticity) [51, 54].

Several technologies are being developed in the field of neuroscience to treat or manipulate neural calls in such a way that can enhance memory or cognition. RNA techniques have been used as therapeutic tools. Although these technologies are helpful, still, some gaps are there. Thus, researchers are moving to the ayurvedic solutions for treating PD by enhancing memory parameters. The mechanism of *B. monnieri* in terms of learning and memory amelioration is still not very clear but some ideas can be depicted from the schematic diagram given below (Fig. **2**).

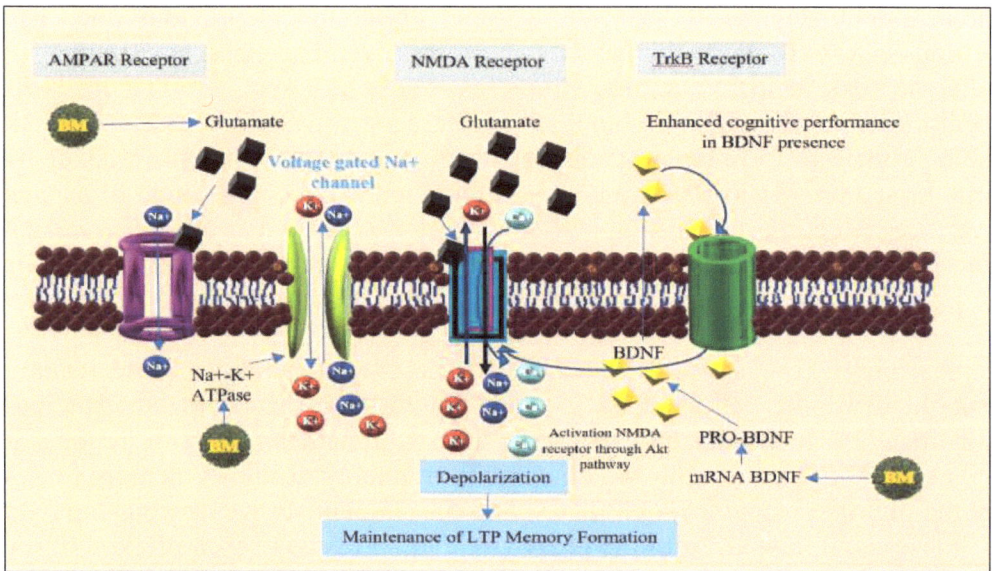

Fig. (2). Diagrammatic representation of *B. monneiri* showing molecular interaction enhancing cognition: Role of *B. monneiri* as a nootropic drug against the PD can be summarized in four pathways (left to right) 1) *B. monneiri* will enhance the level of glutamate, which ultimately will lead to change in flux of sodium ion through AMPAR receptor. 2) *B. monnieri* activates the level Na$^+$K$^+$ ATPase and which will shift the physiology of Na and K ion through Na/K pump towards normal physiology. 3) *B. monnieri* enhances the mRNA level of the BDNF gene, which will further activate the NMDA receptor and TrkB receptor. Activated NMDA will further stabilize the level of ion through the membrane, which will then maintain the LTP memory formation. 4) *B. monnieri* activated TrkB receptor, *via* BDNF, will enhance cognitive performance [128].

CONCLUSION

PD is the second most common cause of neurodegenerative disease, however, various treatment strategies have been designed to cure it. Ayurveda is one such strategy that uses plants and their extract for the treatment of diseases. The ayurvedic herb *B. monneiri* has been used by Indian people for brain-related disorders. Recently, it has shown very potent activity to develop as a nootropic drug. It has reduced major hallmark features of the PD like the reduction of Neuroinflammation through decreasing level of Neuroinflammatory cytokines; antioxidant activity through reducing Oxidative stress; reduction in major hallmark gene α-syn induced degeneration of cells (Fig. **3**). It has shown a high potential to be developed as a nootropic drug but still, its mechanisms of action or mode of action remain to be understood. More research is required to identify the particular compounds responsible for their nootropic action.

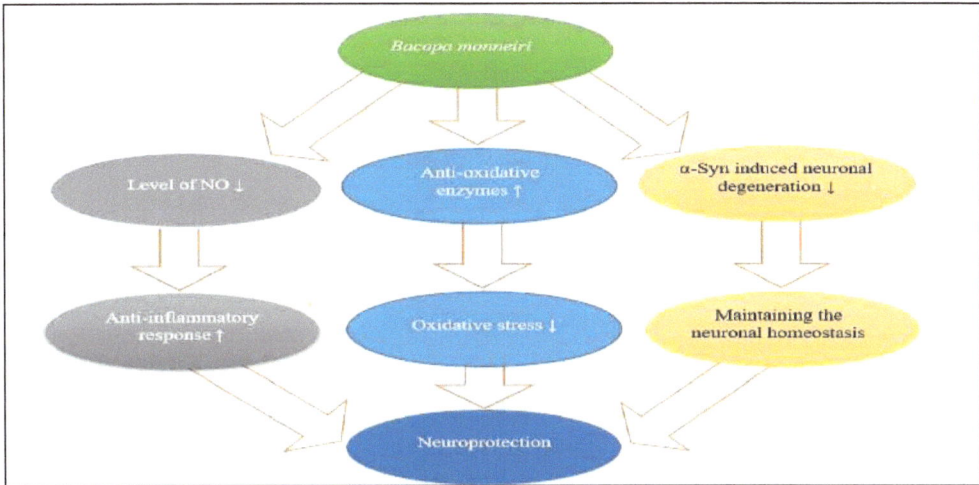

Fig. (3). Major roles of *B. monneiri* in neuroprotection: Role of *B. monneiri* in neuroprotection – it works as a neuroprotective through three pathways-1) it decreases the level of NO, which will reduce oxidative stress. 2) *B. monnieri* also reduces oxidative stress by increasing the level of antioxidant enzymes. 3) Also, it maintains neuronal homeostasis by decreasing the level of α-syn degradation.

CONSENT FOR PUBLICATION

Not applicable.

CONFLICT OF INTEREST

The author declares no conflict of interest, financial or otherwise.

ACKNOWLEDGEMENTS

The preparation of this chapter was financially supported by CSIR-UGC; the Government of India to Vartika Gupta in the form of JRF is highly acknowledged.

REFERENCES

[1]   Verhage M, Maia AS, Plomp JJ, *et al.* Synaptic assembly of the brain in the absence of neurotransmitter secretion. Science 2000; 287(5454): 864-9.
[http://dx.doi.org/10.1126/science.287.5454.864] [PMID: 10657302]

[2]   Toni N, Teng EM, Bushong EA, *et al.* Synapse formation on neurons born in the adult hippocampus. Nat Neurosci 2007; 10(6): 727-34.
[http://dx.doi.org/10.1038/nn1908] [PMID: 17486101]

[3]   Tyler WJ, Alonso M, Bramham CR, Pozzo-Miller LD. From acquisition to consolidation: on the role of brain-derived neurotrophic factor signaling in hippocampal-dependent learning. Learn Mem 2002; 9(5): 224-37.
[http://dx.doi.org/10.1101/lm.51202] [PMID: 12359832]

[4]   Sweatt JD. Mitogen-activated protein kinases in synaptic plasticity and memory. Curr Opin Neurobiol 2004; 14(3): 311-7.
[http://dx.doi.org/10.1016/j.conb.2004.04.001] [PMID: 15194111]

[5]   Nussbaum RL, Ellis CE. Alzheimer's disease and Parkinson's disease. N Engl J Med 2003; 348(14): 1356-64.
[http://dx.doi.org/10.1056/NEJM2003ra020003] [PMID: 12672864]

[6]   Gelb DJ, Oliver E, Gilman S. Diagnostic criteria for Parkinson disease. Arch Neurol 1999; 56(1): 33-9.
[http://dx.doi.org/10.1001/archneur.56.1.33] [PMID: 9923759]

[7]   Poewe W, Seppi K, Tanner CM, *et al.* Parkinson disease. Nat Rev Dis Primers 2017; 3(1): 17013.
[http://dx.doi.org/10.1038/nrdp.2017.13] [PMID: 28332488]

[8]   Armstrong MJ, Okun MS. Diagnosis and treatment of Parkinson disease: a review. JAMA 2020; 323(6): 548-60.
[http://dx.doi.org/10.1001/jama.2019.22360] [PMID: 32044947]

[9]   Kabra A, Sharma R, Kabra R, Baghel US. Emerging and alternative therapies for Parkinson disease: an updated review. Curr Pharm Des 2018; 24(22): 2573-82.
[http://dx.doi.org/10.2174/1381612824666180820150150] [PMID: 30124146]

[10]   Suchowersky O, Gronseth G, Perlmutter J, Reich S, Zesiewicz T, Weiner WJ. Practice Parameter: neuroprotective strategies and alternative therapies for Parkinson disease (an evidence-based review): report of the Quality Standards Subcommittee of the American Academy of Neurology. Neurology 2006; 66(7): 976-82.
[http://dx.doi.org/10.1212/01.wnl.0000206363.57955.1b] [PMID: 16606908]

[11]   Khare CP. Indian herbal remedies: rational Western therapy, ayurvedic, and other traditional usage, Botany: Springer science & business media 2004.
[http://dx.doi.org/10.1007/978-3-642-18659-2]

[12]   Gourie-Devi M, Ramu MG, Venkataram BS. Treatment of Parkinson's disease in 'Ayurveda' (ancient Indian system of medicine): discussion paper. J R Soc Med 1991; 84(8): 491-2.
[http://dx.doi.org/10.1177/014107689108400814] [PMID: 1886119]

[13]   Chopra A, Doiphode VV. Ayurvedic medicine: core concept, therapeutic principles, and current relevance. Med Clin North Am 2002; 86(1): 75-89, vii.
[http://dx.doi.org/10.1016/S0025-7125(03)00073-7] [PMID: 11795092]

[14]   Dubey T, Chinnathambi S. Brahmi (*Bacopa monnieri*): An ayurvedic herb against the Alzheimer's disease. Arch Biochem Biophys 2019; 676: 108153.
        [http://dx.doi.org/10.1016/j.abb.2019.108153] [PMID: 31622587]

[15]   Mehta A, Prabhakar M, Kumar P, Deshmukh R, Sharma PL. Excitotoxicity: Bridge to various triggers in neurodegenerative disorders. Eur J Pharmacol 2013; 698(1-3): 6-18.
        [http://dx.doi.org/10.1016/j.ejphar.2012.10.032] [PMID: 23123057]

[16]   Bartus RT. On neurodegenerative diseases, models, and treatment strategies: lessons learned and lessons forgotten a generation following the cholinergic hypothesis. Exp Neurol 2000; 163(2): 495-529.
        [http://dx.doi.org/10.1006/exnr.2000.7397] [PMID: 10833325]

[17]   Mukherjee PK, Wahile A, Kumar V, Rai S, Mukherjee K, Saha B. Marker profiling of botanicals used for hepatoprotection in Indian system of medicine. Drug information journal: DIJ/Drug Information Association. 2006; 40(2)
        [http://dx.doi.org/10.1177/009286150604000202]

[18]   Tuli R, Sangwan R, Kumar S, *et al.* Ashwagandha (*Withania somnifera*)—a model Indian medicinal plant. Council of Scientific and Industrial Research (CSIR), New Delhi. 2009.

[19]   Vasudevan M, Parle M. Memory enhancing activity of Anwala churna (*Emblica officinalis* Gaertn.): An Ayurvedic preparation. Physiol Behav 2007; 91(1): 46-54.
        [http://dx.doi.org/10.1016/j.physbeh.2007.01.016] [PMID: 17343883]

[20]   Pase MP, Kean J, Sarris J, Neale C, Scholey AB, Stough C. The cognitive-enhancing effects of *Bacopa monnieri*: a systematic review of randomized, controlled human clinical trials. J Altern Complement Med 2012; 18(7): 647-52.
        [http://dx.doi.org/10.1089/acm.2011.0367] [PMID: 22747190]

[21]   Bhalerao SA, Verma DR, Teli NC, Murukate VR. *Eclipta alba* (L): An overview. Int J Bioassays 2013; 2(11): 1443-7p.

[22]   Song XY, Hu JF, Chu SF, *et al.* Ginsenoside Rg1 attenuates okadaic acid induced spatial memory impairment by the GSK3β/tau signaling pathway and the Aβ formation prevention in rats. Eur J Pharmacol 2013; 710(1-3): 29-38.
        [http://dx.doi.org/10.1016/j.ejphar.2013.03.051] [PMID: 23588117]

[23]   Dhama K, Sachan S, Khandia R, *et al.* Medicinal and beneficial health applications of *Tinospora cordifolia* (Guduchi): a miraculous herb countering various diseases/disorders and its Immunomodulatory effects. Recent Pat Endocr Metab Immune Drug Discov 2017; 10(2): 96-111.
        [http://dx.doi.org/10.2174/1872214811666170301105101] [PMID: 28260522]

[24]   Khan MB, Hoda MN, Ishrat T, *et al.* Neuroprotective efficacy of *Nardostachys jatamansi* and crocetin in conjunction with selenium in cognitive impairment. Neurol Sci 2012; 33(5): 1011-20.
        [http://dx.doi.org/10.1007/s10072-011-0880-1] [PMID: 22170092]

[25]   Zeinali M, Zirak MR, Rezaee SA, Karimi G, Hosseinzadeh H. Immunoregulatory and anti-inflammatory properties of *Crocus sativus* (Saffron) and its main active constituents: A review. Iran J Basic Med Sci 2019; 22(4): 334-44.
        [PMID: 31223464]

[26]   Maiti R, Raghavendra M, Kumar S, Acharya SB. Role of aqueous extract of *Azadirachta indica* leaves in an experimental model of Alzheimer's disease in rats. Int J Appl Basic Med Res 2013; 3(1): 37-47.
        [http://dx.doi.org/10.4103/2229-516X.112239] [PMID: 23776838]

[27]   Chonpathompikunlert P, Wattanathorn J, Muchimapura S. Piperine, the main alkaloid of Thai black pepper, protects against neurodegeneration and cognitive impairment in animal model of cognitive deficit like condition of Alzheimer's disease. Food Chem Toxicol 2010; 48(3): 798-802.
        [http://dx.doi.org/10.1016/j.fct.2009.12.009] [PMID: 20034530]

[28]   Bihaqi S, Singh A, Tiwari M. Supplementation of *Convolvulus pluricaulis* attenuates scopolamine-

induced increased tau and Amyloid precursor protein (AβPP) expression in rat brain. Indian J Pharmacol 2012; 44(5): 593-8.
[http://dx.doi.org/10.4103/0253-7613.100383] [PMID: 23112420]

[29]   Parihar MS, Hemnani T. Experimental excitotoxicity provokes oxidative damage in mice brain and attenuation by extract of *Asparagus racemosus*. J Neural Transm (Vienna) 2004; 111(1): 1-12.
[http://dx.doi.org/10.1007/s00702-003-0069-8] [PMID: 14714211]

[30]   Giridharan VV, Thandavarayan RA, Konishi T. *Ocimum sanctum* Linn.(Holy Basil) to Improve Cognition. Diet and Nutrition in Dementia and Cognitive Decline. 2015; 1049-58.
[http://dx.doi.org/10.1016/B978-0-12-407824-6.00098-7]

[31]   Monroy A, Lithgow GJ, Alavez S. Curcumin and neurodegenerative diseases. Biofactors 2013; 39(1): 122-32.
[http://dx.doi.org/10.1002/biof.1063] [PMID: 23303664]

[32]   Parkinson J. An essay on the shaking palsy. 1817. J Neuropsychiatry Clin Neurosci 2002; 14(2): 223-36.
[http://dx.doi.org/10.1176/jnp.14.2.223] [PMID: 11983801]

[33]   Kalia LV, Lang AE. Evolving basic, pathological and clinical concepts in PD. Nat Rev Neurol 2016; 12(2): 65-6.
[http://dx.doi.org/10.1038/nrneurol.2015.249] [PMID: 26782330]

[34]   Marras C, Beck JC, Bower JH, *et al.* Prevalence of Parkinson's disease across North America. NPJ Parkinsons Dis 2018; 4(1): 21.
[http://dx.doi.org/10.1038/s41531-018-0058-0] [PMID: 30003140]

[35]   Dorsey ER, Sherer T, Okun MS, Bloem BR. The emerging evidence of the Parkinson pandemic. J Parkinsons Dis 2018; 8(s1): S3-8.
[http://dx.doi.org/10.3233/JPD-181474] [PMID: 30584159]

[36]   Hobson P, Gallacher J, Meara J. Cross-sectional survey of Parkinson's disease and parkinsonism in a rural area of the United Kingdom. Mov Disord 2005; 20(8): 995-8.
[http://dx.doi.org/10.1002/mds.20489] [PMID: 15852368]

[37]   Kis B, Schrag A, Ben-Shlomo Y, *et al.* Novel three-stage ascertainment method. Neurology 2002; 58(12): 1820-5.
[http://dx.doi.org/10.1212/WNL.58.12.1820] [PMID: 12084883]

[38]   D'Alessandro R, Gamberini G, Granieri E, Benassi G, Naccarato S, Manzaroli D. Prevalence of Parkinson's disease in the Republic of San Marino. Neurology 1987; 37(10): 1679-82.
[http://dx.doi.org/10.1212/WNL.37.10.1679] [PMID: 3658176]

[39]   de Lau LML, Breteler MMB. Epidemiology of Parkinson's disease. Lancet Neurol 2006; 5(6): 525-35.
[http://dx.doi.org/10.1016/S1474-4422(06)70471-9] [PMID: 16713924]

[40]   Lang AE. The progression of Parkinson disease. Neurology 2007; 68(12): 948-52.
[http://dx.doi.org/10.1212/01.wnl.0000257110.91041.5d] [PMID: 17372132]

[41]   Chinta SJ, Andersen JK. Dopaminergic neurons. Int J Biochem Cell Biol 2005; 37(5): 942-6.
[http://dx.doi.org/10.1016/j.biocel.2004.09.009] [PMID: 15743669]

[42]   Keswani C, Dilnashin H, Birla H, Singh S. Re-addressing the commercialization and regulatory hurdles for biopesticides in India. Rhizosphere. 2019; 11(100155): 10.1016.

[43]   Zahra W, Rai SN, Birla H, *et al.* Zahra W, Rai SN, Birla H, Singh SS, Rathore AS, Dilnashin H, Singh R, Keswani C, Singh RK, Singh SP. Neuroprotection of rotenone-induced Parkinsonism by ursolic acid in PD mouse model. CNS & Neurological Disorders-Drug Targets. 2020; 527-540(14)
[http://dx.doi.org/10.2174/1871527319666200812224457]

[44]   Zahra W, Rai SN, Birla H, *et al.* Economic Importance of Medicinal Plants in Asian Countries. Bioeconomy for Sustainable Development. 2020; 359-77.

[http://dx.doi.org/10.1007/978-981-13-9431-7_19]

[45] Adler CH. Nonmotor complications in Parkinson's disease. Mov Disord 2005; 20(S11) (Suppl. 11): S23-9.
[http://dx.doi.org/10.1002/mds.20460] [PMID: 15822106]

[46] Postuma RB, Gagnon JF, Vendette M, Charland K, Montplaisir J. Manifestations of Parkinson disease differ in association with REM sleep behavior disorder. Mov Disord 2008; 23(12): 1665-72.
[http://dx.doi.org/10.1002/mds.22099] [PMID: 18709686]

[47] Hirsch EC, Vyas S, Hunot S. Neuroinflammation in parkinson's disease. Parkinsonism relat disord 2012; 18 (Suppl. 1): S210-2.
[http://dx.doi.org/10.1016/S1353-8020(11)70065-7] [PMID: 22166438]

[48] Singh SS, Rai SN, Birla H, *et al.* Techniques Related to Disease Diagnosis and Therapeutics. Application of Biomedical Engineering in Neuroscience. 2019; 437-56.
[http://dx.doi.org/10.1007/978-981-13-7142-4_22]

[49] Singh S, Rai S, Birla H, Eds., *et al.* Chlorogenic acid protects against MPTP induced neurotoxicity in parkinsonian mice model *via* its anti-apoptotic activity. Journal of Neurochemistry 2019.

[50] Singh SS, Rai SN, Birla H, *et al.* Neuroprotective effect of chlorogenic acid on mitochondrial dysfunction-mediated apoptotic death of DA neurons in a Parkinsonian mouse model. Oxid Med Cell Longev 2020; 2020: 1-14.
[http://dx.doi.org/10.1155/2020/6571484] [PMID: 32566093]

[51] Rathore AS, Birla H, Singh SS, *et al.* Epigenetic Modulation in Parkinson's Disease and Potential Treatment Therapies. Neurochem Res 2021; 46(7): 1618-26.
[http://dx.doi.org/10.1007/s11064-021-03334-w] [PMID: 33900517]

[52] Birla H, Keswani C, Singh SS, *et al.* Unraveling the Neuroprotective Effect of *Tinospora cordifolia* in Parkinsonian Mouse Model Through Proteomics Approach 2021.
[http://dx.doi.org/10.1021/acschemneuro.1c00481]

[53] Keswani C, Dilnashin H, Birla H, Singh SP. Unravelling efficient applications of agriculturally important microorganisms for alleviation of induced inter-cellular oxidative stress in crops. Acta Agric Slov 2019; 114(1): 121-30.
[http://dx.doi.org/10.14720/aas.2019.114.1.14]

[54] Birla H, Keswani C, Rai SN, *et al.* Neuroprotective effects of *Withania somnifera* in BPA induced-cognitive dysfunction and oxidative stress in mice. Behav Brain Funct 2019; 15(1): 9.
[http://dx.doi.org/10.1186/s12993-019-0160-4] [PMID: 31064381]

[55] Rai SN, Birla H, Singh SS, *et al.* Pathophysiology of the Disease Causing Physical Disability. Biomedical Engineering and its Applications in Healthcare. 2019; 573-95.

[56] Rai SN, Singh BK, Rathore AS, *et al.* Quality control in huntington's disease: a therapeutic target. Neurotox Res 2019; 36(3): 612-26.
[http://dx.doi.org/10.1007/s12640-019-00087-x] [PMID: 31297710]

[57] Rai SN, Dilnashin H, Birla H, *et al.* The role of PI3K/Akt and ERK in neurodegenerative disorders. Neurotox Res 2019; 35(3): 775-95.
[http://dx.doi.org/10.1007/s12640-019-0003-y] [PMID: 30707354]

[58] Rai SN, Zahra W, Singh SS, *et al.* Anti-inflammatory activity of ursolic acid in MPTP-induced parkinsonian mouse model. Neurotox Res 2019; 36(3): 452-62.
[http://dx.doi.org/10.1007/s12640-019-00038-6] [PMID: 31016688]

[59] Delamarre A, Meissner WG. Epidemiology, environmental risk factors and genetics of Parkinson's disease. Presse Med 2017; 46(2): 175-81.
[http://dx.doi.org/10.1016/j.lpm.2017.01.001] [PMID: 28189372]

[60] Goedert M. Alpha-synuclein and neurodegenerative diseases. Nat Rev Neurosci 2001; 2(7): 492-501.

[http://dx.doi.org/10.1038/35081564] [PMID: 11433374]

[61] Ruipérez V, Darios F, Davletov B. Alpha-synuclein, lipids and Parkinson's disease. Prog Lipid Res 2010; 49(4): 420-8.
[http://dx.doi.org/10.1016/j.plipres.2010.05.004] [PMID: 20580911]

[62] Baba M, Nakajo S, Tu P-H, *et al.* Aggregation of alpha-synuclein in Lewy bodies of sporadic Parkinson's disease and dementia with Lewy bodies. Am J Pathol 1998; 152(4): 879-84.
[PMID: 9546347]

[63] Wang C, Zhao C, Li D, *et al.* Versatile Structures of α-Synuclein. Front Mol Neurosci 2016; 9: 48.
[http://dx.doi.org/10.3389/fnmol.2016.00048] [PMID: 27378848]

[64] Olanow CW, Brundin P. Parkinson's disease and alpha synuclein: is Parkinson's disease a prion-like disorder? Mov Disord 2013; 28(1): 31-40.
[http://dx.doi.org/10.1002/mds.25373] [PMID: 23390095]

[65] Heman-Ackah SM, Manzano R, Hoozemans JJM, *et al.* Alpha-synuclein induces the unfolded protein response in Parkinson's disease SNCA triplication iPSC-derived neurons. Hum Mol Genet 2017; 26(22): 4441-50.
[http://dx.doi.org/10.1093/hmg/ddx331] [PMID: 28973645]

[66] Kasten M, Klein C. The many faces of alpha-synuclein mutations. Mov Disord 2013; 28(6): 697-701.
[http://dx.doi.org/10.1002/mds.25499] [PMID: 23674458]

[67] Guerrero E, Vasudevaraju P, Hegde ML, Britton GB, Rao KS. Recent advances in α-synuclein functions, advanced glycation, and toxicity: implications for Parkinson's disease. Mol Neurobiol 2013; 47(2): 525-36.
[http://dx.doi.org/10.1007/s12035-012-8328-z] [PMID: 22923367]

[68] Sulzer D. Multiple hit hypotheses for dopamine neuron loss in Parkinson's disease. Trends Neurosci 2007; 30(5): 244-50.
[http://dx.doi.org/10.1016/j.tins.2007.03.009] [PMID: 17418429]

[69] Brown P. Oscillatory nature of human basal ganglia activity: Relationship to the pathophysiology of Parkinson's disease. Mov Disord 2003; 18(4): 357-63.
[http://dx.doi.org/10.1002/mds.10358] [PMID: 12671940]

[70] Hansen C, Angot E, Bergström AL, *et al.* α-Synuclein propagates from mouse brain to grafted dopaminergic neurons and seeds aggregation in cultured human cells. J Clin Invest 2011; 121(2): 715-25.
[http://dx.doi.org/10.1172/JCI43366] [PMID: 21245577]

[71] Lim SY, O'Sullivan SS, Kotschet K, *et al.* Dopamine dysregulation syndrome, impulse control disorders and punding after deep brain stimulation surgery for Parkinson's disease. J Clin Neurosci 2009; 16(9): 1148-52.
[http://dx.doi.org/10.1016/j.jocn.2008.12.010] [PMID: 19553125]

[72] Dauer W, Przedborski S. Parkinson's Disease. Neuron 2003; 39(6): 889-909.
[http://dx.doi.org/10.1016/S0896-6273(03)00568-3] [PMID: 12971891]

[73] Braak H, Ghebremedhin E, Rüb U, Bratzke H, Del Tredici K. Stages in the development of Parkinson's disease-related pathology. Cell Tissue Res 2004; 318(1): 121-34.
[http://dx.doi.org/10.1007/s00441-004-0956-9] [PMID: 15338272]

[74] Russo A, Borrelli F. *Bacopa monniera*, a reputed nootropic plant: an overview. Phytomedicine 2005; 12(4): 305-17.
[http://dx.doi.org/10.1016/j.phymed.2003.12.008] [PMID: 15898709]

[75] Nemetc.hek MD, Stierle AA, Stierle DB, Lurie DI. The Ayurvedic plant *Bacopa monnieri* inhibits inflammatory pathways in the brain. J Ethnopharmacol 2017; 197: 92-100.
[http://dx.doi.org/10.1016/j.jep.2016.07.073] [PMID: 27473605]

[76] Singh RH, Narsimhamurthy K, Singh G. Neuronutrient impact of Ayurvedic Rasayana therapy in brain aging. Biogerontology 2008; 9(6): 369-74.
[http://dx.doi.org/10.1007/s10522-008-9185-z] [PMID: 18931935]

[77] Kongkeaw C, Dilokthornsakul P, Thanarangsarit P, Limpeanchob N, Norman Scholfield C. Meta-analysis of randomized controlled trials on cognitive effects of *Bacopa monnieri* extract. J Ethnopharmacol 2014; 151(1): 528-35.
[http://dx.doi.org/10.1016/j.jep.2013.11.008] [PMID: 24252493]

[78] Devendra P, Patel S, Birwal P, Basu S, Deshmukh G, Datir R. Brahmi (*Bacopa monnieri*) as functional food ingredient in food processing industry. J Pharmacogn Phytochem 2018; 7(3): 189-94.

[79] Barrett SCH, Strother JL. Taxonomy and natural history of *Bacopa* (*Scrophulariaceae*) in California. Syst Bot 1978; 3(4): 408-19.
[http://dx.doi.org/10.2307/2418753]

[80] Elangovan V, Govindasamy S, Ramamoorthy N, Balasubramanian K. *In vitro* studies on the anticancer activity of *Bacopa monnieri*. Fitoterapia (Milano) 1995; 66(3): 211-5.

[81] Aguiar S, Borowski T. Neuropharmacological review of the nootropic herb *Bacopa monnieri*. Rejuvenation Res 2013; 16(4): 313-26.
[http://dx.doi.org/10.1089/rej.2013.1431] [PMID: 23772955]

[82] Nandy S, Dey A, Mukherjeeb A. Advances in dammarane-type triterpenoid saponins from *Bacopa monnieri*: Structure, bioactivity, biotechnology and neuroprotection. Studies in Natural Products Chemistry. 63. 2019; 489-533.

[83] Bhandari P, Sendri N, Devidas SB. Dammarane triterpenoid glycosides in *Bacopa monnieri*: A review on chemical diversity and bioactivity. Phytochemistry 2020; 172: 112276.
[http://dx.doi.org/10.1016/j.phytochem.2020.112276] [PMID: 32058865]

[84] Deepak M, Sangli GK, Arun PC, Amit A. Quantitative determination of the major saponin mixture bacoside A in *Bacopa monnieri* by HPLC. Phytochem Anal 2005; 16(1): 24-9.
[http://dx.doi.org/10.1002/pca.805] [PMID: 15688952]

[85] Rastogi S, Pal R, Kulshreshtha DK. Bacoside A3-A triterpenoid saponin from *Bacopa monniera*. Phytochemistry 1994; 36(1): 133-7.
[http://dx.doi.org/10.1016/S0031-9422(00)97026-2] [PMID: 7764837]

[86] Garai S, Mahato SB, Ohtani K, Yamasaki K. Dammarane-type triterpenoid saponins from *Bacopa monniera*. Phytochemistry 1996; 42(3): 815-20.
[http://dx.doi.org/10.1016/0031-9422(95)00936-1] [PMID: 8768327]

[87] Garai S, Mahato SB, Ohtani K, Yamasaki K. Bacopasaponin D-A pseudojujubogenin glycoside from *Bacopa monniera*. Phytochemistry 1996; 43(2): 447-9.
[http://dx.doi.org/10.1016/0031-9422(96)00250-6] [PMID: 8862037]

[88] Chandel RS, Kulshreshtha DK, Rastogi RP. Bacogenin-A3: A new sapogenin from *Bacopa monniera*. Phytochemistry 1977; 16(1): 141-3.
[http://dx.doi.org/10.1016/0031-9422(77)83039-2]

[89] Kulshreshtha DK, Rastogi R. Bacogenin A2: A new sapogenin from bacosides. Phytochemistry 1974; 13(7): 1205-6.
[http://dx.doi.org/10.1016/0031-9422(74)80101-9]

[90] Kulshreshtha DK, Rastogi RP. Bacogenin-A1: A novel dammarane triterpene sapogenin from *Bacopa monniera*. Phytochemistry 1973; 12(4): 887-92.
[http://dx.doi.org/10.1016/0031-9422(73)80697-1]

[91] Chakravarty AK, Sarkar T, Nakane T, Kawahara N, Masuda K. New phenylethanoid glycosides from *Bacopa monniera*. Chem Pharm Bull (Tokyo) 2002; 50(12): 1616-8.
[http://dx.doi.org/10.1248/cpb.50.1616] [PMID: 12499603]

[92]   Chakravarty AK, Sarkar T, Masuda K, Shiojima K, Nakane T, Kawahara N. Bacopaside I and II: two pseudojujubogenin glycosides from *Bacopa monniera*. Phytochemistry 2001; 58(4): 553-6.
[http://dx.doi.org/10.1016/S0031-9422(01)00275-8] [PMID: 11576596]

[93]   Kumar V. Potential medicinal plants for CNS disorders: an overview. Phytother Res 2006; 20(12): 1023-35.
[http://dx.doi.org/10.1002/ptr.1970] [PMID: 16909441]

[94]   Rajani M, Neeta S, Ravishankara M. Brahmi (*Bacopa monnieri* (L.) Pennell)-a Medhya rasaayana drug of Ayurveda. Biotechnology of medicinal plants: vitalizer and therapeutic. 2004; 89-110.

[95]   Gupta A, Tandon N. Reviews on Indian medicinal plants. 2004.

[96]   Patil D, Bakliwal S, Rane B, Pawar S. A review on *Bacopa monniera*: Brahmi. Pharma Sci Monitor 2012; 3(4)

[97]   Singh H, Dhawan B. Neuropsychopharmacological effects of the Ayurvedic nootropic *Bacopa monniera* Linn.(Brahmi). Indian J Pharmacol 1997; 29(5): 359.
[PMID: 31831931]

[98]   Singh HK, Dhawan BN. Effect of *Bacopa monniera* Linn. (Brāhmi) extract on avoidance responses in rat. J Ethnopharmacol 1982; 5(2): 205-14.
[http://dx.doi.org/10.1016/0378-8741(82)90044-7] [PMID: 7057659]

[99]   Singh H, Dhawan B. Singh H, Dhawan B. Pre-clinical neuro-psychopharmacological investigations on Bacosides: A nootropic memory enhancer. Proceedings of Update Ayurveda. 1994; 94

[100]   Das A, Shanker G, Nath C, Pal R, Singh S, Singh HK. A comparative study in rodents of standardized extracts of *Bacopa monniera* and *Ginkgo biloba*. Pharmacol Biochem Behav 2002; 73(4): 893-900.
[http://dx.doi.org/10.1016/S0091-3057(02)00940-1] [PMID: 12213536]

[101]   Singh HK, Rastogi RP, Srimal RC, Dhawan BN. Effect of bacosides A and B on avoidance responses in rats. Phytother Res 1988; 2(2): 70-5.
[http://dx.doi.org/10.1002/ptr.2650020205]

[102]   Ganguly DK, Malhotra CL. Some behavioural effects of an active fraction from *Herpestis monniera*, Linn. (Brahmi). Indian J Med Res 1967; 55(5): 473-82.
[PMID: 6065425]

[103]   AITHA H. Pharmacological investigation on *Herpestis monniera*. Indian J Pharm 1961; 23: 2-5.

[104]   Bhattacharya SK, Bhattacharya A, Kumar A, Ghosal S. Antioxidant activity of *Bacopa monniera* in rat frontal cortex, striatum and hippocampus. Phytother Res 2000; 14(3): 174-9.
[http://dx.doi.org/10.1002/(SICI)1099-1573(200005)14:3<174::AID-PTR624>3.0.CO;2-O] [PMID: 10815010]

[105]   Tripathi YB, Chaurasia S, Tripathi E, Upadhyay A, Dubey GP. *Bacopa monniera* Linn. as an antioxidant: mechanism of action. Indian J Exp Biol 1996; 34(6): 523-6.
[PMID: 8792640]

[106]   Jyoti A, Sethi P, Sharma D. *Bacopa monniera* prevents from aluminium neurotoxicity in the cerebral cortex of rat brain. J Ethnopharmacol 2007; 111(1): 56-62.
[http://dx.doi.org/10.1016/j.jep.2006.10.037] [PMID: 17189676]

[107]   Kishore K, Singh M. Effect of bacosides, alcoholic extract of *Bacopa monniera* Linn.(brahmi), on experimental amnesia in mice. 2005.

[108]   Malhotra CL, Das PK, Dhalla NS. Some neuro-pharmacological actions of hersaponin - an active principle from *Herpestis monniera*, Linn. Arch Int Pharmacodyn Ther 1960; 129: 290-302.
[PMID: 13765774]

[109]   Jyoti A, Sharma D. Neuroprotective role of *Bacopa monniera* extract against aluminium-induced oxidative stress in the hippocampus of rat brain. Neurotoxicology 2006; 27(4): 451-7.

[http://dx.doi.org/10.1016/j.neuro.2005.12.007] [PMID: 16500707]

[110] Pal R, Sarin JP. Quantitative determination of bacosides by UV-spectrophotometry. Highly accessed article. Indian J Pharm Sci 1992; 54: 1.

[111] Kar A, Panda S, Bharti S. Relative efficacy of three medicinal plant extracts in the alteration of thyroid hormone concentrations in male mice. J Ethnopharmacol 2002; 81(2): 281-5.
[http://dx.doi.org/10.1016/S0378-8741(02)00048-X] [PMID: 12065164]

[112] Handa S. Medicinal plants-priorities in Indian medicines diverse studies and implications. Supplement to Cultivation and Utilization of Medicinal Plants. 1996; 33-511.

[113] Shukia B, Khanna NK, Godhwani JL. Effect of brahmi rasayan on the central nervous system. J Ethnopharmacol 1987; 21(1): 65-74.
[http://dx.doi.org/10.1016/0378-8741(87)90095-X] [PMID: 3695557]

[114] Singh H, Dhawan B. Singh H, Dhawan B. Drugs affecting learning and memory. Lectures in neurobiology. 1992; 1: 189-207.

[115] Singh B, Pandey S, Rumman M, Mahdi AA. Neuroprotective effects of *Bacopa monnieri* in Parkinson's disease model. Metab Brain Dis 2020; 35(3): 517-25.
[http://dx.doi.org/10.1007/s11011-019-00526-w] [PMID: 31834548]

[116] Cedarbaum JM. Clinical pharmacokinetics of anti-parkinsonian drugs. Clin Pharmacokinet 1987; 13(3): 141-78.
[http://dx.doi.org/10.2165/00003088-198713030-00002] [PMID: 3311529]

[117] Bar-Am O, Weinreb O, Amit T, Youdim MBH. The neuroprotective mechanism of 1-(R)-aminoindan, the major metabolite of the anti-parkinsonian drug rasagiline. J Neurochem 2010; 112(5): 1131-7.
[http://dx.doi.org/10.1111/j.1471-4159.2009.06542.x] [PMID: 20002521]

[118] Mazumder MK, Borah A, Choudhury S. Inhibitory potential of plant secondary metabolites on anti-Parkinsonian drug targets: Relevance to pathophysiology, and motor and non-motor behavioural abnormalities. Med Hypotheses 2020; 137: 109544.
[http://dx.doi.org/10.1016/j.mehy.2019.109544] [PMID: 31954292]

[119] Singh B, Pandey S, Yadav SK, Verma R, Singh SP, Mahdi AA. Role of ethanolic extract of *Bacopa monnieri* against 1-methyl-4-phenyl-1,2,3,6-tetrahydropyridine (MPTP) induced mice model *via* inhibition of apoptotic pathways of dopaminergic neurons. Brain Res Bull 2017; 135: 120-8.
[http://dx.doi.org/10.1016/j.brainresbull.2017.10.007] [PMID: 29032054]

[120] Liu J, Li Y, Chen S, *et al.* Biomedical application of reactive oxygen species–responsive nanocarriers in cancer, inflammation, and neurodegenerative diseases. Front Chem 2020; 8: 838.
[http://dx.doi.org/10.3389/fchem.2020.00838] [PMID: 33062637]

[121] Chen X, Guo C, Kong J. Oxidative stress in neurodegenerative diseases. Neural Regen Res 2012; 7(5): 376-85.
[PMID: 25774178]

[122] Zhao Y, Zhao B. Oxidative stress and the pathogenesis of Alzheimer's disease. Oxidative medicine and cellular longevity. 2013.
[http://dx.doi.org/10.1155/2013/316523]

[123] Pandey R, Phulara SC, Shukla V, Tiwari S. *Bacopa monnieri* promotes longevity in Caenorhabditis elegans under stress conditions. Pharmacogn Mag 2015; 11(42): 410-6.
[http://dx.doi.org/10.4103/0973-1296.153097] [PMID: 25829783]

[124] Singh M, Murthy V, Ramassamy C. Modulation of hydrogen peroxide and acrolein-induced oxidative stress, mitochondrial dysfunctions and redox regulated pathways by the *Bacopa monniera* extract: potential implication in Alzheimer's disease. J Alzheimers Dis 2010; 21(1): 229-47.
[http://dx.doi.org/10.3233/JAD-2010-091729] [PMID: 20421692]

[125] Yadav P, Uplanchiwar V, Gahane A, Modi A. Nootropic activity of L33: a polyherbal formulation. Pharmacologyonline 2010; 2: 818-27.

[126] Dwivedi S, Nagarajan R, Hanif K, Siddiqui HH, Nath C, Shukla R. Standardized extract of *Bacopa monniera* attenuates okadaic acid induced memory dysfunction in rats: effect on Nrf2 pathway. 2013.

[127] Jadiya P, Khan A, Sammi SR, Kaur S, Mir SS, Nazir A. Anti-Parkinsonian effects of *Bacopa monnieri*: Insights from transgenic and pharmacological Caenorhabditis elegans models of Parkinson's disease. Biochem Biophys Res Commun 2011; 413(4): 605-10.
[http://dx.doi.org/10.1016/j.bbrc.2011.09.010] [PMID: 21925152]

[128] Sukumaran NP, Amalraj A, Gopi S. Neuropharmacological and cognitive effects of *Bacopa monnieri* (L.) Wettst – A review on its mechanistic aspects. Complement Ther Med 2019; 44: 68-82.
[http://dx.doi.org/10.1016/j.ctim.2019.03.016] [PMID: 31126578]

CHAPTER 9

Diabetic Neuropathy and Neuroprotection by Natural Products

Nilay Solanki[1,*] and **Hardik Koria**[1]

¹ Department of Pharmacology, Ramanbhai Patel College of Pharmacy, Charotar University of Science and Technology, Charusat Campus, Changa-388421(Gujarat), India

Abstract: Diabetic neuropathy (DN) is a serious complication in type-1 diabetes and type-2 diabetes. Animal models show many abnormalities like neuropathy, hyperalgesia, allodynia, slow nerve conduction velocity (NCV), and progressive sensory and motor deficit that are associated with diabetic neuropathy. Various risk factors may be involved in causing DN, such as persistent hyperglycemia, microvascular insufficiency, oxidative stress, nitrosative stress, defective neurotrophism and autoimmune-mediated nerve destruction. Many conventional and newer therapeutic approaches are available. Approaches include effective control of glycemia. Symptoms targeted therapies such as antidepressants, SSRIs, anticonvulsants, opiates, NSAIDs and NMDA receptor antagonists. Therapies targeting particular causes include aldose reductase inhibitors, drugs that act on hexosamine pathways, protein kinase C pathways and AGE receptors. Preclinical studies involving pharmacological agents have shown positive results but were withdrawn at the stage of a clinical study, either due to lack of efficacy or due to their side effects on major organs. Medicinal herbal plants are the richest bio-resource of drugs that have been studied extensively for their neuroprotective effects. Various approaches involving neuroprotection by natural products are discussed here.

Keywords: Diabetic neuropathy, Medicinal plants, Neuroprotection, Treatments.

INTRODUCTION

The incidence of diabetes mellitus is increasing at an alarming rate and rapidly assuming epidemic proportions. India is no exception, and currently, 25 million Indians are estimated to be suffering from diabetes [1]. Further projections indicate that India will have the maximum number of diabetic patients by the year 2025 [2]. Macrovascular complications of diabetes include ischemic heart diseases, peripheral vascular disease, atherosclerosis, myocardial infarction,

* **Corresponding author Nilay Solanki:** Department of Pharmacology, Ramanbhai Patel College of Pharmacy, Charotar University of Science and Technology, Charusat Campus, Changa-388421 (Gujarat), India; E-mail: nivyrx@gmail.com

Surya Pratap Singh, Hagera Dilnashin, Hareram Birla & Chetan Keswani (Eds.)

stroke, and gangrene, whereas microvascular complications include small vessel diseases such as retinopathy, neuropathy, and nephropathy. Neuropathy is a serious complication of type 1 (T1DM) and type two Diabetes (T2DM). Diabetic neuropathy (DN) usually occurs lately in type-1 diabetes, but it could occur early in type-2 diabetes. The prevalence of neuropathy is estimated to be about 8% in newly diagnosed patients and greater than 50% in patients with the long-standing disease [3]. There is increasing evidence that even pre-diabetic conditions are also associated with some forms of neuropathy. Diabetic neuropathy is the leading cause of non-traumatic limb amputation, and it occurs in 50% of diabetic patients. These patients suffer from severe pain. DN patients generally complain about persistent burning or tingling sensation, usually, in the legs and feet, inability to detect heat and cold, loss of vibration sensation, and the loss of pain perception; an estimated 15% of all patients with diabetes are at high risk of development of foot ulcers [4]. The selected animal model of DN should exhibit features present in human pathology. Diabetic animals show many abnormalities that are seen in diabetic patients with neuropathy, hyperalgesia, allodynia, slow nerve conduction velocity (NCV), and progressive sensory and motor deficit. Many causative factors for DN include persistent hyperglycemia, microvascular insufficiency, oxidative stress, nitrosative stress, defective neurotrophism, & autoimmune-mediated nerve destruction [3, 5 - 9]. The annual costs of diabetic neuropathy and related morbidities in the US have been estimated to exceed $10.9 billion [4]. Many approaches for the management of DN have been tested preclinically and clinically. Approaches include effective control of glycemia; Symptoms targeted therapies such as antidepressants, SSRIs, anticonvulsants, opiates, NSAIDs, NMDA receptor antagonists; Therapies targeting particular causes include aldose reductase inhibitors, drugs that act on hexosamine pathways, protein kinase C pathways, AGE receptors. Preclinical studies involving pharmacological agents have shown positive results but were withdrawn at the stage of a clinical study, either due to lack of efficacy or due to their side effects on major organs [10]. Therefore, the development of newer natural approaches for the management of diabetes and associated neuropathic changes is the need of today's world. With advancements in research, our understanding of the biochemical and molecular mechanisms leading to diabetic neuropathy has increased. At the molecular level, Adenosine and adenosine receptor agonists have been shown to have antinociceptive effects in animal models of acute and nerve injury-induced neuropathic pain [11 - 14]. Peroxynitrite mediated nitrosative stress, an initiator of DNA damage and overactivation of poly (ADP-ribose) polymerase (PARP), a nuclear enzyme activated after sensing DNA damage, are two crucial pathogenetic mechanisms in diabetic neuropathy [15]. Hyperglycaemia can induce oxidative stress through various mechanisms, such as glucose autooxidation and the resultant formation of glycation end products, dysregulation of the polyol pathway, modifying eicosanoid metabolism, and reducing eicosanoid metabolism antioxidant defenses in diabetes [16 - 19].

DIABETES MELLITUS AND NEUROLOGICAL COMPLICATIONS

Diabetes mellitus, often simply referred to as diabetes, is a group of metabolic diseases in which a person has high blood sugar, either because the body does not produce enough insulin or because cells do not respond to the insulin produced. This high blood sugar produces the classic symptoms of polyuria (frequent urination), polydipsia (increased thirst), and polyphagia (increased hunger) [20, 21].

Causes of Diabetes

Following is a comprehensive list of causes of diabetes:

  I. Genetic defects of β-cell Function
    a. Maturity onset diabetes of the young (MODY)
    b. Mitochondrial DNA mutations
 II. Genetic defects in insulin processing or insulin action
    a. Defects in proinsulin conversion
    b. Insulin gene mutations
    c. Insulin receptor mutations
III. Exocrine Pancreatic Defects
    a. Chronic pancreatitis
    b. Pancreatectomy
    c. Pancreatic neoplasia
    d. Cystic fibrosis
IV. Endocrinopathies
    a. Growth hormone excess (acromegaly)
    b. Cushing syndrome
    c. Hyperthyroidism
    d. Pheochromocytoma
    e. Glucagonoma
 V. Infections
    a. Cytomegalovirus infection
    b. Coxsackievirus B
VI. Drugs
    a. Glucocorticoids
    b. Thyroid hormone

c. β-adrenergic agonists

Signs and Symptoms

The classic symptoms of diabetes are polyuria (frequent urination), polydipsia (increased thirst), and polyphagia (increased hunger). Symptoms may develop rapidly (weeks or months) in type 1 diabetes, while in type 2 diabetes, they usually develop much more slowly and may be subtle or absent. Prolonged high blood glucose causes glucose absorption, which leads to changes in the shape of the lenses of the eyes, resulting in vision changes; sustained sensible glucose control usually returns the lens to its original shape. Blurred vision is a common complaint leading to a diabetes diagnosis; type 1 should always be suspected in cases of rapid vision change, whereas type 2 changes are generally more gradual but should still be suspected. People (usually with type 1 diabetes) may also present with diabetic ketoacidosis, a state of metabolic dysregulation characterized by the smell of acetone; rapid, deep breathing known as Kussmaul breathing; nausea; vomiting and abdominal pain; and altered states of consciousness [22 - 24].

Diabetic Complications of the Nervous system

Diabetes mellitus (DM) is a systemic disease that can damage any organ in the body. Complications include pathologic changes involving both small and large vessels, cranial and peripheral nerves, skin, and eyes. These organic lesions may lead to hypertension, renal failure, vision loss, autonomic and peripheral neuropathy, peripheral vascular disease, myocardial infarction, and cerebrovascular disease, including stroke [25]. In recent years, significantly more interest has been dedicated to the effect of diabetes on the brain. Along with cerebrovascular disease, diabetes is implicated in the development of other neurological comorbidities. Less addressed and not as well recognized complications of DM are cognitive dysfunction, dementia, metabolic syndrome (MetS), and their possible pathophysiological links with cognitive decline. Cognitive impairment due to diabetes mainly occurs at two main periods: during the first 5–7 years of life when brain systems are in development and the period when the brain undergoes neurodegenerative changes due to aging (older than 65 years) [26 - 29].

DIABETIC NEUROPATHY

Neuropathy is a common and costly complication of both type 1 diabetes mellitus (T1DM) and types two diabetes mellitus (T2DM). The prevalence of neuropathy is estimated to be about 8% in newly diagnosed patients and greater than 50% in patients with long-standing diseases [3, 30]. An estimated 15% of all patients with diabetes are at high risk of the development of foot ulcers [4]. The annual costs of diabetic neuropathy and its associated morbidities in the US have been estimated to exceed $10.9 billion. With advancements in research, our understanding of the biochemical and molecular mechanisms leading to diabetic neuropathy has increased. The main aim of the proposal is to focus on research of diabetes and its complication in the nervous system with special reference to DN with neurodegeneration and the role of selected herbals in the treatment of diabetic neuropathy [31 - 35].

Diabetes mellitus causes diabetic neuropathy by causing damage to peripheral somatic or autonomic neurons. The DN may be categorized under two headings: diffuse neuropathies and focal neuropathies [36 - 38]. The diffuse neuropathies include distal symmetrical sensorimotor polyneuropathy (DPN) and diabetic autonomic neuropathy (DAN). These are common, progressive, and chronic. The focal forms of diabetic neuropathy indicate damage to single or multiple peripheral nerves, cranial nerves, and regions of the brachial or lumbosacral plexuses. The most common peripheral nerve mononeuropathies are medial and ulnar neuropathy. The most common cranial neuropathy affects the third nerve, which causes a unilateral headache, diplopia, and ptosis (diabetic ophthal-moplegia) [5, 36, 39].

Diabetic neuropathy affects all peripheral nerves: pain fibers, motor neurons, and autonomic nerves. Therefore, it can affect all organs and systems since all are innervated. There are several distinct syndromes based on the organ systems and members affected, but these are by no means exclusive. A patient can have sensorimotor and autonomic neuropathy or any other combination [36 - 39]. Symptoms vary depending on the nerve(s) affected and may include symptoms other than those listed. Symptoms usually develop gradually over the years [35, 40].

Symptoms may include:

a. Numbness and tingling of extremities
b. Dysesthesia (abnormal sensation to a body part)
c. Diarrhoea
d. Erectile dysfunction

  e. Urinary incontinence (loss of bladder control)
  f. Facial, mouth, and eyelid drooping
  g. Vision changes
  h. Dizziness
  i. Muscle weakness
  j. Difficulty swallowing
  k. Speech impairment
  l. Fasciculation (muscle contractions)
m. Anorgasmia

Pathophysiology of Diabetic Neuropathy

Multiple etiologic factors may be responsible for the various neuropathic syndromes seen in diabetic patients. Diabetic neuropathy and the other microvascular complications of diabetes occur mainly due to hyperglycemia [34, 41]. Recent investigations mainly focus on glucose metabolic pathways involved in the molecular and biochemical pathophysiology of diabetic neuropathy. These altered pathways responsible for diabetic complications may be targeted for the development of new molecules for the treatment. These pathways most often affect the metabolic and/or redox state of the cell. Pathways and components usually affected include glucose flux through the polyol pathway, the hexosamine pathway, altered activation of protein kinase C (PKC) isoforms and accumulation of glycation end products. Alteration in either single or multiple pathways can cause a disturbance in the mitochondrial redox state of the cell and can lead to an excess generation of reactive oxygen species (ROS). Increased oxidative stress within the cell activates the Poly (ADP-ribose) polymerase (PARP) pathway, which is involved in the regulation of the expression of genes that promote inflammatory reactions and neuronal dysfunction [41]. Each of these mechanisms and the central role of ROS have been discussed here. Diabetic neuropathy is thought to occur from both hyperglycemia-induced damage to nerve cells and from neuronal ischemia caused by hyperglycemia-induced decreases in neurovascular flow. Much of the basic science addressing the etiology/mechanisms of microvascular complications has used non-neuronal derived cells or cell lines, but studies in animal models of neuropathy and/or human clinical studies with specific inhibitors of each pathway suggest that each mechanism can contribute to diabetic neuropathy [30, 34, 35, 40]. Various Pathways/Mechanism involved in the pathophysiology of DN are as follows:

  a. Polyol Pathways
  b. Hexosamine Pathways
  c. Protein Kinase C pathways

d. Advanced glycation end-product pathways
e. Poly (ADP-ribose) polymerase pathway
f. Mechanism of Oxidative stress and Apoptosis
g. Role of Inflammation
h. Role of Growth factors

Therapeutics and Management of Diabetic Neuropathy

Therapies for Diabetic neuropathy may be divided into treatments that target the underlying pathogenetic mechanisms and those aiming to relieve symptoms.

Glycemic Control

Strict glycemic control prevents DPN and DAN and slows progression.

Type 1 Diabetes Mellitus

Diabetes Control and Complications Trial

The DCCT compared intensive treatment with conventional treatment in 1441 patients with T1DM. Intensive treatment involves three or more insulin injections or insulin pumps, while conventional treatment involves 1 or 2 insulin injections in order to normalize HbA1c. Patients were followed up for five years. The prevalence of confirmed clinical neuropathy was 64% lower in patients receiving intensive treatment (HbA1c=7.2%) than in those receiving conventional treatment (HbA1c=9.1%). Further, nerve conduction velocities remained stable in patients receiving intensive treatment and declined significantly in patients receiving conventional treatment.

Continuous Glucose Monitoring

Although HbA1c levels are strong predictors for diabetic complications, there may be other factors apart from average blood glucose levels, which may be responsible for diabetic complications. The prognosis of complications may affect factors other than the average blood-glucose level like HbA1c. The HbA1c level indicated a different correlation with the incidence of diabetic complications in both the conventional therapy group of the DCCT and the intensive therapy group. There was a minimal correlation in the intensive therapy group and a significant correlation in the conventional therapy group. Intense therapy and conventional therapy involved different approaches with respect to multiple insulin injections and blood glucose monitoring. Intensive therapy cohort patients developed less dynamic glycolytic flux. These studies indicate glycemic variability as a better target than average glycemic control (HbA1c) to halt the onset and progression of complications. Diabetes complications can be predicted by oxidative stress, which has a close association with glycemic variability. Real-time tracking and correction of glycemic flux are now possible.

Real-time data from the CGM can be used to check insulin level, and food intake before the occurrence of either hyper- or hypoglycemia occurs. As such, glycemic variability may be minimized by optimizing therapy (insulin/glucose intake) according to glucose trends.

Type 2 Diabetes Mellitus

There is a scarcity of evidence suggesting delay or prevention of the progression of diabetic neuropathy by good glycemic control in patients with T2DM. A most important step for the treatment of patients with diabetic neuropathy is the normalization of both fasting and postprandial glucose levels. In certain circumstances, a rare type of neuropathy can develop in patients with inadequately controlled diabetes after following the start of a rigorous insulin regimen; other cases of abrupt, intense neuropathy have been documented most often in male patients who have faced a decrease insignificant amount of weight. The difference shown from DPN is that of less sensory impairment and uncured weakness. In situations resulting in rapid weight loss, improved glycemic control, and weight restoration contribute to symptomatic remission; in intensive insulin therapy, momentarily relaxing glycemic control provides therapeutic benefits. In this type of neuropathy, complete recovery is typical and usually transpires over six to twenty-four months.

Symptomatic Treatment of Peripheral Neuropathy

To detect high-risk diseases, all diabetic patients should have their feet examined at least once a year. Considering DPN is amongst the most significant antecedents of diabetic foot ulcer, and amputation in neuropathic patients, the necessity of prophylactic foot care cannot be overstated. Every visit to the doctor for neuropathic patients should include a comprehensive foot assessment, and if necessary, a referral to a foot care expert. Patients with sensory impairment should be recommended to investigate thrice regularly to ensure that no sharp artifacts are prevalent. Patient health education on suitable foot treatment, which would include shoe preference, nail clipping, and routine foot monitoring, is crucial if a local infection is detected clinically and surgically.

DIABETIC POLYNEUROPATHY (DPN)

Diabetic neuropathy pain is a frequent condition that develops before diabetes is diagnosed [3]. According to contemporary research, approximately one-third of people with compromised glycemic control (pre-diabetes) require clinical assistance for a persistent pain condition analogous to DPN and DN. An epidemiological investigation of people with T2DM, DPN, and DN is a chronic condition, whereas it is much less prevalent in patients with type 1 diabetes. DPN and DN are accompanied by blistering, stinging and electric-like cramping, which begins in the foot and progresses gradually in an upward direction over time. Allodynia and hyperalgesia are often characteristics of DPN. Allodynia normally occurs when a non-painful stimulus becomes unpleasant, and hyperalgesia arises when the generally painful stimulus becomes excruciating. The discovery of method-specific therapeutics is hampered by a failure to understand the etiology of this condition. As a result, conventional medical therapies are only partly productive and frequently unsuccessful. Anticonvulsants, topical treatments, antidepressants, and opioid-based remedies, for example, have now been reported in patients with DPN and DN in placebo-controlled experiments.

Antidepressants

Tricyclic and Tetracyclic Reagents

Tricyclic and tetracyclic antidepressants (TCA) are considered as the first-line treatment for neuropathic pain. These antidepressants control pain and pain-related symptoms such as insomnia and depression. The therapeutic actions of these agents are mediated by inhibition of the reuptake of norepinephrine and serotonin. Amitriptyline (150 mg/day) is superior to placebo in relieving DPN after 6 weeks of treatment. However, amitriptyline is associated with significant side effects, including dry mouth, sedation, and blurred vision. Desipramine is better tolerated at 111 mg/day and is as effective as amitriptyline in alleviating DPN. Overall, secondary amines (nortriptyline, desipramine) are better tolerated than tertiary amines (amitriptyline, imipramine) [1, 2]. TCAs are not well tolerated in older patients. The TCAs should be used with great caution (or avoided altogether) in patients with cardiac arrhythmias, congestive heart failure, orthostatic hypotension, urinary retention, or angle-closure glaucoma [3].

Selective Serotonin Reuptake Inhibitors and Serotonin-Norepinephrine Reuptake Inhibitors

Selective serotonin reuptake inhibitors (SSRIs) are newer antidepressants that have largely replaced TCAs for the treatment of depression because they are better tolerated. However, in contrast to TCAs, the effects of SSRIs are limited in DPN [4, 5]. Fluoxetine, 40mg/day, is not different from placebo. Nausea, constipation, headache, and dyspepsia were common side effects. The Serotonin-Norepinephrine Reuptake Inhibitors (SNRI) have greater efficacy against DPN than SSRIs. Duloxetine has been approved by the Food and Drug Administration (FDA) for treating DPN following three large randomized placebo control trials [6]. In these trials, duloxetine 60mg and 120 mg daily provided significant relief from DPN. The high dose provides greater relief from DPN but is associated with increased side effects. In general, duloxetine is better tolerated, in terms of gastrointestinal and cardiac side effects, than other Serotonin-Norepinephrine Reuptake Inhibitors [7].

Anticonvulsants

Anticonvulsants control neuronal excitability by blocking sodium and/or calcium channels. Originally developed for preventing seizures, they are in broad use for the treatment of neuropathic pain. Phenytoin and carbamazepine primarily block the voltage-gated sodium channel. At doses between 200 and 600 mg/day, both reduce DPN compared to placebo. Due to side effects and newer improved therapies, these compounds are not recommended [8, 9]. Sodium valproate enhances GABA levels in the central nervous system, inhibits T T-type calcium channels, and increases potassium inward currents. Again, side effects, including hair loss, weight gain, hepatotoxicity, and cognitive dysfunction are not insignificant and increase with long-term use, although a dose of 500 mg/day decreases DPN [10]. Lamotrigine is a new anticonvulsant that blocks voltage-gated sodium channels, decreases presynaptic calcium currents to inhibit the release of glutamate, and increases GABA levels in the brain [11].

Calcium channel α2-δ ligands.

Gabapentin is widely used for neuropathic pain due to its effectiveness and relatively fewer side effects than TCA and other anticonvulsants. Gabapentin produces analgesia *via* binding to the α2-δ site of L-type voltage-gated calcium channels and decreasing calcium influx. Gabapentin ≤2400 mg/day is effective in treating DPN compared to amitriptyline (≤90 mg/day), according to a randomized control trial of 165 patients [12]. However, another study found no difference between gabapentin (900–1800 mg/day) and amitriptyline (25–75 mg/day). Common side effects of gabapentin include dizziness, ataxia, sedation, euphoria, ankle edema, and weight gain. Moreover, it usually takes weeks of titration to reach the maximally effective dose and dosing of 3/day is often necessary. Unlike gabapentin, pregabalin has better GI absorption and can be administered twice per day. Its linear pharmacokinetics provides a rapid (b2 weeks) onset of maximal pain relief [13].

Topical agents.

Capsaicin is an extract of capsicum peppers. Capsaicin binds to the TRPV1 receptor and exhausts substance P in the peripheral nerves to achieve its analgesic effects. In the study published by the Capsaicin Study Group, 0.075% capsaicin cream applied three times a day for 6 weeks was more effective in alleviating DPN than placebo [14]. Burning was the most common side effect, which decreased as therapy continued. The therapeutic effects of capsaicin started weeks after the cream application. Recently, a patch containing high concentrated capsaicin has demonstrated promising effects in treating diabetic pain. Burning was the most common side effect, which tended to decrease as therapy continued. The therapeutic effects of capsaicin started weeks after the cream application. Topical lidocaine 5% patches have been reported by several studies to relieve DPN. In an open-labelled study, up to four 5% lidocaine patches applied for up to 18 h/day are well tolerated in patients with painful diabetic polyneuropathy. Lidocaine patches significantly improved pain and quality-of-life ratings, and may allow tapering of concomitant analgesic therapy [15].

NATURAL PRODUCTS AND NEUROPROTECTION IN DIABETES

There is growing interest in herbal remedies due to the side effects associated with the oral hypoglycaemic agents and other antidiabetic drugs for treating diabetes mellitus and its CNS complications. Therefore, traditional herbal medicines are mainly used, which are obtained from plants, playing an important role in managing diabetes mellitus. A study conducted on ethanol extract (250mg/kg/day) lowered blood glucose levels within 2 weeks in the alloxan diabetic albino rats confirming its hypoglycemic activity [16]. β-sitosterol isolated from the stem bark was found to possess potent hypoglycemic activity compared to other isolated compounds [17]. Another study based on the metabolite of the ethanolic extract of leaves of B. variegata; roseoside demonstrates insulinotropic activity toward pancreatic ß-cells of the INS-1 cell line and may act in conjunction with the chloroplast protein to contribute to the overall anti-diabetic properties [18]. Several studies on diabetic neuropathic (DN) conditions were done to study the role of herbal plants in DN (Fig. **1**). In one study, diabetic neuropathy antioxidants treatment has been tried to combat oxidative stress in both animals and diabetic patients, like vitamin C or α-lipoic acid, free amino acids also improve insulin responses and thus can provide additional benefit to the proposed reduction of oxidative stress in tissues [19]. Vitamin E decreases blood glucose in type 1 diabetic rats through an unknown mechanism [20]. Treatment with herbals (extracts) found to be effective in DN, In the second study with *Enicostemma littorale* Blume (EL) (Gentianaceae) had confirmed its hypoglycemic potential in alloxan-induced diabetic rats [21], the further protective effect of EL against neuropathy found to be due to controlling hyperglycemia and reducing oxidative stress, therefore EL can be used clinically for the management of DN. The management of diabetes and DN without any side effects is still a challenge to the medical system. There is a list of plants and phytoconstituents mentioned with their neuroprotective mechanism below (Tables **1** and **2**).

Table 1. Neuroprotection by Plants.

Sr no.	Medicinal Plants	Protective Phytoconstituents	Findings	Protective Mechanisms/probable Protective Mechanism	Refs.
1.	*Wattakaka volubilis* (L.f.) Stapf root	saponins and glycosides	Increased pain perception observed in different models of analgesia	Preventing nerve damage	[22]
2.	*Momordica cymbalaria* Fenzl	Steroidal saponin	Increased pain sensitivity, improvement in the myelination and degenerative changes of the nerve fiber, delay in the progression of neuropathy	Improvement in myelination and restoration of neuronal integrity, antioxidant activity	[23]
3.	*Artemisia dracunculus* L.	4,5-di-O-caffeoylquinic acid, 6-demethoxycapillarisin, and 2',4'-dihydroxy-4-methoxy dihydrochalcone	Alleviation of nerve conduction slowing and small sensory nerve fiber dysfunction, promotion of small sensory nerve fiber regeneration	Inhibition of oxidative-nitrosative stress and 12/15-LO activation.	[24]

(Table 1) cont.....

Sr no.	Medicinal Plants	Protective Phytoconstituents	Findings	Protective Mechanisms/probable Protective Mechanism	Refs.
4.	*Olea europaea* L.	Phenolic compounds (oleuropein, tyrosol, hydroxytyrosol, and caffeic acid	Attenuation of thermal hyperalgesia, Inhibition of caspase 3 activations, and decrease in Bax/Bcl2 ratio.	Reduction in neuronal apoptosis, free radical scavenging	[25]
5.	*Aegle marmelos*	Aegelin, α and β-sitosterol marmalosin, marmesin	Increased pain sensitivity	Activation of α2 adrenoceptors.	[26]
6.	*Allium sativum*	S-allyl cysteine (SAC) and S-allyl mercaptocysteine (SAMC)	Attenuation of thermal hyperalgesia	Decreasing oxidative stress	[27]
7.	*Gymnema sylvestre*	Gymnemic acids	Attenuation of the elevated levels of cytokines in the serum and sciatic tissues and decrease in oxidative stress markers	Amelioration oxidative stress by blocking the nuclear factor (NF)-κB pathway, Inhibit iNOS activity	[28]
8.	*Coptis chinensis*	Total alkaloids (berberine, palmatine, hydrastine, and copistine)	Reverse pathological changes of the brain, including loss of neurons and Aβ deposition	Regulation of IRS1/PI3K/Akt insulin signaling and GSK3β activity	[29]
9.	*Calotropis procera*	cardenolides, anthocyanins, alkaloids, tannins, saponins and triterpenoids	Attenuated diabetes-induced mechanical hyperalgesia, thermal hyperalgesia, tactile allodynia, regeneration of the β cells of the pancreas, reversal of sensory dysfunction	Decrease in oxidative stress amelioration of axonal degeneration	[30]
10.	*Zingiber officinale Roscoe*	6-shogaol and ginger extract	Alleviation of hyperalgesia and allodynia	Decreased expressions of TRPV1 and NMDAR2B in the spinal cord.	[31]

Table 2. Neuroprotection by Phytoconstituents

Sr no.	Phytoconstituent Name	Findings	Protective mechanisms/Probable Protective mechanism	Ref.
1.	Diosmin	Reduces oxidative damage	Attenuation of increased lipid peroxides, NO concentration, restoration of depleted GSH.	[32]

(Table 2) cont.....

Sr no.	Phytoconstituent Name	Findings	Protective mechanisms/Probable Protective mechanism	Ref.
2.	Hesperidin	Attenuation in neuropathic pain; correction of allodynia and hyperalgesia.	Downregulates generation of free radicals, release of cytokines (TNF-α and IL-1β), elevation in membrane-bound enzymes.	[33]
3.	Kaempferol	Increases level of antioxidant enzymes decreased lipid peroxidation, and advanced glycation end products.	Attenuation of the oxidative stress-mediated release of pro-inflammatory cytokines.	[34]
4.	Naringenin	Attenuation of neuropathic pain.	Modulation of oxidative–nitrosative stress, inflammatory cytokine release, and matrix metalloproteinases inhibition.	[35]
5.	Quercetin	Increases in nerve conduction velocity and a reduction in nociception.	Inhibition of hyperglycemia and modulation of oxidative-nitrosative stress, pro-inflammatory cytokine (TNF- and IL-1) as well as DNA damage.	[36]
6.	Rutin	Increases in nerve conduction velocity and a reduction in nociception.	Inhibition of neuroinflammation, decreasing oxidative stress, augmentation antioxidant defence The system through increasing the levels of H_2S and Nrf2.	[37]
7.	Silibinin	Provides DNA protection and reduces oxidative stress in a brain-specific area	*via* the activation of the HO system	[38]
8.	Proanthocyanidin	Increased nerve conduction velocity	Prevents cell injury, Ca^{2+} overload, and ER stress	[39]
9.	Baicalein	Alleviation of motor and sensory nerve conduction velocity, thermal hypoalgesia, and tactile allodynia characteristic for DPN, slowing down diabetes-associated loss of intraepidermal nerve fibers and promoting their regeneration.	Inhibition of oxidative–nitrosative stress and p38 MAPK activation	[40]
10.	Chrysin	Anti-nociceptive effect and reduction in inflammation-induced pain.	Stimulation of opioid receptor and chrysin-induced downregulation of p-CREB level in the spinal cord.	[41]

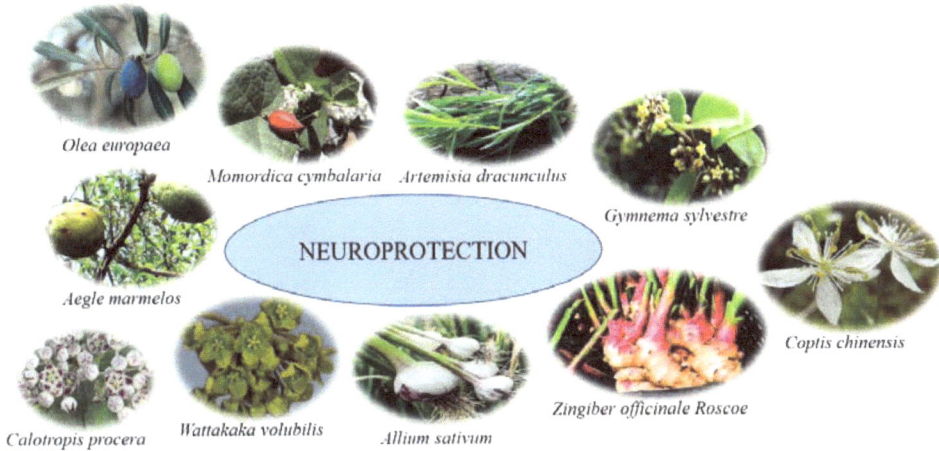

Fig. (1). Medicinal plants showing neuroprotection against diabetic neuropathy.

CONCLUSION

Diabetic neuropathy (DN) is the worst complication associated with hyperalgesia, allodynia, slow nerve conduction velocity, and progressive sensory and motor deficit associated with various causative factors, including persistent hyperglycemia, and microvascular insufficiency, oxidative stress, nitrosative stress, *etc*. Treatment available has limitations due to lots of side effects associated with it. There is a need for an hour to design a natural product-based regimen for neuroprotection in diabetic neuropathy.

CONSENT FOR PUBLICATION

Not applicable.

CONFLICT OF INTEREST

The author declares no conflict of interest, financial or otherwise.

ACKNOWLEDGEMENTS

Declared none.

REFERENCES

[1]   Sindrup SH, Holbech JV, Bach FW, Finnerup NB, Brøsen K, Jensen TS. The impact of serum drug concentration on the efficacy of imipramine, pregabalin, and their combination in painful polyneuropathy. Clin J Pain 2017; 33(12): 1047-52.
[http://dx.doi.org/10.1097/AJP.0000000000000497] [PMID: 28272120]

[2]   Alba-Delgado C, Llorca-Torralba M, Mico JA, Berrocoso E. The onset of treatment with the antidepressant desipramine is critical for the emotional consequences of neuropathic pain. Pain 2018; 159(12): 2606-19.
[http://dx.doi.org/10.1097/j.pain.0000000000001372] [PMID: 30130302]

[3]   Simmons Z, Feldman EL. Treatment of diabetic neuropathy. 2002; 555-76.

[4]   Lochmann D, Richardson T. Selective serotonin reuptake inhibitors. Antidepressants. 2018; 135-44.

[5]   Jakobsen JC, Katakam KK, Schou A, *et al.* Selective serotonin reuptake inhibitors versus placebo in patients with major depressive disorder. A systematic review with meta-analysis and Trial Sequential Analysis. BMC Psychiatry 2017; 17(1): 1-28.
[PMID: 28049496]

[6]   Wernicke JF, Pritchett YL, D'Souza DN, *et al.* A randomized controlled trial of duloxetine in diabetic peripheral neuropathic pain. Neurology 2006; 67(8): 1411-20.
[http://dx.doi.org/10.1212/01.wnl.0000240225.04000.1a] [PMID: 17060567]

[7]   Raouf M, Glogowski AJ, Bettinger JJ, Fudin J. Serotonin-norepinephrine reuptake inhibitors and the influence of binding affinity (Ki) on analgesia. J Clin Pharm Ther 2017; 42(4): 513-7.
[http://dx.doi.org/10.1111/jcpt.12534] [PMID: 28503727]

[8]   Iqbal Z, Azmi S, Yadav R, *et al.* Diabetic peripheral neuropathy: epidemiology, diagnosis, and pharmacotherapy. Clin Ther 2018; 40(6): 828-49.
[http://dx.doi.org/10.1016/j.clinthera.2018.04.001] [PMID: 29709457]

[9]   Khdour MR. Treatment of diabetic peripheral neuropathy: a review. J Pharm Pharmacol 2020; 72(7): 863-72.
[http://dx.doi.org/10.1111/jphp.13241] [PMID: 32067247]

[10]   Kochar DK, Rawat N, Agrawal RP, *et al.* Sodium valproate for painful diabetic neuropathy: a randomized double-blind placebo-controlled study. QJM 2004; 97(1): 33-8.
[http://dx.doi.org/10.1093/qjmed/hch007] [PMID: 14702509]

[11]   Zakin E, Abrams R, Simpson DM, Eds. Diabetic neuropathy. Seminars in neurology. 2019.

[12]   Dallocchio C, Buffa C, Mazzarello P, Chiroli S. Gabapentin vs. amitriptyline in painful diabetic neuropathy: an open-label pilot study. J Pain Symptom Manage 2000; 20(4): 280-5.
[http://dx.doi.org/10.1016/S0885-3924(00)00181-0] [PMID: 11027910]

[13]   Dworkin RH, O'Connor AB, Backonja M, *et al.* Pharmacologic management of neuropathic pain: Evidence-based recommendations. Pain 2007; 132(3): 237-51.
[http://dx.doi.org/10.1016/j.pain.2007.08.033] [PMID: 17920770]

[14]   Group CS. Effect of treatment with capsaicin on daily activities of patients with painful diabetic neuropathy. Diabetes Care 1992; 15(2): 159-65.
[http://dx.doi.org/10.2337/diacare.15.2.159] [PMID: 1547671]

[15]   Barbano RL, Herrmann DN, Hart-Gouleau S, Pennella-Vaughan J, Lodewick PA, Dworkin RH. Effectiveness, tolerability, and impact on quality of life of the 5% lidocaine patch in diabetic polyneuropathy. Arch Neurol 2004; 61(6): 914-8.
[http://dx.doi.org/10.1001/archneur.61.6.914] [PMID: 15210530]

[16]   Kar A, Choudhary BK, Bandyopadhyay NG. Comparative evaluation of hypoglycaemic activity of some Indian medicinal plants in alloxan diabetic rats. J Ethnopharmacol 2003; 84(1): 105-8.
[http://dx.doi.org/10.1016/S0378-8741(02)00144-7] [PMID: 12499084]

[17]   Swain LA, Downum KR. Light-activated toxins of the moraceae. Biochem Syst Ecol 1990; 18(2-3): 153-6.
[http://dx.doi.org/10.1016/0305-1978(90)90052-H]

[18]   Frankish N, De Souza F, Mills C, Sheridan H. Enhancement of Insulin Release from the ß-Cell Line INS-1 by an Ethanolic extract of Buahinia variegate and Its major constituent. Planta Med 2004; 70:

421-6.

[19]   Pop-Busui R, Sima A, Stevens M. Diabetic neuropathy and oxidative stress. Diabetes Metab Res Rev 2006; 22(4): 257-73.
[http://dx.doi.org/10.1002/dmrr.625] [PMID: 16506271]

[20]   Yorek MA, Coppey LJ, Gellett JS, Davidson EP. Sensory nerve innervation of epineurial arterioles of the sciatic nerve containing calcitonin gene-related peptide: effect of streptozotocin-induced diabetes. Exp Diabesity Res 2004; 5(3): 187-93.
[http://dx.doi.org/10.1080/15438600490486732] [PMID: 15512786]

[21]   Maroo J, Vasu VT, Aalinkeel R, Gupta S. Glucose lowering effect of aqueous extract of *Enicostemma littorale* Blume in diabetes: a possible mechanism of action. J Ethnopharmacol 2002; 81(3): 317-20.
[http://dx.doi.org/10.1016/S0378-8741(02)00095-8] [PMID: 12127231]

[22]   Haroon HB, Murali A. Antihyperglycemic and neuroprotective effects of *Wattakaka volubilis* (L.f.) Stapf root against streptozotocin induced diabetes. Braz J Pharm Sci 2016; 52(3): 413-24.
[http://dx.doi.org/10.1590/s1984-82502016000300007]

[23]   Koneri R, Samaddar S, Simi SM, Rao S. Neuroprotective effect of a triterpenoid saponin isolated from *Momordica cymbalaria* Fenzl in diabetic peripheral neuropathy. Indian J Pharmacol 2014; 46(1): 76-81.
[http://dx.doi.org/10.4103/0253-7613.125179] [PMID: 24550589]

[24]   Watcho P, Stavniichuk R, Tane P, *et al.* Evaluation of PMI-5011, an ethanolic extract of *Artemisia dracunculus* L., on peripheral neuropathy in streptozotocin-diabetic mice. Int J Mol Med 2011; 27(3): 299-307.
[PMID: 21225225]

[25]   Kaeidi A, Esmaeili-Mahani S, Sheibani V, *et al.* Olive (*Olea europaea* L.) leaf extract attenuates early diabetic neuropathic pain through prevention of high glucose-induced apoptosis: *In vitro* and *in vivo* studies. J Ethnopharmacol 2011; 136(1): 188-96.
[http://dx.doi.org/10.1016/j.jep.2011.04.038] [PMID: 21540099]

[26]   Bhatti R, Rawal S, Singh J, Ishar M. Effect of Aegle Marmelos Leaf Extract Treatment on Diabetic Neuropathy in Rats: A Possible Involvement of A.

[27]   Shri R, Bhanot A. A comparative profile of methanol extracts of *Allium cepa* and *Allium sativum* in diabetic neuropathy in mice. Pharmacognosy Res 2010; 2(6): 374-84.
[http://dx.doi.org/10.4103/0974-8490.75460] [PMID: 21713142]

[28]   Fatani AJ, Al-Rejaie SS, Abuohashish HM, *et al.* Neuroprotective effects of *Gymnema sylvestre* on streptozotocin-induced diabetic neuropathy in rats. Exp Ther Med 2015; 9(5): 1670-8.
[http://dx.doi.org/10.3892/etm.2015.2305] [PMID: 26136876]

[29]   Li J, Shen X, Shao J, *et al.* The total alkaloids from *Coptis chinensis* Franch improve cognitive deficits in type 2 diabetic rats. Drug Des Devel Ther 2018; 12: 2695-706.
[http://dx.doi.org/10.2147/DDDT.S171025] [PMID: 30214157]

[30]   Yadav SK, Nagori BP, Desai PK. Pharmacological characterization of different fractions of Calotropis procera (Asclepiadaceae) in streptozotocin induced experimental model of diabetic neuropathy. J Ethnopharmacol 2014; 152(2): 349-57.
[http://dx.doi.org/10.1016/j.jep.2014.01.020] [PMID: 24486599]

[31]   Fajrin FA, Nugroho AE, Nurrochmad A, Susilowati R. Ginger extract and its compound, 6-shogaol, attenuates painful diabetic neuropathy in mice *via* reducing TRPV1 and NMDAR2B expressions in the spinal cord. J Ethnopharmacol 2020; 249112396
[http://dx.doi.org/10.1016/j.jep.2019.112396] [PMID: 31743763]

[32]   Jain D, Bansal MK, Dalvi R, Upganlawar A, Somani R. Protective effect of diosmin against diabetic neuropathy in experimental rats. J Integr Med 2014; 12(1): 35-41.
[http://dx.doi.org/10.1016/S2095-4964(14)60001-7] [PMID: 24461593]

[33] Visnagri A, Kandhare AD, Chakravarty S, Ghosh P, Bodhankar SL. Hesperidin, a flavanoglycone attenuates experimental diabetic neuropathy *via* modulation of cellular and biochemical marker to improve nerve functions. Pharm Biol 2014; 52(7): 814-28.
[http://dx.doi.org/10.3109/13880209.2013.870584] [PMID: 24559476]

[34] Kishore L, Kaur N, Singh R. Effect of Kaempferol isolated from seeds of *Eruca sativa* on changes of pain sensitivity in Streptozotocin-induced diabetic neuropathy. Inflammopharmacology 2018; 26(4): 993-1003.
[http://dx.doi.org/10.1007/s10787-017-0416-2] [PMID: 29159712]

[35] Singh P, Bansal S, Kuhad A, Kumar A, Chopra K. Naringenin ameliorates diabetic neuropathic pain by modulation of oxidative-nitrosative stress, cytokines and MMP-9 levels. Food Funct 2020; 11(5): 4548-60.
[http://dx.doi.org/10.1039/C9FO00881K] [PMID: 32400767]

[36] Kandhare AD, Raygude KS, Shiva Kumar V, *et al.* Ameliorative effects quercetin against impaired motor nerve function, inflammatory mediators and apoptosis in neonatal streptozotocin-induced diabetic neuropathy in rats. Biomed Aging Pathol 2012; 2(4): 173-86.
[http://dx.doi.org/10.1016/j.biomag.2012.10.002]

[37] Tian R, Yang W, Xue Q, *et al.* Rutin ameliorates diabetic neuropathy by lowering plasma glucose and decreasing oxidative stress *via* Nrf2 signaling pathway in rats. Eur J Pharmacol 2016; 771: 84-92.
[http://dx.doi.org/10.1016/j.ejphar.2015.12.021] [PMID: 26688570]

[38] Marrazzo G, Bosco P, La Delia F, *et al.* Neuroprotective effect of silibinin in diabetic mice. Neurosci Lett 2011; 504(3): 252-6.
[http://dx.doi.org/10.1016/j.neulet.2011.09.041] [PMID: 21970972]

[39] Ding Y, Dai X, Zhang Z, *et al.* Proanthocyanidins protect against early diabetic peripheral neuropathy by modulating endoplasmic reticulum stress. J Nutr Biochem 2014; 25(7): 765-72.
[http://dx.doi.org/10.1016/j.jnutbio.2014.03.007] [PMID: 24791737]

[40] Stavniichuk R, Drel VR, Shevalye H, *et al.* Baicalein alle*via*tes diabetic peripheral neuropathy through inhibition of oxidative–nitrosative stress and p38 MAPK activation. Exp Neurol 2011; 230(1): 106-13.
[http://dx.doi.org/10.1016/j.expneurol.2011.04.002] [PMID: 21515260]

[41] Hong JS, Feng JH, Park JS, *et al.* Antinociceptive effect of chrysin in diabetic neuropathy and formalin-induced pain models. Anim Cells Syst 2020; 24(3): 143-50.
[http://dx.doi.org/10.1080/19768354.2020.1765019] [PMID: 33209194]

CHAPTER 10

Autism Spectrum Disorder: An Update on the Pathophysiology and Management Strategies

Rubal Singla[1]**, Abhishek Mishra**[1]**, Rupa Joshi**[1]**, Phulen Sarma**[1] **and Bikash Medhi**[1,*]

[1] *Department of Pharmacology, Post Graduate Institute of Medical Education & Research, Chandigarh-160012 (Punjab), India*

Abstract: Autism is a complex neurobehavioral and neurodevelopment disorder with impairments in sociability, language, repetitive, and restrictive stereotypical behaviour as the core symptoms. The term "autism" was first introduced in DSM-III in the year 1980; however, it was changed to autism spectrum disorder (ASD) in DSM-V. It starts in early childhood at the age of around 3 years and persists throughout life. According to data from the Centres for Disease Control and Prevention (CDC), USA, the prevalence of ASD has increased from 1 in 88 (2008 data) to 1 in 59 (2018 data). Being a complex neurological disorder, its etiology is not clear. However, numerous neurochemical pathways have been explicated that may be responsible for the development of this disorder. Besides, it has been evidenced that immune dysfunction and genetic predisposition have a major role in its progression. Some of the major neurochemical systems implicated to be involved in its etiology are glutaminergic and GABAergic as major and others such as DAergic system, adrenergic system, serotonergic system, and the endocannabinoid system. These above-mentioned pathways are crucial in the maturation and development of neurons in different parts of the brain, thus, alteration in any of these pathways enumerates a significant role in the progression of ASD. Current treatment options are antipsychotic medications, which only provide symptomatic relief for behavioral and psychiatric complications such as irritability, anxiety, mood fluctuations,*etc.*. These medications are not effective in treating the core symptoms of ASD. Given the lack of effective treatment options for ASD, drugs targeting the core pathology of the disorder are the need of the hour. Although numerous studies have discussed pharmacotherapy for ASD, the present chapter, more importantly, focuses on the available treatment options for ASD and updates on the recent research approaches for the prevention and treatment of ASD.

Keywords: Autism spectrum disorder, Antipsychotics, GABA, Glutamate, Neurodevelopment, Sociability, Stereotypy.

---

* **Corresponding author Bikash Medhi:** Department of Pharmacology, Post Graduate Institute of Medical Education & Research, Chandigarh-160012 (Panjab), India; E-mail: drbikashus@yahoo.com

INTRODUCTION

Autism spectrum disorder (ASD) is a neurobehavioral and neurodevelopmental disorder marked by impairment in social communication and interaction along with stereotypic/repetitive behaviors [1]. The disease may also be accompanied by a diversity of comorbid conditions like anxiety, memory and learning deficits, seizures, aggressive behaviors, gastrointestinal problems, abnormalities in sensory processing, deficits in motor functioning and sleep disturbances, *etc*. [2]. ASD belongs to the umbrella heading of pervasive developmental disorders, and according to the National Institutes of Health(NIH), "The diagnostic category of pervasive developmental disorders (PDD) refers to a group of disorders that are characterized by delays of the social and communication skills [3]. The ASD includes the following five types:

• **Autistic Disorder:** This is also known as the classic autistic disorder. The children with this disorder show the standard behavioral signs of autism, such as deficits in social behavior, stereotypical patterns, social isolation, problems with communication and understanding, hypersensitivity, and little to no eye contact. They are sensitive to physical touch, high noises, and bright colors.

• **Asperger's Syndrome:** The children with this disorder are often misdiagnosed as obsessive-compulsive disorder or attention deficit disorder, find difficulties in understanding and interpreting social cues, and show an obsessive interest in specific subjects. These children often have high intelligence levels and may often be referred to as "high functioning autism" [4]. They may also suffer from sensory challenges, such as sensitivity from a shirt's tag. This disorder is three times more common in boys than girls.

• **Rett's Disorder**: This disorder only affects girls and starts when the child reaches about 6 months of age [5]. The children with this disorder show similar symptoms to other forms of autism, such as repetitive behaviors and speech and motor activity delay. Moreover, other symptoms such as grinding of the teeth, delays in growth, breathing problems, and mental retardations may aggravate as the age increases.

• **Childhood Disintegrative Disorder:** This form is considered the rarest type of autism. The children with this form of autism seem normal in the initial years but start to suddenly regress after 2 -3 years of age and stop interacting or talking. They suddenly lose multiple areas of function such as social skills, speech, and mental abilities, and the impairment is severe with a very less chance of recovery of the lost functions. This disorder is also linked to the development of seizures.

• **Pervasive Developmental Disorder not Otherwise Specified:** This term is often used for those autistic children that do not properly fit into one criterion of a specific diagnosis. This disorder is characterized as a mild form of autism in which children may show developmental and social-behavioral delays such as delays in walking/ talking than normal children. However, the children with this disorder find it easy to cope with challenges as compared to children with the more severe autism types [6].

HISTORY

Autism was separated from schizophrenia in 1938. A detailed description of autistic disorders was described by Leo Kanner in 1943 [7]. He described the similarities in the behaviors such as autistic aloneness and insistence on the sameness of 11 children to define infantile autism. The broader categories of autism were explained by Rutter [8]. The research by Hans in the Vienna University Hospital led to be known as Asperger syndrome. The milder form of Kanner's autism was then called Asperger syndrome. Then, the other terms like autistic spectrum disorder and Pervasive developmental disorder not otherwise specified came into use.

EPIDEMIOLOGY

The data by the Centre for Disease Control and Prevention (CDC) suggests that1 54 children suffer from ASD [9]. ASD prevalence in 2020 was 18.5 per 1,000 (1 in 54), and it is 4.3 times more common in boys than girls (1 in 37 boys and 1 in 151 girls). According to the CDC2020 report, ASD is the fastest-growing developmental disability. Literature shows 1% in the United Kingdom and 1.5% in the United States, and 2 million children are diagnosed with ASD in India [10].

AUTISM SYMPTOMATOLOGY

Impaired Social Behavior

Impaired social behavior is one of the core diagnostics features as well as an interfering symptom of autism. It includes social exile, difficulty in communication, avoidance of eye contact, and impaired language skills.

Repetitive Stereotypical Behavior

Another diagnostic characteristic of autism and related PDD is repetitive, restrictive, and stereotypic behaviours. Stereotyped motor mannerism, non-adherence to routines, and restrictive patterns of interest often interfere with daily functioning. These phenomena are found to be similar in patients with ASD and obsessive-compulsive disorder (OCD).

Irritability

Irritability is a disruptive symptom often present in patients with autism. It can hamper the daily life and educational access of the affected individuals and is also a cause of major familial distress. Risperidone and Aripiprazole, the currently USFDA-approved medication for ASD, are majorly used to address the irritability symptoms commonly observed in autistic individuals.

Inattention and Hyperactivity

Other common symptoms related to ASD are hyperactivity and inattention. These symptoms are common in children of school-going age. According to DSM-IV, ASD is related to attention deficit hyperactivity disorder (ADHD) in a number of ways having various symptoms in common. The occurrence of any one of these conditions increases the risk of having the other. ADHD can affect social skills and cause trouble in paying attention.

Cognitive Impairments

Cognitive deficits, including mental retardation, are interlinked with communication and social difficulties found in ASD. Many theories of ASD account for the concepts of joint attention and mind involving components of communication, social understanding, and cognition [11].

PATHOPHYSIOLOGY

The etiology of ASD is very complex and not well defined, but the increasing evidence of various scientific studies shows it to be a multifactorial descent combining genetic with environmental factors. Some theories that have been postulated to describe the pathophysiology of ASD are as follows:

Excitatory-Inhibitory Neural Activity

This is one of the most important neurochemical theories of ASD. Evidence of various studies proves that excitatory/inhibitory imbalance may be the underlying cause of ASD [12]. Glutamate (Glu) is one of the major excitatory neurotransmitters in the brain. On the other hand, gamma-aminobutyric acid (GABA) is an essential inhibitory neurotransmitter in the brain [13, 14]. Various scientific evidence enumerates those abnormalities in the excitatory and inhibitory neurotransmitters are extensively found in the brains of individuals with autism. Various genetic studies support this theory [14]. Studies have shown that there is disequilibrium in the glutamate receptor inotropic kainite (GRIK2) and glutamate receptor 6 (GluR6) genes in autistic brains. Also, glutamate decarboxylase (GAD), the enzyme that leads to the metabolism of Glu to GABA, was reduced in the cerebellum as well as the cortex of ASD patients.

N-methyl D-aspartate (NMDA)

A strong association of ASD with the modulation of NMDA has been suggested by various literature studies. Genetic studies reveal variations in the subunit of the NMDA gene [13]. Some findings also suggest a variation of the function of N-methyl D-aspartate receptors (NMDAR) in either direction can lead to developmental changes and thus can contribute to ASD. Thus, targeting NMDAR can be a potential target for ASD, and correcting the dysfunction in NMDAR can be a better option for ASD treatment.

GABA

Various rodent studies have investigated the effect of GABA-R modulation and GABAergic signaling in neural development and behaviors relevant to ASD in different brain regions and at various developmental stages from birth to childhood. The evidence from various studies suggests that the levels of inhibitory neurotransmitter GABA were significantly low in autistic brains. In the early developmental stages, there was a decrease in the expression of GAD67 in the cerebellum and hippocampal regions of autistic rat brains. However, the expression of this enzyme was increased in the pre-frontal cortex from adolescence to adulthood [14, 15]. Some other studies suggest that modulation of GABA-R leads to delayed development of the nervous reflex, abnormalities in motor functions and memory, and anxiety-like behaviours relevant to autism. Thus, the increasing GABAergic signally could be a potential target for the treatment of ASD.

α-amino-3-hydroxy-5-methyl-4-isoxazole propionic acid (AMPA) Receptor

Literature search suggests that one of the major contributors to social deficits in ASD could be the defects in glutamate receptor-interacting proteins. GRIP2-mediated AMPA signalling suggests that modulation of this pathway is a novel therapeutic target for ASD. The role of this signalling has been studied in various other disorders associated with autism, such as fragile X syndrome, Rett's syndrome, Shank2/3 defects,*etc.*. Genetic mutations in the AMPA-linked receptors have also been found to contribute to autism-like defects [16].

Mitochondrial Dysfunction

It has been proposed that one of the major contributing factors in ASD may be the functional abnormalities in the mitochondria [17]. A study by Lombard *et al.* also supported this hypothesis. Various clinical, experimental, and biochemical studies on epilepsy, intellectual disability, and ASD have tried to study a link between nervous system disorders and mitochondrial dysfunction. Despite numerous studies on the dysfunction of mitochondria in various neurological disorders, proper evidence has not been generated supporting this hypothesis.

Synaptic Plasticity

Dysregulation in the long-term synaptic plasticity has been a puzzling observation in the various experimental models of ASD [18]. Several genetic studies have identified high-risk genes in patients with ASD that are the regulators of synaptic. It has been found that long-term potentiation by the mGluR may be impaired in the various regions of the brain, such as the basolateral amygdala and visual cortex. Several changes in synaptic plasticity in the cerebellum and the hippocampus regions in autistic brains have been reported.

Oxidative Stress

The brain has a limited antioxidant capacity and has higher energy requirements making it vulnerable to oxidative stress [19]. There is a strong association between autism and oxidative stress. The brain is highly vulnerable to oxidative stress due to its limited antioxidant capacity, higher energy requirement, and higher amounts of lipids and iron. The levels of various pro and anti-inflammatory markers have been studied in the brain of individuals suffering from ASD. Moreover, lipid peroxidation levels have also been studied in order to find the connection between autism and oxidative stress. The antioxidants can act as a defence system against the reactive oxygen species (ROS) and thus can have a protective action in people with ASDs. Additionally, the antioxidant serum proteins such as transferring and ceruloplasmin are decreased in ASD individuals. Various studies on autism suggest the increased levels of glutathione (GSH), superoxide dismutase (SOD), and catalase (CAT) in autistic patients, which are the major enzymes involved in the generation of ROS.

Neuroinflammation

Neuroinflammation is majorly linked to ASD. Studies suggest that there are marked rise in the inflammatory cytokines' levels of Interleukins such as IL-1β, IL-6, IL-8, tumor necrotic factor-alpha (TNF-α), and interferon-gamma (IFN-γ) in the brain tissues of cerebrospinal fluid in the children with ASD [20]. These increased pro-inflammatory cytokine levels in the ASD brains may be responsible for the social deficits and poor communications in these individuals. The imbalance in the various cytokines during the early stages of development as well as the late stages may be responsible for the amelioration of the neural activity and thus the behavioral symptoms of ASD.

IL-6 is an interleukin that is a pro-inflammatory cytokine [21]. It is one of the most important factors of the neuro-immune system. Various studies suggest the role of IL-6 in physiological brain development as well as various neurological disorders, such as depression, schizophrenia, and Alzheimer's disease. Dysregulation in the IL-6 levels has been found in the plasma, serum, and lymphoblasts of individuals with autism. The stimulation or activation of astrocytes and microglia may be responsible for the elevation of IL-6 levels in the brain. Experimental studies have concluded that if the pregnant mouse were injected with an injection of 1L-6, it could lead to prepulse inhibition and latent inhibition deficits in the adult offspring. IL-1β is another major pro-inflammatory cytokine expressed early in immune responses [22 - 25]. The possible mechanism by which this cytokine induces an inflammatory response in the tissues is by the activation of the vascular endothelium and local immune cells. Studies suggest that disruption in the IL-1β levels can cause various neurological changes linked to autism. IL-1β has a variable action in different CNS regions [26]. It induces the proliferation of neural progenitor cells in some regions and has an inhibitory effect in others. This leads to differential overgrowth and undergrowth patterns characteristically observed in ASD brains.

IL-10 is characteristically the most potent anti-inflammatory cytokine. Various studies have recorded that elevating the levels of IL-10 might be a potential therapeutic target for a number of CNS disorders. Results of various studies show that there is a decrease in the levels of IL-10 in autistic brains. Reports have been reported on the neuroprotective effects of IL-10 elevation [27]. A study suggests that early administration of umbilical cord blood cells to fetal sheep leads to subsequent elevation of IL-10 blood concentrations ad thus has a neuroprotective action.

Neural Connectivity

Early brain overgrowth and neural over connectivity are some of the proposed pathogenesis of ASD. It has been seen that increased neuron numbers leading to overgrowth of the cerebral regions may lead to abnormal wiring and patterning of neurons. This may hinder the long-distance interactions between the different regions of the brain. The reduction in the intra-cortical connectivity leads to a lower degree of integration across multiple regions of the cortex and thus may be responsible for the neuropathological basis of disrupted cognition in ASD [28].

Calcium (Ca^{2+})Signaling

One of the most commonly proposed pathogenesis for ASD is altered Ca^{2+} signaling. Ca^{2+} signalling leads to activity-dependent Ca^{2+} influx into neurons which subsequently regulate numerous cortical excitatory synapses. Alteration in Ca^{2+} signalling could lead to dysfunctional synaptogenesis promotion, which is a major cause of autism [29]. It may be possible that the observed defects in Ca^{2+} signalling are also responsible for the unbalanced excitatory-inhibitory [30 - 32].

Neural Migration

The abnormalities in the neural migration to the cerebral cortex during the first six months of gestation may result in cerebral cortical malformations observed in autism [33]. This subsequent cortical dysgenesis may lead to a thickened cortex, poor grey-white matter boundaries, high neuronal density, and ectopic grey matter.

Neuro-immune Disturbances

The association between ASD and neuro-immune disturbance has a significant impact on autism pathogenesis [34]. This topic is being widely explored in scientific research. It has been found that there are abnormalities in the T-helper cell-mediated immunity in patients with autism. Moreover, abnormal levels of CD4 lymphocytes and reduction in the natural killer cell functions have been recorded in autism. Reduction in the levels of antibodies may also be responsible for the neuroimmune disturbances in patients with autism. Some studies propose that autism may be considered an autoimmune disorder following the findings of autoantibodies against the nervous system proteins in autistic brains. Despite all this evidence, there is still a degree of uncertainty about the possible mechanism by which immune disturbances lead to autism-like conditions.

Dendritic Morphology

This is one surprising theory in the pathogenesis of ASD. It has been found that the brains of autistic patients have increased numbers of long, thin, dendritic spines. Various genetic studies have recorded the changes in the gene encoding the maintenance of dendritic spines [35]. For example, the SHANK3 gene, which is responsible for encoding the synaptic scaffolding and is also involved in dendritic spine maintenance, is deleted in autistic patients [36].

Other Theories

There are several other theories proposed for the pathogenesis of autism. Deficits in cell adhesion molecules, second messenger systems, and secreted molecules have been implicated in the pathogenesis of autism. A decrease in apoptosis may be one cause of ASD [37]. Various studies have also observed that lower levels of Bcl-2 and p53 protein have been reported in the cortical region of autistic brains [38 - 43]. Increased serotonin (5-HT) neurotransmitter levels have also been implicated as one of the theories in the pathogenesis of autism [39 - 42, 44].

ROLE OF DIFFERENT NEUROTRANSMITTERS IN PATHOPHYSIOLOGY OF AUTISM

Numerous neurochemical pathways have been explicated for the development of this disorder [45]. Besides this, it has been evidenced that immune dysfunction and genetic predisposition also have a major role in the development of the disorder. Some of the major neurochemical systems which have been implicated in the development of ASD are the dopaminergic (DAergic) system, adrenergic system, 5-HT system, and endocannabinoid system. As these pathways are crucial in the maturation and development of the neurons in the different parts of the brain, alteration in the above pathways plays a vital role in the progression of ASD. It has been reported that various neurotransmitters like Glu,GABA, 5-HT, and neuropeptides are associated with deficits in autism. Therefore, these are the contributory factors for the advancement of therapeutic interventions primarily in use for alle*via*ting symptoms in ASD.

Monoamines

Monoamines (5-HT, DA, and Norepinephrine) have a major role in the pathophysiology of ASD. 5-HT is distributed throughout the CNS and has a pivotal role as a nerve growth factor in the maturation and development of neurons. The serum 5-HT levels were increased in young subjects with autism as compared to normal controls of the same age in various investigational studies. Genetic variation in the 5-HT system has been reported amongst autistic individuals. Alteration in the synthesis of 5-HT in the cortex region, thalamic region, and cerebellum are observed among people with ASD, as evidenced by clinical neuroimaging studies. The main function of the DAergic system is executive functioning, including planning, analyzing, and prioritizing. There is also evidence that DA level is decreased in ASD due to increased DA transporter level mainly in the cortex region in subjects with high functioning autism. In addition, evidence suggests that alteration of genes involved in the DAergic pathway, *e.g.,* DRD3, DRD4, and DBH (these genes encode for DAreceptors and DA beta-hydroxylase, the enzyme responsible for converting DA to nor-epinephrine) have been related to ASD [36].

Glu and GABA

These are the main imperative neurotransmitters found in the brain. Amongst these, Glu primarily works as an excitatory neurotransmitter, whereas GABA acts as an inhibitory neurotransmitter. GRIP2-mediated AMPA signalling defects contribute to ASD-associated social, behavioral deficits [46]. Recently identified functional GRIP1 mutations that alter GluA2 synaptic trafficking are also found to contribute to the deficits in social interactions associated with ASD. One of the etiologies related to autism is the role of GABA, one of the major inhibitory brain neurotransmitters.

Neuropeptides

Several neuropeptides like oxytocin, vasopressin, melatonin, and secretin are associated with ASD pathogenesis. The essential feature of social recognition in rodents which is social affiliation and parental nurturing behaviour is facilitated by vasopressin and oxytocin. Evidence from the animal studies with oxytocin, vasopressin, and their analogues is suggestive of their implication in neural modulation of human social relationships and are thus promising therapeutic targets for treating disruptions in social behaviors associated with autism and psychiatric disorders.

Endo-cannabinoid

Recently published literature enlightens the key role of the endo-cannabinoid pathway in autism. This lipid signalling pathway comprises a complex network of compounds derived from arachidonic acid and 2-arachidonoyl glycerol, along with CB1 and CB2, which are their G-protein-coupled cannabinoid receptors as well as the associated enzymes [47]. This pathway is the main regulator of various cellular and metabolic pathways involved in autism, such as energy metabolism, food intake, and immune system control. Excessive brain opioid activity during the neonatal period can result in childhood autism which may lead to inhibition of motivation, thus leading to autistic aloofness and isolation. There are three types of arguments strongly supporting this:

a. Induction of exogenous opioid injectionsin young animals and observing similarities withautism such as decreasing social vocalization and increasing social isolation.

b. Biochemical studies such as abnormalities due to peripheral endogenous opioids in autism.

c. Naltrexone, an opioid receptor blocking agent gives long-lasting therapeutic benefits.

Secretin System and Autism

Secretin is widely distributed in the brain. Central secretin is seen to be functionally associated with autism, It is already demonstrated that secretin receptor was present in the brain including cerebellum neuron, supraoptic and periventricular that express these receptor mRNA [48]. Mice having secretin receptor-deficiency were normal and fertile but impairment of the synaptic plasticity in the hippocampal and in CA1 hippocampal region with slightly fewer dendritic spines was seen. Furthermore, these mice also show abnormal cognitive and social behaviors. All the above studies reveal the pivotal role of the secretin receptor in the CNS in social behavior.

CURRENT APPROACHES FOR THE MANAGEMENT OF ASD

For the treatment of ASD, various types of management are available like facilitated communication, vitamin therapy, auditory and sensory training, occupational therapy,*etc.*. These approaches must be individualized depending on the individual potential and capabilities.

The following treatments are used for the management of ASD:

• Pharmacological approach

• Non-Pharmacological approaches

• Curriculum improvement

• Change in dietary habits

• Psychological consultation

• The traditional system of medicines

• Naturopathy and yoga*etc.*.

The improvement in the patient's routine should be implemented as per standard treatment guidelines. The dietary habits should also be reformed as per patient's requirements. The removal of particular food items like gluten and casein-rich food and the addition of multivitamins and a mineral-rich diet can help to cope with the irritability and aggression seen in ASD children. Dietary approaches are focused on food allergies or vitamin and mineral shortages that may be responsible for ASD symptoms [35 - 37, 39, 40, 42, 46, 49].

Many traditional and complementary medicines have been tried to alleviate ASD symptoms. To boost the sleep cycle, it requires specific diets, biological (*e.g.*, secretion) or body-based processes (acupuncture), vitamins such as B12, folic acid, omega-3, and melatonin.

PHARMACOTHERAPY

There are no medications that can relieve the core symptoms of ASD. Risperidone and aripiprazole are the only FDA-approved drugs for the management of ASDs. However, their use is limited only to irritability symptoms associated with this disorder. To date, no intervention targets the underlying pathophysiology of ASD. Various clinical trials have evaluated a bunch of pharmacological treatments that may be useful in the management of ASD [50].

USFDA-APPROVED DRUGS

Risperidone

Risperidone, belonging to the class of antipsychotics, was the first FDA-approved medication for the management of ASD-related irritability by the USFDA in 2006 [51]. It helps reduce deliberate self-injurious behaviors, quick mood changes, and symptoms of aggression of ASD patients towards others. However, the safety and efficacy related to this drug are less established in the pediatric population under the age of 5 years. In a metanalysis by Fung *et al.*, (2016) [52], risperidone use was associated with significant improvement in the aberrant behavioral checklist-irritability (ABC-I) score. The effect size was 0.8 (d=0.8) and adverse effects noted were somnolence or sedation, extrapyramidal symptoms, and weight gain (d=0.8) (But the heterogeneity score among studies for irritability was 52%). Increased weight in patients on risperidone treatment was found in all the studies. In an eight-week placebo-controlled double-blind RCT, McCracken *et al.*, in 101 children (aged 5 to 17 years), risperidone treatment was found to be associated with deletion of the aggressive episodes number, tantrums as well as a decrease in self-injurious behaviors measured using Clinical Global Impressions- Severity (CGI-S) scale and irritability using ABC-I subscale. For long-term therapy, risperidone efficacy was established in many studies. Risperidone is more effective in preventing relapse in the long term.

Aripiprazole

Aripiprazole is another antipsychotic drug, approved in 2009 by the FDA in the symptomatic management of irritability associated with ASD [53]. This antipsychotic drug is also indicated in schizophrenia, Tourette syndrome, bipolar, and major depressive disorder. Aripiprazole is thought to act as a DA type 2 (D2) and serotonin type 1 A (5-HT_{1A}) receptor partial agonist and 5-HT2A receptors antagonist. In a Cochrane review by Hirsch*et al.*, (2016), which included three placebo-controlled trials, meta-analysis results exhibited on average, an improvement of -6.17 (-9.07 to -3.26) concerning the ABC-Irritability subscale, -7.93 (-10.98 to -4.88) on hyperactivity subscale and -2.66 (-3.55 to -1.77) points on the ABC-stereotypy subscale. There was moderate-quality evidence for the efficacy outcome. With a mean rise of 1.13 kg (0.71 to 1.54) in the aripiprazole group as compared to the placebo, children/adolescents on aripiprazole treatment were at greater risk of weight gain as compared to the placebo as well as showed a greater risk ratio (RR) for sedation (RR 4.28, 1.58 to 11.60), and tremor (RR 10.26, 1.37 to 76.63). Chances of relapse were less with aripiprazole when compared to placebo (35% in the aripiprazole group versus 52% in the placebo group, hazard ratio 0.57).

OTHER TREATMENT OPTIONS (REPURPOSING)

Antipsychotics

Olanzapine is an atypical antipsychotic medication that is efficacious in the management of a variety of neuropsychiatric disorders, including schizophrenia, bipolar mania, and depression. This drug has also been tried in the management of children with pervasive developmental disorders. In 2002, Kemner*et al.* [7], in a 3-month study (open-label)reported improvement in ABC checklist parameters (irritability, hyperactivity, excessive speech), and also improvement in the target checklist (it is a five-symptomatology checklist) following therapy with olanzapine in 6-16 years children suffering from autism or PDD-NOS (n=25). However, as per the CGI score, only 3 children were considered as responders. The most common adverse drug reactions reported were increased appetite and weight gain. Extrapyramidal symptoms were seen in three children, but these symptoms disappeared on lowering the dose. In a study by Fido *et al.*, it was found that olanzapine was beneficial in treating behavioral symptoms (irritability, lethargy/withdrawal, and hyperactivity/noncompliance) of ASD.

Clozapine is a second-generation antipsychotic which is found efficacious in aggression-mediated schizophrenia. Zuddas*et al.*, in a case series of three cases, reported the clinical effects of clozapine in ASD as early as 1996 [54]. The dose of clozapine was progressively increased (after 2 months of starting the treatment, the dose of clozapine was 100 mg/day. The child psychiatric rating scale was used for evaluation of efficacy and at 3 months post-treatment, clozapine treatment showed a marked decrease in the child psychiatric rating scale.

Haloperidol is a convincing selective DA receptor antagonist, effective against schizophrenia and Tourette syndrome [55]. A clinical trial conducted in 1982 carefully assessed haloperidol effects on behavioral and learning symptoms. In this study, haloperidol-placebo-haloperidol, as well as placebo-haloperido--placebo treatment, were randomly assigned to the children. The results revealed haloperidol to be statistically more effective than the placebo in reducing behavioral symptoms. Children with haloperidol treatment were seen to learn discrimination in a learning paradigm, while those from a placebo could not. When children who attained discrimination on haloperidol were switched to placebo and discrimination was seen to be retained.

Antidepressants

Sertraline is an antidepressant of the selective 5-HT reuptake inhibitor (SSRI) class. The self-injurious and aggressive behaviour of ASD patients is one of the main reasons for the urgent psychiatric referral of these patients. Sertraline treatment resulted in a decrease in the behaviour of the ASD patients with mental retardation (A). Sertraline also showed efficacy in alleviating behavioral alterations associated with fragile X syndrome (FXS) [56]. Sertraline treatment was associated with an enhanced language development trajectory measured by

Mullen Scales of Early Learning (MSEL). Sertraline-treated groups were seen to have higher mean rates of improvement in the development of both expressive and receptive language (n=34) (C) Polymorphisms of genes involved in the serotonergic pathway seem to be associated with the efficacy of sertraline therapy in young children with FXS. Sertraline also showed efficacy in PDD-NOS. Although the beneficial effect of sertraline may only be temporary in ASD children, short-term sertraline treatment has shown a reduction in behavioral reactions associated with environmental changes and situational transitions in these children.

Fluoxetine is being investigated in adults and children with ASD for treatment of repetitive stereotypical behaviour. Fluoxetine is an antidepressant of SSRI class, widely prescribed for various indications like anxiety, depression, obsessive-compulsive disorder, *etc.* [57]. In a placebo-controlled trial, fluoxetine treatment led to significant improvement in stereotypic behaviors, calculated by the Yale-Brown compulsion subscale as well as the CGI rating of OCD symptoms. There was an overall improvement in the CGI rating. Fluoxetine was found to be tolerated well in trial subjects. For treating repetitive behaviorsin autistic children, a lower dose of a liquid preparation of fluoxetine was superior to placebo. The major problem associated with these studies was their small sample size. Long-term trials with adequate sample sizes are needed to address these issues.

This is another SSRI that is often used in the management of ASD. Martin *et al.*, 2003 reported the effectiveness of treatment with fluvoxamine (low-dose) for PDD children and adolescents.McDougle *et al.,* evaluated fluvoxamine effects in adults with ASD (A 12-week placebo double-blind, controlled trial, 15 in treatment, and 15 in the placebo group). 53% of fluvoxamine-treated patients responded to treatment compared to 0% in placebo. Fluvoxamine effectively reduced repetitive behavior and thoughts, aggression, maladaptive behavior, and some aspects of social relatedness, especially language usage. Adverse effects noted were sedation (mild) and nausea.

Selective 5-HT reuptake inhibitor(SSRI) is the most common medication used in the management of ASD. Citalopram has also shown positive results in ASD patients in various studies. King *et al.*, reported the ineffectiveness of citalopram in managing ASD children (n= 149, age 5-17 years). The use of citalopram was associated with various adverse events, *e.g.*, stereotypy, hyperactivity, impulsiveness, insomnia, decreased concentration, dry skin or pruritus, and diarrhoea.

Escitalopram, is the drug of SSRI class and is often used to improve speech-associated problems in patients with ASD. The use of escitalopram (n=28) led to significant improvement in ABC-CV (Irritability Subscale and subscale) and Clinical Global Improvement Scale severity (CGI-S) ratings. At a dose of <10 mg, 89% of participants responded, but they did not tolerate when the dose was increased to 10 mg. An additional 36% of participants responded at a dose of ≥10 mg. No significant correlation was observed between the final dose and weight and only a weak correlation with age was observed. This study revealed escitalopram to be helpful in the treatment of various difficulties related to PDDs, but the variability in dose could not be accounted for by weight [58]. The information obtained from this study can be used to design a placebo-controlled, double-blind study of escitalopram in PDDs.

Diuretic

Bumetanide is a Na-K-Cl co-transporter (NKCCl) inhibitor. In various animal models of ASD, bumetanide was shown to enhance the GABAergic inhibition, restorethe physiological levels of chloride, and attenuate electrical and behavioral symptoms of ASD. Improvement in the CGI scale and Childhood Autism Rating Scale (CARS) by a minimum of 10 points was associated with bumetanide treatment in a phase 2B trial. Among those who completed the therapy, the CARS score was significantly high when compared to non-completers. Similar results were reported in a study by Lemonnier *et al.*, (2012) in their study with 63 participants, when combined with applied behaviour analysis (ABA), and better outcomes were seen compared to the ABA treatment alone. Adverse effects noted were hypokalemia (mild), loss of appetite, increased urination, asthenia, and dehydration [59].

Hormones

Both 5-HT and oxytocin are important for human effect and sociality and are responsible for many disorders affecting these systems like depression and autism. In a population-based study, significantly lower plasma OT levels were seen in autistic individuals as compared to the normal group. Interaction of these two neuronal systems is important for the regulation of emotion-based behavior. In a study with human healthy volunteers, Mottolese *et al.* [60], demonstrated that OXT regulates the 5-HT_{1A} network in areas like the dorsal raphe nucleus (DRN), amygdala/hippocampal complex, insula, frontal cortex and the regulation of 5-HT by OXT involves centrally amygdala. Genetic variation of the CD38 gene is associated with the defective OT secretion process and is associated with the development of ASD. The Neural and behaviour correlation of social processing was significantly influenced after treatment with intranasal oxytocin in this genotype. Reaction time was slower in homozygotic risk alleles. Moreover, during the visual processing of social stimuli, activation of the left fusiform gyrus was higher in the homozygotic risk allele carriers. During a real-time social interaction in autistic males, improvement in eye contact time was seen with oxytocin administration. Similar results were found in non-autistic males.Althaus *et al.,* in a placebo crossover RCT of oxytocin (OXT) versus placebo, evaluated that OXT, enhanced alignment of social information in male adults with ASD [61]. Participants were administered either OXT or placebo before viewing some affective pictures obtained from the International Affective Picture System (IAPS). Orienting responses evoked by both cortical (late long-lasting parietal positivity) and cardiac (evoked cardiac responses) were measured. Oxytocin was seen to enhance orientation to affective pictures with humans in ASD suffering male adults who were certainly distressed on seeing other people in situations that were stressful and also in healthy normal males who were extremely sensitive to criticism and punishment or have a low goal achievement motivation. Effect on long-term administration of OXT in ASD was evaluated by Tachibana Met *et al.,* In their study, out of eight participants, improvement in communication and social interaction scores was seen in six participants about the autism diagnostic observation schedule-generic (ADOS-G) domains [62]. No significant improvement in Child Behaviour Checklist T-scores and ABC scores could be found, but a mild tendency for improvement was shown in several subcategories. Certain positive effects of oxytocin therapy were reported by caregivers of five of the eight participants. The major effects were observed on the reciprocal communication quality. No side effects were seen in any of the participants and excellent compliance was seen in all.

Vasopressin is also called arginine-vasopressin, primarily synthesized as a pro-hormone in hypothalamic neurons [63]. It plays a vital role in the maintaining of social and affiliative behavior. A strong association was found between prepulse inhibition and Arginine Vasopressin 1a receptor (AVPR1a) on promoter region polymorphism. It improves social sensibility and identifying the ability to assess the familiarity of others, however, the exact mechanism is still unknown.

Melatonin is a neurohormone that is produced in the pineal gland. Various studies suggested that changes in circadian rhythm and abnormalities in the physiology of melatonin were observed in ASD.Tordjman *et al.,* measured the nocturnal urinary excretion of 6-sulphatoxymelatonin in autistic (n=49) as well as normal control (n=88) children and adolescents using radioimmunoassay [64]. Autistic patients show reduced nocturnal melatonin production. Melatonin treatment significantly improved total sleep on an average of 52 min and sleep latency on an average of 47 min when compared to placebo, but did not improve the number of night wakening.

Vitamins

Vitamin D acts as a neuroprotective agent that serves a nutritional role in the CNS, thereby increasing vitamin D receptor (VDR) levels, protecting cortical neurons, and participating in the differentiation, structural formation, and metabolism of neurons. Animal studies demonstrated that early vitamin D deficiency led to permanent brain dysplasia. Physical developments and abnormal social behaviors of autism-like rats were improved after vitamin D supplementation. A case-controlled cross-sectional analysis which was conducted in 122 children with ASD, showed a significant negative correlation with levels of serum 25-OHD. The data was analyzed using the Childhood Autism Rating Scale (CARS) scores. In this study, 57% of patients had a deficiency of vitamin D, and 30% were suffering from vitamin D insufficiency [65].

Tetrahydrobiopterin

Tetrahydrobiopterin is a crucial cofactor in various metabolic pathways that are generally impaired in autism. Thus, this can be a potential candidate for reducing ASD symptoms. In a study by Klaimanet *et al.*, significant improvement in autism mannerism, hyperactivity, and inappropriate speech was associated with tetrahydrobiopterin-treated patients as compared to placebo [66].

Omega-3 Fatty Acid

Omega-3 fatty acids play a crucial role in the normal functioning of the brain. Various reports have revealed the deficiency of these polyunsaturated fatty acids in cases of psychiatric disorders. Thus, regular intake of these fatty acids in the diet can reduce the probability of psychiatric diseases. A 6-week randomized, placebo-controlled double-blind pilot trial investigated the effects of supplementation of 1.5 g/d of omega-3 fatty acids (0.7 g/d docosahexaenoic acids, 0.84 g/d eicosapentaenoic acids) in 13 autistic children having ages between 5 and 17 years that were accompanied by self-injurious behavior and severe aggression. After 6 weeks, the outcomes were measured using the ABC. Omega-3 fatty acids showed significant advantages in hyperactivity and stereotypy related to autism when compared to placebo. The superiority of omega-3 fatty acids over placebo in autism-related hyperactivity was also indicated by repeated-measures ANOVA. Neither of the groups elucidated any clinically significant adverse effects. Evidence collected from the meta-analysis of case-control studies and RCTs published in 2017 revealed that the population with ASD had lower DHA and higher total *n*-6 LCPUFA to *n*-3 LCPUFA ratio. Lower *n*-3 LCPUFA levels were seen in the ASD population. On supplementation with *n*-3 LCPUFA, significant behavioral improvements were seen along with improvement in repetitive and restricted interests and social interaction when compared with placebo [67].

TRADITIONAL MEDICINES

The use of herbal medicines against different diseases has developed in recent years, as they are usually non-toxic and have fewer side effects. The WHO has proposed that plants be used effectively under conditions where modern medicines are not protected. Often when given in conjunction with allopathic medications, herbal preparation provides a strong therapeutic response. India is recognized worldwide as the primary manufacturer of herbal medicines. India accepts the medical use of more than 3000 plants. More than 6000 plants in India are estimated to be used in traditional and herbal medicine systems.

Recently, a variety of human and experimental studies investigated the possible herbs and formulae for ASD and associated conditions in the current research literature. By integrating and systematically analyzing the data obtained from modern and classical literature, the classical literature includes herbal remedies for disorders with symptoms and indications close to those of ASD, it is predicted that natural drugs have the utmost perspective for further studies. Some of the Indian traditional medicines or herbal drugs that have shown efficacy in the management of ASD symptoms include *Bacopa monnieri* which has been used as a memory promoter, antioxidant, anti-inflammatory, antipyretic, analgesic, sedative, and anti-epileptic for decades. *B. Monnieri* is currently regarded as potentially beneficial in the treatment of epilepsy and mental illness. Further, a study by Sandhya *et al.*, has shown *B. Monnieri* to ameliorate the behavioral alterations in the valproic acid model of autism [68]. Further, *Ginkgo biloba* is one of the most commonly studied plants and has shown efficacy in treating a range of circulatory, brain, and nerve conditions. An observational study has found *Ginkgo biloba* at the dose of 100mg/kg twice a day to be effective in ameliorating behavioral irritability, hyperactivity, and inappropriate speech in autism [69]. Another important Indian traditional plant having well-known neuroprotective properties is *Curcuma longa.* This drug has been found to be an active neuro-psycho pharmacotherapeutic adjunct for autism spectrum disorders [70] Also, *Camellia sinensis* (green tea extract) is an important dietary source of polyphenols and has potential antioxidant potential is also recently studied for its beneficial effect for ASD. Literature shows that 300mg/kg of green tea extract has shown neuroprotective potential in the treatment of autism [70]. In addition to all these drugs, numerous other medicinal plants have been tested in autism which include *Withaniasomnifera, Convolvulus pluricaulis, Zingiber officinale, Cannabis sativa, Celastrus paniculatus.*

NEWER TARGETS

Over the years, extensive research on the etiology of ASD, including its specific molecular mechanisms, the brain circuits involved, and genetic testing, has increased our understanding of this disorder. Researchers are now focusing on targeted pharmacotherapy [30, 71 - 74]. Moreover, the role of synaptic plasticity in ASD has gained much consideration. The excitatory and inhibitory imbalance is the most common neurochemical theory of autism, which can be rectified by targeting the NMDA, GABA, mGluR, or GSK-3β signaling. Molecular targets for these receptors have eventually been identified and have entered clinical trials. However, targeting the downstream pathways of these receptors can create new therapeutic options [24, 75, 76]. The pathways like mTOR are other targets that areanticipated to show promising results in clinical trials.The inhibitors of mTOR for treating the core symptoms of ASD are being extensively studied by researchers. Another strategy that has been proposed for correcting the abnormalities and symptoms of ASD isthe studies targeting ROCK1 and ROCK2 kinases [32, 62, 77, 78].

CONCLUSION AND CHALLENGES

The development of disease-modifying drug therapies targeting the neuropathological hallmarks is necessary for improving the quality of life and prognosis in patients with ASD. Although several pharmacological treatments have been reported to be effective for the management of ASD, their benefits are limited because of undesirable adverse effects or their lack of efficacy. Especially, the use of antipsychotics has unfavourable influences on neurocognitive and functional impairment in patients. Given that pharmacological treatments should be performed for ASD as a second step, it is then necessary to identify which ASD sub-symptoms are responsive to each pharmacological treatment. Among several ASD symptoms, irritability, hyperactivity, agitation, respond comparatively well to the pharmacological treatments in patients with ASD. However, these available options are accompanied by various adverse effects such as dizziness, fatigue, drooling, and increased appetite. Thus, extensive research targeting the etiology of ASD and a better understanding of the specific molecular mechanism, genetic testing, and various brain circuits can help in the development of future interventions. The ongoing research and clinical trials have put forward numerous drugs which may have a positive impact on the development of new targets. Since ADHD commonly appears during the progression of ASD, thus the patients might respond to methylphenidate. Various antidepressant drugs, especially SSRIs have shown improvement in the stereotypical behaviours as well as maladaptive behaviours. Additionally, antiepileptics may improve hyperactivity and mood disorders in autistic children. Diuretic bumetanide has been shown to enhance the inhibition of the inhibitory neurotransmitter signaling. NMDA receptor antagonists such as memantine appeared to be beneficial in improving non-verbal communication as well as neuropsychological assessments in ASD children. Moreover, various hormonal therapies have been tried for managing ASD symptoms. Oxytocin treatment was associated with significant improvement in social reciprocity. Finally, the quality of sleep was improved in patients with ASD by the administration of melatonin. Various other interventions such as antioxidants (N-acetyl cysteine), Vitamin D, opioid antagonists have been tried in patients with ASD. However, further research and clinical trials with a larger sample size are required to conclude. Furthermore, these pharmacological treatments for ASD should carefully be used, for a limited duration, and at lower dosages in consideration of undesirable adverse events. Pharmacological treatments for ASD without consideration of the underlying mechanisms may further worsen the ASD symptoms. To avoid this problem, further research is needed to examine the effectiveness of a novel therapeutic strategy such as neuro-modulation techniques, underlying genetics, and molecular mechanisms. These problems concerning the present therapeutic options may provide a good opportunity to develop a long-term treatment strategy and to reconsider and seek alternative treatment options and goals for people with ASD.

CONSENT FOR PUBLICATION

Not applicable.

CONFLICT OF INTEREST

The author declares no conflict of interest, financial or otherwise.

ACKNOWLEDGEMENTS

Declared none.

REFERENCES

[1]   Regier DA, Narrow WE, Kuhl EA, Kupfer DJ. The conceptual development of DSM-V. Am J Psychiatry 2009; 166(6): 645-50.
[http://dx.doi.org/10.1176/appi.ajp.2009.09020279] [PMID: 19487400]

[2]   Argyropoulos A, Gilby KL, Hill-Yardin EL. Studying autism in rodent models: reconciling endophenotypes with comorbidities. Front Hum Neurosci 2013; 7: 417.
[http://dx.doi.org/10.3389/fnhum.2013.00417] [PMID: 23898259]

[3]   Sanchack KE, Thomas CA. Autism spectrum disorder: Primary care principles. Am Fam Physician 2016; 94(12): 972-9.

[PMID: 28075089]

[4]   Mirkovic B, Gérardin P. Asperger's syndrome: What to consider? Encephale 2019; 45(2): 169-74.
        [http://dx.doi.org/10.1016/j.encep.2018.11.005] [PMID: 30736970]

[5]   Kyle SM, Vashi N, Justice MJ. Rett syndrome: a neurological disorder with metabolic components.
        Open Biol 2018; 8(2): 170216.
        [http://dx.doi.org/10.1098/rsob.170216] [PMID: 29445033]

[6]   Sharma SR, Gonda X, Tarazi FI. Autism Spectrum Disorder: Classification, diagnosis and therapy.
        Pharmacol Ther 2018; 190: 91-104.
        [http://dx.doi.org/10.1016/j.pharmthera.2018.05.007] [PMID: 29763648]

[7]   Harris J. Leo Kanner and autism: a 75-year perspective. Int Rev Psychiatry 2018; 30(1): 3-17.
        [http://dx.doi.org/10.1080/09540261.2018.1455646] [PMID: 29667863]

[8]   Hutton J, Goode S, Murphy M, Le Couteur A, Rutter M. New-onset psychiatric disorders in
        individuals with autism. Autism 2008; 12(4): 373-90.
        [http://dx.doi.org/10.1177/1362361308091650] [PMID: 18579645]

[9]   Makushkin EV, Makarov IV, Pashkovskiy VE. The prevalence of autism: genuine and imaginary. Zh
        Nevrol Psikhiatr Im S S Korsakova 2019; 119(2): 80-6.
        [http://dx.doi.org/10.17116/jnevro201911902180] [PMID: 30874532]

[10]   Singh M, Chauhan A, Sahu JK, *et al.* Prevalence of autism spectrum disorder in Indian children: A
        systematic review and meta-analysis. Neurol India 2019; 67(1): 100-4.
        [http://dx.doi.org/10.4103/0028-3886.253970] [PMID: 30860104]

[11]   Faridi F, Khosrowabadi R. Behavioral, Cognitive and Neural Markers of Asperger Syndrome. Basic
        Clin Neurosci 2017; 8(5): 349-60.
        [http://dx.doi.org/10.18869/nirp.bcn.8.5.349] [PMID: 29167722]

[12]   Gao R, Penzes P. Common mechanisms of excitatory and inhibitory imbalance in schizophrenia and
        autism spectrum disorders. Curr Mol Med 2015; 15(2): 146-67.
        [http://dx.doi.org/10.2174/1566524015666150303003028] [PMID: 25732149]

[13]   Lee K, Vyas Y, Garner CC, Montgomery JM. Autism-associated *Shank3* mutations alter mGluR
        expression and mGluR-dependent but not NMDA receptor-dependent long-term depression. Synapse
        2019; 73(8): e22097.
        [http://dx.doi.org/10.1002/syn.22097] [PMID: 30868621]

[14]   Fueta Y, Sekino Y, Yoshida S, Kanda Y, Ueno S. Prenatal exposure to valproic acid alters the
        development of excitability in the postnatal rat hippocampus. Neurotoxicology 2018; 65: 1-8.
        [http://dx.doi.org/10.1016/j.neuro.2018.01.001] [PMID: 29309796]

[15]   Richard E. Frye Mitochondrial dysfunction in autism spectrum disorder: unique abnormalities and
        targeted treatments. Semin Pediatr Neurol 2020; 10: 1016.

[16]   Kim JW, Park K, Kang RJ, Gonzales ELT, Kim DG, Oh HA, *et al.* Pharmacological modulation of
        AMPA receptor rescues social impairments in animal models of autism. 2019.
        [http://dx.doi.org/10.1038/s41386-018-0098-5]

[17]   Rose S, Niyazov DM, Rossignol DA, Goldenthal M, Kahler SG, Frye RE. Clinical and molecular
        characteristics of mitochondrial dysfunction in autism spectrum disorder. Mol Diagn Ther 2018; 22(5):
        571-93.
        [http://dx.doi.org/10.1007/s40291-018-0352-x] [PMID: 30039193]

[18]   Edfawy M, Guedes JR, Pereira MI, *et al.* Abnormal mGluR-mediated synaptic plasticity and autism-
        like behaviours in gprasp2 mutant mice. Nat Commun 2019; 10(1): 1431.
        [http://dx.doi.org/10.1038/s41467-019-09382-9] [PMID: 30926797]

[19]   Manivasagam T, Arunadevi S, Essa MM, *et al.* Role of oxidative stress and antioxidants in autism.
        Adv neurobiol 2020; 24: 193-206.

[http://dx.doi.org/10.1007/978-3-030-30402-7_7] [PMID: 32006361]

[20]   El-Ansary A, Al-Ayadhi L. GABAergic/glutamatergic imbalance relative to excessive neuroinflammation in autism spectrum disorders. J Neuroinflammation 2014; 11(1): 189.
[http://dx.doi.org/10.1186/s12974-014-0189-0] [PMID: 25407263]

[21]   Hodges SL, Nolan SO, Taube JH, Lugo JN. Adult Fmr1 knockout mice present with deficiencies in hippocampal interleukin-6 and tumor necrosis factor-α expression. Neuroreport 2017; 28(18): 1246-9.
[http://dx.doi.org/10.1097/WNR.0000000000000905] [PMID: 28915148]

[22]   Singh SS, Rai SN, Birla H, Zahra W, Rathore AS, Dilnashin H, *et al.* Techniques Related to Disease Diagnosis and Therapeutics. Application of Biomedical Engineering in Neuroscience. 2019; 437-56.
[http://dx.doi.org/10.1007/978-981-13-7142-4_22]

[23]   Singh S, Rai S, Birla H, Zahra W, Rathore A, Dilnashin H, Eds. Chlorogenic acid protects against MPTP induced neurotoxicity in parkinsonian mice model *via* its anti-apoptotic activity. 2019.

[24]   Rai SN, Zahra W, Singh SS, *et al.* Anti-inflammatory activity of ursolic acid in MPTP-induced parkinsonian mouse model. Neurotox Res 2019; 36(3): 452-62.
[http://dx.doi.org/10.1007/s12640-019-00038-6] [PMID: 31016688]

[25]   Singh SS, Rai SN, Birla H, Zahra W, Rathore AS, Dilnashin H, *et al.* Neuroprotective effect of chlorogenic acid on mitochondrial dysfunction-mediated apoptotic death of DA neurons in a Parkinsonian mouse model. 2020.
[http://dx.doi.org/10.1155/2020/6571484]

[26]   Tsilioni I, Theoharides TC. Extracellular vesicles are increased in the serum of children with autism spectrum disorder, contain mitochondrial DNA, and stimulate human microglia to secrete IL-1β. J Neuroinflammation 2018; 15(1): 239.
[http://dx.doi.org/10.1186/s12974-018-1275-5] [PMID: 30149804]

[27]   Leviton A, Joseph RM, Allred EN, *et al.* The risk of neurodevelopmental disorders at age 10 years associated with blood concentrations of interleukins 4 and 10 during the first postnatal month of children born extremely preterm. Cytokine 2018; 110: 181-8.
[http://dx.doi.org/10.1016/j.cyto.2018.05.004] [PMID: 29763840]

[28]   Stoodley CJ, D'Mello AM, Ellegood J, *et al.* Altered cerebellar connectivity in autism and cerebellar-mediated rescue of autism-related behaviors in mice. Nat Neurosci 2017; 20(12): 1744-51.
[http://dx.doi.org/10.1038/s41593-017-0004-1] [PMID: 29184200]

[29]   Liao X, Li Y. Genetic associations between voltage-gated calcium channels and autism spectrum disorder: a systematic review. Mol Brain 2020; 13(1): 96.
[http://dx.doi.org/10.1186/s13041-020-00634-0] [PMID: 32571372]

[30]   Keswani C, Dilnashin H, Birla H, Singh S. Re-addressing the commercialization and regulatory hurdles for biopesticides in India. 2019.

[31]   Rathore AS, Birla H, Singh SS, *et al.* Epigenetic Modulation in Parkinson's Disease and Potential Treatment Therapies. Neurochem Res 2021; 46(7): 1618-26.
[http://dx.doi.org/10.1007/s11064-021-03334-w] [PMID: 33900517]

[32]   Rai SN, Singh BK, Rathore AS, *et al.* Quality control in huntington's disease: a therapeutic target. Neurotox Res 2019; 36(3): 612-26.
[http://dx.doi.org/10.1007/s12640-019-00087-x] [PMID: 31297710]

[33]   Courchesne E, Gazestani VH, Lewis NE. Prenatal Origins of ASD: The When, What, and How of ASD Development. Trends Neurosci 2020; 43(5): 326-42.
[http://dx.doi.org/10.1016/j.tins.2020.03.005] [PMID: 32353336]

[34]   Siniscalco D, Schultz S, Brigida A, Antonucci N. Inflammation and Neuro-immune dysregulations in autism spectrum disorders. Pharmaceuticals (Basel) 2018; 11(2): 56.
[http://dx.doi.org/10.3390/ph11020056] [PMID: 29867038]

[35] Varghese M, Keshav N, Jacot-Descombes S, *et al.* Autism spectrum disorder: neuropathology and animal models. Acta Neuropathol 2017; 134(4): 537-66.
[http://dx.doi.org/10.1007/s00401-017-1736-4] [PMID: 28584888]

[36] Monteiro P, Feng G. SHANK proteins: roles at the synapse and in autism spectrum disorder. Nat Rev Neurosci 2017; 18(3): 147-57.
[http://dx.doi.org/10.1038/nrn.2016.183] [PMID: 28179641]

[37] Eftekharian MM, Komaki A, Oskooie VK, Namvar A, Taheri M, Ghafouri-Fard S. Assessment of Apoptosis Pathway in Peripheral Blood of Autistic Patients 2019.
[http://dx.doi.org/10.1007/s12031-019-01387-9]

[38] Eftekharian MM, Komaki A, Oskooie VK, Namvar A, Taheri M, Ghafouri-Fard S. Assessment of apoptosis pathway in peripheral blood of autistic patients. J Mol Neurosci 2019; 69(4): 588-96.
[http://dx.doi.org/10.1007/s12031-019-01387-9] [PMID: 31363911]

[39] Sadek A, Berk LS, Mainess K, Daher NS. Antioxidants and Autism: Teachers' Perceptions of Behavioral Changes. Adv Mind Body Med 2018; 32(3): 12-7.
[PMID: 29870399]

[40] Gasparotto FM, dos Reis Lívero FA, Tolouei Menegati SEL, Junior AG. Herbal Medicine as an Alternative Treatment in Autism Spectrum Disorder: A Systematic Review. Curr Drug Metab 2018; 19(5): 454-9.
[http://dx.doi.org/10.2174/1389200219666171227202332] [PMID: 29283066]

[41] Zou M, Liu Y, Xie S, *et al.* Alterations of the endocannabinoid system and its therapeutic potential in autism spectrum disorder. Open Biol 2021; 11(2): 200306.
[http://dx.doi.org/10.1098/rsob.200306] [PMID: 33529552]

[42] Gandhi T. Lee Charles. Neural mechanism underlying repetitive behaviors in rodent models of autism spectrum disorders. Front Cell Neurosci 2021; 10: 3389.

[43] Hou Q, Wang Y, Li Y, Chen D, Yang F, Wang S. A developmental study of abnormal behaviors and altered GABAergic signaling in the VPA-treated rat model of autism. Front Behav Neurosci 2018; 12: 182.
[http://dx.doi.org/10.3389/fnbeh.2018.00182] [PMID: 30186123]

[44] Afroze S, Meng F, Jensen K, *et al.* The physiological roles of secretin and its receptors. Ann Transl Med 2012; 10: 3978.

[45] Kardani A, Soltani A, Sewell RDE, Shahrani M, Rafieian-Kopaei M. Neurotransmitter, antioxidant and anti-neuroinflammatory mechanistic potentials of herbal medicines in ameliorating autism spectrum disorder. Curr Pharm Des 2020; 25(41): 4421-9.
[http://dx.doi.org/10.2174/1381612825666191112143940] [PMID: 31721693]

[46] Mejias R, Chiu SL, Han M, *et al.* Purkinje cell-specific Grip1/2 knockout mice show increased repetitive self-grooming and enhanced mGluR5 signaling in cerebellum. Neurobiol Dis 2019; 132: 104602.
[http://dx.doi.org/10.1016/j.nbd.2019.104602] [PMID: 31476380]

[47] Zamberletti E, Gabaglio M, Woolley-Roberts M, Bingham S, Rubino T, Parolaro D. Cannabidivarin treatment ameliorates autism-like behaviors and restores hippocampal endocannabinoid system and glia alterations induced by prenatal valproic acid exposure in rats. Front Cell Neurosci 2019; 13: 367.
[http://dx.doi.org/10.3389/fncel.2019.00367] [PMID: 31447649]

[48] Wang L, Zhang L. Involvement of secretin in the control of cell survival and synaptic plasticity in the central nervous system. Front Neurosci 2020; 14: 387.
[http://dx.doi.org/10.3389/fnins.2020.00387] [PMID: 32435180]

[49] Trudeau MS, Madden RF, Parnell JA, Gibbard WB, Shearer J. Dietary and supplement-based complementary and alternative medicine Use in pediatric autism spectrum Disorder. Nutrients 2019; 11(8): 1783.

[http://dx.doi.org/10.3390/nu11081783] [PMID: 31375014]

[50] Goel R, Hong JS, Findling RL, Ji NY. An update on pharmacotherapy of autism spectrum disorder in children and adolescents. Int Rev Psychiatry 2018; 30(1): 78-95.
[http://dx.doi.org/10.1080/09540261.2018.1458706] [PMID: 29693461]

[51] Vorhees CV, Williams MT. Morris water maze: procedures for assessing spatial and related forms of learning and memory. Nat Protoc 2006; 1(2): 848-58.
[http://dx.doi.org/10.1038/nprot.2006.116] [PMID: 17406317]

[52] Fung LK, Mahajan R, Nozzolillo A, *et al.* Pharmacologic treatment of severe irritability and problem behaviors in autism: A systematic review and meta-analysis. Pediatrics 2016; 137 (Suppl. 2): S124-35.
[http://dx.doi.org/10.1542/peds.2015-2851K] [PMID: 26908468]

[53] Farmer CA, Aman MG. Aripiprazole for the treatment of irritability associated with autism. Expert Opin Pharmacother 2011; 12(4): 635-40.
[http://dx.doi.org/10.1517/14656566.2011.557661] [PMID: 21294670]

[54] Gunes H, Tanidir C, Erdogan A. Effective use of aripiprazole augmentation in a clozapine-treated adolescent with autism spectrum disorder. J Child Adolesc Psychopharmacol 2015; 25(9): 727-8.
[http://dx.doi.org/10.1089/cap.2015.0101] [PMID: 26402582]

[55] Anderson LT, Campbell M, Adams P, Small AM, Perry R, Shell J. The effects of haloperidol on discrimination learning and behavioral symptoms in autistic children. J Autism Dev Disord 1989; 19(2): 227-39.
[http://dx.doi.org/10.1007/BF02211843] [PMID: 2663834]

[56] Achuta VS, Möykkynen T, Peteri UK, *et al.* Functional changes of AMPA responses in human induced pluripotent stem cell–derived neural progenitors in fragile X syndrome. Sci Signal 2018; 11(513): eaan8784.
[http://dx.doi.org/10.1126/scisignal.aan8784] [PMID: 29339535]

[57] Hollander E, Phillips A, Chaplin W, Zagursky K, Novotny S, Wasserman S, *et al.* A placebo controlled crossover trial of liquid fluoxetine on repetitive behaviors in childhood and adolescent autism. 2005.
[http://dx.doi.org/10.1038/sj.npp.1300627]

[58] Owley T, Walton L, Salt J, *et al.* An open-label trial of escitalopram in pervasive developmental disorders. J Am Acad Child Adolesc Psychiatry 2005; 44(4): 343-8.
[http://dx.doi.org/10.1097/01.chi.0000153229.80215.a0] [PMID: 15782081]

[59] Lemonnier E, Degrez C, Phelep M, *et al.* A randomised controlled trial of bumetanide in the treatment of autism in children. Transl Psychiatry 2012; 2(12): e202.
[http://dx.doi.org/10.1038/tp.2012.124] [PMID: 23233021]

[60] Mottolese R, Redouté J, Costes N, Le Bars D, Sirigu A. Switching brain serotonin with oxytocin. Proc Natl Acad Sci USA 2014; 111(23): 8637-42.
[http://dx.doi.org/10.1073/pnas.1319810111] [PMID: 24912179]

[61] Althaus M, Groen Y, Wijers AA, Noltes H, Tucha O, Hoekstra PJ. Oxytocin enhances orienting to social information in a selective group of high-functioning male adults with autism spectrum disorder. 2015.
[http://dx.doi.org/10.1016/j.neuropsychologia.2015.10.025]

[62] Tachibana M, Kagitani-Shimono K, Mohri I, *et al.* Long-term administration of intranasal oxytocin is a safe and promising therapy for early adolescent boys with autism spectrum disorders. J Child Adolesc Psychopharmacol 2013; 23(2): 123-7.
[http://dx.doi.org/10.1089/cap.2012.0048] [PMID: 23480321]

[63] Zink CF, Kempf L, Hakimi S, Rainey CA, Stein JL, Meyer-Lindenberg A. Vasopressin modulates social recognition-related activity in the left temporoparietal junction in humans. Transl Psychiatry 2011; 1(4): e3.

[http://dx.doi.org/10.1038/tp.2011.2] [PMID: 22832391]

[64] Tordjman S, Anderson GM, Pichard N, Charbuy H, Touitou Y. Nocturnal excretion of 6-sulphatoxymelatonin in children and adolescents with autistic disorder. Biol Psychiatry 2005; 57(2): 134-8.
[http://dx.doi.org/10.1016/j.biopsych.2004.11.003] [PMID: 15652871]

[65] Seuter S, Heikkinen S, Carlberg C. Chromatin acetylation at transcription start sites and vitamin D receptor binding regions relates to effects of 1α,25-dihydroxyvitamin D3 and histone deacetylase inhibitors on gene expression. Nucleic Acids Res 2013; 41(1): 110-24.
[http://dx.doi.org/10.1093/nar/gks959] [PMID: 23093607]

[66] Klaiman C, Huffman L, Masaki L, Elliott GR. Tetrahydrobiopterin as a treatment for autism spectrum disorders: a double-blind, placebo-controlled trial. J Child Adolesc Psychopharmacol 2013; 23(5): 320-8.
[http://dx.doi.org/10.1089/cap.2012.0127] [PMID: 23782126]

[67] Amminger GP, Berger GE, Schäfer MR, Klier C, Friedrich MH, Feucht M. Omega-3 fatty acids supplementation in children with autism: a double-blind randomized, placebo-controlled pilot study. Biol Psychiatry 2007; 61(4): 551-3.
[http://dx.doi.org/10.1016/j.biopsych.2006.05.007] [PMID: 16920077]

[68] Sandhya T, Sowjanya J, Veeresh B. *Bacopa monniera* (L.) Wettst ameliorates behavioral alterations and oxidative markers in sodium valproate induced autism in rats. Neurochem Res 2012; 37(5): 1121-31.
[http://dx.doi.org/10.1007/s11064-012-0717-1] [PMID: 22322665]

[69] Deb S, Phukan BC, Dutta A, *et al.* Natural products and their therapeutic effect on autism spectrum disorder. Adv Neurobiol 2020; 24: 601-14.
[http://dx.doi.org/10.1007/978-3-030-30402-7_22] [PMID: 32006376]

[70] Bhandari R, Paliwal JK, Kuhad A. Dietary Phytochemicals as Neurotherapeutics for Autism Spectrum Disorder: Plausible Mechanism and Evidence. Adv Neurobiol 2020; 24: 615-46.
[http://dx.doi.org/10.1007/978-3-030-30402-7_23] [PMID: 32006377]

[71] Zahra W, Rai SN, Birla H, Singh SS, Dilnashin H, Rathore AS, *et al.* The global economic impact of neurodegenerative diseases: Opportunities and challenges. 2020; 333-45.

[72] Zahra W, Rai SN, Birla H, Singh SS, Rathore AS, Dilnashin H, *et al.* Economic Importance of Medicinal Plants in Asian Countries. Bioeconomy for Sustainable Development. 2020; 359-77.
[http://dx.doi.org/10.1007/978-981-13-9431-7_19]

[73] Birla H, Keswani C, Singh SS, Zahra W, Dilnashin H, Rathore AS, *et al.* Unraveling the neuroprotective effect of *tinospora cordifolia* in parkinsonian mouse model through proteomics approach. 2021.
[http://dx.doi.org/10.1021/acschemneuro.1c00481]

[74] Birla H, Keswani C, Rai SN, *et al.* Neuroprotective effects of *Withania somnifera* in BPA induced-cognitive dysfunction and oxidative stress in mice. Behav Brain Funct 2019; 15(1): 9.
[http://dx.doi.org/10.1186/s12993-019-0160-4] [PMID: 31064381]

[75] Keswani C, Dilnashin H, Birla H, Singh SP. Unravelling efficient applications of agriculturally important microorganisms for alleviation of induced inter-cellular oxidative stress in crops. Acta Agric Slov 2019; 114(1): 121-30.
[http://dx.doi.org/10.14720/aas.2019.114.1.14]

[76] Keswani C. Bioeconomy for Sustainable Development. 2020.
[http://dx.doi.org/10.1007/978-981-13-9431-7]

[77] Rai SN, Birla H, Singh SS, Zahra W, Rathore AS, Dilnashin H, *et al.* Pathophysiology of the disease causing physical disability. biomedical engineering and its Applications in Healthcare. 2019; 573-95.

[78]   Rai SN, Dilnashin H, Birla H, *et al.* The role of PI3K/Akt and ERK in neurodegenerative disorders. Neurotox Res 2019; 35(3): 775-95.
[http://dx.doi.org/10.1007/s12640-019-0003-y] [PMID: 30707354]

CHAPTER 11

Neuroprotective Effect of *Ginkgo Biloba* and its Role in Alzheimer's Disease

Divya Raj Prasad[1,*], Bipin Maurya[2,*] and **Aparna Mishra[3]**

[1] *Department of Genetics and Plant Breeding, Institute of Agricultural Sciences, Banaras Hindu University, Varanasi-221005 (U.P.), India*

[2] *Laboratory of Morphogenesis, Centre of Advance Study in Botany, Institute of Science, Banaras Hindu University, Varanasi-221005 (U.P.), India*

[3] *Department of Bioscience and Biotechnology, Banasthali Vidyapith University, Banasthali-304022 (Rajasthan), India*

Abstract: Alzheimer's disease (AD) is a common age-related neurodegenerative disorder that results in cognitive defects. The disease is a progressive, age-associated, irreversible, neurodegenerative disease with severe memory loss, personality changes, unusual behavior and impairment in cognitive function. There is no cure for AD, and the drugs available for the treatment of the disease have limited efficacy. Medicine develops from the extract of medicinal plants have been the single most productive and common source for the development of drugs, and also, more than thousands of new products are already in clinical study. Different types of therapeutic strategies like herbal and synthetic approaches are being used against AD on the basis of understanding AD mechanisms. *Ginkgo biloba* extract (GBE) is the most effective and highly investigated, herbal medicine for AD and other cognitive disorders. One of the famous dietary supplements is GBE, consumed by the elderly population to improve memory and age-related loss of cognitive function. The exact mechanism of action of *Ginkgo* extract in AD is still not very clear. The phytochemical studies of the different plant parts of the *G. biloba* have revealed the presence of many valuable secondary metabolites, such as flavonoids, polyphenols, triterpenes, sterols, and alkaloids that shows a wide spectrum of pharmacological activities like anti-amyloidogenic, anti-inflammatory and antioxidant effects. This book chapter gathers research on the *G. biloba* plant and its neuroprotective and phytochemical effects, which are used against AD. The summarized information concern pharmacological activities, neuroprotective effect, and biological and clinical applications of the *Ginkgo* plant.

Keywords: Alzheimer's disease, *Ginkgo biloba*, Neuroprotective, Phytochemical.

* **Corresponding authors Bipin Maurya & Divya Raj Prasad:** Laboratory of Morphogenesis, Centre of Advance Study in Botany, Institute of Science, Banaras Hindu University, Varanasi-221005 (U.P.), India and Department of Genetics and Plant breeding, Institute of Agricultural Sciences, Banaras Hindu University, Varanasi-221005 (U.P.), India; E-mails: bipinmaurya841@gmail.com and divyarajbhu@gmail.com

Surya Pratap Singh, Hagera Dilnashin, Hareram Birla & Chetan Keswani (Eds.)

INTRODUCTION

Alzheimer's disease (AD) is a progressive neurological disorder of the brain that was first described in the year of 1906 and named after German physician Aloes Alzheimer. It is the most common form of dementia which affects an estimated count of 10 million people across the world [1]. The major symptoms of this disease are impairment of memory and, eventually, the disturbance in language, planning, perception and reasoning, and symptoms appear gradually. AD is an irreversible, age-associated, progressive neurodegenerative, characterized by severe memory loss, personality changes, unusual behavior and a decline in cognitive function [2, 3]. This disease is often seen in people aged 65 and older than that and one-third of those aged 85 or above to this age. The term dementia is generally used for the loss of memory and other cognitive disabilities that seriously interfere with daily routine. There are many different types of dementia, such as Parkinson's disease with dementia, vascular dementia, frontal temporal dementia (FTD), reversible dementia, Korsakoff's syndrome, Posterior cortical atrophy (PCA), Down syndrome dementia and dementia with Lewy bodies. According to a scientific report, an estimated 5.4 million American population was living with AD. In the United States, an estimated population of 930,000 people could be living with Parkinson's disease by the year 2020. The collection of electronic Databases like Pub Med, Cochrane Library, MEDLINE, and Center Watch Trials Database journal articles was used in the research for information and spreading awareness related to the above disease. The database search consoled the terms dementia, AD, phytochemical analysis, etc. The brain is made up of 100 billion nerve cells, and each cell connects to other cells to form huge communication networks. Each group of nerve cells has its unique jobs [4 - 6].

Some cells are active in learning, thinking, and memory; another group helps us smell, sight, hear, and coordinate our muscles when to move. Our brain cells operate like tiny factories that further receive the supplies, construct equipment, generate energy, and eliminate waste. Many functions are controlled by the brain and body, which needs a large amount of fuel and oxygen and coordination between organs. Extracellular deposits of aggregated amyloid-protein (Aβ) in the brain parenchyma and Cerebral blood vessels, cerebral amyloid angiopathy (CAA) is one of the pathological hallmarks of AD [7]. Due to the deposition of high levels of fibrillar Aβ in AD, the brain is associated with loss of synapses, impairment of neuronal functions, and loss of neurons. Aβ was sequenced from meningeal vessels and senile plaques of AD patients and individuals with Down's syndrome [8]. Scientists still have not discovered a complete treatment and cure for AD. Neuropathological genetic and biochemical data suggest that Aβ aggregation is the main reason for the initiation of AD pathogenesis, neurofibrillary pathogen strongly related to neuronal dysfunction and development of the clinical phase of AD. The clinical phase of AD is also recognized by neurotransmitter loss, synaptic loss, and neuroinflammation selective neuronal death [9]. That's why AD creates a serious problem in the whole world. It believes that therapeutic intervention that could postpone the onset or progression of AD would reduce the number of cases in the upcoming next 50 years. In the current scenario, scientists need more accurate scientific knowledge for awareness, prevention and treatment of diseases like AD and dementia [3, 10 - 12].

Herbal medicine offers several options to control the method of symptoms diagnosis, prevention and progression of AD. There has been a new trend coming for the preparation and marketing of herbal drugs based on medicinal herbs, so the scientific and commercial significance of those drugs appear to be gaining momentum in the health system. These plant-derived herbal drugs were carefully standardized, and their efficacy and safety for a specific health problems have been identified [13, 14].

The past decade has also increased awareness and intensified the interest in herbal drugs in which phytochemicals constitute can have long-term benefits for human health. Medicinal herbs are well known for their potent source of many antioxidants and phenolic compounds. Among these organic compounds in herbal plants, polyphenols have been recognized for their antioxidant activity and many more health benefits. Natural antioxidants and free radical scavengers like phenolic compounds and flavonoids have become of substantial interest among scientists due to their health benefits in the food and pharmacological industry [15 - 18].

Many Phytochemicals found in vegetables and fruits are believed to reduce the risk of several diseases like cancers, cardiovascular diseases and neurodegenerative disorders. Therefore, those populations who consume a high amount of vegetables and fruits have a reduced risk for such diseases that are caused due to neuronal dysfunction [19]. Herbal medicines have been used for a long time to treat neural disorders [5, 20, 21].

Ginkgo biloba (Ginkgoaceae) is the best and most well-known herb for AD and its associated symptoms. *G. biloba* tree, also called "a living fossil," has a life span of approx. 4000 years, possibly because of its resistance to infections and high tolerance to pollution [22]. *G. biloba* is generally called a living fossil, maidenhair tree, ginkyo, kew tree, yinhsing and is considered native to China, Japan and Korea. Now, it is widely cultivated for its leaves and nuts for commercial use [6, 12].

The dry leave extracts of *G. biloba* have been used for 5000 years in traditional Chinese medicine for various medicinal purposes. Studies on the biological activity of different components of the *Ginkgo* leaf began with the advent of modern scientific methods about 20 years ago, and its true pharmaceutical value has been realized recently [23]. This medicinal herb reveals memory-enhancing action by increasing the supply of oxygen, and helps the body eliminate free radicals, thereby improving memory. Leaf extract of *Ginkgo* contains 6% of terpenoid lactones and 24% flavonoids providing its unique polyvalent pharmacological action. The fraction of flavonoid is mostly composed of three types of flavonols, quercetin, keampferol and isorhamnetin whereas terpenic derivatives are marked by diterpenic lactones and the ginkgolides A, B, C, J, M [24]. Bilobalide and ginkgolides present in *G. biloba* have been categorized as nootropic (memory enhancer) agents [14]. EGb761 (*G. biloba* extract) mainly protects from Ab-induced neurotoxicity by glucose uptake, mitochondrial dysfunction, blocking ROS accumulation, activation of JNK & ERK pathways and preventing neuronal apoptosis. Another research suggests that EGb761 has the potential to deviate amyloid precursor protein (APP) metabolism to a secretase pathway and that further increases the release of a soluble form of APP [25]. The aim of this book chapter is to summarize the antioxidant and neuroprotective effects of the *G. biloba* extract, a popularly used herbal extract in the experimental and clinical studies.

LEAF EXTRACT OF *G. BILOBA*

The leaves of the *G. biloba* have been used for medical purposes for a long time. At the beginning of the 1970s, Dr. Willmar Schwabe Pharmaceuticals (Karlsruhe, Germany) effectively developed a method for the extraction and standardization of *G. biloba* extract preparation and produced highly concentrated and stable extracts from leaves [26]. There is number of flavonoids such as kaempferol, quercetin, and isohammnetin derivatves, and terpenes like gingolides and biobalide present in leaves of Ginkgo. It contains a specific concentration of the substance, which varies with season. The leaf extract of *G. biloba* (GBE) contains important medicinal compounds, among them important components are 6% terpenoids (have 3.1% are ginkgolides A, B, C, J and 2.9% is bilobalide), 24% flavonoid glycosides (isorhamnetin, quercetin, kaempferol), and 5–10% organic acids. Active constituents of GBE are flavonoids and terpenoids (19, 20) (Fig. **1**). Several studies suggest the neuroprotective effects of GBE in animal-based and cell models [27 - 30].

G. biloba leaf is often taken orally for memory and thought problems, anxiety, and many other conditions, but most scientific evidence does not support these uses. GBE is extensively used in multiple disorders and diseases, such as multi-infarct dementia, cerebral insufficiency (symptoms such as memory impairment, poor concentration, anxiety, and confusion), depressed mood, myocardial ischemia, thrombosis, stroke, and peripheral occlusive arterial disease (POAD). It is also effective in antidepressant-induced sexual dysfunction [31].

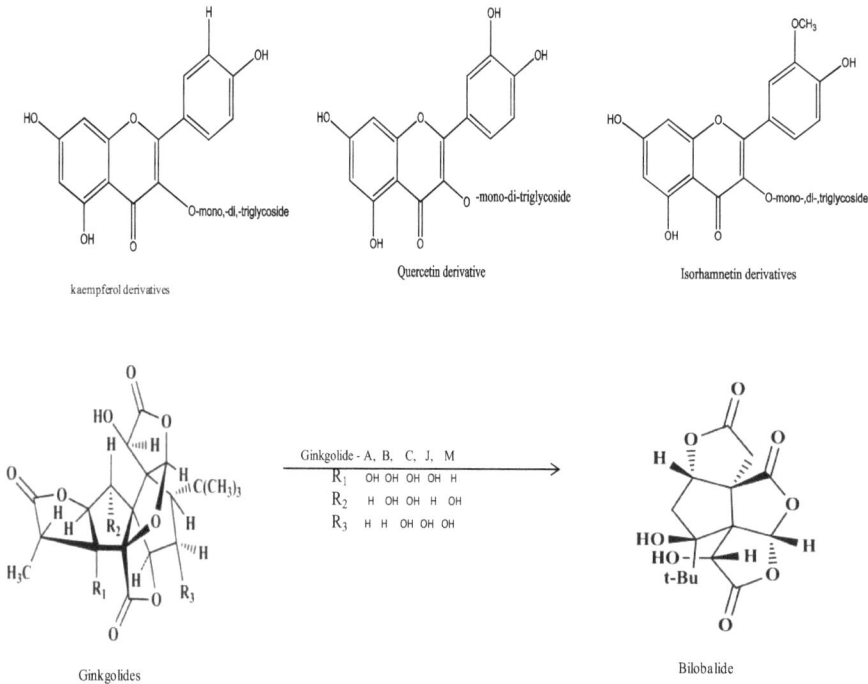

Fig. (1). Chemical compounds present in *G. biloba* leaf extract.

PHARMACOLOGICAL IMPORTANCE

Although the *G. biloba* tree has been around for 200 million years, its true value has been recognized only during the last couple of decades. Pharmacological Treatment through *G. biloba* leaves extract can be outlined with Chinese traditional medicines and modern Chinese medicine, fruit and leaves are yet suggested for the treatment of other diseases like asthma, and Heart problems. The use of boiled *G. biloba* leaves effective in inflammation and also used for hazardous conditions of the disease may have a poor moment as a common indication, such as vertigo, tinnitus, and inner ear hearing loss [32]. *G. biloba* leaves reducing Alzheimer's or another disease is unproven, nowadays, it is controversial. In addition, pure antioxidants may further disrupt tightly regulated stress responses. The positive effect of the *G. biloba* plant has been reported on AD, memory enhancement, dementia of vascular origin, cognitive disorders, and its antioxidative effects in combination with other drugs, which enhance their effects or decrease their psychiatric side effects [33]. *G. biloba* leaves can be used as a neuroprotective drug in brain injuries and support antidepressant agents. Several studies show its effect on many different neurotransmitters of the central nervous system. The anti-anxiety and mild anti-depression property of GBE is accounted from the reversible inhibition of two MAOA and MAOB enzymes [34], while the antioxidant, anti-inflammatory, and neuroprotective effects are contributed mainly by the flavonoids and terpenoids content in GBE. *G. biloba* has a positive effect on cognitive and neurological function through vascular flow regulation and platelet-activating antagonism factors that protect the brain from ischemic injuries [35]. *G. biloba* has positive effects on psychosis, anxiety, schizophrenia, and depression. It stimulates cerebral blood circulation and improves problems caused by the failure of blood circulation in the brain, including anxiety, stress, low memory, hearing problems, low concentration, thinking, social behaviour, and dementia in AD [36].

NEUROPROTECTIVE IMPORTANCE

The 'Green' movement has changed the attitudes of the general population in Western society, who now conceive naturally derived substances and herbal extracts as being inherently safer and more desirable than synthetic chemical products, with the net effect of an increase in sales of herbal preparations. In the traditional system of medicine, numerous plants have been used to treat cognitive disorders, including neurodegenerative diseases such as AD and other memory-related disorders. Herbal products contain complicated mixtures of organic chemicals, which may include fatty acids, sterols, alkaloids, flavonoids, glycosides, saponins, tannins, and terpenes [37]. The neuroprotective effect of GBE has been described on the basis of scientific studies (Table **1**).

Table 1. Examples of studies in which *G. biloba* extracts have been shown to promote the recovery from neural damage.

Extract	Species	Model	Dose/route/frequency	Reference
EGB 761 Non-terpenic	CATS	Vestibular compensation	25mg/kg (i.p.) per day, 40 days	Tighilet and Lacour (1995)
EGB 761	RATS	Electroconvulsive shock	100mg/kg (os) per day, 14 days	Rodriguez de Turco et. al (1993)
EGB 761	CATS	Vestibular compensation	50mg/kg (i.p.) per day, 30days	Lacour et. al (1991)

(Table 1) cont.....

Extract	Species	Model	Dose/route/frequency	Reference
EGB 761	MICE	Passive avoidance learned helplessness	100mg/kg (oral) per day, 5 days	Winter (1991)
EGB 761	RATS, MICE	Operant task	50,100mg/kg (oral) per day, 14-18 weeks	Porsolt et. al (1990)
EGB 761	RATS	Frontal cortex lesions	100mg/kg (i.p.) per day, 60 days	Attella et. al(1990)
EGB 761	RATS	Vestibular compensation	50mg/kg (i.p.) per day, 10 days	Denise and Bustany (1989)
EGB 761	HUMAN	Sternberg scanning test	120,240, 600 mg (oral), single	Subhan and Hindmarch (1984)
EGB 761	RATS	Hypoxin	200mg/kg (i.p.) per day, 14 days	Karcher et. al (1984)
EGB 761	[41]RATS	Hypoxin	100mg/kg (i.p.) per, single	Karcher et. al (1984)
EGB 761	RATS	Microembolization	100mg/kg (os) per day, 21 days	Le Poncin Lafitte et. al (1980)

Rodriguez de Turco (1993) examined the effects of EGB 761 treatment (100 mg/kg per day, oesophageally, for 14 days) on the neurochemical effects of electroconvulsive shock treatment (ECS) in rats. Sham control animals received identical treatment except that they received vehicle (6.6 ml/kg 5% ethanol) rather than EGB 761. ECS caused a rapid accumulation of free fatty acids and an increase in diacylglycerols in both the hippocampus and cerebral cortex. EGB 761 treatment reduced free fatty acid levels in the hippocampus and delayed the increase in diacylglycerol concentrations in the hippocampus and cerebral cortex [42]. He concludes that the effect with higher selectivity those neuronal circuitries contributing to the FFA pool during the clonic seizure.

Le Poncin Lafitte (1980) used the microembolization technique to investigate the effects of EGB 761 on cerebral blood flow and energy metabolism following microinfarctions in rats. EGB 761 treatment (100 mg/kg per day) for 21 days prior to microembolization resulted in an increase in blood flow, and in an increase in ATP, glucose and lactate levels in the embolized hemisphere, relative to controls (which received an injection of NaCl) [38].

Karcher (1984) examined and concluded that EGB is able to protect against hypoxia. Brain energy metabolism might be involved in this effect because EGB elevated the glucose level of the cortical brain and inhibited the breakdown of the energy metabolism under hypoxic conditions. He also explains the effects of EGB 761 (100 mg/kg) single injection 30 days pre-treatment on cerebral energy metabolism in rats exposed to hypobaric or hypoxic hypoxia. Animals treated with EGB 761 survived hypobaric hypoxia for a longer period of time than controls; they also retained higher cerebral glucose levels and exhibited a slower breakdown of high-energy phosphates relative to controls. In a second experiment, *Karcher (1984)* pre-treated rats with an average daily oral dose of

200 mg/kg EGB 761 for 14 days prior to hypobaric hypoxia. In this case, the EGB 761-treated animals survived the hypoxia for a longer period of time, however, brain energy metabolism was not significantly affected [39].

Attella (1989) studied the effects of EGB761 on recovery from a penetrating brain injury in rats. Animals received 100 mg/kg per day for 30 days, were trained on a delayed spatial alternation task and then subjected either to a sham operation or to bilateral frontal cortex lesions using aspiration. Sham-operated animals then received daily saline injections for 30 days, while the frontal cortex lessoned animals received either daily saline injections or EGB 761 (100 mg/kg i.p) for 30 days post-op [40]. Histological examination showed that GBE reduced the extent of brain swelling in response to the injury.

Kleijnen and Knipschild (1992) reviewed 40 studies in which *Ginkgo* was used to treat cerebral insufficiency in humans. The majority of these studies involved EGB 761; the remaining ones used another *Ginkgo* extract containing 25% *Ginkgo*-flavone glycosides and 6% terpenoids. Of the 40 trials evaluated, Kleijnen and Knipschild found 8 that were, in their view, well designed and conducted. Common shortcomings in the other studies included small numbers of patients, lack of double-blind procedures, and poor measurement techniques. The authors concluded that, on the basis of the 8 well-controlled studies, there is ample justification for further assessment of *G. biloba* extracts in relation to the treatment of cerebral insufficiency in humans [43].

Tighilet and Lacour (1995) compared the effects of EGB 761 with and without the terpene component, which contains PAF antagonists such as *Ginkgo*lide B. They reported that administration of non-terpenic EGB 761 (25 mg/kg per day, i.p) for up to 40 days following UVD resulted in an acceleration of vestibular compensation which was comparable to the same dose of the standard EGB 761 extract. The authors concluded that the non-terpenic fraction of EGB 761, containing flavonol heterosides, is mainly responsible for the beneficial effects of EGB 761 on vestibular compensation [44] (Table **10.1**). On the mg/kg basis, the neuroprotective effects of *Ginkgo* in animal studies are generally larger than in human studies. *Ginkgo* leaves extract contains 24% of flavonoids and 6% of terpenic lactose, which is mainly used in pharmacological properties. *Ginkgo* leaf (EGb761) is used as a medicine for memory and age-related deterioration.

The neuroprotective effect of GBE has been validated in several *in vitro* and *in vivo* models studies. *in vitro* studies revealed that GBE protected cultured neurons against death induced by hydrogen peroxide, hypoxia, glutamate, verapamil, amyloid-β, 1-methyl-4-phenyl-1,2,3,6- tetrahydropyridine (MPTP), nitric oxide (NO), and cyanide [45]. Also, *in vivo* effect, reduction of neuronal damage by

EGb761 (10–100 mg/kg, per os or intraperitoneally has been observed after transient middle cerebral artery occlusion (MCAO) in rats and gerbils focal cerebral ischemia in mice and rats hypoxia heat stress sub-chronic cold stress and amphetamine-induced behavioral sensitization and in a transgenic mouse model of amyotrophic lateral sclerosis [46]. At a recent meeting of the Society for Neuroscience, two groups of investigators, working on different systems, reported on a possible role of EGb761 in neuroregeneration *Ginkgo*lide B (BN52021), a component of EGb761, may protect neurons by being an antagonist of a receptor for the platelet-activating factor (PAF). PAF is an alkyl phospholipid produced by a variety of cells; it is one of the most potent lipid mediators known [47, 48]. Therefore, it can be used as a preferable choice for the prevention of AD and many neurodegenerative diseases.

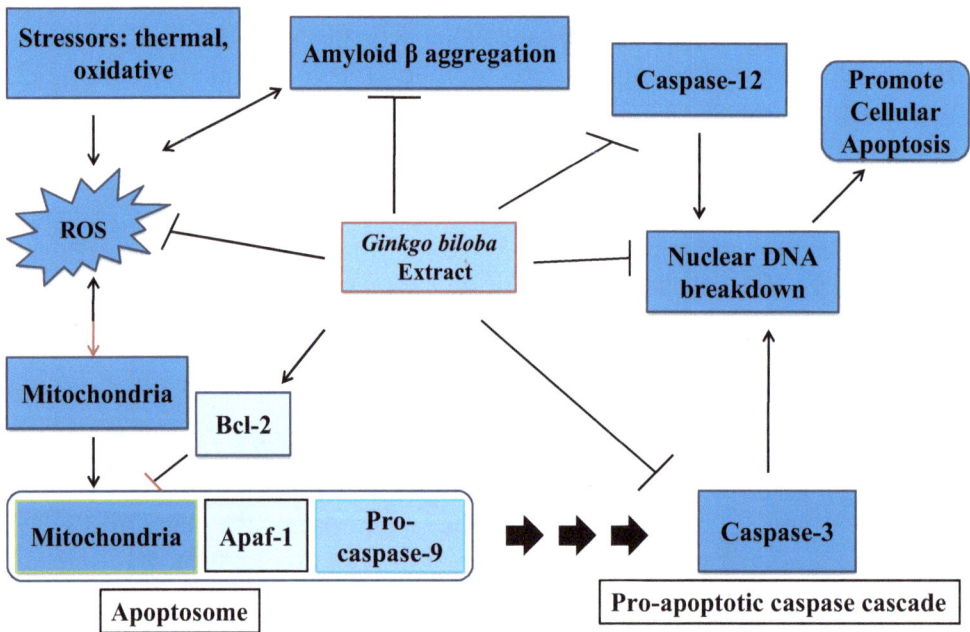

Fig. (2). Neuroprotective mechanism of *G.biloba.*

Fig. (**2**) shows the anti-apoptotic properties of EGb761, *in vitro* via the maintenance of the mitochondrial membrane potential, up-regulation of antiapoptotic Bcl-2 protein, and subsequent inhibition of both the formation of the apoptosome and activation of the pro-apoptotic protein. Caspase-cascade leads to programmed cell death, by nuclear DNA fragmentation. Additionally, the expression of caspase 12, an endoplasmic reticulum-stress specific protease, is down-regulated by EGb 761 treatment [49]. The anti-oxidative effect of EGb 761 in transgenic cells and *C. elegans* models through direct attenuation of hydroxyl radicals-related reactive oxygen species (ROS) levels, and imparting increased stress resistance and longevity in model organisms. Anti-Aβ aggregation properties of EGb 761 through decreased Aβ aggregation in the conditioned medium of an Aβ-secreting cell line, and also by directly inhibiting the aggregation of Aβ fibrils in a cell-free solution *in vitro* [50].

PHYTOCHEMICAL PROPERTIES OF *G. BILOBA*

One of the most popular studies and clinical effects relevant to AD is *G. biloba*, which may have an emphasis on the standardized extract EG761. *Ginkgo's* therapeutic uses were based on macerated plant leaves, which contain known active compounds. However, not all these components were useful as therapeutic compounds. The *G. biloba* has been reported to have memory-enhancing properties by increasing the supply of oxygen and helping to eliminate free radicals from the system, thereby improving memory. *Ginkgo* (EGb761) Phytochemicals include terpenoids (bilobalide, Ginkgolides), flavonoids (quercetin, kaempferol, and isorhamnetin), steroids (sitosterol and stigmasterol), and organic acids (ascorbic, benzoic shikimic, and vanillic acid). Egb761 was extracted from dry and mashed leaves. Major bioactive constituents are diterpenic lactones, Ginkgolides A, B, C, J, and M, and a sesquiterpene trilactone, the bilobalide [24]. Many clinical trials of EGb761 have suggested that daily treatment for 3–6 months may provide mild cognitive benefit over placebo in elderly demented patients [51 - 53]. One study found that *G. biloba* extract was as effective as the pharmaceutical AChE inhibitor donepezil [54]. The flavonoid fraction in this extract stops lipid peroxidation, acting as a free-radical scavenger, and helping in the prevention of oxidative stress. In addition, flavonoids increase the release and reuptake of serotonin [55], stop the reduction of cholinergic muscarinic receptors related to age, and stimulate its reuptake in the hippocampus [56]. Flavanones such as hesperetin, naringenin, and their *in vivo* metabolites, along with some dietary anthocyanins, cyanidin-3-rutinoside, and pelargonidin- 3-glucoside, have been shown to traverse the BBB in relevant *in-vitro* and *in-situ* models [57]. Currently, the famous scientist also studies and describes the photochemical component in *Ginkgo*, according to Liu *et al.*, more than 34 flavonoids have been isolated from *Ginkgo* leaves, and more than 70 flavonoids have been tentatively identified by mass spectrometry. The major flavanol glycosides in *Ginkgo* are the derivatives of quercetin, kaempferol, and isorhamnetin linked with glucose and rhamnose in different linkage forms and numbers [58]. Kobus *et al.,* determined qualitatively the composition of flavanols in the aqueous acetonic, ethanolic, and water infusion extracts of green and yellow *G. biloba* leaves. These authors found a significantly (p < 0.05) higher content of flavanol aglycones in the extracts from yellow *Ginkgo* leaves. The highest amounts of these components were determined in the aqueous acetonic extract from yellow leaves (4938 _g/g DM) and the water infusion extract from yellow leaves (3146 _g/g DM), while the lowest was detected in the water infusion extract from green leaves (878 _g/g DM) and the ethanolic extract from green leaves (512 _g/g DM). Regarding the extract preparations from yellow *G. biloba* leaves, the dominant flavanol was myricetin accounting for 1683, 1116, and 680 g/g DM in the yellow water, aqueous acetonic, and ethanolic extracts, respectively [59]. Recently many studies have demonstrated the neuroprotective role of *Ginkgo*. In one of the studies, plant extract has been shown, protect the hippocampal neurons from neurotoxicity induced by nitric oxide or beta-amyloi--derived peptide [60].

Flavonoids are responsible for health awareness due to their high antioxidant capacity in both *in-vivo* and *in-vitro* systems. These compounds can raise human protective enzyme systems. Several clinical studies have confirmed the protective effects of flavonoids against many infectious (bacterial and viral) and civilization diseases, such as cardiovascular and digestive disorders, cancers, and other age-related health problems [61].

Ginkgolide B is another important active principle in the EGb761 extract that acts as an antagonist of the platelet-activating factor (PAF) receptor, and thus, inhibits platelet aggregation and improves cognitive and memory function [62]. The active compounds, bilobalide (1), Ginkgolide A (2), and Ginkgolide B (3) found in the EGb761 extract, have been reported to induce the reduction of peripheral benzodiazepine receptors, that are involved in many biological processes, however, with unknown functions [62].

BENEFITS OF *G. BILOBA*

Alzheimer's and dementia are treated by a herb known as extract of *G. biloba* leaf (EGb761). Meta-analysis of clinical studies discovered the hepatoprotective effect and photo-protective effect. It also enhances the repairing mechanism of DNA and also reveals the free radical scavenging and anti-inflammatory effect. It also inhibits the formation of cancer [63]. *G. biloba* had modest effects on improving the symptoms of dementia and cerebral insufficiency, equivalent to pharmacologic therapy. Many meta-analysis articles examine the effect of *G. biloba* on object measures of cognitive function in patients with neurodegenerative disease. A study of at least six months in duration demonstrated that *G. biloba* extract and second-generation cholinesterase inhibitors were equally effective in treating mild to moderate Alzheimer's dementia. Another study on *G. biloba* use showed a safe and positive effect beyond placebo, but the investigators remained tentative in recommending it for the treatment of dementia until better studies were conducted [64].

One of the studies analyzed in the Cochrane review was a Dutch study of 214 patients over 24 weeks using a medium dosage of *G. biloba* (160 mg per day), a high dosage of *G. biloba* (240 mg per day), or placebo in a crossover design. This study failed to show improvement in age-associated memory impairment or mild or moderate dementia in several neuropsychologic and behavior outcome measures [65]. However, this study included patients with age-associated memory impairment rather than just persons with dementia, which may have limited the statistical power of its conclusions about the role of *G. biloba* in dementia [66].

G. biloba is licensed in Germany for the treatment of cerebral dysfunction, for example, the following symptoms: difficulties of memory, headaches, dizziness, and emotional instability with anxiety. It is also licensed as a supportive treatment for hearing loss due to cervical syndrome and for peripheral arterial circulatory disturbances with intact circulatory reserve (intermittent claudicating) [67]. *G. biloba* is also used in tablet form. *G. biloba* leaf extracts can vary significantly in quantity and quality, but they must be standardized on the basis of the active ingredients.

The United States Pharmacopeia (USP) 32 and the European Pharmacopoeia 6.1 also published monographs for *G. biloba* extract and formulations, providing standards for herbal preparations. Both of the pharmacopeias list the standardized dry extracts that are produced with acetone 60% and a drug/ extract ratio of 35:37:1, such as EGb 761 and Li 1370, both of which have a defined composition. Variations in the levels of the active ingredients are likely due to the multistep extraction and concentration process used [68]. These authors also stated that *G. biloba* is used to treat cognitive impairment in various types of dementia, peripheral arterial diseases, tinnitus, ischemic stroke, and autism, and to moderate the undesirable effect of some cancer therapies. EGb761 has been shown to have anti-stress effects, which support its use in preventing or impeding the development of psychiatric disorders in which stress is a pathogenic factor [69].

World Health Organization (WHO) recommended *G. biloba* for Raynaud's disease. The WHO has also accepted the standardized extracts like EGb761 and Li 1370 as anti-dementia drugs based on the pharmacological studies done *in vitro* and *in vivo* and the numerous clinical trials supporting the efficacy of EGb761 in the central nervous system (CNS) when taking a 240-mg daily dose [60]. Described current uses in medical applications, include improving brain function, strengthening the cerebrovascular and cardiovascular systems by inhibition of platelet aggregation and the increase of blood flow and oxygen supply, neutralizing free radicals, stabilizing cellular energy production, and suppressing hemorrhoids, inflammation, migraines, allergies, and asthma.

G. biloba leave extract can improve blood flow by increasing red blood cell deformability and decreasing red cell aggregation, thus, improving red blood cell fluidity and decreasing whole blood viscosity. *G. biloba* extract resulted in decreases in platelet aggregation, allergic reaction, general inflammatory response, oxygen radical discharge, and other proinflammatory functions of macrophages. EGb 761 significantly decreased plasma concentrations of adrenocorticotrophic hormone, corticosterone, norepinephrine, and epinephrine and the hypophysial portal blood concentration in rats. The flavanol glycosides and proanthocyanidins have free radical-scavenging activity and thus may play a protective role in the prevention of the atherosclerotic processes and improving conditions resulting from oxidative stress.

EGb761 inhibits the functional and morphological retina impairments observed after lipoperoxide release and protects pancreatic cells against the toxic effects of alloxan, probably by scavenging free radicals and stimulation of glucose utilization. Emerit *et al.* reported that the clastogenic factors in the plasma of persons irradiated accidentally or therapeutically were suppressed by EGb 761. EGB (100 mg/kg) given prior to irradiation of transplanted fibrosarcoma in C3H mice enhanced the radio-sensitivity of tumor cells. Biloblide has insecticidal properties and may be involved in protecting *Ginkgo* against herbivorous insects or mammals.

G. biloba and its derivatives have been used in cosmetics to protect the skin against ravages caused by UV radiation and to prevent signs of aging. Hairless mice treated with topical application of *G. biloba* and green tea were subjected to UV radiation to evaluate different parameters like erythema, skin barrier damage, histological alteration, and sunburn cell formation. The results compared after 20 h of UV exposure revealed that formulations containing EGB provided total protection against UV radiation damage, such as skin barrier damage and erythema [70, 71]. *G. biloba* leaf extract has seemed to improve eNOS development and, hence, NO bioavailability in human endothelial cells [72]; it has been the cardioprotective property of GBE against Adriamycin-started exceptional cardiotoxicity has been represented by the rule of provocative and NO hailing pathways [73].

ECONOMICAL IMPORTANCE OF *G. BILOBA*

G. biloba has grown significantly since the 1980s owing to its potent action on the cardiovascular system of human beings, particularly on cerebral vascular activity.

Over 7 billion dollars are spent annually on botanical medicines. *Ginkgo* ranks first among herbal medications. Fifty million *G. biloba* trees are grown, especially in China, France, and South Carolina, USA, producing 8000 tons of dried leaves each year to meet the commercial demand for *G. biloba* products. The use of *Ginkgo* has been growing very instant worldwide and per year open in the world commercial market [74].

G. biloba is a dicot, and its wood is "pycnoxylic." It is compact and dense, with narrow rays, pith, and cortex, and hence commercially very useful. The commercially useful woods are called "timbers," and timber used for building purposes is called "lumber." *Tectona grandis* (teak) and *Cedrus deodara* (deodar) are, respectively, considered the best angiospermic and gymnospermic timbers in the world, respectively [75].

G. biloba is among the most sold medicinal plants, and the annual consumption in 2001 was between 4.5 million pounds and 5.1 million pounds of dried leaves. Presently, there are around 142 *G. biloba* products on the global market, and it is estimated that in the coming five years, its utilization is expected to grow threefold. *G. biloba* is sold in the form of leaf, powder extract, and as a tincture to pharmaceutical and herbal companies [76]. The extract of the *Ginkgo* leaves contains flavonoids, glycosides, and terpenoids (Ginkgolides, bilobalides) and has been used pharmaceutically and also nut-like gametophyte is consumed in China.

MARKETING ANALYSIS OF *G. BILOBA*

G. biloba is found in Asian countries regions such as Japan and China, now grown in the U.S.A. and some regions of European countries. As a dietary supplement, *G. biloba* extract is being consumed. The *G. biloba* extract is used for the treatment of several types of diseases, which includes patients who are suffering from memory disorders like AD. In the global market, *Ginkgo* extract usage is separated into three different categories such as food, cosmetics, and pharmaceuticals. Among the application segments, the food segment contributes a major market share, and the research on the *G. biloba* extract is also influencing the pharmaceutical sector. In this above sector, the market of *G. biloba* extract is categorized into liquid form, capsule, and tablet. The tablet form of *G. biloba* extract is the most popular one [41].

The extract of *G. biloba* is a great source of flavonoids. The other characteristics that the *G. biloba* extract contains are scent property, antioxidant property, anti-influenza property, anti-neoplastic property, anti-inflammatory property, anti-bacterial property, and also helps in reducing the effect of Raynaud's syndrome. Some other benefits of the extract are in the treatment of the disorders related to the central nervous system, slowing down the process of aging, and helpful for the treatment of bronchitis and asthma. Due to these benefits, *G. biloba* extract is in high demand in the pharmaceutical sector, further driving the global growth of the market. The awareness about the health benefits of the *G. biloba* extracts is increasing among consumers day by day, which further contributes to the global market growth of this sector.

The study of different regions of the global market for the *G. biloba* extract is diversified into the Asia Pacific, the Middle East, Africa, Western Europe, Eastern Europe, North America, and Latin America. The dominating region for the *G. biloba* extract market is the Asia Pacific because that region is the largest producer and consumer of that extract.

WARNING AND ADVERSE EFFECT OF *G. BILOBA*

G. biloba extract seems to be a relatively safer option. Extremely high doses of this extract have been given to animals and human beings for a long time and do not show any serious consequences on any type of organism [77, 78]. Safety for pregnant or nursing women, young children, or patients that suffer from severe liver or kidney disease has not been established. Up to 1991, the clinical trials of *G. biloba*, including a total of almost 10,000 participants, showed that the incidence of side effects produced by *G. biloba* extract was extremely small. A total number of 21 cases of gastrointestinal discomfort and cases of dizziness, headaches & allergic skin reactions had occurred. The most serious complication of *G. biloba* extract is the internal bleeding that showed in many trial patients [79].

G. biloba should not be consumed by patients with bleeding problems like haemophilia before or after baby delivery, surgery or labour and during the periods. It also seems reasonable to hypothesize that *G. biloba* might obstruct blood-thinning drugs, amplifying their effects on coagulation. Another two studies reveal the opposite result of the previous study. According to this result, the interaction between *G. biloba* and warfarin (Coumadin) does not occur, and no interaction with clopidogrel was found. The active ingredients in *G. biloba* extract account for its antioxidant property and its ability to inhibit platelet aggregation. Subsequently, this herbal extract is promoted for use in improvising blood flow and cognitive function in the human body. According to a study, a 70-year-old man who suffered from internal bleeds from the iris into the anterior chamber of the eye one week after beginning a self-prescribed regimen consisting of a *G. biloba* concentrated extract (Ginkoba), in a dosage of 40 mg twice daily was reported. The medical history of the patient included coronary artery bypass surgery, performed three years before. His only medication was aspirin, in a dosage of 325 mg per day, which he had taken since his bypass surgery. After the spontaneous bleeding episode, he continued to take aspirin but discontinued the *G. biloba* product. Over a three-month follow-up period, he had no further bleeding episodes. Interaction of the *G. biloba* product and aspirin was considered the cause of his ocular haemorrhage [80].

One study found that when a high concentration of *G. biloba* was placed in a test tube with hamster sperm and ova, the sperm was less able to penetrate the ova. However, we have no idea whether this much *G. biloba* in our human body can come into contact with sperm and ovum or not. This case is not clear from the above experiment [81].

The above experimental results may not be as important and meaningful in the real world as when they are in the human body rather than in a test tube. Recently, the best-designed studies have failed to find any such actions. People suffering from diabetes should take *G. biloba* only under the supervision of a physician until the situation gets clarified. A 33-year-old woman was diagnosed with bilateral subdural hematomas after almost two years of ingesting *G. biloba*, in a dosage of 60 mg twice daily. She briefly used the preparation of acetaminophen and an ergotamine-caffeine. As she stopped taking *G. biloba* extract, her bleeding period became normal after 35 days, from 9.5 - 15 minutes [82].

CONCLUSION

This book chapter briefly discusses the neuroprotective effect of *G. biloba* and its phytochemical preparation in AD. The phytochemical studies of different parts of *Ginkgo* extract reveal the presence of many more secondary metabolites like alkaloids, flavonoids, polyphenols, triterpenes, and sterols that show a wide spectrum of pharmacological activities like anti-inflammatory, anti-amyloidogenic, anti-oxidant effects, neuroprotective, and vasotropic effects. *G. biloba* is used for enhancing memory power and age-related memory deterioration problems like degenerative dementia of the AD type in western countries like the United States and Europe. The substantial experiment revealed that EGb761 (*G. biloba* extract) has the potential to treat some types of nerve damage like peripheral, ischemia, etc. This extract is also used for enhancing both the cerebral and peripheral blood flows as their therapeutic treatment.

Further, we summarize the pharmacological, phytochemical, and neurological importance of *G. biloba* extract. After that, we discuss the mechanism of action induced by standardized extract of *G. biloba* leaves and their constituents. The effects of extract experimented on animals mostly include those on cellular redox state, cerebral blood flow, neurotransmitter systems, and nitric oxide level. Then, the current status of clinical trials and undesired side effects of *G. biloba* extract are discussed.

This chapter focuses on cellular and molecular approaches towards understanding the polyvalent action of 'EGb761' *Ginkgo* extract on neuroprotective effect. There are two potential mechanisms of action, i.e., stimulating machinery and reducing oxidative damage. The mechanism of this extract is partially unknown because the composition of that extract is quite a complex chemical. The action of that complex chemical is called "polyvalent action".

The understanding of neuroprotective action mechanisms, *G. biloba* extract will contribute to stimulation for possible combinational therapies and local mechanism-based strategies that target the goal of age-related neurodegeneration and AD. Thus, our book reveals the summary of the neuroprotective and pharmacological importance of the extract, which is further explored for possible clinical intervention.

A better understanding of the neuroprotective mechanisms of the 'EGb761' extract will provide the impetus for possible combination therapies and for the design of rational, mechanism-based strategies that target age-related neurodegeneration and AD.

Overall, a better understanding of the mechanisms underlying the neuroprotective effects of EGb761 may contribute to a better understanding of the effectiveness and complexity of this drug and may also help design therapeutic strategies in future clinical practice.

CONSENT FOR PUBLICATION

Not applicable.

CONFLICT OF INTEREST

The author declares no conflict of interest, financial or otherwise.

ACKNOWLEDGMENTS

The authors thank the Central Library, Banaras Hindu University, Varanasi, India, for providing the facilities required to access relevant papers.

REFERENCES

[1]   Singhal A, Bangar OP, Naithani V. Medicinal plants with a potential to treat Alzheimer and associated symptoms. Int J Nutr Pharmacol Neurol Dis 2012; 2(2): 84.
[http://dx.doi.org/10.4103/2231-0738.95927]

[2]   Perrotta G. General Overview of "Human Dementia Diseases". 2020.

[3]   Zahra W, Rai SN, Birla H, *et al.* Neuroprotection of rotenone-induced Parkinsonism by ursolic acid in PD mouse model. CNS & Neurological Disorders-Drug Targets 2020; (14): 527-40.
        [http://dx.doi.org/10.2174/1871527319666200812224457]

[4]   Singh SS, Rai SN, Birla H, *et al.* Techniques related to disease diagnosis and therapeutics. Application of biomedical engineering in neuroscience. 2019; 437-56.
        [http://dx.doi.org/10.1007/978-981-13-7142-4_22]

[5]   Singh SS, Rai SN, Birla H, *et al.* Neuroprotective effect of chlorogenic acid on mitochondrial dysfunction-mediated apoptotic death of DA neurons in a Parkinsonian mouse model. Oxid Med Cell Longev 2020; 2020: 1-14.
        [http://dx.doi.org/10.1155/2020/6571484] [PMID: 32566093]

[6]   Zahra W, Rai SN, Birla H, *et al.* The global economic impact of neurodegenerative diseases: Opportunities and challenges. 2020; 333-45.

[7]   Toledo JB, Zetterberg H, van Harten AC, *et al.* Alzheimer's disease cerebrospinal fluid biomarker in cognitively normal subjects. Brain 2015; 138(9): 2701-15.
        [http://dx.doi.org/10.1093/brain/awv199] [PMID: 26220940]

[8]   Hartmann T, Bieger SC, Brühl B, *et al.* Distinct sites of intracellular production for Alzheimer's disease Aβ40/42 amyloid peptides. Nat Med 1997; 3(9): 1016-20.
        [http://dx.doi.org/10.1038/nm0997-1016] [PMID: 9288729]

[9]   Karch CM, Goate AM. Alzheimer's disease risk genes and mechanisms of disease pathogenesis. Biol Psychiatry 2015; 77(1): 43-51.
        [http://dx.doi.org/10.1016/j.biopsych.2014.05.006] [PMID: 24951455]

[10]   Keswani C, Dilnashin H, Birla H, Singh S. Re-addressing the commercialization and regulatory hurdles for biopesticides in India Rhizosphere 2019; 11(100155): 10.

[11]   Rai SN, Dilnashin H, Birla H, *et al.* The role of PI3K/Akt and ERK in neurodegenerative disorders. Neurotox Res 2019; 35(3): 775-95.
        [http://dx.doi.org/10.1007/s12640-019-0003-y] [PMID: 30707354]

[12]   Zahra W, Rai SN, Birla H, *et al.* Economic importance of medicinal plants in asian countries. Bioeconomy for sustainable development.2020; 359-77.
        [http://dx.doi.org/10.1007/978-981-13-9431-7_19]

[13]   Abascal K, Yarnell E. Alzheimer's Disease: Part 2—A Botanical Treatment Plan. Altern Complement Ther 2004; 10(2): 67-72.
        [http://dx.doi.org/10.1089/107628004773933299]

[14]   Kumar V. Potential medicinal plants for CNS disorders: an overview. Phytother Res 2006; 20(12): 1023-35.
        [http://dx.doi.org/10.1002/ptr.1970] [PMID: 16909441]

[15]   Pandey KB, Rizvi SI. Plant polyphenols as dietary antioxidants in human health and disease. Oxid Med Cell Longev 2009; 2(5): 270-8.
        [http://dx.doi.org/10.4161/oxim.2.5.9498] [PMID: 20716914]

[16]   Birla H, Keswani C, Rai SN, *et al.* Neuroprotective effects of *Withania somnifera* in BPA induced-cognitive dysfunction and oxidative stress in mice. Behav Brain Funct 2019; 15(1): 9.
        [http://dx.doi.org/10.1186/s12993-019-0160-4] [PMID: 31064381]

[17]   Birla H, Keswani C, Singh SS, *et al.* Unraveling the Neuroprotective Effect of *Tinospora cordifolia* in Parkinsonian Mouse Model Through Proteomics Approach. 2021.
        [http://dx.doi.org/10.1021/acschemneuro.1c00481]

[18]   Keswani C, Dilnashin H, Birla H, Singh SP. Unravelling efficient applications of agriculturally important microorganisms for alleviation of induced inter-cellular oxidative stress in crops. Acta Agric

Slov 2019; 114(1): 121-30.
[http://dx.doi.org/10.14720/aas.2019.114.1.14]

[19]   Selvam A. Inventory of vegetable crude drug samples housed in botanical survey of India, Howrah. Pharmacogn Rev 2008; 2(3): 61.

[20]   Rai SN, Zahra W, Singh SS, *et al.* Anti-inflammatory activity of ursolic acid in MPTP-induced parkinsonian mouse model. Neurotox Res 2019; 36(3): 452-62.
[http://dx.doi.org/10.1007/s12640-019-00038-6] [PMID: 31016688]

[21]   Singh S, Rai S, Birla H, Eds., *et al.* Chlorogenic acid protects against MPTP induced neurotoxicity in parkinsonian mice model via its anti-apoptotic activity. 2019.

[22]   DeFeudis FV. Ginkgo biloba extract (EGb 761): from chemistry to the clinic: Ullstein Medical Wiesbaden; 1998.

[23]   Mohanta TK, Tamboli Y, Zubaidha PK. Phytochemical and medicinal importance of *Ginkgo biloba* L. Nat Prod Res 2014; 28(10): 746-52.
[http://dx.doi.org/10.1080/14786419.2013.879303] [PMID: 24499319]

[24]   Chandrasekaran K, Mehrabian Z, Spinnewyn B, Drieu K, Fiskum G. Neuroprotective effects of bilobalide, a component of the *Ginkgo biloba* extract (EGb 761), in gerbil global brain ischemia. Brain Res 2001; 922(2): 282-92.
[http://dx.doi.org/10.1016/S0006-8993(01)03188-2] [PMID: 11743961]

[25]   Braidy N, Grant R, Adams S, Guillemin GJ. Neuroprotective effects of naturally occurring polyphenols on quinolinic acid-induced excitotoxicity in human neurons. FEBS J 2010; 277(2): 368-82.
[http://dx.doi.org/10.1111/j.1742-4658.2009.07487.x] [PMID: 20015232]

[26]   Le Bars P. Magnitude of effect and special approach to *Ginkgo biloba* extract EGb 761® in cognitive disorders. Pharmacopsychiatry. 2003; 36(S 1): 44-9.

[27]   Ahlemeyer B, Krieglstein J. Neuroprotective effects of *Ginkgo biloba* extract. Cell Mol Life Sci 2003; 60(9): 1779-92.
[http://dx.doi.org/10.1007/s00018-003-3080-1] [PMID: 14523543]

[28]   Diamond BJ, Shiflett SC, Feiwel N, *et al. Ginkgo biloba* extract: Mechanisms and clinical indications. Arch Phys Med Rehabil 2000; 81(5): 668-78.
[http://dx.doi.org/10.1016/S0003-9993(00)90052-2] [PMID: 10807109]

[29]   Rai SN, Birla H, Singh SS, *et al.* Pathophysiology of the disease causing physical disability. Biomedical engineering and its applications in healthcare. Springer 2019; 573-95.

[30]   Rai SN, Singh BK, Rathore AS, *et al.* Quality control in huntington's disease: a therapeutic target. Neurotox Res 2019; 36(3): 612-26.
[http://dx.doi.org/10.1007/s12640-019-00087-x] [PMID: 31297710]

[31]   Wheatley D. *Ginkgo biloba* in the treatment of sexual dysfunction due to antidepressant drugs. Hum Psychopharmacol 1999; 14(7): 512-3.
[http://dx.doi.org/10.1002/(SICI)1099-1077(199910)14:7,512:AID-HUP127>3.0.CO;2-P]

[32]   Jahanshahi M, Nickmahzar EG, Babakordi F. The effect of *Ginkgo biloba* extract on scopolamine-induced apoptosis in the hippocampus of rats. Anat Sci Int 2013; 88(4): 217-22.
[http://dx.doi.org/10.1007/s12565-013-0188-8] [PMID: 23828103]

[33]   Dower JI, Geleijnse JM, Gijsbers L, Schalkwijk C, Kromhout D, Hollman PC. Supplementation of the pure flavonoids epicatechin and quercetin affects some biomarkers of endothelial dysfunction and inflammation in (pre) hypertensive adults: a randomized double-blind, placebo-controlled, crossover trial. J Nutr 2015; 145(7): 1459-63.
[http://dx.doi.org/10.3945/jn.115.211888] [PMID: 25972527]

[34]   White HL, Scates PW, Cooper BR. Extracts of *Ginkgo biloba* leaves inhibit monoamine oxidase. Life

Sci 1996; 58(16): 1315-21.
[http://dx.doi.org/10.1016/0024-3205(96)00097-5] [PMID: 8614288]

[35]   Nourbala A, Akhoundzadeh S. Attention-deficit/hyperactivity disorder: etiology and pharmacotherapy 2006.

[36]   Singh S, Barreto G, Aliev G, Echeverria V. E Barreto G, Aliev G, Echeverria V. *Ginkgo biloba* as an alternative medicine in the treatment of anxiety in dementia and other psychiatric disorders. Curr Drug Metab 2017; 18(2): 112-9.
[http://dx.doi.org/10.2174/1389200217666161201112206] [PMID: 27908257]

[37]   Kumar GP, Khanum F. Neuroprotective potential of phytochemicals. Pharmacogn Rev 2012; 6(12): 81-90.
[http://dx.doi.org/10.4103/0973-7847.99898] [PMID: 23055633]

[38]   Le Poncin Lafitte M, Rapin J, Rapin JR. Effects of *Ginkgo biloba* on changes induced by quantitative cerebral microembolization in rats. Arch Int Pharmacodyn Ther 1980; 243(2): 236-44.
[PMID: 7377897]

[39]   Karcher L, Zagermann P, Krieglstein J. Effect of an extract of *Ginkgo biloba* on rat brain energy metabolism in hypoxia. Naunyn Schmiedebergs Arch Pharmacol 1984; 327(1): 31-5.
[http://dx.doi.org/10.1007/BF00504988] [PMID: 6493348]

[40]   Attella MJ, Hoffman SW, Stasio MJ, Stein DG. *Ginkgo biloba* extract facilitates recovery from penetrating brain injury in adult male rats. Exp Neurol 1989; 105(1): 62-71.
[http://dx.doi.org/10.1016/0014-4886(89)90172-6] [PMID: 2744128]

[41]   Isah T. Rethinking *Ginkgo biloba* L.: Medicinal uses and conservation. Pharmacogn Rev 2015; 9(18): 140-8.
[http://dx.doi.org/10.4103/0973-7847.162137] [PMID: 26392712]

[42]   Rodriguez de Turco EB, Droy-Lefaix MT, Bazan NG. Decreased electroconvulsive shock-induced diacylglycerols and free fatty acid accumulation in the rat brain by *Ginkgo biloba* extract (EGb 761): selective effect in hippocampus as compared with cerebral cortex. J Neurochem 1993; 61(4): 1438-44.
[http://dx.doi.org/10.1111/j.1471-4159.1993.tb13638.x] [PMID: 8376997]

[43]   Kleijnen J, Knipschild P. *Ginkgo biloba* for cerebral insufficiency. Br J Clin Pharmacol 1992; 34(4): 352-8.
[http://dx.doi.org/10.1111/j.1365-2125.1992.tb05642.x] [PMID: 1457269]

[44]   Tighilet B, Lacour M. Pharmacological activity of the *Ginkgo biloba* extract (EGb 761) on equilibrium function recovery in the unilateral vestibular neurectomized cat. J Vestib Res 1995; 5(3): 187-200.
[http://dx.doi.org/10.3233/VES-1995-5303] [PMID: 7627378]

[45]   Bauer R. Phytomedicines of Europe: chemistry and biological activity. 1998.

[46]   Krieglstein J, Ausmeier F, El-Abhar H, *et al.* Neuroprotective effects of *Ginkgo biloba* constituents. Eur J Pharm Sci 1995; 3(1): 39-48.
[http://dx.doi.org/10.1016/0928-0987(94)00073-9]

[47]   Cheung Z, So K, Yip H, Wu W. Cheung Z, So K, Yip H, Wu W. Mixture of American ginseng extract, ginkgo biloba extract and St. John's wort extract enhances the survival of axotomized retinal ganglion cells. Neuroscience 2000 2000.

[48]   Luo Y. *Ginkgo biloba* neuroprotection: Therapeutic implications in Alzheimer's disease. J Alzheimers Dis 2001; 3(4): 401-7.
[http://dx.doi.org/10.3233/JAD-2001-3407] [PMID: 12214044]

[49]   Smith JV, Burdick AJ, Golik P, Khan I, Wallace D, Luo Y. Anti-apoptotic properties of *Ginkgo biloba* extract EGb 761 in differentiated PC12 cells. Cell Mol Biol 2002; 48(6): 699-707.
[PMID: 12396082]

[50]   Luo Y, Smith JV, Paramasivam V, *et al.* Inhibition of amyloid-β aggregation and caspase-3 activation

by the *Ginkgo biloba* extract EGb761. Proc Natl Acad Sci USA 2002; 99(19): 12197-202.
[http://dx.doi.org/10.1073/pnas.182425199] [PMID: 12213959]

[51] Kanowski S, Herrmann W, Stephan K, Wierich W, Hörr R. Proof of efficacy of the ginkgo biloba special extract EGb 761 in outpatients suffering from mild to moderate primary degenerative dementia of the Alzheimer type or multi-infarct dementia. Pharmacopsychiatry 1996; 29(2): 47-56.
[http://dx.doi.org/10.1055/s-2007-979544] [PMID: 8741021]

[52] Maurer K, Ihl R, Dierks T, Frölich L. Clinical efficacy of *Ginkgo biloba* special extract EGb 761 in dementia of the Alzheimer type. J Psychiatr Res 1997; 31(6): 645-55.
[http://dx.doi.org/10.1016/S0022-3956(97)00022-8] [PMID: 9447569]

[53] Keswani C. Bioeconomy for Sustainable Development. 2020.
[http://dx.doi.org/10.1007/978-981-13-9431-7]

[54] Mazza M, Capuano A, Bria P, Mazza S. *Ginkgo biloba* and donepezil: a comparison in the treatment of Alzheimer's dementia in a randomized placebo-controlled double-blind study. Eur J Neurol 2006; 13(9): 981-5.
[http://dx.doi.org/10.1111/j.1468-1331.2006.01409.x] [PMID: 16930364]

[55] da Silva RR, de Oliveira TT, Nagem TJ, Leão MA. Efeito de flavonóides no metabolismo do ácido araquidônico. 2002.
[http://dx.doi.org/10.11606/issn.2176-7262.v35i2p127-133]

[56] DeFeudis FV. *Ginkgo biloba* extract (EGb 761): pharmacological activities and clinical applications. 1991.

[57] Youdim KA, Qaiser MZ, Begley DJ, Rice-Evans CA, Abbott NJ. Flavonoid permeability across an in situ model of the blood–brain barrier. Free Radic Biol Med 2004; 36(5): 592-604.
[http://dx.doi.org/10.1016/j.freeradbiomed.2003.11.023] [PMID: 14980703]

[58] Liu XG, Wu SQ, Li P, Yang H. Advancement in the chemical analysis and quality control of flavonoid in *Ginkgo biloba*. J Pharm Biomed Anal 2015; 113: 212-25.
[http://dx.doi.org/10.1016/j.jpba.2015.03.006] [PMID: 25812435]

[59] Kobus J, Flaczyk E, Siger A, Nogala-Kałucka M, Korczak J, Pegg RB. Phenolic compounds and antioxidant activity of extracts of *Ginkgo* leaves. Eur J Lipid Sci Technol 2009; 111(11): 1150-60.
[http://dx.doi.org/10.1002/ejlt.200800299]

[60] Chan PC, Xia Q, Fu PP. *Ginkgo biloba* leave extract: biological, medicinal, and toxicological effects. J Environ Sci Health Part C Environ Carcinog Ecotoxicol Rev 2007; 25(3): 211-44.
[http://dx.doi.org/10.1080/10590500701569414] [PMID: 17763047]

[61] Kumar S, Pandey AK. Chemistry and biological activities of flavonoids: an overview. 2013.
[http://dx.doi.org/10.1155/2013/162750]

[62] Amri H, Ogwuegbu SO, Boujrad N, Drieu K, Papadopoulos V. *in vivo* regulation of peripheral-type benzodiazepine receptor and glucocorticoid synthesis by *Ginkgo biloba* extract EGb 761 and isolated ginkgolides. Endocrinology 1996; 137(12): 5707-18.
[http://dx.doi.org/10.1210/endo.137.12.8940403] [PMID: 8940403]

[63] Tan MS, Yu JT, Tan CC, *et al.* Efficacy and adverse effects of *Ginkgo biloba* for cognitive impairment and dementia: a systematic review and meta-analysis. J Alzheimers Dis 2014; 43(2): 589-603.
[http://dx.doi.org/10.3233/JAD-140837] [PMID: 25114079]

[64] Wettstein A. Cholinesterase inhibitors and *Gingko* extracts--are they comparable in the treatment of dementia? Comparison of published placebo-controlled efficacy studies of at least six months' duration. Phytomedicine 2000; 6(6): 393-401.
[http://dx.doi.org/10.1016/S0944-7113(00)80066-5] [PMID: 10755847]

[65] van Dongen MCJM, van Rossum E, Kessels AGH, Sielhorst HJG, Knipschild PG. The efficacy of ginkgo for elderly people with dementia and age-associated memory impairment: new results of a randomized clinical trial. J Am Geriatr Soc 2000; 48(10): 1183-94.

[http://dx.doi.org/10.1111/j.1532-5415.2000.tb02589.x] [PMID: 11037003]

[66]   Weber W. *Ginkgo* not effective for memory loss in elderly. Lancet 2000; 356(9238): 1333.
[http://dx.doi.org/10.1016/S0140-6736(05)74241-0]

[67]   Kleijnen J, Knipschild P. *Ginkgo biloba.* Lancet 1992; 340(8828): 1136-9.
[http://dx.doi.org/10.1016/0140-6736(92)93158-J] [PMID: 1359218]

[68]   Heinonen T, Gaus W. Cross matching observations on toxicological and clinical data for the assessment of tolerability and safety of *Ginkgo biloba* leaf extract. Toxicology 2015; 327: 95-115.
[http://dx.doi.org/10.1016/j.tox.2014.10.013] [PMID: 25446328]

[69]   Montes P, Ruiz-Sanchez E, Rojas C, Rojas P. Montes P, Ruiz-Sanchez E, Rojas C, Rojas P. *Ginkgo biloba* extract 761: a review of basic studies and potential clinical use in psychiatric disorders. CNS & Neurological Disorders-Drug Targets 2015; 14(1): 132-49.

[70]   Nishizawa Y, Kanazawa S, Hotsuta M, Kidena H, Kobayashi H. Nishizawa Y, Kanazawa S, Hotsuta M, Kidena H, Kobayashi H. Hair growth stimulants containing plant extracts and other agents for synergistic effects. Patent Jpn Kokai Tokkyo Koho JP. 1999; 8(73,324): 96.

[71]   Belo SED, Gaspar LR, Campos PMBGM. Photoprotective effects of topical formulations containing a combination of *Ginkgo biloba* and green tea extracts. Phytother Res 2011; 25(12): 1854-60.
[http://dx.doi.org/10.1002/ptr.3507] [PMID: 21520309]

[72]   Koltermann A, Hartkorn A, Koch E, Fürst R, Vollmar AM, Zahler S. *Ginkgo biloba* extract EGb® 761 increases endothelial nitric oxide production *in vitro* and *in vivo*. Cell Mol Life Sci 2007; 64(13): 1715-22.
[http://dx.doi.org/10.1007/s00018-007-7085-z] [PMID: 17497242]

[73]   El-Boghdady NA. Increased cardiac endothelin-1 and nitric oxide in adriamycin-induced acute cardiotoxicity: protective effect of *Ginkgo biloba* extract. 2013.

[74]   Kato E, Howitt R, Dzyuba SV, Nakanishi K. Synthesis of novel ginkgolide photoaffinity–biotin probes. Org Biomol Chem 2007; 5(23): 3758-61.
[http://dx.doi.org/10.1039/b713333b] [PMID: 18004454]

[75]   Seth MK. Trees and their economic importance. Bot Rev 2003; 69(4): 321-76.
[http://dx.doi.org/10.1663/0006-8101(2004)069[0321:TATEI]2.0.CO;2]

[76]   DeFeudis F, Drieu K. *Ginkgo biloba*: medicinal and aromatic plants: industrial profiles. Adaptive effects of ginkgo biloba extract (EGb 761). 2000; 279-301.

[77]   Lechat P, Thesleff S, Bowman WC. Lechat P, Thesleff S, Bowman WC. Aminopyridines and Similarly Acting Drugs: Effects on Nerves, Muscles and Synapses: Proceedings of a IUPHAR Satellite Symposium in Conjunction with the 8th International Congress of Pharmacology, Paris, France, July 27-29, 1981: Elsevier 2013.

[78]   Kalus JS, Piotrowski AA, Fortier CR, Liu X, Kluger J, White CM. Hemodynamic and electrocardiographic effects of short-term *Ginkgo biloba*. Ann Pharmacother 2003; 37(3): 345-9.
[http://dx.doi.org/10.1345/aph.1C254] [PMID: 12639160]

[79]   Le Bars PL, Katz MM, Berman N, Itil TM, Freedman AM, Schatzberg AF. A placebo-controlled, double-blind, randomized trial of an extract of *Ginkgo biloba* for dementia. North American EGb Study Group. JAMA 1997; 278(16): 1327-32.
[http://dx.doi.org/10.1001/jama.1997.03550160047037] [PMID: 9343463]

[80]   Rosenblatt M, Mindel J. Spontaneous hyphema associated with ingestion of *Ginkgo biloba* extract. N Engl J Med 1997; 336(15): 1108.
[http://dx.doi.org/10.1056/NEJM199704103361518] [PMID: 9091822]

[81]   Ondrizek RR, Chan PJ, Patton WC, King A. An alternative medicine study of herbal effects on the penetration of zona-free hamster oocytes and the integrity of sperm deoxyribonucleic acid. Fertil Steril 1999; 71(3): 517-22.

[http://dx.doi.org/10.1016/S0015-0282(98)00476-2] [PMID: 10065791]

[82] Rowin J, Lewis SL. Spontaneous bilateral subdural hematomas associated with chronic *Ginkgo biloba* ingestion. Neurology 1996; 46(6): 1775-6.
[http://dx.doi.org/10.1212/WNL.46.6.1775] [PMID: 8649594]

CHAPTER 12

Role of *Withania somnifera* (Ashwagandha) in Neuronal Health

Ambarish Kumar Sinha[1], **Hagera Dilnashin**[2], **Hareram Birla**[2] and **Gaurav Kumar**[1,*]

[1] *Department of Clinical Research, School of Biosciences and Biomedical Engineering, Galgotias University, Greater Noida, Uttar Pradesh, India*

[2] *Department of Biochemistry, Institute of Science, Banaras Hindu University, Varanasi 221005(U.P.), India*

Abstract: Neurodegenerative disease refers to the progressive deterioration of neurologic function which leads to loss of speech, vision, hearing, and movement. It is also associated with seizures, eating difficulties, and memory impairment. Natural products have emerged as potential neuroprotective agents for the treatment of neurodegenerative diseases due to the enormous adverse effects associated with pharmacological drugs. *Withania somnifera* (Ashwagandha) is a traditional Ayurvedic medicine, used in India as a general tonic. It contains withanolides, and phytochemicals that may have adaptogenic properties. Studies show that *W. somnifera* is a neuroprotective agent and can protect the brain from oxidative stress and inflammation. This explains its ability to protect from mood disorders. In this review, we have reviewed the available evidence of *W. somnifera* and its phytochemicals for neurodegenerative disorders.

Keywords: Ayurvedic medicine, Chinese medicine, Neurological diseases, Phytochemicals, *Withania somnifera*.

INTRODUCTION

Neurodegenerative diseases are a heterogeneous group of disorders that are characterized by the progressive degeneration of the structure and function of the central nervous system (CNS) or peripheral nervous system (PNS). Neurodegenerative diseases are incurable and debilitating conditions that result in progressive degeneration and/or death of nerve cells. Neurodegenerative diseases represent a major threat to human health. Most common neurodegenerative

* ***Corresponding author Gaurav Kumar:** Department of Clinical Research, School of Biosciences and Biomedical Engineering, Galgotias University, Greater Noida (U.P.), India; E-mail: gaurav.rs.bme14@iitbhu.ac.in

diseases include Alzheimer's disease (AD), Parkinson's disease (PD), Huntington's disease (HD), amyotrophic lateral sclerosis (ALS), frontotemporal dementia, and, the spinocerebellar ataxias. *Withania somnifera* (Ashwagandha) is one of the most potent and most versatile drugs used in traditional systems of medicine. *W. somnifera* has been traditionally used for the treatment of general debility, nervous exhaustion, insomnia, memory loss, etc. Ashwagandha has been reported to be used in over 300 formulations in the traditional systems of medicine such as Ayurveda, Siddha, and Unani [1 - 5]. These traditional uses suggest that Ashwagandha might help treat neurodegenerative diseases and brain health in general (Fig. **1**). Several studies have reported the anti-inflammatory, anti-tumor, antioxidant, immunomodulatory, and anti-neuropsychiatric activity of Ashwagandha (Fig. **2**). In this chapter, we discuss the evidence of various health benefits of Ashwagandha in neurological diseases.

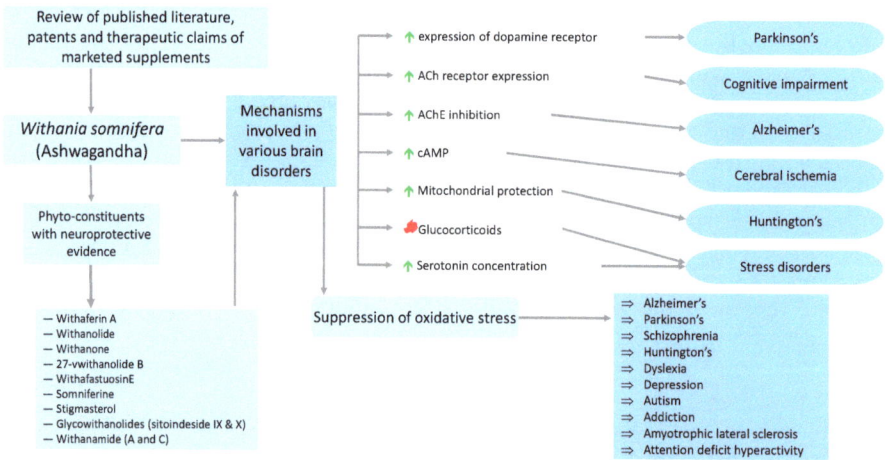

Fig. (1). Summary of neuroprotective constituents of Ashwagandha and related mechanism in brain disorder.

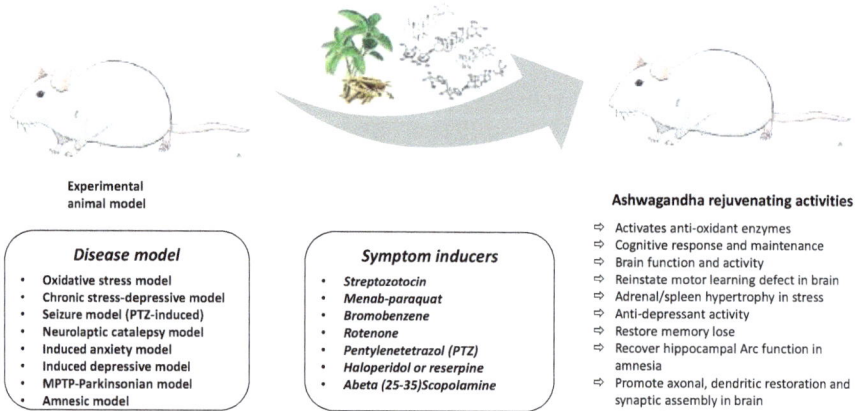

Fig. (2). Molecular activities of Ashwagandha have been validated in various animal models.

CHEMICAL COMPOSITION OF ASHWAGANDHA

Natural products have been used since ancient times for their therapeutic properties and have emerged as a preferred choice of treatment due to the large number of safety concerns associated with pharmacological drugs. Ashwagandha (*Withania somnifera*) also known as "Indian winter cherry" is a perennial plant that belongs to the *Solanaceae* family. The roots of Ashwagandha smell like a horse ("ashwa" in Sanskrit), therefore it is named Ashwagandha. Herbalists also call Ashwagandha "Indian ginseng" because in the Ayurvedic system of medicine, it is used similarly as the Panax ginseng is used in the Traditional Chinese Medicine (TCM). Table **1** lists the mechanism of Ashwagandha and its phytochemicals used in neurological disease models. The major constituents of the Ashwagandha are steroidal alkaloids and steroidal lactones which are collectively called withanolides. Withanolides are naturally occurring C-28 steroidal lactones built on an intact ergostane structure, in which C-22 and C-26 are oxidized to form a six-membered lactone ring. The basic structure of withanolides is made up of 22-hydroxy-ergostan-26-oic acid-26, 22-lactone, and is called the "withanolide skeleton" [5 - 10]. To date, twelve alkaloids, thirty-five withanolides, and a few sitoindos have been identified and investigated in neurological disease. Apart from withanolides, other alkaloid constituents of Ashwagandha include: somniferine, somnine, somniferinine, withananine, pseudo-withanine, tropine, pseudotropine, 3-a-gloyloxytropane, choline, cuscohygrine, isopelletierine, and anaferine andanahydrine. To date, various products/formulations of Ashwagandha are developed and commercially available. Table **2** outlines some commercially available formulations of Ashwagandha and their associated health claims.

Table 1. Some commercially available formulations of Ashwagandha and associated health claims

S. No.	Product	Manufacturer	Health Claim
1	Neuro Response™	INNATE Response	Support for stress
2	Adrenal Response®	INNATE Response	Support for stress
3	Mito2Max	doTERRA International	Supports healthy cellular energy production and optimal mitochondrial function
4	Integrative Therapeutics® HPA Adapt™	Integrative Therapeutics	Support for stress
5	Ashwagandha	Pure Encapsulations®	Support for occasional stress
6	Daily Stress Formula	Pure Encapsulations®	Promotes mental relaxation and moderates the effects of occasional stress

S. No.	Product	Manufacturer	Health Claim
7	Energy Xtra	Pure Encapsulations®	Adaptogen formula for physical and mental stamina
8	PureCell	Pure Encapsulations®	Supports cell and tissue health
9	Adreno Calm	Genestra Brands®	Promotes healthy stress management
10	Adreno Restore	Genestra Brands®	Phytonutrient support for mental and physical well-being during stress
11	Rhodiola Ashwagandha Ginseng Complex	Genestra Brands®	Supports healthy adrenal function and energy metabolism
12	Phytisone	Thorne Research, Inc.	Support brain/nerves
13	Ashwagandha 500 MG	RB Health (US) LLC	Better sleep for better days
14	FORMULA W™	Oregon's Wild Harvest	Helps the body adapt to stress
15	Ultimate Ashwagandha	Nature Made	Clinically proven ashwagandha to reduce stress, and magnesium to help relax the body
16	Beyond Raw Anabolic Testosterone System - Infinite Test™	General Nutrition Centers, Inc. (GNC)	Dual-release stress, sleep & recovery support
17	Ashwagandha	Health Thru Nutrition	Manage Symptoms of Daily Stress, Promote Body & Mind Relaxation, Trusted Ayurvedic to Balance Mental & Physical Vitality
18	Ashwagandha *Ginkgo*	Oregon's Wild Harvest	Helps the body adapt to stress
19	Herbal Sleep	Oregon's Wild Harvest	Calms and soothes the nerves

CEREBRAL ISCHEMIA

A stroke occurs when a blood vessel carrying oxygen and nutrients to the brain is obstructed or ruptures. Thus, the brain does not receive the necessary nutrients and begins to die. Stroke is the leading cause of brain injury and disability in millions of people worldwide. Researchers examined the neuroprotective properties of an aqueous extract of Ashwagandha in both pre-and post-stroke treatment regimens in a mouse model of permanent distal middle cerebral artery occlusion (pMCAO). Ashwagandha supplementation (200 mg/kg) improved functional recovery and significantly reduced the infarct volume in mice. Ashwagandha up-regulated the expression of heme oxygenase 1 (HO1) and downregulated the expression of the proapoptotic protein poly (ADP-ribose) polymerase-1 (PARP1) *via* the PARP1-AIF pathway, thus preventing the nuclear translocation of apoptosis-inducing factor (AIF), and subsequent apoptosis. Also, Semaphorin-3A (Sema3A) expression was reduced in the Ashwagandha-treated group, whereas Wnt, pGSK3β, and pCRMP2 expression levels were almost unchanged. These results suggest that Ashwagandha exerts neuroprotective effects by mediating the interaction of anti-oxidant/ anti-apoptotic pathways [11]. In a rat model produced by unilateral internal carotid artery ligation, Ashwagandha was shown to exert neuroprotective and antioxidant properties [12]. In another rat model of bilateral common carotid artery occlusion, Ashwagandha pre-supplementation (50 mg/kg p.o. for 5 days) decreased the reperfusion injury-induced biochemical and histopathological alterations [13]. In a middle cerebral artery occlusion (MCAO) model of stroke, Ashwagandha supplementation was shown to reduce oxidative stress, reduce lesion volume and reestablish neurological damage [14]. In another study on the MCAO model, Ashwagandha supplementation was shown to be effective in restoring the acetylcholinesterase activity, lipid peroxidation, thiols, and attenuated MCAO induced behavioral deficits. In addition to this Ashwagandha supplementation significantly reduced the cerebral infarct volume and ameliorated histopathological alterations. Improved blood flow was also observed in the brain regions of ischemic rats [15]. Glutamate toxicity has been implicated in stroke, head trauma, multiple sclerosis, and neurodegenerative disorders [16]. Researchers investigated the neuroprotective role of Ashwagandha against glutamate-induced toxicity in the retinoic acid differentiated rat glioma (C6) and human neuroblastoma (IMR-32) cells. Results showed that pre-treatment with Ashwagandha water extract inhibited glutamate-induced cell death and was able to revert glutamate-induced changes in HSP70. In addition to this, the supplementation also induced the neuronal plasticity markers, NCAM (Neural cell adhesion molecule), and its polysialylated form, PSA-NCAM which are known to play an important role in neuronal regeneration and repair [17]. Nrf2, a transcriptional factor is a key regulator of cellular and organismal defense mechanisms that offer protection from endogenous and exogenous stresses by coordinating basal and stress-inducible activation of multiple cytoprotective genes [18]. In a study, the ameliorative effect of withanolide A for hypoxia-induced memory impairment in male Sprague Dawley rats was investigated. Results showed that withanolide A reduces neurodegeneration by restoring hypoxia-induced glutathione depletion in the hippocampus. Further, Withanolide A increases glutathione biosynthesis in neuronal cells by upregulating the GCLC level through the Nrf2 pathway in a corticosterone-dependent manner [19]. In another study, Ashwagandha supplementation (25, 50, and 100 mg/kg) in Sprague Dawley rats exerted neuroprotection by activating the PI3K/Akt signaling pathway, modulation of the expression of MMPs, and by inhibiting the migration of VSMCs [10, 20 - 25].

Table 2. Mechanism of Ashwagandha and its phytochemicals in neurological disease models.

Disease Models	Materials	Mechanism
Alzheimer's disease/Dementia	Extract	Neurite outgrowth *in vitro* Memory improvement Neuroprotective effects *in vitro* Aβ clearance *in vivo*
	Withanolide A	Neurite outgrowth *in vitro* Axonal regeneration and synaptic reconstruction *in vitro* and *in vivo* Memory improvement Upregulation of BACE1, ADAM10, and IDE *in vitro*
	Withanoside IV	Neurite outgrowth *in vitro* Axonal regeneration and synaptic reconstruction *in vitro* and *in vivo* Memory improvement
	Withanoside VI	Neurite outgrowth *in vitro* Axonal regeneration and synaptic reconstruction *in vitro* and *in vivo* Memory improvement
	Sominone	Axonal regeneration and synaptic reconstruction *in-vitro* Axonal growth *in-vivo* Memory improvement and memory enhancement
Spinal cord injury	Withanoside IV	Axonal growth *in-vivo* and functional recovery
	Denosomin	Axonal growth *in-vivo* and functional recovery
Parkinson's disease	Extract	Anti-oxidant effect *in-vivo* Neuroprotective effect *in-vivo* Functional recovery
Huntington's disease	Extract	Functional recovery Huntington's disease Extract Anti-oxidant effect *in-vivo*

TRAUMATIC BRAIN INJURY

Traumatic brain injury (TBI) is associated with increased morbidity and mortality and makes it a major public health concern globally. In TBI mice, Withaferin A significantly improved neurobehavioral functions and diminished histological changes of tissue injury. Additionally, Withaferin A was shown to reduce blood-brain barrier disruption and brain edema in the brain which was believed to be mediated by a decrease in apoptosis in endothelial cells. Furthermore, Withaferin A was shown to reduce the number of mediators of neuroinflammation such as TNF-α, IL-1β, and IL-6 [26]. These results imply that Withaferin A offers neuroprotection by regulating the activation of microglia and inhibition of apoptosis in endothelial cells. In another study, Ashwagandha supplementation reduced the expression of cell death factor Bax by 2 folds thereby reducing cell death in the model neuron TBI system. It also led to an increase in neurite [27].

EPILEPSY

Epilepsy is one of the most common and serious neurological disorders which affects approx. 50 million people globally. Epilepsy is a chronic, heterogeneous disease characterized by recurrent and unprovoked seizures. It mainly results from a disturbance in the balance of inhibitory and stimulatory neurotransmitters. Glutamate and GABA are known to play an important role in epilepsy. In a rat model of temporal lobe epilepsy Ashwagandha root extract decreased the muscarinic receptor expression and reduced oxidative stress and led to the restoration of cell signaling [28]. In another study in the epileptic rats, Ashwagandha treatment corrected spatial memory deficits by enhancing the antioxidant system and restoring NMDA receptor expression to physiological levels [29]. Ashwagandha root extract (100 mg/kg) demonstrated significant protection against PTZ-induced chemical kindling, and the effects were equivalent to 1mg/kg diazepam [30]. Few researchers have also proposed that the anticonvulsant mechanism of Ashwagandha is mediated by stimulation of benzodiazepine receptors, thereby enhancing the GABAergic system in the brain [31]. A study evaluated the effects of aqueous extract of Ashwagandha in pilocarpine-induced convulsions in rats. Ashwagandha increased latencies of the first convulsion and decreased serum Ca^{2+} level and increased TAC and Na+/K+-ATPase activity. Additionally, it resulted in elevated GSH content and reduction in MDA and NO contents in the hippocampus. Furthermore, Ashwagandha modulated serotonin and dopamine in the hippocampus. In a mouse model of pilocarpine-induced status epilepticus, the Ashwagandha treatment ameliorated neuronal cell death in the hippocampus as well as decreased the release of pro-inflammatory factors such as interleukin-1 β, and tumor necrosis factor in the hippocampus, which resulted in neuroprotection [32].

HUNTINGTON'S DISEASE (HD)

HD s a neurodegenerative disease caused by a mutation in the HTT gene, which encodes for the Huntington protein. Mutated Huntington protein aggregates in neurons causing neuronal death.

HD is characterized by progressive motor, cognitive, and psychiatric decline, eventually leading to death. There are no approved drugs for HD. Austedo (deutetrahenazines) and Xenazine (tetrabenazine) are oral VMAT2 inhibitors that are FDA-approved to treat chorea associated with HD. In a study, researchers evaluated the effects of Ashwagandha root extract in gait abnormalities, oxidative stress, and mitochondrial dysfunction induced by 3-Nitropropionic acid (3-NP), a potent neurotoxin. Treatment with Ashwagandha root extract resulted in significant improvement in cognitive function and motor functions in the 3-NP induced rat model of HD. The neuroprotective effects of Ashwagandha were attributed to the reduction of oxidative stress and enrichment of acetylcholinesterase enzyme activity [33].

AMYOTROPHIC LATERAL SCLEROSIS (ALS)

ALS is a rare, fatal neurodegenerative disorder characterized by stiff muscles, muscle twitching, and gradually worsening weakness due to muscles decreasing in size. ALS attacks neurons responsible for controlling voluntary muscles, resulting in muscle weakness in limbs, and impacts speaking, chewing, swallowing, and breathing, leading to progressive disability and eventually death, typically from respiratory failure and aspiration pneumonia. In addition, up to 50% of ALS patients develop cognitive impairment associated with frontotemporal dementia. There are no effective therapies and average survival is 3-5 years after initial symptom onset. ALS symptoms include muscle twitches in the arm, leg, shoulder, or tongue, muscle cramps, muscle weakness, slurred speech, and difficulty chewing or swallowing. In the advanced disease, patients lose voluntary muscle control leading to an inability to speak, move, and breathe. In the SOD1 mice model, early-stage treatment with Ashwagandha resulted in improvement in neuroinflammation, decreased levels of SOD1 misfolded in the spinal cord, and reduction in motor neurons loss which delayed the disease progression and mortality. Furthermore, Ashwagandha treatment led to significant upregulation of heat shock protein 25 (Hsp25). This implies that Ashwagandha offers neuroprotection through induction of Hsp25 and reduction of SOD1 misfolds [34]. In another SOD1 mice model, Ashwagandha treatment led to an improvement in motor functions and delay in disease progression. Additionally, Ashwagandha treatment led to a reduction in levels of SOD1 misfold and phosphorylation of NF-κB [35].

ALZHEIMER'S DISEASE (AD)

AD is the most common form of dementia, it is responsible for 80% of all dementia cases worldwide. Around 24 million are estimated to have Alzheimer's disease worldwide, with increasing prevalence as we get into the older populations. Symptoms of AD include short-term memory impairment to the point of interference with daily activities, impairments in other cognitive domains such as language, executive functions, and orientation that occur later. The hallmark biological characteristics of AD include the accumulation of amyloid B plaques and intraneuronal deposits of neurofibrillary tangles (NFTS). NFTS is composed of aggregated tau protein, which leads to microtubule and axonal transport destabilization. Ashwagandha extract has been shown to reverse the behavioral deficits and pathological clues involved in experimental models of AD [36, 37]. In an *in vitro* study using neuronal cell lines, Ashwagandha mediated the reversal of β-amyloid-induced toxicity in SK-N-MC neuronal cells and also prevented the amyloid-induced reduction in spine density, spine area, spine length, and several spines suggesting a protective effect of Ashwagandha in AD. Further, β-amyloid treated neuronal cultures increased acetylcholinesterase activity and increased the internalization of amyloid-beta, which was reversed on Ashwagandha supplementation [36]. Molecular docking studies have revealed that withanolide A has a high binding affinity with human acetylcholinesterase involving Thr78, Trp81, Ser120, and His442 residues all of which fall under one or other active sites/subsites of the enzyme which may be critical to its inhibitory action on acetylcholinesterase and suggesting the likely mechanism involved in its potential therapeutic effect against AD [38]. Active constituents of Ashwagandha (withanamides) have been reported to prevent fibril formation and protect cells from amyloid-beta toxicity by unique binding of withanamides-A and -C to the active motif of amyloid-beta (25–35) [39]. Withanolide A has been shown to modulate multiple targets associated with amyloid-beta precursor protein processing and amyloid-beta protein clearance by specifically downregulating beta-secretase 1 (BACE1) and upregulating a disintegrin and metalloprotease 10 (ADAM10) [40]. BACE1 is a rate-limiting enzyme in the production of beta from amyloid-beta precursor protein (AbetaPP), while ADAM10 is involved in the non-amyloidogenic processing of AbetaPP. Researchers have suggested increased efflux of amyloid peptides through activation of P-glycoprotein [41]. In another study, an active metabolite of Withanoside-IV, sominone had been reported to attenuate amyloid-beta (25–35)-induced neurodegeneration by regeneration of axons, dendrites, and synapses [42]. In another study, oral administration with a semi-purified extract of the roots of *Ashwagandha* (containing withanolides and withanosides) was shown to reverse behavioral deficits, plaque pathology, accumulation of β-amyloid peptides and oligomers in the brains of middle-aged and old APP/PS1 transgenic AD mice [42]. This effect of *Ashwagandha* supplementation in rapidly clearing β-amyloid peptides was shown to be related to the ability of *Ashwagandha* to increase the levels of liver low-density lipoprotein receptor-related protein (LRP) in brain microvessels and the β-amyloid-degrading protease neprilysin (NEP) in the liver. Liver LRP mediates endocytosis of β-amyloid peptides present in the plasma, which are then cleared through NEP and other proteases present in the liver. This ability of *Ashwagandha* to induce liver LRP could be a useful tool since the cell surface LRP in the liver is required for the rapid systemic clearance of the toxic β-amyloid peptide and subsequent degradation of this peptide by proteases in the liver. Moreover, high-resolution Q-TOF/ MS studies have been shown to demonstrate that the withanamide peaks in *Ashwagandha* fruit extract crossed the blood-brain barrier in the mouse after intraperitoneal administration, suggesting that an oral administration of the extract could give similar results since the extract has lipophilic and hydrophilic functionalities and easily crosses membranes [43]. Another study has reported that withanolide A promotes neuritogenic and inhibits secretase activity which may contribute towards its beneficial role in AD [44].

PARKINSON'S DISEASE (PD)

PD is a neurodegenerative condition, which is characterized by muscle rigidity, tremor, and bradykinesia [45]. Reduction in dopamine levels in brain regions involved in control motor functions is responsible for the development of PD [46, 47]. Oxidative stress is the major contributing factor in neurodegeneration in the PD brain [48]. Ashwagandha has been reported to show therapeutic effects in experimental models of PD [49, 50]. Ashwagandha extract was reported to reverse neurobehavioral deficits, increased lipid peroxidation, reduced glutathione content, activities of glutathione-S-transferase, glutathione reductase, glutathione peroxidase, superoxide dismutase, and catalase, catecholamine content, dopaminergic D2 receptor binding, and tyrosine hydroxylase expression in the 6-Hydroxydopamine-induced model of PD in a dose-dependent manner [51]. Oral administration of Ashwagandha root extract (100 mg/kg) in PD mice resulted in improved dopamine, 3,4-dihydroxy-phenylacetic acid, and homovanillic acid levels, along with normalization of thiobarbituric reactive substances levels (a marker of oxidative stress) in the corpus striatum. The reduction in oxidative was accompanied by an increase in glutathione levels and glutathione peroxidase activity in brain regions of PD animals [52]. Another study further demonstrated the anti-apoptotic and anti-inflammatory properties of Ashwagandha, which could be involved in beneficial effects in PD. In addition, supplementation with ethanolic root extract of Ashwagandha (100 mg/kg, i.p) for 9 weeks, inhibited the expression of inducible nitric oxide synthase (iNOS) and astroglial activation marker glial fibrillary acidic protein (GFAP) in Maneb (MB) and paraquat (PQ) induced model of PD. MB and PQ are environmental toxins that have been experimentally used to induce selective damage of dopaminergic neurons leading to the development of PD. In another study, Ashwagandha was shown to inhibit apoptotic cell death in PD by reducing the level of the pro-apoptotic (Bax) proteins and increase in the level of anti-apoptotic (Bcl-2) proteins in the MB–PQ model [49]. A group of researchers has proposed that the neuromodulatory effect of Ashwagandha against the rotenone-induced PD model in *Drosophila melanogaster* is mediated *via* suppression of oxidative stress and its potential to attenuate mitochondrial dysfunctions [50]. Supplementation of Ashwagandha to leucine-rich-repeat-kinase-2 mutants (LRRK2) loss-of-function model of PD in *Drosophila* resulted in increasing their lifespan, improved motor function, and mitochondrial morphology [53]. These studies suggest the therapeutic potential of Ashwagandha in patients with PD.

SPINAL CORD INJURY (SCI)

Spinal cord injuries (SCI) are damage to the spinal cord, and nerves in the spinal canal following a sudden, traumatic blow to the spine that fractures or dislocates the vertebrae. The damage begins at the moment of injury when displaced bone fragments, disc material, or ligaments bruise or tear into spinal cord tissue. Symptoms include loss of voluntary muscle movement in the chest, arms, or legs, loss of sensation, including the ability to feel heat, cold, and touch, loss of bowel or bladder control, exaggerated reflex activities or spasms, pain, or an intense stinging sensation caused by damage to the nerve fibers in the spinal cord, difficulty in breathing, coughing or clearing secretions from lungs and muscle weakness. In a mouse model of SCI, oral administration of Ashwagandha led to improvement in hindlimb function, and promoted axonal extension and increase in PNS myelin level [54]. In another study on the mice model, denosomin an analogous derivative of sominone which in turn is a sapogenin metabolized from withanoside IV, improved hind limb motor dysfunction and axonal growth, especially in the 5-HT-positive tracts across the scar and increased the density of astrocytes. Denosomin increased astrocyte proliferation, inhibited astrocytic death, and increased the expression and secretion of vimentin in cultured astrocytes. Furthermore, vimentin increased axonal outgrowth in cultured neurons, even in the presence of inhibitory CSPG. Denosomin increased the number of vimentin-expressing astrocytes inside glial scars of SCI mice, and 5-HT-positive axonal growth occurred in a vimentin-associated manner [55].

OTHER NEUROLOGICAL CONDITIONS

Researchers have demonstrated that therapeutic effects of Ashwagandha in scopolamine dementia involved upregulation of activity-regulated cytoskeletal-associated protein (Arc), a member of the immediate-early gene (IEG) family protein which plays key role in memory and learning [56]. An in-silico study showed that anaferine, beta-sitosterol, withaferin A, withanolide A, withanolide B and withanolide D, inhibit GluN2B containing NMDARs through allosteric mode suggesting the beneficial effect of Ashwagandha in treating multiple neurodegenerative diseases mediated through glutamate excitoxicity [57]. Results from another study suggested that Ashwagandha possesses glycine mimetic activities, which can be the potential target for inducing memory in hippocampal CA1 neurons [20]. Another study has suggested that Ashwagandha can be a potential agent to suppress the effect of sleep loss on memory impairments [58]. Ashwagandha reduced the intracranial tumor volumes *in vivo* and suppressed the tumor-promoting proteins p-nuclear factor kappa B (NF-κB), p-Akt, vascular endothelial growth factor (VEGF), a heat shock protein 70 (HSP70), PSA-NCAM, and cyclin D1 in the rat model of orthotopic glioma allograft. Further, reduction in glial fibrillary acidic protein (GFAP) and upregulation of mortalin and neural cell adhesion molecule (NCAM) expression specifically in tumor-bearing tissue further indicated the anti-glioma efficacy of Ashwagandha *in vivo* [59]. In another study, researchers observed that key constituents in Ashwagandha have an important role in neurological disorders associated with altered GABAergic signaling that include anxiety disorders, sleep disturbances, muscle spasms, and seizures. It was suggested that differential activation of GABA receptor subtypes elucidates a potential mechanism by which Ashwagandha accomplishes its reported adaptogenic properties [60]. One study reported oral administration of Ashwagandha root extract stabilized mitochondrial functions and prevented oxidative damage in the hypothalamus of diabetic rats [61]. Withanolide A has also been shown to increase glutathione biosynthesis in neuronal cells by upregulating γ-glutamylcysteinyl ligase (GCLC) levels through Nrf2 pathway in a corticosterone dependent manner [20]. Ashwagandha was shown to attenuate lipid peroxidation and accentuate antioxidant enzymes; catalase and superoxide dismutase in brain as well as liver and kidney, suggesting its ability to act as a free radical scavenger protecting cells against lead induced toxic insult [62]. Another study found GABA-mimetic actions of Ashwagandha on substantia gelatinosa neurons of the trigeminal subnucleus caudalis in mice suggesting Ashwagandha may be affecting the modulatiom of orofacial pain processing [63, 64]. Ashwagandha has been shown to prevent downregulation of neuronal cell markers NF-H, MAP2, PSD-95, GAP-43, BDNF and glial cell marker GFAP and upregulation of DNA damage and oxidative stress following scopolamine induced effect on the brain or brain derived cells. Sominone, an aglycone of withanoside IV, identified as an active metabolite after oral administration of withanoside IV was observed to increase phosphorylation of RET (a receptor for the glial cell line-derived neurotrophic factor, GDNF) in hippocampal neurons without affecting the synthesis and secretion of GDNF. The densities of axons and dendrites were increased in the hippocampus by sominone administration [65]. Ashwagandha has been shown to be effective in reversing haloperidol induced catalepsy, which is believed to be due its antioxidant properties [66]. In another study, researchers found withanolide A-treated cells, had increased length of NF-H-positive processes compared with vehicle-treated cells, whereas, the length of MAP2-positive processes was increased by withanosides IV and VI suggesting that axons are predominantly extended by withanolide A, and dendrites by withanosides IV and VI [67].

CONCLUSION

Ashwagandha and its constituents have demonstrated various activities against neurodegenerative disease including Alzheimer's disease and spinal cord injury. In addition, pharmacological analyses of Ashwagandha extracts and related compounds offer novel insights into the treatment of neurodegenerative diseases. However, direct target molecules of Ashwagandha-related compounds have not been identified as yet. Also, more research is needed to determine a potential dosage range for achieving its multipurpose drug properties. Further studies of Ashwagandha will contribute to resolving an urgent unmet medical need which is "efficacious treatments that may offer cure of neurodegenerative diseases".

CONSENT FOR PUBLICATION

Not applicable.

CONFLICT OF INTEREST

The author declares no conflict of interest, financial or otherwise.

ACKNOWLEDGEMENTS

Declared none.

REFERENCES

[1]   Tavhare SD, Nishteswar K. Collection practices of medicinal plants-Vedic, Ayurvedic and modern perspectives. Int J Pharm Biol Arch 2014; 5: 54-61.

[2]   Zahra W, Rai SN, Birla H, *et al*. Economic Importance of Medicinal Plants in Asian Countries. Bioeconomy for Sustainable Development. Bioeconomy for Sustainable Development. Springer 2020; pp. 359-77.
[http://dx.doi.org/10.1007/978-981-13-9431-7_19]

[3]   Birla H, Keswani C, Singh SS, *et al*. Unraveling the Neuroprotective Effect of *Tinospora cordifolia* in Parkinsonian Mouse Model Through Proteomics Approach. 2021.
[http://dx.doi.org/10.1021/acschemneuro.1c00481]

[4]   Keswani C, Dilnashin H, Birla H, Singh SP. Unravelling efficient applications of agriculturally important microorganisms for alleviation of induced inter-cellular oxidative stress in crops. Acta Agric Slov 2019; 114(1): 121-30.
[http://dx.doi.org/10.14720/aas.2019.114.1.14]

[5]   Birla H, Keswani C, Rai SN, *et al*. Neuroprotective effects of *Withania somnifera* in BPA induced-cognitive dysfunction and oxidative stress in mice. Behav Brain Funct 2019; 15(1): 9.
[http://dx.doi.org/10.1186/s12993-019-0160-4] [PMID: 31064381]

[6]   Keswani C, Dilnashin H, Birla H, Singh S. Re-addressing the commercialization and regulatory hurdles for biopesticides in India. Rhizosphere 2019; 11(100155): 1016.

[7]   Rathore AS, Birla H, Singh SS, *et al.* Epigenetic Modulation in Parkinson's Disease and Potential Treatment Therapies. Neurochem Res 2021; 46(7): 1618-26.
[http://dx.doi.org/10.1007/s11064-021-03334-w] [PMID: 33900517]

[8]   Singh SS, Rai SN, Birla H, *et al.* Techniques Related to Disease Diagnosis and Therapeutics Application of Biomedical Engineering in Neuroscience:. Springer 2019; pp. 437-56.
[http://dx.doi.org/10.1007/978-981-13-7142-4_22]

[9]   Zahra W, Rai SN, Birla H, *et al.* The global economic impact of neurodegenerative diseases: Opportunities and challenges Bioeconomy for Sustainable Development 2020; pp. 333-45.

[10]   Rai SN, Dilnashin H, Birla H, *et al.* The role of PI3K/Akt and ERK in neurodegenerative disorders. Neurotox Res 2019; 35(3): 775-95.
[http://dx.doi.org/10.1007/s12640-019-0003-y] [PMID: 30707354]

[11]   Raghavan A, Shah ZA. *Withania somnifera* improves ischemic stroke outcomes by attenuating PARP1-AIF-mediated caspase-independent apoptosis. Mol Neurobiol 2015; 52(3): 1093-105.
[http://dx.doi.org/10.1007/s12035-014-8907-2] [PMID: 25294638]

[12]   Koirala S, Shah S, Rouniar G, Koirala B, Khanal L. Role of *Withania somnifera* (Ashwagandha) in Ischemic Stroke Rat Model Produced by Unilateral Internal Carotid Artery Ligation: A Histological Staining with 2, 3, 5 Triphenyltetrazolium Chloride and a Behavior Analysis. Austin J Anat 2017; 4(3): 1074.

[13]   Trigunayat A, Raghavendra M, Singh R, Bhattacharya A, Acharya S. Neuroprotective effect of *Withania somnifera* (WS) in cerebral ischemia-reperfusion and long-term hypoperfusion induced alterations in rats. J Nat Rem 2007; 7(2): 234-46.

[14]   Chaudhary G, Sharma U, Jagannathan NR, Gupta YK. Evaluation of *Withania somnifera* in a middle cerebral artery occlusion model of stroke in rats. Clin Exp Pharmacol Physiol 2003; 30(5-6): 399-404.
[http://dx.doi.org/10.1046/j.1440-1681.2003.03849.x] [PMID: 12859433]

[15]   Sood A, Kumar A, Dhawan DK, Sandhir R. Propensity of *Withania somnifera* to attenuate behavioural, biochemical, and histological alterations in experimental model of stroke. Cell Mol Neurobiol 2016; 36(7): 1123-38.
[http://dx.doi.org/10.1007/s10571-015-0305-4] [PMID: 26718711]

[16]   Lewerenz J, Maher P. Chronic glutamate toxicity in neurodegenerative diseases—what is the evidence? Front Neurosci 2015; 9: 469.
[http://dx.doi.org/10.3389/fnins.2015.00469] [PMID: 26733784]

[17]   Kataria H, Wadhwa R, Kaul SC, Kaur G. Water extract from the leaves of *Withania somnifera* protect RA differentiated C6 and IMR-32 cells against glutamate-induced excitotoxicity. PLoS One 2012; 7(5): e37080.
[http://dx.doi.org/10.1371/journal.pone.0037080] [PMID: 22606332]

[18]   Liu L, Locascio LM, Doré S. Critical role of Nrf2 in experimental ischemic stroke. Front Pharmacol 2019; 10: 153.
[http://dx.doi.org/10.3389/fphar.2019.00153] [PMID: 30890934]

[19]   Baitharu I, Jain V, Deep SN, *et al.* Withanolide A prevents neurodegeneration by modulating hippocampal glutathione biosynthesis during hypoxia. PLoS One 2014; 9(10): e105311.
[http://dx.doi.org/10.1371/journal.pone.0105311] [PMID: 25310001]

[20]   Zhang QZ, Guo YD, Li HM, Wang RZ, Guo SG, Du YF. Protection against cerebral infarction by Withaferin A involves inhibition of neuronal apoptosis, activation of PI3K/Akt signaling pathway, and reduced intimal hyperplasia *via* inhibition of VSMC migration and matrix metalloproteinases. Adv Med Sci 2017; 62(1): 186-92.
[http://dx.doi.org/10.1016/j.advms.2016.09.003] [PMID: 28282606]

[21]   Singh S, Rai S, Birla H, Eds., *et al.* Chlorogenic acid protects against MPTP induced neurotoxicity in parkinsonian mice model *via* its anti-apoptotic activity. Journal of Neurochemistry. NJ USA: Wiley 111 River St, Hoboken 2019.

[22]   Rai SN, Birla H, Singh SS, *et al.* Pathophysiology of the Disease Causing Physical Disability Biomedical Engineering and its Applications in Healthcare. Springer 2019; pp. 573-95.

[23]   Rai SN, Singh BK, Rathore AS, *et al.* Quality control in huntington's disease: a therapeutic target. Neurotox Res 2019; 36(3): 612-26.
[http://dx.doi.org/10.1007/s12640-019-00087-x] [PMID: 31297710]

[24]   Zahra W, Rai SN, Birla H, *et al.* Neuroprotection of rotenone-induced Parkinsonism by ursolic acid in PD mouse model. CNS & Neurological Disorders-Drug Targets 2020; 14: 527-40.
[http://dx.doi.org/10.2174/1871527319666200812224457]

[25]   Rai SN, Zahra W, Singh SS, *et al.* Anti-inflammatory activity of ursolic acid in MPTP-induced parkinsonian mouse model. Neurotox Res 2019; 36(3): 452-62.
[http://dx.doi.org/10.1007/s12640-019-00038-6] [PMID: 31016688]

[26]   Zhou Z, Xiang W, Jiang Y, *et al.* Withaferin A alleviates traumatic brain injury induced secondary brain injury *via* suppressing apoptosis in endothelia cells and modulating activation in the microglia. Eur J Pharmacol 2020; 874: 172988.
[http://dx.doi.org/10.1016/j.ejphar.2020.172988] [PMID: 32032599]

[27]   Saykally JN, Hatic H, Keeley KL, Jain SC, Ravindranath V, Citron BA. *Withania somnifera* extract protects model neurons from in vitro traumatic injury. Cell Transplant 2017; 26(7): 1193-201.
[http://dx.doi.org/10.1177/0963689717714320] [PMID: 28933215]

[28]   Anju TR, Smijin S, Jobin M, Paulose CS. Altered muscarinic receptor expression in the cerebral cortex of epileptic rats: restorative role of *Withania somnifera*. Biochem Cell Biol 2018; 96(4): 433-40.
[http://dx.doi.org/10.1139/bcb-2017-0198] [PMID: 29216436]

[29]   Soman S, Korah PK, Jayanarayanan S, Mathew J, Paulose CS. Oxidative stress induced NMDA receptor alteration leads to spatial memory deficits in temporal lobe epilepsy: ameliorative effects of *Withania somnifera* and Withanolide A. Neurochem Res 2012; 37(9): 1915-27.
[http://dx.doi.org/10.1007/s11064-012-0810-5] [PMID: 22700086]

[30]   Kulkarni SK, George B. Anticonvulsant action of *Withania Somnifera* (Aswaganda) root extract against pentylenetetrazol☐induced kindling in mice. Phytother Res 1996; 10(5): 447-9.
[http://dx.doi.org/10.1002/(SICI)1099-1573(199608)10:5<447::AID-PTR869>3.0.CO;2-M]

[31]   Roshanaei K, Nazif N. Effect of withania somnifera root extract on PTZ-induced seizure threshold in mice. Res J Fish Hydrobiol 2015; 10(10): 719-23.

[32]   Salamaa AA, El-Kassabyb M, Elhadidyc ME, Raoufc ERA, Abdallad AM, Farrage ARH. Effects of the Aqueous Seed Extract of *Withania somnifera* (Ashwagandha) against Pilocarpine-induced Convulsions in Rats. Int J Pharm Sci Rev Res 2016; 41(1): 116-21.

[33]   Kumar P, Kumar A. Possible neuroprotective effect of *Withania somnifera* root extract against 3-nitropropionic acid-induced behavioral, biochemical, and mitochondrial dysfunction in an animal model of Huntington's disease. J Med Food 2009; 12(3): 591-600.
[http://dx.doi.org/10.1089/jmf.2008.0028] [PMID: 19627208]

[34]   Patel P, Julien JP, Kriz J. Early-stage treatment with Withaferin A reduces levels of misfolded superoxide dismutase 1 and extends lifespan in a mouse model of amyotrophic lateral sclerosis. Neurotherapeutics 2015; 12(1): 217-33.
[http://dx.doi.org/10.1007/s13311-014-0311-0] [PMID: 25404049]

[35]   Dutta K, Patel P, Julien JP. Protective effects of *Withania somnifera* extract in SOD1^{G93A} mouse model of amyotrophic lateral sclerosis. Exp Neurol 2018; 309: 193-204.
[http://dx.doi.org/10.1016/j.expneurol.2018.08.008] [PMID: 30134145]

[36] Kurapati KRV, Atluri VSR, Samikkannu T, Nair MPN. Ashwagandha (*Withania somnifera*) reverses β-amyloid1-42 induced toxicity in human neuronal cells: implications in HIV-associated neurocognitive disorders (HAND). PLoS One 2013; 8(10): e77624.
[http://dx.doi.org/10.1371/journal.pone.0077624] [PMID: 24147038]

[37] Sehgal N, Gupta A, Valli RK, *et al. Withania somnifera* reverses Alzheimer's disease pathology by enhancing low-density lipoprotein receptor-related protein in liver. Proc Natl Acad Sci USA 2012; 109(9): 3510-5.
[http://dx.doi.org/10.1073/pnas.1112209109] [PMID: 22308347]

[38] Grover A, Shandilya A, Agrawal V, Bisaria VS, Sundar D. Computational evidence to inhibition of human acetyl cholinesterase by withanolide a for Alzheimer treatment. J Biomol Struct Dyn 2012; 29(4): 651-62.
[http://dx.doi.org/10.1080/07391102.2012.10507408] [PMID: 22208270]

[39] Jayaprakasam B, Padmanabhan K, Nair MG. Withanamides in *Withania somnifera* fruit protect PC-12 cells from β-amyloid responsible for Alzheimer's disease. Phytother Res 2010; 24(6): 859-63.
[http://dx.doi.org/10.1002/ptr.3033] [PMID: 19957250]

[40] Patil SP, Maki S, Khedkar SA, Rigby AC, Chan C. Withanolide A and asiatic acid modulate multiple targets associated with amyloid-β precursor protein processing and amyloid-β protein clearance. J Nat Prod 2010; 73(7): 1196-202.
[http://dx.doi.org/10.1021/np900633j] [PMID: 20553006]

[41] Shinde P, Vidyasagar N, Dhulap S, Dhulap A, Hirwani R. Natural Products based P-glycoprotein Activators for Improved β-amyloid Clearance in Alzheimer's Disease: An *in silico* Approach Central Nervous System Agents in Medicinal Chemistry (Formerly Current Medicinal Chemistry-Central Nervous System Agents) 2016; 16(1): 50-9.

[42] Kuboyama T, Tohda C, Komatsu K. Withanoside IV and its active metabolite, sominone, attenuate Aβ(25-35)-induced neurodegeneration. Eur J Neurosci 2006; 23(6): 1417-26.
[http://dx.doi.org/10.1111/j.1460-9568.2006.04664.x] [PMID: 16553605]

[43] Vareed SK, Bauer AK, Nair KM, Liu Y, Jayaprakasam B, Nair MG. Blood-brain barrier permeability of bioactive withanamides present in *Withania somnifera* fruit extract. Phytother Res 2014; 28(8): 1260-4.
[http://dx.doi.org/10.1002/ptr.5118] [PMID: 24458838]

[44] Jana CK, Hoecker J, Woods TM, Jessen HJ, Neuburger M, Gademann K. Synthesis of withanolide A, biological evaluation of its neuritogenic properties, and studies on secretase inhibition. Angew Chem Int Ed 2011; 50(36): 8407-11.
[http://dx.doi.org/10.1002/anie.201101869] [PMID: 21766402]

[45] Rascol O. "Disease-modification" trials in Parkinson disease: Target populations, endpoints and study design. Neurology 2009; 72(7, Supplement 2) (Suppl.): S51-8.
[http://dx.doi.org/10.1212/WNL.0b013e318199049e] [PMID: 19221315]

[46] Piggott MA, Marshall EF, Thomas N, *et al.* Striatal dopaminergic markers in dementia with Lewy bodies, Alzheimer's and Parkinson's diseases: rostrocaudal distribution. Brain 1999; 122(8): 1449-68.
[http://dx.doi.org/10.1093/brain/122.8.1449] [PMID: 10430831]

[47] Hinterberger H. The biochemistry of catecholamines in relation to Parkinson's disease. Aust N Z J Med 1971; 1: 14-18, 14-18.
[http://dx.doi.org/10.1111/j.1445-5994.1971.tb02560.x] [PMID: 5292808]

[48] Olanow CW. The pathogenesis of cell death in Parkinson's disease – 2007. Mov Disord 2007; 22(S17) (Suppl. 17): S335-42.
[http://dx.doi.org/10.1002/mds.21675] [PMID: 18175394]

[49] Prakash J, Chouhan S, Yadav SK, Westfall S, Rai SN, Singh SP. *Withania somnifera* alleviates parkinsonian phenotypes by inhibiting apoptotic pathways in dopaminergic neurons. Neurochem Res

2014; 39(12): 2527-36.
[http://dx.doi.org/10.1007/s11064-014-1443-7] [PMID: 25403619]

[50]   Manjunath MJ, Muralidhara . Standardized extract of *Withania somnifera* (Ashwagandha) markedly offsets rotenone-induced locomotor deficits, oxidative impairments and neurotoxicity in Drosophila melanogaster. J Food Sci Technol 2015; 52(4): 1971-81.
[http://dx.doi.org/10.1007/s13197-013-1219-0] [PMID: 25829577]

[51]   Ahmad M, Saleem S, Ahmad AS, *et al.* Neuroprotective effects of *Withania somnifera* on 6-hydroxydopamine induced Parkinsonism in rats. Hum Exp Toxicol 2005; 24(3): 137-47.
[http://dx.doi.org/10.1191/0960327105ht509oa] [PMID: 15901053]

[52]   RajaSankar S, Manivasagam T, Sankar V, *et al. Withania somnifera* root extract improves catecholamines and physiological abnormalities seen in a Parkinson's disease model mouse. J Ethnopharmacol 2009; 125(3): 369-73.
[http://dx.doi.org/10.1016/j.jep.2009.08.003] [PMID: 19666100]

[53]   De Rose F, Marotta R, Poddighe S, *et al.* Functional and morphological correlates in the *Drosophila* LRRK2 loss-of-function model of Parkinson's disease: drug effects of *Withania somnifera* (Dunal) administration. PLoS One 2016; 11(1): e0146140.
[http://dx.doi.org/10.1371/journal.pone.0146140] [PMID: 26727265]

[54]   Nakayama N, Tohda C. Withanoside IV improves hindlimb function by facilitating axonal growth and increase in peripheral nervous system myelin level after spinal cord injury. Neurosci Res 2007; 58(2): 176-82.
[http://dx.doi.org/10.1016/j.neures.2007.02.014] [PMID: 17386954]

[55]   Teshigawara K, Kuboyama T, Shigyo M, *et al.* A novel compound, denosomin, ameliorates spinal cord injury *via* axonal growth associated with astrocyte-secreted vimentin. Br J Pharmacol 2013; 168(4): 903-19.
[http://dx.doi.org/10.1111/j.1476-5381.2012.02211.x] [PMID: 22978525]

[56]   Gautam A, Wadhwa R, Thakur MK. Involvement of hippocampal Arc in amnesia and its recovery by alcoholic extract of Ashwagandha leaves. Neurobiol Learn Mem 2013; 106: 177-84.
[http://dx.doi.org/10.1016/j.nlm.2013.08.009] [PMID: 24012642]

[57]   Kumar G, Patnaik R. Exploring neuroprotective potential of *Withania somnifera* phytochemicals by inhibition of GluN2B-containing NMDA receptors: An *in silico* study. Med Hypotheses 2016; 92: 35-43.
[http://dx.doi.org/10.1016/j.mehy.2016.04.034] [PMID: 27241252]

[58]   Manchanda S, Mishra R, Singh R, Kaur T, Kaur G. Aqueous leaf extract of *Withania somnifera* as a potential neuroprotective agent in sleep-deprived rats: a mechanistic study. Mol Neurobiol 2017; 54(4): 3050-61.
[http://dx.doi.org/10.1007/s12035-016-9883-5] [PMID: 27037574]

[59]   Kataria H, Kumar S, Chaudhary H, Kaur G. *Withania somnifera* suppresses tumor growth of intracranial allograft of glioma cells. Mol Neurobiol 2016; 53(6): 4143-58.
[http://dx.doi.org/10.1007/s12035-015-9320-1] [PMID: 26208698]

[60]   Candelario M, Cuellar E, Reyes-Ruiz JM, *et al.* Direct evidence for GABAergic activity of *Withania somnifera* on mammalian ionotropic GABAA and GABAρ receptors. J Ethnopharmacol 2015; 171: 264-72.
[http://dx.doi.org/10.1016/j.jep.2015.05.058] [PMID: 26068424]

[61]   Parihar P, Shetty R, Ghafourifar P, Parihar MS. Increase in oxidative stress and mitochondrial impairment in hypothalamus of streptozotocin treated diabetic rat: Antioxidative effect of *Withania somnifera*. Cell Mol Biol 2016; 62(1): 73-83.
[PMID: 26828992]

[62]   Kumar P, Singh R, Nazmi A, Lakhanpal D, Kataria H, Kaur G. Glioprotective effects of Ashwagandha leaf extract against lead induced toxicity. Biomed Res Int. 2014;2014..

[63]   Yin H, Cho DH, Park SJ, Han SK. GABA-mimetic actions of *Withania somnifera* on substantia gelatinosa neurons of the trigeminal subnucleus caudalis in mice. Am J Chin Med 2013; 41(5): 1043-51.
[http://dx.doi.org/10.1142/S0192415X13500705] [PMID: 24117067]

[64]   Keswani C. Bioeconomy for Sustainable Development. Springer 2020.
[http://dx.doi.org/10.1007/978-981-13-9431-7]

[65]   Konar A, Shah N, Singh R, *et al.* Protective role of Ashwagandha leaf extract and its component withanone on scopolamine-induced changes in the brain and brain-derived cells. PLoS One 2011; 6(11): e27265.
[http://dx.doi.org/10.1371/journal.pone.0027265] [PMID: 22096544]

[66]   Nair V, Arjuman A, Gopalakrishna HN, Nandini M. Effect of*Withania somnifera* root extract on haloperidol-induced catalepsy in albino mice. Phytother Res 2008; 22(2): 243-6.
[http://dx.doi.org/10.1002/ptr.2299] [PMID: 17886228]

[67]   Kuboyama T, Tohda C, Zhao J, Nakamura N, Hattori M, Komatsu K. Axon- or dendrite-predominant outgrowth induced by constituents from Ashwagandha. Neuroreport 2002; 13(14): 1715-20.
[http://dx.doi.org/10.1097/00001756-200210070-00005] [PMID: 12395110]

CHAPTER 13

Modulation of Proinflammatory Cytokines by Flavonoids in the Main Age-related Neurodegenerative Diseases

Héctor Eduardo López-Valdés[1,*] and **Hilda Martínez-Coria[1]**

[1] Departamento de Fisiología, Facultad de Medicina, Universidad Nacional Autónoma de México (UNAM), Ciudad de México, México

Abstract: Aging is a process associated with distinctive changes in physiological functions and physical appearance that result from progressive tissue degeneration, harming the structure and function of vital organs. Illnesses that are particularly frequent in people 65 years of age and older are generally grouped as age-related diseases or aging-related diseases and include neurodegenerative diseases such as Alzheimer's disease (AD) and Parkinson's disease (PD), which are caused by progressive degeneration and/or neuronal death to produce debilitating conditions, and they have no cure. For these illnesses, the most important risk factor is aging. Aging involves changes in neuroendocrine and inflammatory responses and presents a stage with chronic and low-grade inflammation, characterized by a general increase in the production of proinflammatory cytokines, inflammatory markers, and cellular senescence. Herbal medicine, as well as various components of the human diet, including vegetables, cereals, and fruits, contain widely varied phytochemicals including flavonoids, which are the most common polyphenolic compounds. Epidemiological studies suggest that a higher intake of flavonoid-rich foods and beverages is associated with better cognitive outcomes, lower dementia rates, and reduced risk of neurodegenerative diseases. Moreover, numerous preclinical studies have shown that these compounds have a therapeutic effect on animal models of human degenerative diseases and highlight the anti-inflammatory effect of flavonoids by decreasing the activated glial cells and several proinflammatory mediators. Much modern scientific research has focused on establishing biological activities of purified single compounds to provide an evidence base for the rationale of traditional practice, and also to integrate these into modern medical practice.

Keywords: Aging, Age-related diseases, Flavonoids, Neurodegenerative diseases.

---

* **Corresponding author Hector Eduardo Lopez Valdes:** Departamento de Fisiología, Facultad de Medicina, Universidad Nacional Autónoma de México (UNAM), Ciudad de México, México; E-mail: helopezv@gmail.com

Surya Pratap Singh, Hagera Dilnashin, Hareram Birla & Chetan Keswani (Eds.)

INTRODUCTION

Aging is an irreversible and inevitable process associated with distinctive changes in physiological functions and physical appearance, that result from progressive tissue degeneration, harming the structure and function of vital organs [1]. For the vast majority of chronic diseases, including chronic obstructive pulmonary disease (COPD), atherosclerosis, hypertension, osteoporosis, osteoarthritis cardiac failure, type 2 diabetes, metabolic syndrome, chronic renal disease, neurodegenerative diseases, and cancer, the most important risk factor is aging [2, 3]. Neurodegenerative diseases are a heterogeneous group of conditions caused by progressive degeneration and/or neuronal death to produce debilitating conditions and have no cure. These groups include Alzheimer's disease (AD), vascular dementia (VaD), Lewy body dementia (LBD), Parkinson's disease (PD) Huntington's disease (HD), amyotrophic lateral sclerosis (ALS), and frontotemporal dementia [4, 5]. Herbal medicine, as well as components of the human diet, including teas, wine, vegetables, cereals and fruits, contains varied phytochemicals including flavonoids, which are the most common polyphenolic compounds [6]. Numerous preclinical studies have shown that these compounds have a therapeutic effect on animal models of human degenerative diseases. The mechanism and active compounds for most of the herbs used in medicine are still not well-defined because they contain multiple bioactive molecules and consequently can modulate multiple pharmacologic targets. This rich source of bioactive molecules has been the subject of much modern scientific research, concentrating mainly on establishing biological activities of purified single compounds to provide an evidence base for the rationale of traditional practice, and also to integrate them into modern medical practice [7].

In the sections below, we will describe the basic knowledge of flavonoids, aging, neuroinflammation, AD, PD, and HD, and we will provide an overview of the evidence relating to the anti-inflammatory effects of single flavonoids in different model systems of these diseases.

FLAVONOIDS

Flavonoids are the most common group of plant polyphenols, they are present in all vascular plants and have a wide range of functions in plant biochemistry, physiology, and ecologies, such as coloration of flower petals, fertility, and pollen germination, and in protection against ultraviolet light. Moreover, a single plant will often contain several dozens of different flavonoids [8]. Flavonoids are low-molecular-weight phenolic compounds that are widely distributed in the plant kingdom and are the main phytochemicals found in more than 6000 species of plants, and they also are abundantly found in foods and beverages of plant origin, including vegetables, fruits, grains roots, wine, tea and cocoa [9].

Structurally, flavonoids occur as glycosides, methylated derivatives, and aglycones, and the latter of which represent the basic structure that has a shared C6–C3–C6 structure containing two aromatic rings (A and B rings) that are linked by a three-carbon bridge (Fig. **1**), creating an oxygenated heterocycle. This type of structure is commonly divided into subclasses based on the connection of the B ring to the C ring, as well as the oxidation state and functional groups of the C ring [10]. Depending on the carbon of the C ring on which the B ring is attached and the degree of unsaturation and oxidation, flavonoids can be subdivided into different subgroups such as flavones, flavonols, flavanones, flavanonols, flavanols (or catechins), anthocyanins, chalcones, and isoflavonoids [9] (Fig. **1**).

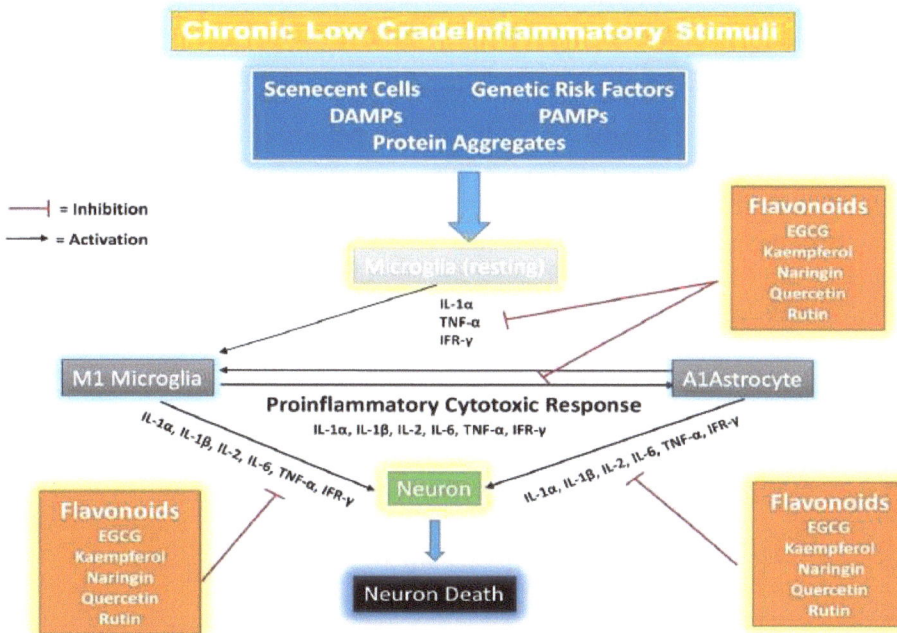

Fig. (1). Basic structure of flavonoid and flavonoids subgroups. Below of each flavonoid subgroup, some representative compounds.

To be absorbed from the small intestine upon ingestion, the flavonoids contained in foods and beverages must be in the aglycones form to allow them to pass from the gut lumen into the circulatory system. Except for catechins, all flavonoids are in the form of glycosides, therefore, the attached sugar must be removed. One mechanism to remove the sugar and release the aglycone form is by hydrolysis performed by lactase phlorizin hydrolase (LPH) in the brush-border of the small intestine epithelial cells and after it has been released, the molecule can enter into epithelial cells. An alternative mechanism to remove sugar by hydrolysis is the cytosolic β-glucosidase (CBG). For that to happen, the polar glycosides must be transported into the epithelial cells, possibly with the involvement of the active sodium-dependent glucose transporter. Before passing into the bloodstream, the flavonoid aglycones undergo conjugation reactions forming sulfate, glucuronide, and/or methylated metabolites (conjugates) that can be subjected to additional phase II metabolism in the liver, and then returned to the circulatory system, but some conjugates may be exported into the bile duct. Conjugates can be excreted by the kidney and the flavonoids not absorbed from the small intestine will be degraded in the colon [11]. Apart from catechins, all flavonoids in plasma and urine are mainly conjugated forms. Thus, cells in the body are usually exposed to less active flavonoid metabolites and conjugates rather than aglycones [12]. However, an *in vivo* study showed that glucuronidated quercetin metabolites were deconjugated quercetin in its aglycone form in the mesenteric vasculature of rats, from the action of a β-glucuronidase, and this effect was inhibited when a β-glucuronidase inhibitor was present [13], which suggests that deconjugation may occur in situ, to produce a more effective aglycone form. Members of ATP-binding-cassette (ABC) transport systems, which translocate solutes across cell membranes, are responsible for most of the absorption and distribution of flavonoids around the body as well as their excretion in urine [11]. The absorption of the flavonoids will depend on their physicochemical properties such as molecular size, lipophilicity, solubility, configuration, and pKa value [14]. Between flavonoids, there is great variability in the magnitude and velocity of absorption, the rate of elimination, plasma half-life, bioavailability, and plasma kinetics, but in general, they have low bioavailability and rapid urinary and biliary excretion and it has been suggested that with a regular diet, their plasma concentration rarely exceeds 1 μM after the consumption of 10-100 mg of a single phenolic compound [15]. Also analyzing 97 bioavailability studies on humans, Manach *et al.* [16], found that plasma concentrations of total metabolites ranged from 0 to 4 μmol/L with an intake of 50 mg aglycone equivalents, and the relative urinary excretion ranged from 0.3% to 43% of the ingested dose, depending on the polyphenol. They also found that among the 97 flavonoids analyzed, gallic acid and isoflavones had the best rate of absorption, followed by catechins, flavanones, and quercetin glycosides, and that proanthocyanidins and anthocyanins had very low bioavailability. There is some evidence that flavonoids and/or their metabolites can enter the brain, for example, anthocyanins and (−)-

epicatechin and some of their metabolites [17 - 19]. Flavonoids have received much attention because of their potential to exert beneficial health effects and this is due to their extensive range of biological activities in the prevention of several diseases including cancer, gastrointestinal disorders, and neurodegenerative diseases, among others. The beneficial effects of flavonoids are related to several effects including antioxidant, antibacterial, antiviral and anti-inflammatory activities [20]. However, the majority of the studies on anti-inflammatory activities were performed *in-vitro*, using generally the aglycone form and usually with supraphysiological concentration, while research involving flavonoid conjugates, animal models and human studies has been limited [21].

AGING

Aging is an inevitable and complex process that results from the interaction of many factors, including genetic, epigenetic, and environmental, causing a progressive reduction of homeostasis with age, characterized by progressive degeneration of tissue and functions of several vital organs which contributes to increasing the risk of disease and death [22, 23]. Aging affects brain regions, cell types, and cellular structures differently, with considerable individual variations, but in general, there is a decrease in the grey and white matter density, focal abnormalities in the white matter and basal ganglia, and atrophy of specific brain regions including the hippocampus [24]. A diverse group of illnesses that increase their frequency in people 65 years of age and older are grouped as age-related diseases or aging-related diseases, and this group includes illnesses such as cancer, hypertension, arthritis, type 2 diabetes, stroke, and many neurodegenerative diseases including AD and PD [25]. In the nervous system, there are alterations associated with normal aging that include structural and functional changes. Structural changes include cerebral atrophy, blood flow reductions, neuronal loss and enlargement of the ventricles. Functional changes include a decrease in synapses and neurotransmitter release. Moreover, aging affects the brain's structures differently and the most commonly affected is the hippocampus [26]. Major alterations or hallmarks in aging, include telomere attrition, genomic instability, mitochondrial dysfunction, loss of proteostasis, cellular senescence, epigenetic alterations, deregulated nutrient-sensing, stem cell exhaustion, and altered intercellular communication [23]. In the latter, aging involves changes in neuroendocrine and inflammatory responses and a noticeable alteration known as 'inflammaging', a stage with chronic and low-grade inflammation, characterized by a general increase in the production of proinflammatory cytokines and inflammatory markers [27]. Another important feature in aging is the cellular senescence in tissues and organs including the immune system (immunosenescence), which is characterized by reduced humoral immune responses and a decrease in cell-mediated immune function for both innate and adaptive immune systems [28]. Senescent cells are characterized by a failure to re-enter the cell cycle in response to mitogenic stimuli, increased activity of senescence-associated β-galactosidase (SA-β-GAL), a pro-inflammatory secretome, called senescence-associated secretory phenotype (SASP), and resistance to cell death [29, 30]. Cellular senescence can be induced by several common factors in aging including oxidative stress, neuroinflammation and DNA damage, and, due to their increased presence in different neurodegenerative diseases, it has been suggested that cellular senescence contributes to the pathophysiology of these disorders [31]. In the age-related diseases, some of the inflammaging characteristics are observed in blood, for example, monocytes exhibit impaired phagocytosis and higher intracellular levels of TNF-α [32], presence of senescent T cells [33], impaired macrophage polarization, antibody production by the activated B cells [34], impaired M1 and M2 macrophages [35], and high levels of proinflammatory cytokines (*e.g.*, IL-1β, IL-6, IL-8, IL-10) in sera [36]. These circulating proinflammatory molecules can interact with a receptor on endothelial cells from cerebral vasculature, which leads to the release of more cytokines that can induce impairment of BBB integrity [37], and thus systemic inflammation may contribute to neuroinflammation in age-related neurodegeneration disorders. Another factor that is present in neurodegenerative age-related diseases is oxidative stress. Oxidative stress and neuroinflammation are strongly related. Oxidative stress is the result of excessive production of a group of unstable molecules that contains oxygen called reactive oxygen species (ROS), and the antioxidant system in the cells and tissues is not able to neutralize them. The imbalance in this protective mechanism can lead to the damage of cellular molecules, including DNA, proteins, and lipids [38]. Mitochondrial oxidative metabolism in cells produces ROS species in the process of cell respiration and it has been shown that a proinflammatory cytokine such as TNF-α promotes over-production of ROS in mitochondria to cause oxidative stress [39]. On the other hand, mitochondrial dysfunction can result in the release of the damage-associated molecular pattern (DAMPs) within the cytosol or the extracellular environment thereby instigating innate immune activation and can also activate the NLRP3 inflammasome, which leads to the production of IL1-β [40, 41]. Different counter regulatory mechanisms have been identified and include proteins that inhibit signal transduction pathways such as the suppressor of cytokine signaling proteins (SOCS), induction of transcriptional repressors (*e.g.*, ATF3), and production of mediators with anti-inflammatory activities (*e.g.*, IL-10 and transforming growth factor-beta or TGF-β). However, it is not well understood how these negative feedback pathways are integrated with pro-inflammatory signaling pathways [42].

NEUROINFLAMMATION

Neuroinflammation is a complex inflammatory reaction in the central nervous system (CNS) and is typically induced when innate immune cells detect tissue damage or infection. This response is essential to isolate damaged tissue from uninjured areas and to clean and repair the extracellular matrix, while in general; acute inflammation is beneficial and promotes regeneration. However, prolonged and excessive inflammation, as well as stable low-grade, can lead to the onset or exacerbation of cell injury [5], and it is widely accepted that low-grade neuroinflammation is the key factor in the onset and progression of several neurological diseases. The CNS glial cell presents different activities under different situations of neuroinflammation, and thus it can contribute to protecting or exacerbating the damage, depending on the period and particular environments of inflammation. The major sources for low-grade chronic inflammation in aging, are endogenous host-derived cell debris that accumulate with age as a consequence of both impaired elimination and increased production, senescent cells, and immunosenescence, but these processes are not typically the initiating factor of neurodegenerative diseases, nevertheless, the production of neurotoxic factors by inflammatory cells amplifying the disease states, would suggest that neuroinflammation plays an important role in neuronal dysfunction and death [43, 44]. All glial cells including microglia, astrocytes, oligodendrocytes, and glial antigen-2 (NG2) glial cells (also known as oligodendrocyte precursor cells; OPCs), play a role in the immune response, but the most important are the microglia and astrocytes. Microglia is the resident innate immune cell in the CNS, the most motile cell, continuously scanning the microenvironment of parenchyma, and it is the first cell that responds to any damage stimulation [45]. Astrocytes are the most abundant cell type in the CNS and have diverse homeostatic functions, for example, extracellular K^+ buffering, control of extracellular pH is due to several H^+ and HCO^{3-} transporting enzymes, neurotransmitter uptake, and recycling of glutamate and GABA, they regulate cerebral blood flow and the blood-brain barrier (BBB) antioxidant functions, promote synaptogenesis, supply energy metabolites to neurons and form part of the innate immune system of the CNS [46, 47]. During injury or disease, glial cells can recognize molecules present in pathogens (pathogen-associated molecular patterns; PAMPs) and endogenous molecules released by damaged or dead cells (DAMPs) through the pattern recognition receptors (PRR), which are formed by four major subfamilies: the C-type lectin receptors (CLRs), the retinoic acid-inducible gene 1 (RIG-1) - like receptors (RLR; aka RIG-1-like helicases—RLH), the nucleotide-binding oligomerization domain (NOD)- Leucine Rich Repeats (LRR)-containing receptors (NLR) and the Toll-like receptors (TLRs) [48]. TLRs are the best-known member of PRR and are type 1 transmembrane glycoproteins that are extensively expressed in microglia and astrocytes, with specific members expressed in neurons in the CNS [49]. Each TLR recognizes different DAMPs or PAMPs, for example, TLR4 recognizes accumulated misfolded proteins, including α-synuclein and Aβ present in PD and AD, respectively [50, 51]. DAMPs include a wide range of molecules such as cytokine IL-1α, uric acid, ATP and cytoplasmic and nuclear proteins released during necrosis, and it also has been suggested that those other members of the extended IL-1 cytokine family including IL-1β, IL-18, IL-33, IL-36α, IL-36β, and IL-36γ also act as DAMPs and stimulate the sterile inflammation induced by necrosis [30]. The binding of ligands to the TLR of the host cell activates an intracellular signaling cascade that leads to the release of inflammatory cytokines and immune modulators, as a mechanism against invaders and to repair the damaged tissue, but excessive TLR activation disturbs the immune homeostasis inducing sustained proinflammatory cytokines and chemokine production, which contributes to the development and progression of many diseases [52]. After TLR recognition of specific stimulus, the TLR activates one of the several signal transduction pathways such as mitogen-activated protein kinase (MAPK), phosphoinositide 3-kinase/protein kinase B (PI3K/AKT), or mammalian target of rapamycin (mTOR), which leads to activation of different transcription factors including nuclear factor kappa-B (NF-κB), activator protein 1 (AP-1) and interferon regulatory factor 3 (IRF3), which mediate the production of chemokines and inducible enzymes, proinflammatory cytokines, and induce nitric oxide synthase (iNOS) and cyclooxygenase-2 (COX-2), which all result in neuroinflammation (44,52). Activation of different TLR receptors can produce activation of different signaling pathways including PI3K/AKT/mTOR, which activate the transcription factor NF-κB and promote the expression of proinflammatory molecules including cytokines (*e.g.* IL-6 and TNF-α), iNOS, and COX-2, while other receptors activate MAPK (p38 MAPK or SAPK/JNK), which then activate the transcription factor AP-1 and promote the expression of proinflammatory molecules including cytokines (e. g. IL-6), iNOS and COX-2 [44]. Another well-known PRR is a member of the NOD subfamily, the cytosolic NOD-like receptor 3, which is part of the inflammasome NLRP3, together with procaspase 1 and the adaptor protein apoptosis-associated speck-like protein comprising a caspase recruitment domain (ASC), which together form an oligomer when stimuli activate the receptor and induce the active precursors of proinflammatory cytokines, such as IL-1β, IL-1α and IL-18 [30, 53]. These cytokines are polypeptides and glycoproteins synthesized by immune cells and constitute the major communication mechanism used by the immune system and include interleukins (IL), lymphokines, chemokines, interferons (IFN), and tumor necrosis factor (TNF), which can act as pro-and anti-inflammatory molecules [54]. Proinflammatory cytokines include: IL-1α and IL-1β, IL-2, IL-6, IL-12, IL-15, IL-16, IL-17, IL-18, IL-22, IL-23, IL-27, TNF-α and IFN, while the anti-inflammatory cytokines include: IL-1 Rα, IL-10, IL-11 and heat-shock proteins

[55]. Once released to the extracellular space, cytokines interact with cytokine receptors to initiate intracellular signaling, which regulates a diverse range of biological functions. Cytokine receptors share the feature of activating the JAK-STAT pathway [56]. The main proinflammatory cytokines, such as IL-6, TNF-α, and IL-1α, contribute significantly to the phenomenon of inflammaging in healthy elderly individuals and play a major role in many age-related diseases, including neurodegenerative age-related diseases [30]. Moreover, TNF-α also induces apoptosis by activating receptors containing a homologous cytoplasmic sequence identifying an intracellular death domain including tumor necrosis factor receptor 1 (TNFR1), 2 (p75), and CD95 (APO-1/Fas) [44]. Microglia and astrocytes can release pro and anti-inflammatory responses and the character of the neuroinflammation is related to the phenotypes of the glial cells and their interaction with each other. The different phenotypes that show glial cells are the result of transcriptional and functional changes that are generally known as activation or reactivity. Although several different phenotypes have been observed, the reactivity of microglia generally is referred to as M1 for detrimental and neurotoxic inflammation functions and M2 for pro reparative and anti-inflammation functions. Similarly, the A1 astrocytes phenotype is toxic to neurons and oligodendrocytes, and A2 astrocytes promote neuroprotection [57, 58]. M1 microglia as well astrocytes A1 are highly present in human neurodegenerative illnesses including PD, AD, and HD, and it has been proposed that M1 microglia induces the A1 astrocyte phenotype in this illness [57, 59]. Proinflammatory cytokines releasing from M1 microglia and A1 astrocytes can induce apoptosis through activation of extrinsic pathways and also induce DNA damage, overproduction of ROS, mitochondrial dysfunction, and production of larger amounts of inflammatory mediators that promote cell aging, inducing the permeabilization of the BBB, and the infiltration of peripheral leukocytes that may contribute to a harmful brain inflammatory reaction [44, 60]. Activated microglia and astrocytes have been found in most types of CNS diseases, all of which have a neuroinflammatory component [42, 57].

NEURODEGENERATIVE AGE-RELATED DISEASES

During aging, glial cells gradually lose some homeostatic functions and cannot provide pathogen clearance to neuron support and defensive responses, leading to susceptibility of the CNS to damages. Also, some neurodegenerative age-related diseases show the aggregation of toxic proteins such as Aβ in AD, α-synuclein in PD, and polyQ in HD. These toxic protein aggregates induce glial cell activation leading to chronic CNS inflammation [49, 61]. In the following sections, we will briefly describe the pathology of AD, PD, and HD.

Alzheimer's Disease (AD)

AD is a chronic disease manifesting as loss of memory, language, cognition, and problem-solving skills and changes in behavior, and ultimately death. AD is a progressive neurodegenerative disorder that results in synapse loss and neuronal atrophy from wide areas of the cerebral cortex and hippocampus [62]. The pathology appears to start within the hippocampus and entorhinal regions and spreads subsequently throughout the frontotemporal cortices [63]. Clinically, AD is commonly divided into idiopathic or sporadic AD (SAD) and familial AD (FAD). SAD is the most common type and has a mean onset age of 80 years. Another classification takes into account the lifetime because age is considered to be the principal risk factor for AD, and it is used as a categorical marker. The two main disease categories include early-onset and late-onset AD, based on the age when individuals start to present symptoms. Early-onset accounts for 3% of the reported cases of AD, occurring before age 65, and most of the cases are FAD. FAD is due to dominant genetic mutations in the amyloid-beta (Aβ) A4 precursor protein (APP), presenilin 1 (PSEN1), and presenilin 2 (PSEN2), while most late-onset AD is sporadic, has no single genetic cause, and represents over 95% of all AD cases [64, 65]. In addition to these three genes (APP, PSEN1, and PSEN2), the strongest genetic risk factor for AD is the ε4 allele of apolipoprotein E (ApoE). ApoE is a class of proteins involved in lipid metabolism and is immunochemically colocalized to senile plaques, vascular amyloid deposits, and neurofibrillary tangles (NFTs) in AD [66]. Environmental and metabolic risk factors such as diabetes, cerebrovascular disease, poor diet, head injury, and stress are linked to an increased risk of dementia [62]. AD is associated with the accumulation of insoluble forms of Aβ in plaques and intraneuronal deposition of NFTs composed of hyperphosphorylated tau protein. Aβ is derived from the proteolytic cleavage of the APP by a complex family of enzymes, which include PSEN1 and PSEN2 [67]. The amyloid hypothesis suggests that APP mis-metabolism and Aβ deposition are the primary events in AD. APP is cleaved in two ways: α and β pathways. In the α pathway, APP is hydrolyzed by α-secretase and then by γ-secretase. This process does not produce insoluble Aβ. The β pathway is through the hydrolyzed APP by β-secretase (BACE1) and then by γ-secretase to produce insoluble Aβ and some mutations are prone to hydrolysis by the β pathway, resulting in an excessive accumulation of insoluble Aβ and eventually the development of AD [68]. The tau propagation hypothesis suggests that aggregates of fibrillar and misfolded tau may propagate through cells in a prion-like way, eventually spreading through the brains of AD patients. The main function of tau is to stabilize microtubules. The alterations in the function of tau phosphorylation may be due to changes in the activities of kinases or phosphatases that target tau, and thus, the toxicity of tau can be augmented as a result [69]. The pathological hallmarks (Aβ plaques and NFTs) are often complemented by additional morphological changes including synaptic loss, neuronal loss, microglial activation, reactive astrocytes, neurovascular dysfunction, disruption of the blood-brain barrier, and brain atrophy [70]. The inflammatory responses of microglia and astrocytes in the CNS also play important roles in the development of AD. The fibrillar conformation of Aβ seems to be crucial to the cytokine-induced activation of microglia. Aβ can bind to microglia cells through the CD36-TLR4-TLR6 receptor complex and the NLRP3 inflammatory complex, destroy cells, release inflammation-inducing factors, such as TNF-α, and cause immune responses. In addition to increased levels of TNF-α, increased levels of the inflammatory cytokines IL-1β, TGF-β, IL-12, and IL-18 in the CNS are also correlated with AD progression and increased damage in the brains of AD patients [71]. Moreover, Aβ activates the NF-κB pathway in astrocytes to release complement C3 and, since high levels of C3 expression are related to cognitive impairment, and antagonist treatment rescues the alterations, this would suggest that this dysregulation contributes to neuroinflammation [72, 73]. Proinflammatory cytokines (IL-1α, C1q, and TNF) released by activated microglia induce a proinflammatory A1 astrocytes phenotype, which may result in the implication of inflammation [57]. In post-mortem analyses of AD patients, microglia shows alterations in its morphology, such as reduced branching and arborized area, and immunoreactivity to ionized calcium-binding adaptor molecule 1 (Iba 1), which is a microglia/macrophage-specific calcium-binding protein that is upregulated in activated microglia [74]. Activated microglia have been detected in several imaging studies in humans, taking advantage of the increase in the density of the target translocator protein (TSPO) on the external mitochondrial membrane on active microglia and the availability of labeled molecules that bind selectively to these proteins, which are used as markers (*e.g.,* [11]PK11195) in positron emission tomography (PET) studies. Activated microglia were observed in the entorhinal, temporoparietal, and cingulate cortex [75]. Moreover, microglial activation was confirmed in other studies using only activated microglia markers (*e.g.,* [11] PK11195 and [11] PBR28) or in combination with Aβ plaques markers (*e.g.,* [18] F-flutemetamol) and/or tau (*e.g.,* [18] F-AV145). Activated microglia were found in the occipital lobe in AD patients [76]. Another study found that AD patients increases microglial activation and Aβ in the frontal, temporal, parietal, occipital, and cingulate cortices [77].

Microglial activation, tau aggregation, and Aβ deposition were found in similar areas of the association cortex [78]. The results of a longitudinal PET study (14 months) to evaluate the change in microglia activation in mild cognitive impairment (MCI) and AD patients showed that activated microglia in MCI patients was reduced in contrast to AD patients that presented activated microglia [79]. In another study, the researchers used 11 PK11195 PET in combination with structural magnetic resonance imaging (structural MRI) to estimate brain atrophy, and they found tau in the temporoparietal area and activated microglia in the anterior temporal and grey matter atrophy [80]. A similar study found that activated microglia were observed in temporal cortices and related to parieto-occipital atrophy and cortical thinning [81].

Parkinson's Disease (PD)

PD is a multifactorial and age-related neurodegenerative disorder, characterized by the presence of tremors at rest, rigidity, postural instability, and bradykinesia symptoms, and it shares the Lewy body (LB) inclusions in neuron and glial cells, composed mainly of α-synuclein protein with other clinical syndromes referred to as "Parkinsonism" Disorders [82]. The other pathological characteristic in PD is the degeneration of neurons in one of the basal ganglia, the substantia nigra pars compacta (SNpc), where these cells are involved in the transmission of dopamine (DA) to the other basal ganglia nucleus and the striatum [83]. The basal ganglia process the signal from the cerebral cortex to perform accurate voluntary movements and are also involved in cognitive functions [84]. Along with the alterations previously mentioned, some PD patients also show olfactory dysfunction, sleep disorders, autonomic dysfunction, pain, fatigue, depression, anxiety, and dementia [85]. Idiopathic PD is the most common form of this disease and together with aging, several environmental or behavioral factors increase the risk of PD, such as consumption of dairy products, exposure to pesticides, history of melanoma, and traumatic brain injury [86]. Genetic forms of PD include monogenic mutations in eight genes that encode proteins, including DJ-1, PTEN-induced putative, Parkin, Coiled-coil-helix-coiled-coil-helix (CHCHD10), Receptor-mediated endocytosis 8 (REM-8) domain containing 2, Eukaryotic translation initiation factor 4-γ 1 kinase 1, Vacuolar protein sorting 35, Leucine-rich repeat kinase 2, and α-synuclein, in which missense mutations have been found, as well as gene duplications and triplications [87]. In its physiological condition, α-synuclein has two conformations, as soluble unfolded monomer and multimeric membrane-bound helical α-synuclein. It participates in vesicle trafficking, DA synthesis, transport neurotransmitter release, and synaptic plasticity. Still, under pathological conditions, the soluble unfolded monomer forms βsheet-like oligomers (protofibrils), which convert into amyloid fibrils and eventually deposit into LBs. Also, the protofibrils and fibrils may propagate by a transcellular mechanism from neuron to neuron [88]. LB inclusions are not only present in neurons of the substantia nigra (SN), but also in other structures such as the basal nucleus of Meynert, raphe nuclei, mesopontine tegmentum, dorsal motor nucleus of the vagus, locus ceruleus, amygdala, and neocortex. Moreover, oligodendroglial also shows inclusions in the midbrain and basal ganglia [82].

Cellular damage in PD is related to neuroinflammation. Gerhard *et al.*, used ((11)C)(R)-(1-(2-chlorophenyl)-N-methyl-N-(1-methyl   propyl)-3-isoquinoline carboxamide) (PK11195) positron emission tomography (PET) in PD patients and found increased activation of microglia on the caudate nucleus, putamen, SN, pons, pre-and postcentral gyrus, and the frontal lobe which corresponds well with the known distribution of neuropathological changes [89]. Furthermore, post-mortem studies on PD patients' brains found increased pro-inflammatory mediators (*e.g.*, TNF-β) and active microglia and astrocytes in the SN [90, 91]. Postmortem studies of PD patients have reported TNF in glial cells in the SN [92]. The 1-methyl-4-phenyl-1,2,3,6tetrahydropyridine (MPTP) animal model of PD, as well as human brains, showed an increase of pro-inflammatory molecules such as COX-2 in nigrostriatal dopaminergic (DAergic) neurons [93]. *In vitro* studies also show that IL-1 increases the alpha-synuclein (α-syn) in neuronal cultures [94] and also that microglia exposed to α-syn induce microglial activation and increase the production of TNF and IL1β [95]. There is evidence that the adaptive immune system also participates in the pathology. The presence of CD4+ and CD8+ T cells has been reported in SN from postmortem studies of PD patients and animal models [96]. This information on neuroinflammation, when analyzed together, shows that inflammatory responses are involved in the pathophysiology of PD.

Huntington's Disease (HD)

HD is an incurable, rare, progressive, and severe neurodegenerative disorder that shows a combination of alterations in the motor, behavior, and cognitive functions that are manifested as uncontrolled movements, emotional problems, and loss of thinking ability that appear at a mean age of 45 years [97]. HD is due to an autosomal dominant inheritance mutation of the *HTT* gene which is located at chromosome 4p16.3 and encodes the protein huntingtin (HTT) [98]. The normal HTT participates in several functions such as endocytosis, intracellular vesicular trafficking, synapses, autophagy, and transcription [99]. The mutated *HTT* gene contains a segment of cytosine, adenine, and guanine repeat known as CAG trinucleotide repeat that appears unusually multiple times (typically 40 - 55 repeats), which causes an abnormally long glutamine stretch or polyglutamine (poly Q) in the mutated protein's N′terminus, which is toxic and causes dysfunction such as oxidative stress, autophagy, disruption of transcription, aggregate formation and cellular death [99, 100]. The most characteristic neuropathological feature of HD includes a shrinking of the neostriatum, atrophy of the caudate nucleus and putamen, reduction in the size of the caudate nucleus, and enlargement of ventricles [101]. At the cellular level, the pathological cascade starts after translocation of the N-terminal of the huntingtin fragment into the nucleus, which takes place after selective proteolysis of polyQ. This protein fragment, together with ubiquitin (which mediates the protein degradation), forms spherical amyloid-like inclusions [102]. These inclusion bodies have been found in different parts of the brain, including the cerebral cortex, striatum, cerebellum, brain stem, and spinal cord [99]. HD also shows other pathologic mechanisms, including oxidative stress and neuroinflammation. In the latter, evidence from post-mortem studies of HD patients and animal models has reported a significant increase in the IL-1β level, activated microglia, and astrogliosis [103, 104]. Moreover, the use of [(11)C)(R)-(1-(2-chlorophenyl)-N-methyl-N-(1-methyl propyl)-3-isoquinoline carboxamide] (PK11195) positron emission tomography (PET) showed activated microglia in HD patients [105, 106]. Microglia activation happens many years before the onset of clinical signs, and the level of microglial activation correlates with HD severity [106, 107]. Furthermore, HD mouse models (R6/2 mouse) have shown that caspase 1 promotes the conversion of inactive pro-IL-1β to active IL1β [104]. In the same mouse model, the expression of proinflammatory factors, such as TNF-α, IFN-γ, and TGFβ1 has been observed in the striatal region [108]. It has also been reported that mHTT is expressed at high levels in microglia and monocytes in human patients [109] and this mutated protein can activate the NF-kB signaling pathway, inducing the release of inflammatory cytokines including IL-6 and IL-8 [110], and also stimulate the enzyme kynurenine 3-monooxygenase (KMO) to increase the production of tryptophan-derived neurotoxins [111]. On the other hand, animal models and clinical studies provide substantial evidence of peripheral inflammation implications in HD. Blood levels of several proinflammatory cytokines, including IL-4, IL-6, IL-8, IL-10, IL-1β, and TNF-α, and also in some organs such as the kidney, heart, liver, and spleen have been reported [112].

EFFECTS OF FLAVONOIDS IN AD, PD, AND HD

The general neuroprotective effects of flavonoids are related to anti-inflammatory and antioxidant activity, which can increase the protection of neurons and glial cells against neurotoxins-induced injury and improve CNS functions. Modulation of molecular pathways involved in neuroinflammation and their modulation by flavonoids have been mainly described in cell cultures, particularly microglia cultures exposed to lipopolysaccharides which have been used as a model of neuroinflammation to explore the general mechanism involved in the anti-inflammatory effects of flavonoids. Activated microglia and astrocytes have been described in AD, PD, and HD, and the *in vitro* studies that show modulatory effects on activation or production of cytokines may apply to AD, PD, and HD.

In-vitro Studies

Flavonoids can produce anti-inflammatory effects through different modulate mechanisms but almost all studies have been conducted with cell cultures using the flavonoid aglycone, therefore these results must be considered carefully. However, they may be used to show a general view of the possible molecular pathways of neuroinflammation modulated by flavonoids in neurodegenerative age-related diseases, and only a few studies using cell cultures of brain neurons and glial cells have been included to illustrate the effects of flavonoids. A well-established method to stimulate the activation of microglia and the production of proinflammatory cytokines *in vitro* as well as *in vivo* is stimulation with lipopolysaccharides (LPS), a toxin from gram-negative bacteria. This toxin is a PAMP that binds the Toll-like receptor 4 (TLR4) to induce the productions of proinflammatory cytokines such as IL-1β, IL-6, and TNF-α, activating several intracellular signaling pathways that include the NF-κB pathway and three mitogen-activated protein kinase (MAPK) pathways: extracellular signal-regulated kinases (ERK) 1 and 2, c-Jun N-terminal kinase (JNK) and p38 to finally activate transcription factors including NF-κB and AP-1 [113]. LPS activates microglia through TNF-α signaling [114]. This activated microglia *in vitro* model has demonstrated that several flavonoids decrease the production of different proinflammatory cytokines. Apigenin, luteolin, naringenin, and quercetin decrease the activation of the transcription factor STAT1 and the production of IL-6 and luteolin also decreases the activation of AP-1 [115, 116]. Scutellarin inhibits the activation of NF-κB, and STAT1, and the expression of TNF-α, and IL-1β [117]. Similar results were obtained with quercetin in the inhibition of the activation of NF-κB and STAT1 [118]. Wooing decreases the production of TNF-α in activated microglia and comparable results were obtained in a co-culture of microglia and astrocytes stimulated with LPS and treated with naringenin, hesperetin, (+)-catechin, and (-)-epicatechin [119, 120]. Icariin inhibits the expression of TNF-α, interleukin (IL)-1beta, and IL-6 in activated microglia [121]. Tangeretin reduces the expression of TNF-α, IL-1β, and IL-6 and inhibits the activation of NF-κB in activated microglia [122]. Numerous flavonoids decrease the production of proinflammatory cytokines in immune cells, such as TNF-α, IL-1β, and IL-6, through the inhibition of several elements of the TLR4-dependent MyD88/IKK/NF-κB signaling pathway and some also decrease iNOS and COX-2. Some examples of flavonoids that have these effects are schisandrin B [123], genistein [124], luteolin [116], tangeretin [125], chrysin [126], epigallocatechin-3-Gallate [127], and hesperetin [128]. The abovementioned studies illustrate the reduction induced by flavonoids of the pro-inflammatory molecules such as TNF-α, IL-1β, and IL-6 through modulation at different levels of PI3K/AKT/mTOR and MAPK pathways, resulting in the inactivation of the transcriptor factors, including NF-κB and AP-1 in neurons and activated microglia and astrocytes (Fig. **2**).

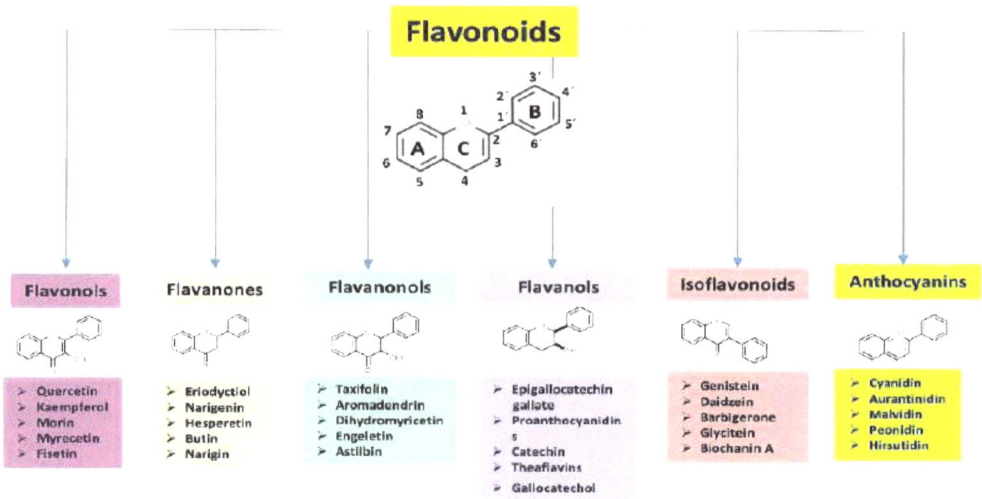

Fig. (2). Proinflammatory cytokines inhibited by flavonoids.

MODULATORY EFFECTS OF FLAVONOID IN AD.

In-vitro Studies

Several *in vitro* studies evaluate the formation of Aβ oligomer and its assembly into aggregates, and different flavonoids inhibit the oligomer formation and aggregation. (-)-epi-gallocatechin gallate remodel Aβ fibrils into smaller protein aggregates that are non-toxic to mammalian cells [129], inhibits the fibrillogenesis of Aβ [130], and in cultured hippocampal neuronal cells has protective effects against Aβ-induced neuronal apoptosis through scavenging reactive oxygen species [131]. Pretreatment of primary hippocampal cultures with quercetin significantly attenuated Aβ (1-42)-induced cytotoxicity, protein oxidation, lipid peroxidation, and apoptosis [132]. Myricetin inhibits the fibrillogenesis of Aβ [133]. Cyanidin 3-O-β-glucopyranoside decreases the cytotoxicity of Aβ (25–35) and its aggregation in the neuroblastoma SH-SY5Y cells [134]. Luteolin and diosmetin reduce Aβ (1–40 and 1-42) in SweAPP N2a cells and primary neuronal cells [135]. In the SH-SY5Y neuroblastoma cells, wogonin decreased Aβ aggregation and phosphorylated Tau [136]. In a cell system overexpressing APP Swedish mutation (APPswe), quercetin and rutin inhibit the formation of Aβ fibrils and disaggregate Aβ fibrils [137]. Baicalein inhibits the aggregation of human tau protein [138, 139].

Animal Models

There are different animal models for AD, including the spontaneous (*e.g.,* senescence-accelerated mouse), chemically induced (*e.g.,* amyloid infusion and streptozotocin), and numerous transgenic mice and some transgenic rats that express mutant human genes involved in the production of amyloid plaques and neurofibrillary tangles (*e.g.,* TG2576, APP/PS1, 3×Tg and 5×FAD) [140]. These AD familial transgenic models incompletely recapitulate the idiopathic or typical late-onset AD, and one of the factors that limit their use in neuroinflammation research is that most of these models do not develop neurodegeneration, but apart from expressing amyloid plaques and neurofibrillary tangles, they all manifest deficits in memory [140, 141]. Because these animal models do not develop neurodegeneration, the main interest of the research in these animals has been focused on the effects of flavonoids in the impairment of cognition function and Aβ aggregation. In the streptozotocin model, kaempferol improves memory and increases the density of intact neurons in the CA1 area of the hippocampus [142]. In the mouse model of memory deficits induced by scopolamine, isorhamnetin prevents learning and memory deficits and induces an increase of brain-derived neurotrophic factor (BDNF) level in the prefrontal cortex and hippocampus [143]. In the transgenic (h-APPswe, h-Tau P301L, and h-PS1 M146V) mice, wogonin improves memory. In the scopolamine-induced memory deficit rat model, naringin and rutin improve memory [144]. In scopolamine-induced memory, hesperidin pretreatment improves memory and decreases inflammatory markers like NF-κB, iNOS, COX-2, and astrogliosis [145]. In the streptozotocin rat model, luteolin improves memory [146]. In the APP-SL 7-5 transgenic mice, nobiletin reduces the quantity of soluble Aβ (1-40 and 1-42) and Aβ plaques in the hippocampus [147]. In the 3xTg mice, diosmin and its bioactive metabolite of diosmetin decrease Aβ generation and tau hyperphosphorylation [148]. In the transgenic APP/PS1 mice, hesperidin restores social interaction, reduces Aβ plaque in the hippocampus and cortex, and decreases microglial activation and astrogliosis [149]. In the Tg2576 transgenic mouse model, luteolin and diosmin reduce Aβ (1-40 and 1-42) [135]. In the APPsw transgenic mice, (---epigallocatechin-3-gallate reduces the quantity of soluble Aβ (1-40 and 1-42) and Aβ deposits in the hippocampal and cortical brain regions [150], and in the Aβ infusion model, it inhibits memory dysfunction, decreases Aβ (1–42) level, decreases alpha-secretase and increases beta- and gamma-secretase, in both the cortex and hippocampus, and similar results were obtained in the presenilin 2 (PS2) mutant mice [151], and in the APPsw transgenic mouse model, memory improved [152]. Nobiletin decreases Aβ plaques in the hippocampus and improves memory deficits in the APP-SL 7-5 transgenic mice [147] and the 3XTg mice, it reversed the impairment of memory and reduced the levels of Aβ (1-40) [153]. In the senescence-accelerated mouse (SAMP8), nobiletin reverses memory impairment in the hippocampus [154]. In the 3XTg mice, quercetin improves memory, active behaviors and decreases plaques of Aβ and hyperphosphorylated tau in the CA1 area of the hippocampus [155]. Cyanidin 3-O-glucoside reverses memory impairment and reduces tau phosphorylation in the hippocampus in the Aβ infusion rat [156], and with the APP(Swe)/PS1(ΔE9) mouse model, it improved learning and memory [134]. In the APPswe/PS1dE9 double transgenic mice, fisetin prevents the development of learning and memory deficits through modulation of the cyclin-dependent kinase 5 (Cdk5), reporting hyperactivity leading to neuroinflammation and neurodegeneration [157]. Most of the studies mentioned were focused on amyloidopathy and cognitive deficits, while studies on the effects of flavonoids on tauopathy are scarce.

Clinical

A double-blind study has shown that cocoa flavanol consumption improves cognitive function in aging subjects [158], and in mild cognitive impairment patients, cocoa flavanol for 8 weeks improves cognitive function [159]. Moreover, in healthy 50-69-year-old subjects, consumption of cocoa flavanol 3 by months improves dentate gyrus functions evaluated by cognitive test and a high-resolution variant of functional magnetic resonance imaging (fMRI) [160].

MODULATORY EFFECTS OF FLAVONOIDS IN PD

In-vitro Studies

In a series of *in vitro* studies to evaluate the formation of α-syn oligomer and assembly into aggregates, different flavonoids were found to inhibit the oligomer formation and aggregation. These flavonoids include: morin, quercetin, apigenin, baicalein, (−)-Epigallocatechin gallate, myricetin and Scutellarein [161 - 163]. Apigenin and luteolin decease tumor necrosis factor-alpha (TNF-α) and IL-6 production in activated microglia induced by LPS [115], while in the same model, nobiletin inhibits the release of the proinflammatory cytokines TNF-α and IL-1β [164], naringenin inhibits iNOS and COX-2, induce the expression of the suppressor of cytokine signaling 3 (SOCS-2), a negative regulator of cytokines, and inhibits the activation of NF-κB in activated microglia [165, 166]. Daidzein downregulates the production of IL-6 and the activation of NF-κB [167] and its metabolite Equol (7-hydroxy-3-(4'-hydroxyphenyl)-chroman) inhibits the secretion of TNF-α, IL-6, and NF-κB activation [168]. Luteolin attenuates the decrease of DA induced by LPS in a co-culture of neuron and glial cells, inhibiting the activation of microglia and the activation of NF-κB [169]. Morin reduces cell mortality and apoptosis in PC12 cells exposed to the neurotoxic MPP$^+$ [170] and reduces astrogliosis and nuclear translocation of NF-κB in primary cultured astrocytes exposed to the neurotoxic MPP^+ [171]. Fustin, fisetin, sulfuretin, butein, and butin protect the murine hippocampal HT22 cells against glutamate-induced neurotoxicity and decrease the induced nitric oxide (NO) production in BV2 cells microglial BV2 cell lines, and butein suppresses the expression of iNOS and COX-2 [172].

Animal Models Studies

Two of the most widely used animal models of PD are the chemically induced MPTP and 6-hydroxydopamine (6-OHDA) rat. Both MPTP and 6-OHDA are neurotoxic and are substrates for the DA transporter (DAT) and have strong face validity for both the loss of DAergic neurons and the elicited motor phenotype [173]. Moreover, the systemic rotenone model of PD also shows the main pathological hallmarks of PD [174]. On the rotenone mouse model of PD, baicalein decreased the formation and accumulation of α-syn oligomers and protected DAergic neurons [175]. In the 1-methyl-4-phenylpyridinium (MPP^+) induced rat model, this flavonoid attenuates α-syn aggregation and inhibits inflammasome activation [176], while in the MPTP mouse model, it improves motor ability, decreases activated microglia, and astrocytes, and increases DA and serotonin neurotransmitters in the striatum [177 - 179]. In the rat rotenone model, apigenin decreases the expression of NF-κB, increases the expression of DA D2 receptor (D2R), and decreases the α-syn aggregation [180]. Nobiletin inhibited microglial activation and preserved the expression of the glial cell line-derived neurotrophic factor (GDNF) [181] and improved motor deficits and, DA contents in the striatum and hippocampal CA1 region [182]. Naringin decreases the TNF-α expression and increases the GDNF in SN in an MPP^+ rat model [183] and protects the nigrostriatal DA projection but does not change the DA phenotypes in the SN and striatum [184]. (-)-epigallocatechin-3-gallate decreases DA neuronal loss in SN [185]. Apigenin and luteolin improved the locomotor behavior, decreased the GFAP, and increased the brain-derived neurotrophic factor (BDNF) in SN in an MPTP mice model [186]. Quercetin reduced DAergic neuronal loss and increased striatal DA [24]. In the MitoPark transgenic mouse models of PD, quercetin treatment reverses behavioral deficits, striatal DA depletion, and DAergic neuronal loss [187]. Quercetin and kaempferol in an MTPT mouse model improve motor coordination and striatal DA [188, 189]. In the same model, hesperidin improves motor coordination and glial cells and the expression of IL-1 β, TNF-α, and IL-6 [190, 191]. In the 6-OHDA lesion rat model of PD, tangeretin protects the striatal DAergic neurons [192], rutin improves motor coordination and protects DAergic neurons [193], troxerutin decreases striatal lipoperoxidation, astrogliosis, and neuronal loss [194], and myricitrin protects DAergic neurons from SN and inhibits the expression of TNF-α [195]. In the MPTP mouse model, pretreatment with morin reduces behavioral deficits, DAergic neuronal death, and striatal DA depletion [170], and improves motor dysfunction, decreasing DAergic neuronal losses and astrogliosis [171]. Dihydromyricetin treatment in two different transgenic mouse models (TG2576 and TG-SwDI) improves exploratory and locomotor activity, decreases anxiety, improves memory, and reverses Aβ accumulation [196].

MODULATORY EFFECTS OF FLAVONOID IN HD

In-vitro Studies

A modified PC12 cell line containing the mutated huntingtin protein exon 1 that expresses polyQ is an *in vitro* system of HD that screens the ability of compounds to protect this cell from death caused by polyQ [197]. In this system, fisetin increases cell survival [198]. Baicalein disaggregates α-syn and inhibits oligomer formation [199]. Meng *et al.* analyzed the capability of numerous flavonoids to inhibit the fibrils formation of α-syn, and they found that quercetin, gossypetin, myricetin, 6,2',3'- Trihydroxyflavone, 2',3'- Dihydroxyflavone, 5,6-Dihydroxy-7-Methoxyflavone, tricetin, 7,3',4',5'- Tetrahydroxyflavone, 7,3',4'-Trihydroxyisoflavone and epigalloCatechin Gallate completely inhibit α-syn fibril formation [200].

In-vivo Studies

A chemical-induced animal model of HD is produced by systemic administration at low doses of 3-nitropropionic acid (3-NP) to rats or mice to induce selective degeneration of striatal neurons [201]. In this model, quercetin decreases motor deficits, astrogliosis, and microglial proliferation [202, 203]. Rutin improves motor coordination and activity, and memory and decreases astrogliosis in the striatum [204]. Kaempferol reduces cell death in the striatal, gliosis, motor deficit, and delayed mortality [205]. Hesperidin pretreatment causes an increase in locomotor activity and coordination and a decrease in iNOS [206, 207]. Naringin pretreatment improves locomotor activity and coordination [207]. Epigallocatechin-3-gallate improves memory [208]. Chrysin improves memory, motor coordination, and activity, and increases the surviving cells in the striatum [209]. Genistein improves motor activity and decreases COX-2 and iNOS expression [210]. Other common animal models of HD are the R6/1 and R6/2, both expressing the mutant *exon* 1 of the human huntingtin gene carrying CAG repeat expansion and mimic many features of HD [211]. In the R6/1 model, chronic treatment with 7,8-Dihydroxyflavone reverses memory deficit in the novel object recognition test, delays motor deficits, improves striatal levels of enkephalin, and prevents striatal volume loss [212]. In the R6/2 model, fisetin improves motor coordination and increases lifespan [198].

CONCLUSION

Sustained low grade of neuroinflammation is a major characteristic of neurodegenerative age-related disorders, such as AD, PD, and HD. This inflammatory reaction results in tissue damage, and the factors that activate this process can be environmental or endogenous (*e.g.*, protein aggregates). Sustained inflammation may result in the production of neurotoxic factors that amplify underlying disease states. Until now, there has been no treatment to cure these diseases, rather treatments have been symptomatic. Flavonoids are consumed in the human diet *via* vegetables, cereals, fruits, herbs and spices, and other plant-based products, and epidemiological studies suggest that a higher intake of flavonoid-rich foods and beverages is associated with better cognitive outcomes, lower dementia rates, and reduced risk of neurodegenerative diseases [213 - 215]. Interventional studies in humans using a single flavonoid molecule to evaluate the impact on health are scares, and there is no research data on whether a single flavonoid can modulate inflammatory markers in the blood. However, some studies evaluate those markers after consuming flavonoids-rich foods and beverages that show a decrease in pro-inflammatory molecules, including C-reactive protein and IL-6 [216 - 221]. Furthermore, numerous preclinical studies highlight the anti-inflammatory effect of flavonoids by decreasing the activated glial cells (microglia and astrocytes) and the pro-inflammatory mediators, including TNF-α, IL-1β, IL-6, COX-2, and iNOS, through indirect or direct inactivation of transcription factors such as NF-κB and AP-1 and also through inactivation of the inflammasome. Although these studies have shown that flavonoids (Table **1**) can downregulate several pro-inflammatory pathways, these effects need further confirmation using conjugated flavonoids in both *in vitro* and *in vivo* models. Moreover, several flavonoids have anti-aggregation effects (*in vitro* and *in vivo*) in the different proteins involved in AD, PD, and HD and improve the alteration in motor coordination and cognition in animal models of those diseases. Although no randomized clinical trials are evaluating the efficacy of the single flavonoid as an anti-inflammatory agent in neurodegenerative diseases, searching the clinical trial data set at ClinicalTrails.gov revealed several ongoing studies looking at the effects of flavonoids in cognition performance, risk of dementia and endothelial dysfunction, suggesting an interest in translating the preclinical knowledge into clinical trials. Moreover, a recent pilot phase 1 study showed that a combination of the anti-leukemic drug Dasatinib and quercetin reduced adipose senescent cells [222]. Taking into consideration the relevance of neuroinflammation in neurodegenerative age-related diseases, and the substantial evidence that supports the anti-inflammatory and antioxidant effects of this group of molecules, it is reasonable to assume that these molecules have the potential to be a therapeutic agent to treat neurodegenerative age-related diseases, alone or in combination with drugs used in allopathic medicine. Future research must be oriented not only to validate the anti-inflammatory effects of flavonoids in animal models and interventional studies but also to allow better knowledge about bioavailability, BBB penetration, and other modulatory effects *in vivo*.

Table 1. Flavonoids that have shown therapeutic effects in preclinical models of Alzheimer's disease (AD), Parkinson's disease (PD), and Huntington's disease (HD).

Flavonoid	AD	PD	HD
7,8-Dihydroxyflavone			•
Apigenin		•	
Baicalein		•	
Cyanidin 3-O-glucoside	•		
Chrysin			•
Dihydromyricetin		•	
Diosmin	•		
Epi-gallocatechin gallate	•	•	•
Fisetin			•
Fisetin	•		
Genistein			•
Hesperidin		•	•
Isorhamnetin	•		
Kaempferol	•	•	•
Luteolin	•	•	
Morin		•	
Myricitrin		•	
Naringin	•	•	•
Nobiletin	•	•	
Quercetin	•	•	
Rutin	•	•	•
Tangeretin		•	
Troxerutin		•	
Wogonin	•		

CONSENT FOR PUBLICATION

Not applicable.

CONFLICT OF INTEREST

The author declares no conflict of interest, financial or otherwise.

ACKNOWLEDGEMENTS

Declared none.

REFERENCES

[1]   Kirkwood TBL. Understanding the odd science of aging. Cell 2005; 120(4): 437-47.
        [http://dx.doi.org/10.1016/j.cell.2005.01.027] [PMID: 15734677]

[2]   Harris RE. Harris, R.E. Global Epidemiology of Chronic Diseases: The Epidemiologic Transition. In
        Epidemiology of Chronic Disease: Global Perspectives: Global Perspectives; Burlington, MA, 2019.

[3]   Barnes PJ. Mechanisms of development of multimorbidity in the elderly. Eur Respir J 2015; 45(3):
        790-806.
        [http://dx.doi.org/10.1183/09031936.00229714] [PMID: 25614163]

[4]   Dugger BN, Dickson DW. Pathology of Neurodegenerative Diseases. Cold Spring Harb Perspect Biol
        2017; 9(7): a028035.
        [http://dx.doi.org/10.1101/cshperspect.a028035] [PMID: 28062563]

[5]   López-Valdés HE, Martínez-Coria H. The Role of Neuroinflammation in Age-Related Dementias.
        Rev. Investig. Clínica Organo Hosp. Enfermedades Nutr 2016; 68: 40-8.

[6]   Beecher GR. Overview of dietary flavonoids: nomenclature, occurrence and intake. J Nutr 2003;
        133(10): 3248S-54S.
        [http://dx.doi.org/10.1093/jn/133.10.3248S] [PMID: 14519822]

[7]   Ramzan I, Li GQ. Phytotherapies—Past, Present, and Future. Phytotherapies 2015; 1-17.
        [http://dx.doi.org/10.1002/9781119006039.ch1]

[8]   Forkmann G, Heller W. Biosynthesis of flavonoids. Comprehensive Natural Products Chemistry 1ˢᵗ ed.
        1999; 714-46.
        [http://dx.doi.org/10.1016/B978-0-08-091283-7.00028-X]

[9]   Panche AN, Diwan AD, Chandra SR. Flavonoids: an overview. J Nutr Sci 2016; 5: e47.
        [http://dx.doi.org/10.1017/jns.2016.41] [PMID: 28620474]

[10]   Dwivedi S, Malik C, Chhokar V. Molecular Structure, Biological Functions, and Metabolic Regulation
        of Flavonoids. In: Gahlawat SK, Salar RK, Siwach P, Duhan JS, Kumar S, Kaur P, Eds. Plant
        Biotechnology: Recent Advancements and Developments 2017; 171-88.
        [http://dx.doi.org/10.1007/978-981-10-4732-9_9]

[11]   Williamson G, Kay CD, Crozier A. The bioavailability, transport, and bioactivity of dietary
        flavonoids: a review from a historical perspective. Compr Rev Food Sci Food Saf 2018; 17(5): 1054-
        112.
        [http://dx.doi.org/10.1111/1541-4337.12351] [PMID: 33350159]

[12]   Akhlaghi M, Foshati S. Bioavailability and Metabolism of Flavonoids: A Review. Int J Nurs Sci 2017;
        2: 180-4.

[13]   Menendez C, Dueñas M, Galindo P, *et al.* Vascular deconjugation of quercetin glucuronide: The

flavonoid paradox revealed? Mol Nutr Food Res 2011; 55(12): 1780-90.
[http://dx.doi.org/10.1002/mnfr.201100378] [PMID: 22144045]

[14]   Hollman PCH. Absorption, Bioavailability, and Metabolism of Flavonoids. Pharm Biol 2004; 42(sup1): 74-83.
[http://dx.doi.org/10.3109/13880200490893492]

[15]   Scalbert A, Williamson G. Dietary intake and bioavailability of polyphenols. J Nutr 2000; 130(8) (Suppl.): 2073S-85S.
[http://dx.doi.org/10.1093/jn/130.8.2073S] [PMID: 10917926]

[16]   Manach C, Williamson G, Morand C, Scalbert A, Rémésy C. Bioavailability and bioefficacy of polyphenols in humans. I. Review of 97 bioavailability studies. Am J Clin Nutr 2005; 81(1) (Suppl.): 230S-42S.
[http://dx.doi.org/10.1093/ajcn/81.1.230S] [PMID: 15640486]

[17]   El Mohsen MA, Marks J, Kuhnle G, *et al.* Absorption, tissue distribution and excretion of pelargonidin and its metabolites following oral administration to rats. Br J Nutr 2006; 95(1): 51-8.
[http://dx.doi.org/10.1079/BJN20051596] [PMID: 16441916]

[18]   Talavéra S, Felgines C, Texier O, *et al.* Anthocyanin metabolism in rats and their distribution to digestive area, kidney, and brain. J Agric Food Chem 2005; 53(10): 3902-8.
[http://dx.doi.org/10.1021/jf050145v] [PMID: 15884815]

[19]   Abd El Mohsen MM, Kuhnle G, Rechner AR, *et al.* Uptake and metabolism of epicatechin and its access to the brain after oral ingestion. Free Radic Biol Med 2002; 33(12): 1693-702.
[http://dx.doi.org/10.1016/S0891-5849(02)01137-1] [PMID: 12488137]

[20]   Kumar S, Pandey AK. Chemistry and biological activities of flavonoids: an overview. ScientificWorldJournal 2013; 2013: 1-16.
[http://dx.doi.org/10.1155/2013/162750] [PMID: 24470791]

[21]   Tuñón M, García-Mediavilla M, Sánchez-Campos S, González-Gallego J. Potential of flavonoids as anti-inflammatory agents: modulation of pro-inflammatory gene expression and signal transduction pathways. Curr Drug Metab 2009; 10(3): 256-71.
[http://dx.doi.org/10.2174/138920009787846369] [PMID: 19442088]

[22]   MacNee W, Rabinovich RA, Choudhury G. Ageing and the border between health and disease. Eur Respir J 2014; 44(5): 1332-52.
[http://dx.doi.org/10.1183/09031936.00134014] [PMID: 25323246]

[23]   López-Otín C, Blasco MA, Partridge L, Serrano M, Kroemer G. The hallmarks of aging. Cell 2013; 153(6): 1194-217.
[http://dx.doi.org/10.1016/j.cell.2013.05.039] [PMID: 23746838]

[24]   Haleagrahara N, Siew CJ, Mitra NK, Kumari M. Neuroprotective effect of bioflavonoid quercetin in 6-hydroxydopamine-induced oxidative stress biomarkers in the rat striatum. Neurosci Lett 2011; 500(2): 139-43.
[http://dx.doi.org/10.1016/j.neulet.2011.06.021] [PMID: 21704673]

[25]   Figueira I, Fernandes A, Mladenovic Djordjevic A, *et al.* Interventions for age-related diseases: Shifting the paradigm. Mech Ageing Dev 2016; 160: 69-92.
[http://dx.doi.org/10.1016/j.mad.2016.09.009] [PMID: 27693441]

[26]   Nagaratnam N, Nagaratnam K, Cheuk G. Neurological Disorders and Related Problems in the Elderly. In: Nagaratnam N, Nagaratnam K, Cheuk G, Eds. Diseases in the Elderly: Age-Related Changes and Pathophysiology 2016; 151-213.
[http://dx.doi.org/10.1007/978-3-319-25787-7_7]

[27]   Cevenini E, Caruso C, Candore G, *et al.* Age-related inflammation: the contribution of different organs, tissues and systems. How to face it for therapeutic approaches. Curr Pharm Des 2010; 16(6): 609-18.

[http://dx.doi.org/10.2174/138161210790883840] [PMID: 20388071]

[28] Weiskopf D, Weinberger B, Grubeck-Loebenstein B. The aging of the immune system. Transpl Int 2009; 22(11): 1041-50.
[http://dx.doi.org/10.1111/j.1432-2277.2009.00927.x] [PMID: 19624493]

[29] Calcinotto A, Kohli J, Zagato E, Pellegrini L, Demaria M, Alimonti A. Cellular Senescence: Aging, Cancer, and Injury. Physiol Rev 2019; 99(2): 1047-78.
[http://dx.doi.org/10.1152/physrev.00020.2018] [PMID: 30648461]

[30] Rea IM, Gibson DS, McGilligan V, McNerlan SE, Alexander HD, Ross OA. Age and Age-Related Diseases: Role of Inflammation Triggers and Cytokines. Front Immunol 2018; 9: 586.
[http://dx.doi.org/10.3389/fimmu.2018.00586] [PMID: 29686666]

[31] Martínez-Cué C, Rueda N. Cellular Senescence in Neurodegenerative Diseases. Front Cell Neurosci 2020; 14: 16.
[http://dx.doi.org/10.3389/fncel.2020.00016] [PMID: 32116562]

[32] Hearps AC, Martin GE, Angelovich TA, *et al.* Aging is associated with chronic innate immune activation and dysregulation of monocyte phenotype and function. Aging Cell 2012; 11(5): 867-75.
[http://dx.doi.org/10.1111/j.1474-9726.2012.00851.x] [PMID: 22708967]

[33] Effros R. Replicative senescence: the final stage of memory T cell differentiation? Curr HIV Res 2003; 1(2): 153-65.
[http://dx.doi.org/10.2174/1570162033485348] [PMID: 15043200]

[34] Frasca D, Diaz A, Romero M, Landin AM, Blomberg BB. Age effects on B cells and humoral immunity in humans. Ageing Res Rev 2011; 10(3): 330-5.
[http://dx.doi.org/10.1016/j.arr.2010.08.004] [PMID: 20728581]

[35] Mahbub S, Deburghgraeve CR, Kovacs EJ. Advanced age impairs macrophage polarization. J Interferon Cytokine Res 2012; 32(1): 18-26.
[http://dx.doi.org/10.1089/jir.2011.0058] [PMID: 22175541]

[36] Trollor JN, Smith E, Agars E, *et al.* The association between systemic inflammation and cognitive performance in the elderly: the Sydney Memory and Ageing Study. Age (Omaha) 2012; 34(5): 1295-308.
[http://dx.doi.org/10.1007/s11357-011-9301-x] [PMID: 21853262]

[37] Anthony D, Bolton SJ, Fearn S, Perry VH. Age-related effects of interleukin-1 beta on polymorphonuclear neutrophil-dependent increases in blood-brain barrier permeability in rats. Brain 1997; 120(3): 435-44.
[http://dx.doi.org/10.1093/brain/120.3.435] [PMID: 9126055]

[38] Ďuračková Z. Some current insights into oxidative stress. Physiol Res 2010; 59(4): 459-69.
[http://dx.doi.org/10.33549/physiolres.931844] [PMID: 19929132]

[39] Fernández-Checa JC, Kaplowitz N, García-Ruiz C, *et al.* GSH transport in mitochondria: defense against TNF-induced oxidative stress and alcohol-induced defect. Am J Physiol Gastrointest Liver Physiol 1997; 273(1): G7-G17.
[http://dx.doi.org/10.1152/ajpgi.1997.273.1.G7] [PMID: 9252504]

[40] Chen GY, Nuñez G. Sterile inflammation: sensing and reacting to damage. Nat Rev Immunol 2010; 10(12): 826-37.
[http://dx.doi.org/10.1038/nri2873] [PMID: 21088683]

[41] Zhou R, Yazdi AS, Menu P, Tschopp J. A role for mitochondria in NLRP3 inflammasome activation. Nature 2011; 469(7329): 221-5.
[http://dx.doi.org/10.1038/nature09663] [PMID: 21124315]

[42] Glass CK, Saijo K, Winner B, Marchetto MC, Gage FH. Mechanisms underlying inflammation in neurodegeneration. Cell 2010; 140(6): 918-34.
[http://dx.doi.org/10.1016/j.cell.2010.02.016] [PMID: 20303880]

[43] Franceschi C, Campisi J. Chronic inflammation (inflammaging) and its potential contribution to age-associated diseases. J Gerontol A Biol Sci Med Sci 2014; 69 (Suppl. 1): S4-9.
[http://dx.doi.org/10.1093/gerona/glu057] [PMID: 24833586]

[44] Shabab T, Khanabdali R, Moghadamtousi SZ, Kadir HA, Mohan G. Neuroinflammation pathways: a general review. Int J Neurosci 2017; 127(7): 624-33.
[http://dx.doi.org/10.1080/00207454.2016.1212854] [PMID: 27412492]

[45] Nimmerjahn A, Kirchhoff F, Helmchen F. Resting microglial cells are highly dynamic surveillants of brain parenchyma *in vivo*. Science 2005; 308(5726): 1314-8.
[http://dx.doi.org/10.1126/science.1110647] [PMID: 15831717]

[46] Rossi D. Astrocyte physiopathology: At the crossroads of intercellular networking, inflammation and cell death. Prog Neurobiol 2015; 130: 86-120.
[http://dx.doi.org/10.1016/j.pneurobio.2015.04.003] [PMID: 25930681]

[47] Kimelberg HK, Nedergaard M. Functions of astrocytes and their potential as therapeutic targets. Neurotherapeutics 2010; 7(4): 338-53.
[http://dx.doi.org/10.1016/j.nurt.2010.07.006] [PMID: 20880499]

[48] Amarante-Mendes GP, Adjemian S, Branco LM, Zanetti LC, Weinlich R, Bortoluci KR. Pattern Recognition Receptors and the Host Cell Death Molecular Machinery. Front Immunol 2018; 9: 2379.
[http://dx.doi.org/10.3389/fimmu.2018.02379] [PMID: 30459758]

[49] Yang Q, Zhou J. Neuroinflammation in the central nervous system: Symphony of glial cells. Glia 2019; 67(6): 1017-35.
[http://dx.doi.org/10.1002/glia.23571] [PMID: 30548343]

[50] Hughes C, Choi ML, Yi JH, *et al.* Beta amyloid aggregates induce sensitised TLR4 signalling causing long-term potentiation deficit and rat neuronal cell death. Commun Biol 2020; 3(1): 79.
[http://dx.doi.org/10.1038/s42003-020-0792-9] [PMID: 32071389]

[51] Fellner L, Irschick R, Schanda K, *et al.* Toll☐like receptor 4 is required for α☐synuclein dependent activation of microglia and astroglia. Glia 2013; 61(3): 349-60.
[http://dx.doi.org/10.1002/glia.22437] [PMID: 23108585]

[52] El-Zayat SR, Sibaii H, Mannaa FA. Toll-like receptors activation, signaling, and targeting: an overview. Bull Natl Res Cent 2019; 43(1): 187.
[http://dx.doi.org/10.1186/s42269-019-0227-2]

[53] Kelley N, Jeltema D, Duan Y, He Y. The NLRP3 Inflammasome: An Overview of Mechanisms of Activation and Regulation. Int J Mol Sci 2019; 20(13): 3328.
[http://dx.doi.org/10.3390/ijms20133328] [PMID: 31284572]

[54] Ferreira VL, Borba HHL, Bonetti A de F, Leonart P. L.; Pontarolo, R. Cytokines and Interferons: Types and Functions. 2018.
[http://dx.doi.org/10.5772/intechopen.74550]

[55] Musolino C, Allegra A, Innao V, Allegra AG, Pioggia G, Gangemi S. Inflammatory and Anti-Inflammatory Equilibrium, Proliferative and Antiproliferative Balance: The Role of Cytokines in Multiple Myeloma. Mediators Inflamm 2017; 2017: 1-24.
[http://dx.doi.org/10.1155/2017/1852517] [PMID: 29089667]

[56] Brooks AJ, Dehkhoda F, Kragelund BB. Cytokine Receptors. 2018.
[http://dx.doi.org/10.1007/978-3-319-44675-2_8]

[57] Liddelow SA, Guttenplan KA, Clarke LE, *et al.* Neurotoxic reactive astrocytes are induced by activated microglia. Nature 2017; 541(7638): 481-7.
[http://dx.doi.org/10.1038/nature21029] [PMID: 28099414]

[58] Tang Y, Le W. Differential Roles of M1 and M2 Microglia in Neurodegenerative Diseases. Mol Neurobiol 2016; 53(2): 1181-94.

[http://dx.doi.org/10.1007/s12035-014-9070-5] [PMID: 25598354]

[59]   Du L, Zhang Y, Chen Y, Zhu J, Yang Y, Zhang HL. Role of microglia in neurological disorders and their potentials as a therapeutic target. Mol Neurobiol 2017; 54(10): 7567-84.
[http://dx.doi.org/10.1007/s12035-016-0245-0] [PMID: 27830532]

[60]   Chen WW, Zhang X, Huang WJ. Role of neuroinflammation in neurodegenerative diseases (Review). Mol Med Rep 2016; 13(4): 3391-6.
[http://dx.doi.org/10.3892/mmr.2016.4948] [PMID: 26935478]

[61]   Becher B, Spath S, Goverman J. Cytokine networks in neuroinflammation. Nat Rev Immunol 2017; 17(1): 49-59.
[http://dx.doi.org/10.1038/nri.2016.123] [PMID: 27916979]

[62]   Polis B, Samson AO. A New Perspective on Alzheimer's Disease as a Brain Expression of a Complex Metabolic Disorder. 2019.
[http://dx.doi.org/10.15586/alzheimersdisease.2019.ch1]

[63]   McDonald CR, McEvoy LK, Gharapetian L, *et al.* Regional rates of neocortical atrophy from normal aging to early Alzheimer disease. Neurology 2009; 73(6): 457-65.
[http://dx.doi.org/10.1212/WNL.0b013e3181b16431] [PMID: 19667321]

[64]   2019 Alzheimer's disease facts and figures. Alzheimers Dement 2019; 15(3): 321-87.
[http://dx.doi.org/10.1016/j.jalz.2019.01.010]

[65]   Wingo TS, Lah JJ, Levey AI, Cutler DJ. Autosomal recessive causes likely in early-onset Alzheimer disease. Arch Neurol 2012; 69(1): 59-64.
[http://dx.doi.org/10.1001/archneurol.2011.221] [PMID: 21911656]

[66]   Liu CC, Kanekiyo T, Xu H, Bu G, Bu G. Apolipoprotein E and Alzheimer disease: risk, mechanisms and therapy. Nat Rev Neurol 2013; 9(2): 106-18.
[http://dx.doi.org/10.1038/nrneurol.2012.263] [PMID: 23296339]

[67]   Kelleher RJ III, Shen J. Presenilin-1 mutations and Alzheimer's disease. Proc Natl Acad Sci USA 2017; 114(4): 629-31.
[http://dx.doi.org/10.1073/pnas.1619574114] [PMID: 28082723]

[68]   Karran E, Mercken M, Strooper BD. The amyloid cascade hypothesis for Alzheimer's disease: an appraisal for the development of therapeutics. Nat Rev Drug Discov 2011; 10(9): 698-712.
[http://dx.doi.org/10.1038/nrd3505] [PMID: 21852788]

[69]   Frost B, Jacks RL, Diamond MI. Propagation of tau misfolding from the outside to the inside of a cell. J Biol Chem 2009; 284(19): 12845-52.
[http://dx.doi.org/10.1074/jbc.M808759200] [PMID: 19282288]

[70]   Henstridge CM, Hyman BT, Spires-Jones TL. Beyond the neuron–cellular interactions early in Alzheimer disease pathogenesis. Nat Rev Neurosci 2019; 20(2): 94-108.
[http://dx.doi.org/10.1038/s41583-018-0113-1] [PMID: 30643230]

[71]   Michaud M, Balardy L, Moulis G, *et al.* Proinflammatory cytokines, aging, and age-related diseases. J Am Med Dir Assoc 2013; 14(12): 877-82.
[http://dx.doi.org/10.1016/j.jamda.2013.05.009] [PMID: 23792036]

[72]   Lian H, Yang L, Cole A, *et al.* NFκB-activated astroglial release of complement C3 compromises neuronal morphology and function associated with Alzheimer's disease. Neuron 2015; 85(1): 101-15.
[http://dx.doi.org/10.1016/j.neuron.2014.11.018] [PMID: 25533482]

[73]   Lian H, Litvinchuk A, Chiang ACA, Aithmitti N, Jankowsky JL, Zheng H. Astrocyte-microglia cross talk through complement activation modulates amyloid pathology in mouse models of alzheimer's disease. J Neurosci 2016; 36(2): 577-89.
[http://dx.doi.org/10.1523/JNEUROSCI.2117-15.2016] [PMID: 26758846]

[74]   Davies DS, Ma J, Jegathees T, Goldsbury C. Microglia show altered morphology and reduced

arborization in human brain during aging and Alzheimer's disease. Brain Pathol 2017; 27(6): 795-808.
[http://dx.doi.org/10.1111/bpa.12456] [PMID: 27862631]

[75]   Cagnin A, Brooks DJ, Kennedy AM, *et al. In-vivo* measurement of activated microglia in dementia. Lancet 2001; 358(9280): 461-7.
[http://dx.doi.org/10.1016/S0140-6736(01)05625-2] [PMID: 11513911]

[76]   Schuitemaker A, Kropholler MA, Boellaard R, *et al.* Microglial activation in Alzheimer's disease: an (R)-[11C]PK11195 positron emission tomography study. Neurobiol Aging 2013; 34(1): 128-36.
[http://dx.doi.org/10.1016/j.neurobiolaging.2012.04.021] [PMID: 22840559]

[77]   Edison P, Archer HA, Gerhard A, *et al.* Microglia, amyloid, and cognition in Alzheimer's disease: An [11C](R)PK11195-PET and [11C]PIB-PET study. Neurobiol Dis 2008; 32(3): 412-9.
[http://dx.doi.org/10.1016/j.nbd.2008.08.001] [PMID: 18786637]

[78]   Dani M, Wood M, Mizoguchi R, *et al.* Microglial activation correlates *in vivo* with both tau and amyloid in Alzheimer's disease. Brain 2018; 141(9): 2740-54.
[http://dx.doi.org/10.1093/brain/awy188] [PMID: 30052812]

[79]   Fan Z, Brooks DJ, Okello A, Edison P. An early and late peak in microglial activation in Alzheimer's disease trajectory. Brain 2017; 140(3): aww349.
[http://dx.doi.org/10.1093/brain/aww349] [PMID: 28122877]

[80]   Malpetti M, Kievit RA, Passamonti L, *et al.* Microglial activation and tau burden predict cognitive decline in Alzheimer's disease. Brain 2020; 143(5): 1588-602.
[http://dx.doi.org/10.1093/brain/awaa088] [PMID: 32380523]

[81]   Nicastro N, Malpetti M, Mak E, *et al.* Gray matter changes related to microglial activation in Alzheimer's disease. Neurobiol Aging 2020; 94: 236-42.
[http://dx.doi.org/10.1016/j.neurobiolaging.2020.06.010] [PMID: 32663716]

[82]   Dickson DW. Neuropathology of Parkinson disease. Parkinsonism Relat Disord 2018; 46 (Suppl. 1): S30-3.
[http://dx.doi.org/10.1016/j.parkreldis.2017.07.033] [PMID: 28780180]

[83]   Lotankar S, Prabhavalkar KS, Bhatt LK. Biomarkers for Parkinson's Disease: Recent Advancement. Neurosci Bull 2017; 33(5): 585-97.
[http://dx.doi.org/10.1007/s12264-017-0183-5] [PMID: 28936761]

[84]   Prakash KG, Bannur BM, Chavan M, Saniya K, Sailesh K, Rajagopalan A. Neuroanatomical changes in Parkinson's disease in relation to cognition: An update. J Adv Pharm Technol Res 2016; 7(4): 123-6.
[http://dx.doi.org/10.4103/2231-4040.191416] [PMID: 27833890]

[85]   Weintraub D, Burn DJ. Parkinson's disease: The quintessential neuropsychiatric disorder. Mov Disord 2011; 26(6): 1022-31.
[http://dx.doi.org/10.1002/mds.23664] [PMID: 21626547]

[86]   Ascherio A, Schwarzschild MA. The epidemiology of Parkinson's disease: risk factors and prevention. Lancet Neurol 2016; 15(12): 1257-72.
[http://dx.doi.org/10.1016/S1474-4422(16)30230-7] [PMID: 27751556]

[87]   Kalia LV, Lang AE. Parkinson's disease. Lancet 2015; 386(9996): 896-912.
[http://dx.doi.org/10.1016/S0140-6736(14)61393-3] [PMID: 25904081]

[88]   Burré J, Sharma M, Südhof TC. Cell Biology and Pathophysiology of α-Synuclein. Cold Spring Harb Perspect Med 2018; 8(3): a024091.
[http://dx.doi.org/10.1101/cshperspect.a024091] [PMID: 28108534]

[89]   Gerhard A, Watts J, Trender-Gerhard I, *et al.* In vivo imaging of microglial activation with [11C](R)-PK11195 PET in corticobasal degeneration. Mov Disord 2004; 19(10): 1221-6.
[http://dx.doi.org/10.1002/mds.20162] [PMID: 15390000]

[90]   Banati RB, Daniel SE, Blunt SB. Glial pathology but absence of apoptotic nigral neurons in long-standing Parkinson's disease. Mov Disord 1998; 13(2): 221-7.
[http://dx.doi.org/10.1002/mds.870130205] [PMID: 9539333]

[91]   Vawter MP, Dillon-Carter O, Tourtellotte WW, Carvey P, Freed WJ. TGFbeta1 and TGFbeta2 concentrations are elevated in Parkinson's disease in ventricular cerebrospinal fluid. Exp Neurol 1996; 142(2): 313-22.
[http://dx.doi.org/10.1006/exnr.1996.0200] [PMID: 8934562]

[92]   Boka G, Anglade P, Wallach D, Javoy-Agid F, Agid Y, Hirsch EC. Immunocytochemical analysis of tumor necrosis factor and its receptors in Parkinson's disease. Neurosci Lett 1994; 172(1-2): 151-4.
[http://dx.doi.org/10.1016/0304-3940(94)90684-X] [PMID: 8084523]

[93]   Teismann P, Tieu K, Choi DK, *et al.* Cyclooxygenase-2 is instrumental in Parkinson's disease neurodegeneration. Proc Natl Acad Sci USA 2003; 100(9): 5473-8.
[http://dx.doi.org/10.1073/pnas.0837397100] [PMID: 12702778]

[94]   Griffin WST, Liu L, Li Y, Mrak RE, Barger SW. Interleukin-1 mediates Alzheimer and Lewy body pathologies. J Neuroinflammation 2006; 3(1): 5.
[http://dx.doi.org/10.1186/1742-2094-3-5] [PMID: 16542445]

[95]   Klegeris A, Pelech S, Giasson BI, *et al.* α-Synuclein activates stress signaling protein kinases in THP-1 cells and microglia. Neurobiol Aging 2008; 29(5): 739-52.
[http://dx.doi.org/10.1016/j.neurobiolaging.2006.11.013] [PMID: 17166628]

[96]   Brochard V, Combadière B, Prigent A, *et al.* Infiltration of CD4+ lymphocytes into the brain contributes to neurodegeneration in a mouse model of Parkinson disease. J Clin Invest 2008; 119(1): 182-92.
[http://dx.doi.org/10.1172/JCI36470] [PMID: 19104149]

[97]   Bates GP, Dorsey R, Gusella JF, *et al.* Huntington disease. Nat Rev Dis Primers 2015; 1(1): 15005.
[http://dx.doi.org/10.1038/nrdp.2015.5] [PMID: 27188817]

[98]   MacDonald M, Ambrose CM, Duyao MP, *et al.* A novel gene containing a trinucleotide repeat that is expanded and unstable on Huntington's disease chromosomes. Cell 1993; 72(6): 971-83.
[http://dx.doi.org/10.1016/0092-8674(93)90585-E] [PMID: 8458085]

[99]   Pandey M, Rajamma U. Huntington's disease: the coming of age. J Genet 2018; 97(3): 649-64.
[http://dx.doi.org/10.1007/s12041-018-0957-1] [PMID: 30027901]

[100] Huang WJ, Chen WW, Zhang X. Huntington's disease: Molecular basis of pathology and status of current therapeutic approaches. Exp Ther Med 2016; 12(4): 1951-6.
[http://dx.doi.org/10.3892/etm.2016.3566] [PMID: 27698679]

[101] Vonsattel JP, Myers RH, Stevens TJ, Ferrante RJ, Bird ED, Richardson EP Jr. Neuropathological classification of Huntington's disease. J Neuropathol Exp Neurol 1985; 44(6): 559-77.
[http://dx.doi.org/10.1097/00005072-198511000-00003] [PMID: 2932539]

[102] Illarioshkin SN, Klyushnikov SA, Vigont VA, Seliverstov YA, Kaznacheyeva EV. Molecular Pathogenesis in Huntington's Disease. Biochemistry (Mosc) 2018; 83(9): 1030-9.
[http://dx.doi.org/10.1134/S0006297918090043] [PMID: 30472941]

[103] Singhrao SK, Neal JW, Morgan BP, Gasque P. Increased complement biosynthesis by microglia and complement activation on neurons in Huntington's disease. Exp Neurol 1999; 159(2): 362-76.
[http://dx.doi.org/10.1006/exnr.1999.7170] [PMID: 10506508]

[104] Ona VO, Li M, Vonsattel JPG, *et al.* Inhibition of caspase-1 slows disease progression in a mouse model of Huntington's disease. Nature 1999; 399(6733): 263-7.
[http://dx.doi.org/10.1038/20446] [PMID: 10353249]

[105] Banati RB. Visualising microglial activation *in vivo.* Glia 2002; 40(2): 206-17.
[http://dx.doi.org/10.1002/glia.10144] [PMID: 12379908]

[106] Pavese N, Gerhard A, Tai YF, *et al.* Microglial activation correlates with severity in Huntington disease: A clinical and PET study. Neurology 2006; 66(11): 1638-43.
[http://dx.doi.org/10.1212/01.wnl.0000222734.56412.17] [PMID: 16769933]

[107] Crotti A, Glass CK. The choreography of neuroinflammation in Huntington's disease. Trends Immunol 2015; 36(6): 364-73.
[http://dx.doi.org/10.1016/j.it.2015.04.007] [PMID: 26001312]

[108] Crocker SF, Costain WJ, Robertson HA. DNA microarray analysis of striatal gene expression in symptomatic transgenic Huntington's mice (R6/2) reveals neuroinflammation and insulin associations. Brain Res 2006; 1088(1): 176-86.
[http://dx.doi.org/10.1016/j.brainres.2006.02.102] [PMID: 16626669]

[109] Moscovitch-Lopatin M, Weiss A, Rosas HD, Ritch J, Doros G, Kegel KB. Marian; Kuhn, R.; Bilbe, G.; Paganetti, P.; et al. Optimization of an HTRF Assay for the Detection of Soluble Mutant Huntingtin in Human Buffy Coats: A Potential Biomarker in Blood for Huntington Disease. PLOS Curr. Huntingt. Dis . 2010.
[http://dx.doi.org/10.1371/currents.RRN1205]

[110] Khoshnan A, Ko J, Watkin EE, Paige LA, Reinhart PH, Patterson PH. Activation of the IkappaB kinase complex and nuclear factor-kappaB contributes to mutant huntingtin neurotoxicity. J Neurosci 2004; 24(37): 7999-8008.
[http://dx.doi.org/10.1523/JNEUROSCI.2675-04.2004] [PMID: 15371500]

[111] Giorgini F, Guidetti P, Nguyen Q, Bennett SC, Muchowski PJ. A genomic screen in yeast implicates kynurenine 3-monooxygenase as a therapeutic target for Huntington disease. Nat Genet 2005; 37(5): 526-31.
[http://dx.doi.org/10.1038/ng1542] [PMID: 15806102]

[112] Valadão PAC, Santos KBS, Ferreira e Vieira TH, *et al.* Inflammation in Huntington's disease: A few new twists on an old tale. J Neuroimmunol 2020; 348: 577380.
[http://dx.doi.org/10.1016/j.jneuroim.2020.577380] [PMID: 32896821]

[113] Guha M, Mackman N. LPS induction of gene expression in human monocytes. Cell Signal 2001; 13(2): 85-94.
[http://dx.doi.org/10.1016/S0898-6568(00)00149-2] [PMID: 11257452]

[114] Xing B, Bachstetter AD, Van Eldik LJ. Microglial p38α MAPK is critical for LPS-induced neuron degeneration, through a mechanism involving TNFα. Mol Neurodegener 2011; 6(1): 84.
[http://dx.doi.org/10.1186/1750-1326-6-84] [PMID: 22185458]

[115] Rezai-Zadeh K, Ehrhart J, Bai Y, *et al.* Apigenin and luteolin modulate microglial activation via inhibition of STAT1-induced CD40 expression. J Neuroinflammation 2008; 5(1): 41.
[http://dx.doi.org/10.1186/1742-2094-5-41] [PMID: 18817573]

[116] Jang S, Kelley KW, Johnson RW. Luteolin reduces IL-6 production in microglia by inhibiting JNK phosphorylation and activation of AP-1. Proc Natl Acad Sci USA 2008; 105(21): 7534-9.
[http://dx.doi.org/10.1073/pnas.0802865105] [PMID: 18490655]

[117] Wang S, Wang H, Guo H, Kang L, Gao X, Hu L. Neuroprotection of Scutellarin is mediated by inhibition of microglial inflammatory activation. Neuroscience 2011; 185: 150-60.
[http://dx.doi.org/10.1016/j.neuroscience.2011.04.005] [PMID: 21524691]

[118] Chen JC, Ho FM, Chen C-P, *et al.* Inhibition of iNOS gene expression by quercetin is mediated by the inhibition of IκB kinase, nuclear factor-kappa B and STAT1, and depends on heme oxygenase-1 induction in mouse BV-2 microglia. Eur J Pharmacol 2005; 521(1-3): 9-20.
[http://dx.doi.org/10.1016/j.ejphar.2005.08.005] [PMID: 16171798]

[119] Vafeiadou K, Vauzour D, Lee HY, Rodriguez-Mateos A, Williams RJ, Spencer JPE. The citrus flavanone naringenin inhibits inflammatory signalling in glial cells and protects against neuroinflammatory injury. Arch Biochem Biophys 2009; 484(1): 100-9.

[http://dx.doi.org/10.1016/j.abb.2009.01.016] [PMID: 19467635]

[120] Lee H, Kim YO, Kim H, *et al.* Flavonoid wogonin from medicinal herb is neuroprotective by inhibiting inflammatory activation of microglia. FASEB J 2003; 17(13): 1-21.
[http://dx.doi.org/10.1096/fj.03-0057fje] [PMID: 12897065]

[121] Zeng KW, Fu H, Liu GX, Wang XM. Icariin attenuates lipopolysaccharide-induced microglial activation and resultant death of neurons by inhibiting TAK1/IKK/NF-κB and JNK/p38 MAPK pathways. Int Immunopharmacol 2010; 10(6): 668-78.
[http://dx.doi.org/10.1016/j.intimp.2010.03.010] [PMID: 20347053]

[122] Shu Z, Yang B, Zhao H, *et al.* Tangeretin exerts anti-neuroinflammatory effects via NF-κB modulation in lipopolysaccharide-stimulated microglial cells. Int Immunopharmacol 2014; 19(2): 275-82.
[http://dx.doi.org/10.1016/j.intimp.2014.01.011] [PMID: 24462494]

[123] Zeng K-W, Zhang T, Fu H, Liu G-X, Wang X-M, Schisandrin B. Exerts Anti-Neuroinflammatory Activity by Inhibiting the Toll-like Receptor 4-Dependent MyD88/IKK/NF-KB Signaling Pathway in Lipopolysaccharide-Induced Microglia. Eur J Pharmacol 2012; 692: 29-37.
[http://dx.doi.org/10.1016/j.ejphar.2012.05.030] [PMID: 22698579]

[124] Jeong JW, Lee HH, Han MH, Kim GY, Kim WJ, Choi YH. Anti-inflammatory effects of genistein via suppression of the toll-like receptor 4-mediated signaling pathway in lipopolysaccharide-stimulated BV2 microglia. Chem Biol Interact 2014; 212: 30-9.
[http://dx.doi.org/10.1016/j.cbi.2014.01.012] [PMID: 24491678]

[125] Lee YY, Lee EJ, Park JS, Jang SE, Kim DH, Kim HS. Anti-inflammatory and antioxidant mechanism of tangeretin in activated microglia. J Neuroimmune Pharmacol 2016; 11(2): 294-305.
[http://dx.doi.org/10.1007/s11481-016-9657-x] [PMID: 26899309]

[126] Ha SK, Moon E, Kim SY. Chrysin suppresses LPS-stimulated proinflammatory responses by blocking NF-κB and JNK activations in microglia cells. Neurosci Lett 2010; 485(3): 143-7.
[http://dx.doi.org/10.1016/j.neulet.2010.08.064] [PMID: 20813161]

[127] Zhong X, Liu M, Yao W, *et al.* Epigallocatechin-3-Gallate Attenuates Microglial Inflammation and Neurotoxicity by Suppressing the Activation of Canonical and Noncanonical Inflammasome via TLR4/NF□κB Pathway. Mol Nutr Food Res 2019; 63(21): 1801230.
[http://dx.doi.org/10.1002/mnfr.201801230] [PMID: 31374144]

[128] Muhammad T, Ikram M, Ullah R, Rehman S, Kim M. Hesperetin, a Citrus Flavonoid, Attenuates LPS-Induced Neuroinflammation, Apoptosis and Memory Impairments by Modulating TLR4/NF-κB Signaling. Nutrients 2019; 11(3): 648.
[http://dx.doi.org/10.3390/nu11030648] [PMID: 30884890]

[129] Bieschke J, Russ J, Friedrich RP, *et al.* EGCG remodels mature α-synuclein and amyloid-β fibrils and reduces cellular toxicity. Proc Natl Acad Sci USA 2010; 107(17): 7710-5.
[http://dx.doi.org/10.1073/pnas.0910723107] [PMID: 20385841]

[130] Ehrnhoefer DE, Bieschke J, Boeddrich A, *et al.* EGCG redirects amyloidogenic polypeptides into unstructured, off-pathway oligomers. Nat Struct Mol Biol 2008; 15(6): 558-66.
[http://dx.doi.org/10.1038/nsmb.1437] [PMID: 18511942]

[131] Choi YT, Jung CH, Lee SR, *et al.* The green tea polyphenol (−)-epigallocatechin gallate attenuates β-amyloid-induced neurotoxicity in cultured hippocampal neurons. Life Sci 2001; 70(5): 603-14.
[http://dx.doi.org/10.1016/S0024-3205(01)01438-2] [PMID: 11811904]

[132] Ansari MA, Abdul HM, Joshi G, Opii WO, Butterfield DA. Protective effect of quercetin in primary neurons against Aβ(1–42): relevance to Alzheimer's disease. J Nutr Biochem 2009; 20(4): 269-75.
[http://dx.doi.org/10.1016/j.jnutbio.2008.03.002] [PMID: 18602817]

[133] Hirohata M, Hasegawa K, Tsutsumi-Yasuhara S, *et al.* The anti-amyloidogenic effect is exerted against Alzheimer's beta-amyloid fibrils *in vitro* by preferential and reversible binding of flavonoids to the amyloid fibril structure. Biochemistry 2007; 46(7): 1888-99.

[http://dx.doi.org/10.1021/bi061540x] [PMID: 17253770]

[134]   Song N, Zhang L, Chen W, *et al.* Cyanidin 3- O -β-glucopyranoside activates peroxisome proliferator-activated receptor-γ and alleviates cognitive impairment in the APP swe /PS1 ΔE9 mouse model. Biochim Biophys Acta Mol Basis Dis 2016; 1862(9): 1786-800.
[http://dx.doi.org/10.1016/j.bbadis.2016.05.016] [PMID: 27240542]

[135]   Rezai-Zadeh K, Douglas Shytle R, Bai Y, *et al.* Flavonoid-mediated presenilin-1 phosphorylation reduces Alzheimer's disease β-amyloid production. J Cell Mol Med 2009; 13(3): 574-88.
[http://dx.doi.org/10.1111/j.1582-4934.2008.00344.x] [PMID: 18410522]

[136]   Huang D-S, Yu Y-C, Wu C-H, Lin J-Y. Protective Effects of Wogonin against Alzheimer's Disease by Inhibition of Amyloidogenic Pathway Available online https://www.hindawi.com/journals/ecam/2017/3545169/
[http://dx.doi.org/10.1155/2017/3545169]

[137]   Jiménez-Aliaga K, Bermejo-Bescós P, Benedí J, Martín-Aragón S. Quercetin and rutin exhibit antiamyloidogenic and fibril-disaggregating effects *in vitro* and potent antioxidant activity in APPswe cells. Life Sci 2011; 89(25-26): 939-45.
[http://dx.doi.org/10.1016/j.lfs.2011.09.023] [PMID: 22008478]

[138]   Sonawane SK, Uversky VN, Chinnathambi S. Baicalein inhibits heparin-induced Tau aggregation by initializing non-toxic Tau oligomer formation. Cell Commun Signal 2021; 19(1): 16.
[http://dx.doi.org/10.1186/s12964-021-00704-3] [PMID: 33579328]

[139]   Sonawane SK, Balmik AA, Boral D, Ramasamy S, Chinnathambi S. Baicalein suppresses Repeat Tau fibrillization by sequestering oligomers. Arch Biochem Biophys 2019; 675: 108119.
[http://dx.doi.org/10.1016/j.abb.2019.108119] [PMID: 31568753]

[140]   Mullane K, Williams M. Preclinical Models of Alzheimer's Disease: Relevance and Translational Validity. Curr Protocols Pharmacol 2019; 84(1): e57.
[http://dx.doi.org/10.1002/cpph.57] [PMID: 30802363]

[141]   Vitek MP, Araujo JA, Fossel M, *et al.* Translational Animal Models for Alzheimer's Disease: An Alzheimer's Association Business Consortium Think Tank. Alzheimers Dement. Transl. Res. Clin. Interv. 2020; 6: e12114.
[http://dx.doi.org/10.1002/trc2.12114]

[142]   Darbandi N, Ramezani M, Khodagholi F, Noori M. Kaempferol promotes memory retention and density of hippocampal CA1 neurons in intra-cerebroventricular STZ-induced experimental AD model in Wistar rats. Biologija (Vilnius) 2016; 62(3)
[http://dx.doi.org/10.6001/biologija.v62i3.3368]

[143]   Ishola IO, Osele MO, Chijioke MC, Adeyemi OO. Isorhamnetin enhanced cortico-hippocampal learning and memory capability in mice with scopolamine-induced amnesia: Role of antioxidant defense, cholinergic and BDNF signaling. Brain Res 2019; 1712: 188-96.
[http://dx.doi.org/10.1016/j.brainres.2019.02.017] [PMID: 30772273]

[144]   Nandakumar K, Ramalingayya GV, Nampoothiri M, *et al.* Naringin and rutin alleviates episodic memory deficits in two differentially challenged object recognition tasks. Pharmacogn Mag 2016; 12(45) (Suppl. 1): 63.
[http://dx.doi.org/10.4103/0973-1296.176104] [PMID: 27041861]

[145]   Javed H, Vaibhav K, Ahmed ME, *et al.* Effect of hesperidin on neurobehavioral, neuroinflammation, oxidative stress and lipid alteration in intracerebroventricular streptozotocin induced cognitive impairment in mice. J Neurol Sci 2015; 348(1-2): 51-9.
[http://dx.doi.org/10.1016/j.jns.2014.10.044] [PMID: 25434716]

[146]   Wang H, Wang H, Cheng H, Che Z. Ameliorating effect of luteolin on memory impairment in an Alzheimer's disease model. Mol Med Rep 2016; 13(5): 4215-20.
[http://dx.doi.org/10.3892/mmr.2016.5052] [PMID: 27035793]

[147] Onozuka H, Nakajima A, Matsuzaki K, *et al*. Nobiletin, a citrus flavonoid, improves memory impairment and Abeta pathology in a transgenic mouse model of Alzheimer's disease. J Pharmacol Exp Ther 2008; 326(3): 739-44.
[http://dx.doi.org/10.1124/jpet.108.140293] [PMID: 18544674]

[148] Sawmiller D, Habib A, Li S, *et al*. Diosmin reduces cerebral Aβ levels, tau hyperphosphorylation, neuroinflammation, and cognitive impairment in the 3xTg-AD mice. J Neuroimmunol 2016; 299: 98-106.
[http://dx.doi.org/10.1016/j.jneuroim.2016.08.018] [PMID: 27725131]

[149] Li C, Zug C, Qu H, Schluesener H, Zhang Z. Hesperidin ameliorates behavioral impairments and neuropathology of transgenic APP/PS1 mice. Behav Brain Res 2015; 281: 32-42.
[http://dx.doi.org/10.1016/j.bbr.2014.12.012] [PMID: 25510196]

[150] Rezai-Zadeh K, Shytle D, Sun N, *et al*. Green tea epigallocatechin-3-gallate (EGCG) modulates amyloid precursor protein cleavage and reduces cerebral amyloidosis in Alzheimer transgenic mice. J Neurosci 2005; 25(38): 8807-14.
[http://dx.doi.org/10.1523/JNEUROSCI.1521-05.2005] [PMID: 16177050]

[151] Lee JW, Lee YK, Ban JO, *et al*. Green tea (-)-epigallocatechin-3-gallate inhibits beta-amyloid-induced cognitive dysfunction through modification of secretase activity via inhibition of ERK and NF-kappaB pathways in mice. J Nutr 2009; 139(10): 1987-93.
[http://dx.doi.org/10.3945/jn.109.109785] [PMID: 19656855]

[152] Rezai-Zadeh K, Arendash GW, Hou H, *et al*. Green tea epigallocatechin-3-gallate (EGCG) reduces β-amyloid mediated cognitive impairment and modulates tau pathology in Alzheimer transgenic mice. Brain Res 2008; 1214: 177-87.
[http://dx.doi.org/10.1016/j.brainres.2008.02.107] [PMID: 18457818]

[153] Nakajima A, Aoyama Y, Shin EJ, *et al*. Nobiletin, a citrus flavonoid, improves cognitive impairment and reduces soluble Aβ levels in a triple transgenic mouse model of Alzheimer's disease (3XTg-AD). Behav Brain Res 2015; 289: 69-77.
[http://dx.doi.org/10.1016/j.bbr.2015.04.028] [PMID: 25913833]

[154] Nakajima A, Aoyama Y, Nguyen TTL, *et al*. Nobiletin, a citrus flavonoid, ameliorates cognitive impairment, oxidative burden, and hyperphosphorylation of tau in senescence-accelerated mouse. Behav Brain Res 2013; 250: 351-60.
[http://dx.doi.org/10.1016/j.bbr.2013.05.025] [PMID: 23714077]

[155] Paula PC, Angelica Maria SG, Luis CH, Gloria Patricia CG. Preventive Effect of Quercetin in a Triple Transgenic Alzheimer's Disease Mice Model. Molecules 2019; 24(12): 2287.
[http://dx.doi.org/10.3390/molecules24122287] [PMID: 31226738]

[156] Qin L, Zhang J, Qin M. Protective effect of cyanidin 3-O-glucoside on beta-amyloid peptide-induced cognitive impairment in rats. Neurosci Lett 2013; 534: 285-8.
[http://dx.doi.org/10.1016/j.neulet.2012.12.023] [PMID: 23274703]

[157] Currais A, Prior M, Dargusch R, *et al*. Modulation of p25 and inflammatory pathways by fisetin maintains cognitive function in A lzheimer's disease transgenic mice. Aging Cell 2014; 13(2): 379-90.
[http://dx.doi.org/10.1111/acel.12185] [PMID: 24341874]

[158] Mastroiacovo D, Kwik-Uribe C, Grassi D, *et al*. Cocoa flavanol consumption improves cognitive function, blood pressure control, and metabolic profile in elderly subjects: the Cocoa, Cognition, and Aging (CoCoA) Study—a randomized controlled trial. Am J Clin Nutr 2015; 101(3): 538-48.
[http://dx.doi.org/10.3945/ajcn.114.092189] [PMID: 25733639]

[159] Desideri G, Kwik-Uribe C, Grassi D, *et al*. Benefits in Cognitive Function, Blood Pressure, and Insulin Resistance through Cocoa Flavanol Consumption in Elderly Subjects with Mild Cognitive Impairment: The Cocoa, Cognition, and Aging (CoCoA) Study. Hypertens. Dallas Tex 1979 2012; 60: 794-801.
[http://dx.doi.org/10.1161/HYPERTENSIONAHA.112.193060]

[160] Brickman AM, Khan UA, Provenzano FA, *et al.* Enhancing dentate gyrus function with dietary flavanols improves cognition in older adults. Nat Neurosci 2014; 17(12): 1798-803.
[http://dx.doi.org/10.1038/nn.3850] [PMID: 25344629]

[161] Caruana M, Neuner J, Högen T, *et al.* Polyphenolic compounds are novel protective agents against lipid membrane damage by α-synuclein aggregates *in vitro*. Biochim Biophys Acta Biomembr 2012; 1818(11): 2502-10.
[http://dx.doi.org/10.1016/j.bbamem.2012.05.019] [PMID: 22634381]

[162] Takahashi R, Ono K, Takamura Y, *et al.* Phenolic compounds prevent the oligomerization of α-synuclein and reduce synaptic toxicity. J Neurochem 2015; 134(5): 943-55.
[http://dx.doi.org/10.1111/jnc.13180] [PMID: 26016728]

[163] Xu Y, Zhang Y, Quan Z, *et al.* Epigallocatechin Gallate (EGCG) Inhibits Alpha-Synuclein Aggregation: A Potential Agent for Parkinson's Disease. Neurochem Res 2016; 41(10): 2788-96.
[http://dx.doi.org/10.1007/s11064-016-1995-9] [PMID: 27364962]

[164] Cui Y, Wu J, Jung SC, *et al.* Anti-neuroinflammatory activity of nobiletin on suppression of microglial activation. Biol Pharm Bull 2010; 33(11): 1814-21.
[http://dx.doi.org/10.1248/bpb.33.1814] [PMID: 21048305]

[165] Wu LH, Lin C, Lin HY, *et al.* Naringenin Suppresses Neuroinflammatory Responses Through Inducing Suppressor of Cytokine Signaling 3 Expression. Mol Neurobiol 2016; 53(2): 1080-91.
[http://dx.doi.org/10.1007/s12035-014-9042-9] [PMID: 25579382]

[166] Choi YH, Kim G-Y, Choi YH. Naringenin attenuates the release of pro-inflammatory mediators from lipopolysaccharide-stimulated BV2 microglia by inactivating nuclear factor-κB and inhibiting mitogen-activated protein kinases. Int J Mol Med 2012; 30(1): 204-10.
[http://dx.doi.org/10.3892/ijmm.2012.979] [PMID: 22552813]

[167] Chinta SJ, Ganesan A, Reis-Rodrigues P, Lithgow GJ, Andersen JK. Anti-inflammatory role of the isoflavone diadzein in lipopolysaccharide-stimulated microglia: implications for Parkinson's disease. Neurotox Res 2013; 23(2): 145-53.
[http://dx.doi.org/10.1007/s12640-012-9328-5] [PMID: 22573480]

[168] Subedi L, Ji E, Shin D, Jin J, Yeo J, Kim S. Equol, a Dietary Daidzein Gut Metabolite Attenuates Microglial Activation and Potentiates Neuroprotection *In Vitro*. Nutrients 2017; 9(3): 207.
[http://dx.doi.org/10.3390/nu9030207] [PMID: 28264445]

[169] Chen HQ, Jin ZY, Wang XJ, Xu XM, Deng L, Zhao JW. Luteolin protects dopaminergic neurons from inflammation-induced injury through inhibition of microglial activation. Neurosci Lett 2008; 448(2): 175-9.
[http://dx.doi.org/10.1016/j.neulet.2008.10.046] [PMID: 18952146]

[170] Zhang Z, Cao X, Xiong N, *et al.* Morin exerts neuroprotective actions in Parkinson disease models in vitro and *in vivo*. Acta Pharmacol Sin 2010; 31(8): 900-6.
[http://dx.doi.org/10.1038/aps.2010.77] [PMID: 20644549]

[171] Lee KM, Lee Y, Chun HJ, *et al.* Neuroprotective and anti-inflammatory effects of morin in a murine model of Parkinson's disease. J Neurosci Res 2016; 94(10): 865-78.
[http://dx.doi.org/10.1002/jnr.23764] [PMID: 27265894]

[172] Cho N, Choi JH, Yang H, *et al.* Neuroprotective and anti-inflammatory effects of flavonoids isolated from Rhus verniciflua in neuronal HT22 and microglial BV2 cell lines. Food Chem Toxicol 2012; 50(6): 1940-5.
[http://dx.doi.org/10.1016/j.fct.2012.03.052] [PMID: 22465834]

[173] Blandini F, Armentero MT. Animal models of Parkinson's disease. FEBS J 2012; 279(7): 1156-66.
[http://dx.doi.org/10.1111/j.1742-4658.2012.08491.x] [PMID: 22251459]

[174] Johnson ME, Bobrovskaya L. An update on the rotenone models of Parkinson's disease: Their ability to reproduce the features of clinical disease and model gene–environment interactions.

Neurotoxicology 2015; 46: 101-16.
[http://dx.doi.org/10.1016/j.neuro.2014.12.002] [PMID: 25514659]

[175] Hu Q, Uversky VN, Huang M, *et al.* Baicalein inhibits α-synuclein oligomer formation and prevents progression of α-synuclein accumulation in a rotenone mouse model of Parkinson's disease. Biochim Biophys Acta Mol Basis Dis 2016; 1862(10): 1883-90.
[http://dx.doi.org/10.1016/j.bbadis.2016.07.008] [PMID: 27425033]

[176] Hung KC, Huang HJ, Wang YT, Lin AMY. Baicalein attenuates α-synuclein aggregation, inflammasome activation and autophagy in the MPP⁻-treated nigrostriatal dopaminergic system in vivo. J Ethnopharmacol 2016; 194: 522-9.
[http://dx.doi.org/10.1016/j.jep.2016.10.040] [PMID: 27742410]

[177] Lee E, Park HR, Ji ST, Lee Y, Lee J. Baicalein attenuates astroglial activation in the 1-methyl-4-phenyl-1,2,3,4-tetrahydropyridine-induced Parkinson's disease model by downregulating the activations of nuclear factor-κB, ERK, and JNK. J Neurosci Res 2014; 92(1): 130-9.
[http://dx.doi.org/10.1002/jnr.23307] [PMID: 24166733]

[178] Mu X, He GR, Yuan X, Li XX, Du GH. Baicalein protects the brain against neuron impairments induced by MPTP in C57BL/6 mice. Pharmacol Biochem Behav 2011; 98(2): 286-91.
[http://dx.doi.org/10.1016/j.pbb.2011.01.011] [PMID: 21262257]

[179] Cheng Y, He G, Mu X, *et al.* Neuroprotective effect of baicalein against MPTP neurotoxicity: Behavioral, biochemical and immunohistochemical profile. Neurosci Lett 2008; 441(1): 16-20.
[http://dx.doi.org/10.1016/j.neulet.2008.05.116] [PMID: 18586394]

[180] Anusha C, Sumathi T, Joseph LD. Protective role of apigenin on rotenone induced rat model of Parkinson's disease: Suppression of neuroinflammation and oxidative stress mediated apoptosis. Chem Biol Interact 2017; 269: 67-79.
[http://dx.doi.org/10.1016/j.cbi.2017.03.016] [PMID: 28389404]

[181] Jeong KH, Jeon MT, Kim HD, *et al.* Nobiletin protects dopaminergic neurons in the 1-methyl-4-phenylpyridinium-treated rat model of Parkinson's disease. J Med Food 2015; 18(4): 409-14.
[http://dx.doi.org/10.1089/jmf.2014.3241] [PMID: 25325362]

[182] Yabuki Y, Ohizumi Y, Yokosuka A, Mimaki Y, Fukunaga K. Nobiletin treatment improves motor and cognitive deficits seen in MPTP-induced Parkinson model mice. Neuroscience 2014; 259: 126-41.
[http://dx.doi.org/10.1016/j.neuroscience.2013.11.051] [PMID: 24316474]

[183] Leem E, Nam JH, Jeon MT, *et al.* Naringin protects the nigrostriatal dopaminergic projection through induction of GDNF in a neurotoxin model of Parkinson's disease. J Nutr Biochem 2014; 25(7): 801-6.
[http://dx.doi.org/10.1016/j.jnutbio.2014.03.006] [PMID: 24797334]

[184] Kim HD, Jeong KH, Jung UJ, Kim SR. Naringin treatment induces neuroprotective effects in a mouse model of Parkinson's disease *in vivo*, but not enough to restore the lesioned dopaminergic system. J Nutr Biochem 2016; 28: 140-6.
[http://dx.doi.org/10.1016/j.jnutbio.2015.10.013] [PMID: 26878791]

[185] Levites Y, Weinreb O, Maor G, Youdim MBH, Mandel S. Green tea polyphenol (-)-epigallocatech-n-3-gallate prevents N-methyl-4-phenyl-1,2,3,6-tetrahydropyridine-induced dopaminergic neurodegeneration. J Neurochem 2001; 78(5): 1073-82.
[http://dx.doi.org/10.1046/j.1471-4159.2001.00490.x] [PMID: 11553681]

[186] Patil SP, Jain PD, Sancheti JS, Ghumatkar PJ, Tambe R, Sathaye S. RETRACTED: Neuroprotective and neurotrophic effects of Apigenin and Luteolin in MPTP induced parkinsonism in mice. Neuropharmacology 2014; 86: 192-202.
[http://dx.doi.org/10.1016/j.neuropharm.2014.07.012] [PMID: 25087727]

[187] Ay M, Luo J, Langley M, *et al.* Molecular mechanisms underlying protective effects of quercetin against mitochondrial dysfunction and progressive dopaminergic neurodegeneration in cell culture and MitoPark transgenic mouse models of Parkinson's Disease. J Neurochem 2017; 141(5): 766-82.
[http://dx.doi.org/10.1111/jnc.14033] [PMID: 28376279]

[188] Li S, Pu XP. Neuroprotective effect of kaempferol against a 1-methyl-4-phenyl-1,2-3,6-tetrahydropyridine-induced mouse model of Parkinson's disease. Biol Pharm Bull 2011; 34(8): 1291-6.
[http://dx.doi.org/10.1248/bpb.34.1291] [PMID: 21804220]

[189] Lv C, Hong T, Yang Z, *et al.* Effect of Quercetin in the 1-Methyl-4-phenyl-1, 2, 3, 6-tetrahydropyridine-Induced Mouse Model of Parkinson's Disease. Evid Based Complement Alternat Med 2012; 2012: 1-6.
[http://dx.doi.org/10.1155/2012/928643] [PMID: 22454690]

[190] Manivasagam T, Nataraj J, Tamilselvam K, Essa MM, Janakiraman U. Antioxidant and anti-inflammatory potential of hesperidin against 1-methyl-4-phenyl-1, 2, 3, 6-tetrahydropyridine-induced experimental Parkinson's disease in mice. Int J Nutr Pharmacol Neurol Dis 2013; 3(3): 294.
[http://dx.doi.org/10.4103/2231-0738.114875]

[191] Baluchnejadmojarad T, Roghani M. The Flavonoid Hesperetin Alleviates Behavioral Abnormality in 6-Hydroxydopamine Rat Model of Hemi-Parkinsonism. Basic Clin Neurosci 2010; 2: 20-3.

[192] Datla KP, Christidou M, Widmer WW, Rooprai HK, Dexter DT. Tissue distribution and neuroprotective effects of citrus flavonoid tangeretin in a rat model of Parkinson's disease. Neuroreport 2001; 12(17): 3871-5.
[http://dx.doi.org/10.1097/00001756-200112040-00053] [PMID: 11726811]

[193] Moshahid Khan M, Raza SS, Javed H, *et al.* Rutin protects dopaminergic neurons from oxidative stress in an animal model of Parkinson's disease. Neurotox Res 2012; 22(1): 1-15.
[http://dx.doi.org/10.1007/s12640-011-9295-2] [PMID: 22194158]

[194] Baluchnejadmojarad T, Jamali-Raeufy N, Zabihnejad S, Rabiee N, Roghani M. Troxerutin exerts neuroprotection in 6-hydroxydopamine lesion rat model of Parkinson's disease: Possible involvement of PI3K/ERβ signaling. Eur J Pharmacol 2017; 801: 72-8.
[http://dx.doi.org/10.1016/j.ejphar.2017.03.002] [PMID: 28284752]

[195] Kim HD, Jeong KH, Jung UJ, Kim SR. Myricitrin Ameliorates 6-Hydroxydopamine-Induced Dopaminergic Neuronal Loss in the Substantia Nigra of Mouse Brain. J Med Food 2016; 19(4): 374-82.
[http://dx.doi.org/10.1089/jmf.2015.3581] [PMID: 26991235]

[196] Liang J, López-Valdés HE, Martínez-Coria H, *et al.* Erratum to: Dihydromyricetin Ameliorates Behavioral Deficits and Reverses Neuropathology of Transgenic Mouse Models of Alzheimer's Disease. Neurochem Res 2014; 39(7): 1403-3.
[http://dx.doi.org/10.1007/s11064-014-1358-3]

[197] Aiken CT, Tobin AJ, Schweitzer ES. A cell-based screen for drugs to treat Huntington's disease. Neurobiol Dis 2004; 16(3): 546-55.
[http://dx.doi.org/10.1016/j.nbd.2004.04.001] [PMID: 15262266]

[198] Maher P, Dargusch R, Bodai L, Gerard PE, Purcell JM, Marsh JL. ERK activation by the polyphenols fisetin and resveratrol provides neuroprotection in multiple models of Huntington's disease. Hum Mol Genet 2011; 20(2): 261-70.
[http://dx.doi.org/10.1093/hmg/ddq460] [PMID: 20952447]

[199] Zhu M, Rajamani S, Kaylor J, Han S, Zhou F, Fink AL. The flavonoid baicalein inhibits fibrillation of alpha-synuclein and disaggregates existing fibrils. J Biol Chem 2004; 279(26): 26846-57.
[http://dx.doi.org/10.1074/jbc.M403129200] [PMID: 15096521]

[200] Meng X, Munishkina LA, Fink AL, Uversky VN. Effects of various flavonoids on the α-synuclein fibrillation process. Parkinsons Dis 2010; 2010: 1-16.
[http://dx.doi.org/10.4061/2010/650794] [PMID: 20976092]

[201] Borlongan CV, Koutouzis TK, Sanberg PR. 3-Nitropropionic acid animal model and Huntington's disease. Neurosci Biobehav Rev 1997; 21(3): 289-93.

[http://dx.doi.org/10.1016/S0149-7634(96)00027-9] [PMID: 9168265]

[202] Chakraborty J, Singh R, Dutta D, Naskar A, Rajamma U, Mohanakumar KP. Quercetin improves behavioral deficiencies, restores astrocytes and microglia, and reduces serotonin metabolism in 3-nitropropionic acid-induced rat model of Huntington's Disease. CNS Neurosci Ther 2014; 20(1): 10-9.
[http://dx.doi.org/10.1111/cns.12189] [PMID: 24188794]

[203] Sandhir R, Mehrotra A. Quercetin supplementation is effective in improving mitochondrial dysfunctions induced by 3-nitropropionic acid: Implications in Huntington's disease. Biochim Biophys Acta Mol Basis Dis 2013; 1832(3): 421-30.
[http://dx.doi.org/10.1016/j.bbadis.2012.11.018] [PMID: 23220257]

[204] Suganya SN, Sumathi T. Effect of rutin against a mitochondrial toxin, 3-nitropropionicacid induced biochemical, behavioral and histological alterations-a pilot study on Huntington's disease model in rats. Metab Brain Dis 2017; 32(2): 471-81.
[http://dx.doi.org/10.1007/s11011-016-9929-4] [PMID: 27928694]

[205] Lagoa R, Lopez-Sanchez C, Samhan-Arias AK, Gañan CM, Garcia-Martinez V, Gutierrez-Merino C. Kaempferol protects against rat striatal degeneration induced by 3-nitropropionic acid. J Neurochem 2009; 111(2): 473-87.
[http://dx.doi.org/10.1111/j.1471-4159.2009.06331.x] [PMID: 19682208]

[206] Menze ET, Tadros MG, Abdel-Tawab AM, Khalifa AE. Potential neuroprotective effects of hesperidin on 3-nitropropionic acid-induced neurotoxicity in rats. Neurotoxicology 2012; 33(5): 1265-75.
[http://dx.doi.org/10.1016/j.neuro.2012.07.007] [PMID: 22850463]

[207] Kumar P, Kumar A. Protective effect of hesperidin and naringin against 3-nitropropionic acid induced Huntington's like symptoms in rats: Possible role of nitric oxide. Behav Brain Res 2010; 206(1): 38-46.
[http://dx.doi.org/10.1016/j.bbr.2009.08.028] [PMID: 19716383]

[208] Kumar P, Kumar A. Effect of lycopene and epigallocatechin-3-gallate against 3-nitropropionic acid induced cognitive dysfunction and glutathione depletion in rat: A novel nitric oxide mechanism. Food Chem Toxicol 2009; 47(10): 2522-30.
[http://dx.doi.org/10.1016/j.fct.2009.07.011] [PMID: 19616597]

[209] Thangarajan S, Ramachandran S, Krishnamurthy P. Chrysin exerts neuroprotective effects against 3-Nitropropionic acid induced behavioral despair—Mitochondrial dysfunction and striatal apoptosis via upregulating Bcl-2 gene and downregulating Bax—Bad genes in male wistar rats. Biomed Pharmacother 2016; 84: 514-25.
[http://dx.doi.org/10.1016/j.biopha.2016.09.070] [PMID: 27690136]

[210] Menze ET, Esmat A, Tadros MG, Khalifa AE, Abdel-Naim AB. Genistein improves sensorimotor gating: Mechanisms related to its neuroprotective effects on the striatum. Neuropharmacology 2016; 105: 35-46.
[http://dx.doi.org/10.1016/j.neuropharm.2016.01.007] [PMID: 26764242]

[211] Li JY, Popovic N, Brundin P. The use of the R6 transgenic mouse models of Huntington's disease in attempts to develop novel therapeutic strategies. NeuroRx 2005; 2(3): 447-64.
[http://dx.doi.org/10.1602/neurorx.2.3.447] [PMID: 16389308]

[212] García-Díaz Barriga G, Giralt A, Anglada-Huguet M, *et al.* 7,8-dihydroxyflavone ameliorates cognitive and motor deficits in a Huntington's disease mouse model through specific activation of the PLCγ1 pathway. Hum Mol Genet 2017; 26(16): 3144-60.
[http://dx.doi.org/10.1093/hmg/ddx198] [PMID: 28541476]

[213] Vauzour D, Rodriguez-Mateos A, Corona G, Oruna-Concha MJ, Spencer JPE. Polyphenols and human health: prevention of disease and mechanisms of action. Nutrients 2010; 2(11): 1106-31.
[http://dx.doi.org/10.3390/nu2111106] [PMID: 22254000]

[214] Jaeger BN, Parylak SL, Gage FH. Mechanisms of dietary flavonoid action in neuronal function and neuroinflammation. Mol Aspects Med 2018; 61: 50-62.

[http://dx.doi.org/10.1016/j.mam.2017.11.003] [PMID: 29117513]

[215] Beking K, Vieira A. Flavonoid intake and disability-adjusted life years due to Alzheimer's and related dementias: a population-based study involving twenty-three developed countries. Public Health Nutr 2010; 13(9): 1403-9.
[http://dx.doi.org/10.1017/S1368980009992990] [PMID: 20059796]

[216] Holt EM, Steffen LM, Moran A, *et al.* Fruit and vegetable consumption and its relation to markers of inflammation and oxidative stress in adolescents. J Am Diet Assoc 2009; 109(3): 414-21.
[http://dx.doi.org/10.1016/j.jada.2008.11.036] [PMID: 19248856]

[217] Kelley DS, Rasooly R, Jacob RA, Kader AA, Mackey BE. Consumption of Bing sweet cherries lowers circulating concentrations of inflammation markers in healthy men and women. J Nutr 2006; 136(4): 981-6.
[http://dx.doi.org/10.1093/jn/136.4.981] [PMID: 16549461]

[218] Nantz MP, Rowe CA, Nieves C Jr, Percival SS. Immunity and antioxidant capacity in humans is enhanced by consumption of a dried, encapsulated fruit and vegetable juice concentrate. J Nutr 2006; 136(10): 2606-10.
[http://dx.doi.org/10.1093/jn/136.10.2606] [PMID: 16988134]

[219] De Bacquer D, Clays E, Delanghe J, De Backer G. Epidemiological evidence for an association between habitual tea consumption and markers of chronic inflammation. Atherosclerosis 2006; 189(2): 428-35.
[http://dx.doi.org/10.1016/j.atherosclerosis.2005.12.028] [PMID: 16442546]

[220] Steptoe A, Gibson EL, Vuononvirta R, *et al.* The effects of chronic tea intake on platelet activation and inflammation: A double-blind placebo controlled trial. Atherosclerosis 2007; 193(2): 277-82.
[http://dx.doi.org/10.1016/j.atherosclerosis.2006.08.054] [PMID: 17010979]

[221] Widlansky ME, Duffy SJ, Hamburg NM, *et al.* Effects of black tea consumption on plasma catechins and markers of oxidative stress and inflammation in patients with coronary artery disease. Free Radic Biol Med 2005; 38(4): 499-506.
[http://dx.doi.org/10.1016/j.freeradbiomed.2004.11.013] [PMID: 15649652]

[222] Hickson LJ, Langhi Prata LGP, Bobart SA, *et al.* Senolytics decrease senescent cells in humans: Preliminary report from a clinical trial of Dasatinib plus Quercetin in individuals with diabetic kidney disease. EBioMedicine 2019; 47: 446-56.
[http://dx.doi.org/10.1016/j.ebiom.2019.08.069] [PMID: 31542391]

CHAPTER 14

Utilization of Nutraceuticals and Ayurvedic Drugs in the Management of Parkinson's Disease

Shilpa Negi[1] and Sarika Singh[1,*]

[1] Department of Neuroscience and Ageing Biology and Division of Toxicology and Experimental Medicine, CSIR-Central Drug Research Institute, Lucknow-226031, (U.P.), India

Abstract: Age-related degeneration of dopaminergic (DAergic) neurons may be either genetic or due to exposure to environmental toxins that mark the onset of Parkinson's disease (PD) pathology. Treatments like surgery and symptoms relieving drugs are available, but they have their side effects during prolonged consumption. Recent studies have shown that the use of food-derived compounds offers significant prevention and treatment of many neurological disorders. These compounds, commonly known as nutraceuticals, show immense importance in mitigating neuronal disease as there is a strong correlation between food and mental health. Accumulation of α-synuclein protein in the degenerated neurons and concomitant oxidative stress-related pathological events are critical and known pathological markers of PD therefore, food-derived compounds containing antioxidative capacity may offer therapeutic implications. In addition, nutraceuticals are comparatively cost-effective and the safest alternatives of drugs available. Indian medicine system of Ayurveda has long been incorporating the use of herbs to cure PD. This chapter focuses on the utilization of nutraceuticals and ayurvedic preparations in PD pathology.

Keywords: Ayurvedic drugs, DA agonists, Nutraceuticals, Therapeutics, PD.

INTRODUCTION

Parkinson's Disease (PD) is a neuropathological condition associated with progressive deterioration of dopamine (DA) secreting neurons in the substantia nigra pars compacta (SNpc) region of the midbrain [1]. Extensive research has identified various genetic mutations that induce the PD, however, the majority of the PD cases are sporadic or idiopathic, therefore, environmental exposure also plays a critical role in disease onset [2]. Idiopathic PD is induced due to exposure to several chemical and environmental toxins, such as rotenone, paraquat, *etc.*

---
[*] **Corresponding authors Sarika Singh:** Department of Neuroscience and Ageing Biology and Division of Toxicology and Experimental Medicine, CSIR-Central Drug Research Institute, Lucknow-226031, (U.P.), India;
E-mail: sarika_singh@cdri.res.in

Rotenone, 1-Methyl-4-Phenyl-1, 2, 3, 6-Tetrahydroxypyridiine (MPTP), 6-Hydroxydopamine (6-OHDA) etc., are successfully being utilized in research to induce PD-related pathology in both cellular and rodent models to elucidate the disease mechanisms [3]. These toxins interact with and modulate the functions of various genes like SNCA/alpha-synuclein (α-syn), Ubiquitin carboxy-terminal Hydrolase-1 (UCHL1), Leucine Rich Repeat Kinase-2 (LRRK-2), Serine Protease (HTRA2), Parkin (PRKN), PTEN-Induced Putative Kinase 1(PINK), Lysosomal ATPase and Glucocerebrosidase (GBA) whose mutation or alteration in protein structure & function is responsible for the induction of disease pathology [4]. Symptomatically PD pathology involves tremor, rigidity, bradykinesia (slowness of movement), and postural instability [5]. Including these motor disabilities, various non-motor clinical features are also associated with the disease and advancing age. These non-motor symptoms include neuropsychiatric symptoms (depression, dementia, panic attacks, hallucinations etc.), sleep disorders (insomnia, restless legs, periodic limb movement, etc.), nausea, constipation, dry eyes, etc [6 - 10]. Biochemical pathogenesis of PD involves the misfolding and aggregation of protein alpha-synuclein (which accumulate along with chaperones and ubiquitin residues in the Lewy bodies found in DAergic neurons undergoing degeneration), unfolded protein response (UPR) and endoplasmic reticulum-associated degradation (ERAD), oxidative & nitrosative stress, mitochondrial dysfunction and altered bioenergetics which disturbs the neuronal physiological functions and promote the mitophagy and apoptosis. Although, SNpc has neuromelanin that offers neuroprotective effects, the high level of iron in SNpc activates the monoamine oxidase B (MAO-B), which participates in DA metabolism and forms the neurotoxic H_2O_2 [3, 11]. Downstream cellular signalling or mechanisms of PD are not intensively known, nonetheless, pathways involving oxidative stress and protein misfolding work in a feedback route and induce the apoptosis of neurons. Current treatment of PD includes drugs like Levodopa (L-Dopa), DA agonists (pramipexole, lisuride, cabergoline), and MAO-B inhibitors (selegiline and rasagiline), while deep brain surgery and implantation of embryonic DAergic neurons (gene therapy) are also employed but limited to very few patients due to its high cost [4]. Despite the available complicated surgeries and various medications, no therapeutic strategy could modify the disease status and prevent neuronal degeneration. Therefore, further review of available research and the therapeutic molecule is needed. Since synthetic drugs are not offering the disease modifications now, researchers are looking for nutraceuticals that may have comparatively fewer side effects and better therapeutic implications. Nutraceuticals are the top priority in this category as they are readily available, comparatively have fewer side effects, and are cost-effective. The term Nutraceutical was coined by Dr. De Felice, which refers to food or bioactive compounds derived from food that has therapeutic benefits in the prevention and/or in the treatment of chronic diseases like PD [1, 2, 12 - 14]. These nutraceuticals are crucial as they have Antioxidative capacity. Since PD pathology involves oxidative neuronal apoptosis, these nutraceuticals offer therapeutic implications but still, the pre-clinical studies are limited and further explorations are required.

NUTRACEUTICALS USED IN PD THERAPEUTICS

Various nutraceuticals have been tested for their effects on cell culture and animal models in the perspective of PD pathology, mainly targeting the mechanisms including (a) reactive oxygen species (ROS) scavenging (b) anti-inflammation (c) iron-chelation (d) modulation of cell signaling pathway (e) mitochondrial function restoration and (f) anti-apoptosis (Fig. **1**) [3]. L-Dopa is the potential synthetic drug given to PD patients along with carbidopa, however, it shows significant side effects after chronic consumption [4, 15 - 19]. Nutraceuticals on the basis of their natural resource, may be of different types, and three key terms are being used for them 1. Nutrients 2. Herbals 3. Dietary supplements/fibers. Globally, the most rapidly growing segment of the industry is dietary supplements, and they also offer significant health improvements [20 - 25]. In a study by Zhao *et al.* (2007), the twenty-four genera of plants have been reviewed and suggested to have therapeutic implications in PD and readers may refer to the article [26, 27]. Phytochemicals like ginsenosides, curcumin, asiatic acid, etc., have well-known therapeutic potentials. Also, nutrients like co-enzyme Q_{10}, Nicotinamide adenine dinucleotide (NADH), vitamin C, etc., can be obtained from fruits or other parts of plants and act as anti-oxidants. Extracts of *Panax ginseng* contain ginsenosides Rb_1, Rg_1, Re, and Rd, known for their neuroprotection, anti-inflammatory, anti-oxidant and anti-apoptotic properties [26]. *Gastrodia*, an herbal medicine used in oriental countries, has anti-oxidative properties due its constituents like vanillyl alcohol, 4-hydroxybenzaldehyde, etc. and can cross the blood-brain barrier, which is the most important concern during drug development for neurodegenerative disorders [28]. Resveratrol obtained from grapes, peanuts, berries, and pines acts as a ROS scavenger [28]. Catechins from green tea act as anti-oxidant and restore catalase activity [29]. The details of various nutraceuticals are given in Table **1**.

Table 1. Neutraceutical explored in experimental models of PD.

Bioactive Compound	Model	Mechanism of Action	Refs.
Omega-3-Polyunsaturated Fatty acid from fish	MPTP-induced mice	Reduce DA oxidation and important modulators of DAergic neurons in basal ganglia.	[3]
Coenzyme Q_{10}	MPTP-induced rodent	Maintains Electron Transport Chain of mitochondria.	[3, 4]

Bioactive Compound	Model	Mechanism of Action	Refs.
Creatine	MPTP-induced mouse	Neuroprotective as counters ATP depletion by increasing intracellular phosphocreatine.	[4]
Vitamin D	6-OHDA-induced and MPTP-induced rodent	Upregulates Glial Derived Neurotrophic Factor (GDNF), glutathione, anti-apoptotic and reduces Nitric Oxide Synthase (NOS).	[3]
Vitamin C and Vitamin D	-	Free radical scavenger and anti-oxidant.	[3]
Lycopene	MPTP-induced mouse	Increases activity of Superoxide Dismutase (SOD), NADH, and glutathione.	[2]
Vitamin B complex	MPTP-induced mice	Regulates homocysteine levels and restores mitochondrial functioning.	[3]
Nucleoprotein from salmon	MPTP-induced mouse	ROS scavenger and prevent lipofuscin-like substance.	[3]
Quercetin from onion, broccoli, apple.	6-OHDA-induced rat	Antioxidant, and anti-inflammatory.	[3]
Ginsenosides (Rb1, Rg1, Re and Rd) Saponins	MPP^+-induced SH-SY5Y DAergic cell culture PC12 cells Rat model	Neuroprotective. Attenuates neuro-inflammation. Suppresses oxidative stress and cell death by inhibiting Nuclear factor-kappa B (NF-κB). Decreases neuro-inflammation.	[30, 31, 32, 33]
Catechins (*Epicatechin* Gallate, Epigallatoca-techin, Epicatechin, Epigallocate-chin 3 gallate) Thioflavin	6-OHDA-induced SH-SY5Y cells MPTP-induced mice	Downregulation of inducible NO synthase and Tumor necrosis factor-alpha (TNF-α). Anti-apoptotic as it attenuates caspase-3,8,9 and increases Tyrosine Hydroxylase (TH) and level of anti-oxidants.	[34, 35]
Bilobalide, Quercetine and Kaempferol	MPTP-induced mice	Relieves oxidative stress and activates the NF-κB pathway.	[2, 36]
Stilbene, hypaphori-ne, proanthocy-nidine, catechins and gallic acid.	Paraquat-induced mice	Anti-oxidant, free radical scavenger and inhibits MAO-B activity.	[37]
Gastrodin, vinyllyl alcohol, vanillin.	MPP^+-induced SH-SY5Y cells	Anti-apoptotic by maintaining Bax/Bcl-2 ratio, anti-oxidant, and free radical scavenger.	[38]
Baicalein, wogonin	Rotenone-induced PC12 cells	Anti-apoptotic as attenuates caspase-3/7 prevents ROS accumulation and restores mitochondrial functioning.	[39]

Bioactive Compound	Model	Mechanism of Action	Refs.
Pinostilbene (Reversatol)	6- OHDA-induced rat	Decreases cyclooxygenase-2 (COX-2) and TNF-α levels and neuroprotective.	[40, 41]
Glycosides (Echinacoside), Acteoside	MPTP-induced mouse	Inhibition of caspase-3,8 and increase in TH expression. Increase in GDNF.	[42, 43]
Paeoniflorin	MPP$^+$-induced PC12 cells	Induces chaperone-mediated autophagy pathway	[44]
Tenuigenin	6-OHDA-induced PC12 cells	Anti-oxidant and anti-apoptotic as it reduces ROS, nitric oxide (NO), and caspase-3 activity.	[27]
Protocatechuic acid	6-OHDA-induced PC12 cells	Inhibits induced Nitric Oxide Synthase (iNOS), downregulates TNF-α and modulates PI3K/AKT pathway.	[45]
Peurarin, daidzein, genistein	MPTP-induced SH-SY5Y cells	PI3K/AKT pathway activation and inhibits expression of Bax and caspase-3.	[46]
Sesamin, Eleutheroside B	MPP$^+$-induced PC12 cells	Modulates TH, SOD, Catalase (CAT), iNOS and interleukin.	[47]
Astragaloside 4, Polysaccharides	MPP$^+$-induced SH-SY5Y cells	Inhibits Bax mediated pathway and ROS production.	[48]
Tetramethylpyrazine	LPS-induced N9 microglial cells	Antioxidant.	[49]
S-Allylcycteine	MPTP-induced mice	Inhibition of TNF-α, iNOS, and Glial Fibrillary Acidic Protein (GFAP).	[50]
Alkaloids, tannins, saponins, glycosides	MPTP-induced PC12 cells	Suppress glutathione peroxidase expression and microglia	[51]
Luteolin, quinic acid	MPTP mouse model	neuroprotective	[52]
Fraxetin, Esculin, liriodendrin	DA-induced and MPP$^+$-induced SH-SY5Y cells	Anti-apoptotic	[53]
Saponins, glycpenosides	MPP$^+$-induced mouse	Antioxidant	[54]
Hyperoside, flavonoids	MPTP-induced mice	Antioxidant enzyme upregulation.	[55]
salidroside	MPP$^+$-induced PC12 cells	Anti-apoptotic inhibits NO pathway and activates PI3K/AKT pathway.	[56]
Salvianic acid A, salvianolic acid A and Salvianolic acid B	6-OHDA-induced SH-SY5Y cells	Anti- apoptotic	[57]
Triptolide, tripcholoro-lide	6-OHDA-induced rats	Immunosuppressive action due to inactivation of TNF-α and interleukin-2 (IL-2).	[58]

(Table 1) cont.....

Bioactive Compound	Model	Mechanism of Action	Refs.
Polyphenols, flavonoids	6-MPTP-induced mice	Neuroprotection against lipid peroxidation decreases oxidative stress.	[59]
Flavonoids (Pelargonium)	6-OHDA-induced rats	Antioxidant	[60]
Alkaloids, phenols, saponins, flavonoids, tannins	6-OHDA-induced rats	Increases the amount of antioxidant enzymes and glutathione.	[61]
Hydroxysafflor Yellow (HYSA)	6-OHDA-induced rats	Upregulates GDNF and Brain-derived neurotrophic factor (BDNF).	[62]
Chalcones, tannins	6-OHDA-induced rats	TH upregulation.	[63]
Tripenes, flavonoids, lignans, amino acid	MPTP-induced rats	Anti-oxidant	[64]
Alkaloids, flavonoids, steroids, berberine	6-OHDA-induced mouse	neuroprotection	[65]
crocin	6-OHDA-induced rat	Decreases NO and prevents nitrosative stress.	[66]

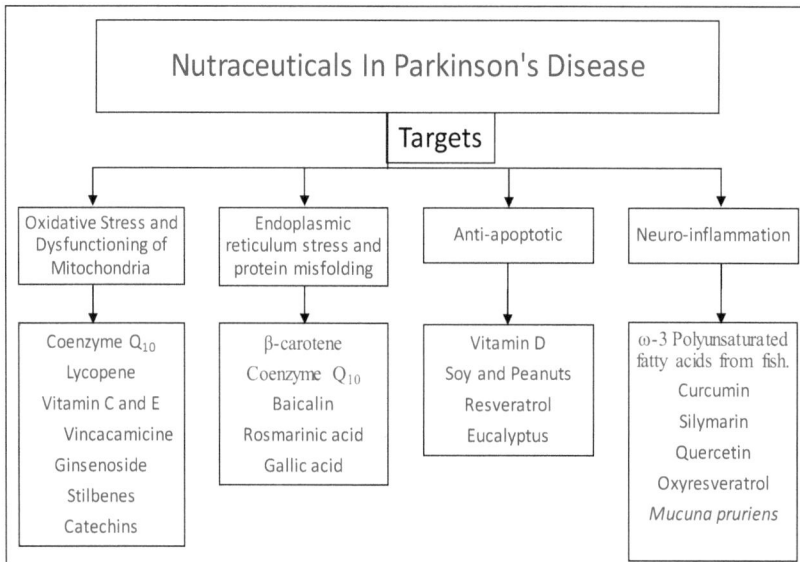

Fig. (1). Indicating the various targets of nutraceuticals and nutraceuticals offer neuroprotection in PD pathology [2, 4].

AYURVEDIC PREPARATIONS IN PD THERAPEUTICS

Ayurveda is the ancient Indian medicine system that classifies bio-entities into 3 aspects – "Vata" (Psychomotor), "Pitta" (digestive and metabolic), and "Kapha" (growth). Under "Vata" there are 3 symptoms – "Kampa" (Tremors), "Stambha" (stiffness), and "vishada" (depression) [67]. Thus, PD with respect to Ayurveda is known as "Kampavata". To treat a PD, one of the first strategies is "Yukti Vyapshryaya" which involves "shaman" (diet drugs) and "shodhan" (balancing procedures) [68]. For "Shaman", "Rasayanas" is used, which are drugs given to restore and replenish specific tissues, body systems or in general [49]. "Rasayana" is any medicine that improves the quality of life, i.e., strengthens or promotes the health of all tissues of the body [69]. "Shodhan" treatments (Panchkarma) involve treatment of PD with herbs or "Rasayanas" through oleation, sudation, purgation, enema, and errhines [70]. "Basti" (enemas with oils and decoctions) and "Nasya"/smoking (nasal instillation of oil-based and aqueous liquids and smoking herbs) are effective against tremors [68]. Pharmaceutical company "Zhandu" developed a standardized product – HP200 from *Mucuna pruriens* seeds with ± 4% L-Dopa [68]. In Ayurveda, the seeds of *M. pruriens*, *Vicia faba*, are being used as a therapeutic option for PD patients as these contain the L-Dopa required for the synthesis of DA, however, limited studies are available. Few contradictory studies showed that L–Dopa accelerates the loss of nigrostriatal DA nerve terminals and thus its potential long-term effects remain uncertain and need to be explored in long-term studies [71]. However, to date, the chronic utilization of neutraceutical or ayurvedic preparations did not show significant side effects and could be utilized clinically subjected to detailed efficacy and toxicity studies in experimental models and further clinical trials (Table **2**).

Table 2. Indicate various Ayurvedic preparations evaluated in experimental models of PD and also in PD patients.

Ayurvedic Herb	Bioactive Compounds	Experimental Model	Mechanism of Action	Refs.
Atmagupta (*M. pruriens*) Zandopa	Ethanolic extract(L-Dopa, NADH, CoQ_{10})	*Drosophila* Parkinson's patients	Enhanced locomotor activities. Anti-oxidant and iron chelator. Symptoms like pain, tremors, bradykinesia, *etc.* improved when given along with palliative therapy.	[72, 73, 69]
Ashwagandha (*Withania somnifera*)	Leaf extract, ethanolic extract (alkaloids and lactone steroids, catecholamines-serotonin)	MPTP-induced mice	Increases glutathione and glutathione peroxidase.	[74]

(Table 2) cont.....

Ayurvedic Herb	Bioactive Compounds	Experimental Model	Mechanism of Action	Refs.
Haridra (*Curcuma longa*)	Curcuminoides (Curcumin, Demethoxy-Curcumin, Bisdemethoxy-Curcumin)	6-OHDA-induced MES23.5 cells 6-OHDA-induced mouse	Antioxidant inhibits translocation of NF-κB translocation. Iron chelation	[75, 76]
Bala (*Sida cardifolia)* and **Parasika Yavani** (*Hyocyamus)*	The concoction in milk (hyoscyamine, somniferin, ephedrine, etc.)	Parkinson's patients	Neuroprotective when given with *M. pruriens* after palliative therapy.	[70]
Tulsi (*Ocimum sativum)*	Leaf extract (alkaloids, glycosides, saponins, tannins, ascorbic acid, carotene)	*Drosophila*	Neuroprotective and antioxidant.	[77]
Neelgiri (*Eucalyptus citriodora*)	Acetone extract (terpenoids)	*Drosophila*	Antioxidant	[78]
Brahmi (*Bacopa monnieri)*	Saponins- Bacoside A Bacoside B	*Drosophila Caenorhabditis elegans*	Protects against oxidative stress. Reduce α-syn aggregation.	[72, 79]
Gotu Kola (*Centella asiatica)*	Asiaticoside Asiatic acid	MPTP-induced rat.	Maintains Bcl-z/Bax ratio and prevents apoptosis. Increases free radical scavenging enzymes.	[80, 2]
Aloe vera (*Aloe arborescens)*		Copper-intoxicated rats	Neuroprotective effect by adjustment of oxidative state disequilibrium.	[81]

CONCLUSION

Lifestyle and food have a great impact on the mental health of people, therefore, they must be attentively improved in PD patients. Since PD pathology is progressive but slow thus, the stringent effort in the improvement of lifestyle and food may offer significant delay the independence of patients on caretakers. Since it's known that the PD onset is related to genetic mutations and environmental toxins, the family members of PD patients may take preventive measures and may successfully delay the disease onset. Also, the disease pathology is related to specific types of environmental toxins thus, awareness of the same in the public domain may also help people to take preventive measures. The above-given details of various neutraceuticals show the available option and opportunities for researchers and industries to provide economical treatment to patients. However, detailed preclinical studies and regulated clinical trials are mandatory for their clinical use and recommendations.

CONSENT FOR PUBLICATION

Not applicable.

CONFLICT OF INTEREST

The author declares no conflict of interest, financial or otherwise.

ACKNOWLEDGEMENTS

Declared none.

REFERENCES

[1]　Bhowmik D, Gopinath H, Kumar BP, Duraivel S, Kumar KS. Nutraceutical-a bright scope and opportunity of Indian healthcare market. Pharma Innov 2013; 1 (11, Part A): 29.

[2]　Makkar R, Behl T, Bungau S, *et al.* Nutraceuticals in neurological disorders. Int J Mol Sci 2020; 21(12): 4424.
[http://dx.doi.org/10.3390/ijms21124424] [PMID: 32580329]

[3]　Hang L, Basil AH, Lim KL. Nutraceuticals in Parkinson's disease. Neuromolecular Med 2016; 18(3): 306-21.
[http://dx.doi.org/10.1007/s12017-016-8398-6] [PMID: 27147525]

[4]　Chao J, Leung Y, Wang M, Chang RCC. Nutraceuticals and their preventive or potential therapeutic value in Parkinson's disease. Nutr Rev 2012; 70(7): 373-86.
[http://dx.doi.org/10.1111/j.1753-4887.2012.00484.x] [PMID: 22747840]

[5]　Blochberger A, Jones S. Clinical Focus-Parkinson's Disease-Clinical features and diagnosis. Clin Pharm 2011; 3(11): 361.

[6]　Chaudhuri KR, Healy DG, Schapira AHV. National Institute for Clinical Excellence. Non-motor symptoms of Parkinson's disease: diagnosis and management. Lancet Neurol 2006; 5(3): 235-45.
[http://dx.doi.org/10.1016/S1474-4422(06)70373-8] [PMID: 16488379]

[7]　Zahra W, Rai SN, Birla H, *et al.* Economic Importance of Medicinal Plants in Asian Countries. Bioeconomy for Sustainable Development. Springer 2020; pp. 359-77.
[http://dx.doi.org/10.1007/978-981-13-9431-7_19]

[8]　Birla H, Keswani C, Singh SS, *et al.* Unraveling the Neuroprotective Effect of *Tinospora cordifolia* in Parkinsonian Mouse Model Through Proteomics Approach. 2021.

[9]　Keswani C, Dilnashin H, Birla H, Singh SP. Unravelling efficient applications of agriculturally important microorganisms for alleviation of induced inter-cellular oxidative stress in crops. Acta Agric Slov 2019; 114(1): 121-30.
[http://dx.doi.org/10.14720/aas.2019.114.1.14]

[10]　Birla H, Keswani C, Rai SN, *et al.* Neuroprotective effects of *Withania somnifera* in BPA induced-cognitive dysfunction and oxidative stress in mice. Behav Brain Funct 2019; 15(1): 9.
[http://dx.doi.org/10.1186/s12993-019-0160-4] [PMID: 31064381]

[11]　Dauer W, Przedborski S. Parkinson's Disease. Neuron 2003; 39(6): 889-909.
[http://dx.doi.org/10.1016/S0896-6273(03)00568-3] [PMID: 12971891]

[12]　Keswani C, Singh HB, Hermosa R, *et al.* Antimicrobial secondary metabolites from agriculturally important fungi as next biocontrol agents. Appl Microbiol Biotechnol 2019; 103(23-24): 9287-303.
[http://dx.doi.org/10.1007/s00253-019-10209-2] [PMID: 31707442]

[13] Keswani C. Bioeconomy for Sustainable Development. Springer 2020.
[http://dx.doi.org/10.1007/978-981-13-9431-7]

[14] Keswani C, Bisen K, Singh S, Singh H. Traditional knowledge and medicinal plants of India in intellectual property landscape. Med Plants Int J Phytomed Relat Ind 2017; 9.

[15] Keswani C, Dilnashin H, Birla H, Singh S. Re-addressing the commercialization and regulatory hurdles for biopesticides in India 2019.

[16] Rathore AS, Birla H, Singh SS, *et al.* Epigenetic modulation in parkinson's disease and potential treatment therapies. Neurochem Res 2021; 46(7): 1618-26.
[http://dx.doi.org/10.1007/s11064-021-03334-w] [PMID: 33900517]

[17] Singh SS, Rai SN, Birla H, *et al.* Techniques Related to Disease Diagnosis and Therapeutics. Application of Biomedical Engineering in Neuroscience. Springer 2019; pp. 437-56.
[http://dx.doi.org/10.1007/978-981-13-7142-4_22]

[18] Zahra W, Rai SN, Birla H, *et al.* The global economic impact of neurodegenerative diseases: Opportunities and challenges. Bioeconomy for Sustainable Development 2020; pp. 333-45.

[19] Singh S, Rai S, Birla H, Eds., *et al.* Chlorogenic acid protects against MPTP induced neurotoxicity in parkinsonian mice model *via* its anti-apoptotic activity. Journal of Neurochemistry. NJ USA.: Wiley 111 River St, Hoboken 2019.

[20] Rai SN, Birla H, Singh SS, *et al.* Pathophysiology of the Disease Causing Physical Disability. Biomedical Engineering and its Applications in Healthcare. Springer 2019; pp. 573-95.

[21] Rai SN, Singh BK, Rathore AS, *et al.* Quality control in huntington's disease: a therapeutic target. Neurotox Res 2019; 36(3): 612-26.
[http://dx.doi.org/10.1007/s12640-019-00087-x] [PMID: 31297710]

[22] Rai SN, Dilnashin H, Birla H, *et al.* The role of PI3K/Akt and ERK in neurodegenerative disorders. Neurotox Res 2019; 35(3): 775-95.
[http://dx.doi.org/10.1007/s12640-019-0003-y] [PMID: 30707354]

[23] Zahra W, Rai SN, Birla H, *et al.* Neuroprotection of rotenone-induced Parkinsonism by ursolic acid in PD mouse model. CNS & Neurological Disorders-Drug Targets 2020; (14): 527-40.
[http://dx.doi.org/10.2174/1871527319666200812224457]

[24] Rai SN, Zahra W, Singh SS, *et al.* Anti-inflammatory activity of ursolic acid in MPTP-induced parkinsonian mouse model. Neurotox Res 2019; 36(3): 452-62.
[http://dx.doi.org/10.1007/s12640-019-00038-6] [PMID: 31016688]

[25] Singh SS, Rai SN, Birla H, *et al.* Neuroprotective effect of chlorogenic acid on mitochondrial dysfunction-mediated apoptotic death of DA neurons in a Parkinsonian mouse model. Oxid Med Cell Longev 2020; 2020: 1-14.
[http://dx.doi.org/10.1155/2020/6571484] [PMID: 32566093]

[26] Li X, Zhang S, Liu S, Lu F. Recent advances in herbal medicines treating Parkinson's disease. Fitoterapia 2013; 84: 273-85.
[http://dx.doi.org/10.1016/j.fitote.2012.12.009] [PMID: 23266574]

[27] Feng Z, Wei HB, Guo Y, *et al.* From rainforest to herbland: New insights into land plant responses to the end-Permian mass extinction. Earth Sci Rev 2020; 204: 103153.
[http://dx.doi.org/10.1016/j.earscirev.2020.103153]

[28] More SV, Kumar H, Kang SM, Song SY, Lee K, Choi DK. Advances in neuroprotective ingredients of medicinal herbs by using cellular and animal models of Parkinson's disease. Evidence-based complementary and alternative medicine 2013; 2013
[http://dx.doi.org/10.1155/2013/957875]

[29] Kim TH, Cho KH, Jung WS, Lee MS. Herbal medicines for Parkinson's disease: a systematic review of randomized controlled trials. PLoS One 2012; 7(5): e35695.

[http://dx.doi.org/10.1371/journal.pone.0035695] [PMID: 22615738]

[30]   Hu S, Han R, Mak S, Han Y. Protection against 1-methyl-4-phenylpyridinium ion (MPP+)-induced apoptosis by water extract of ginseng (Panax ginseng C.A. Meyer) in SH-SY5Y cells. J Ethnopharmacol 2011; 135(1): 34-42.
[http://dx.doi.org/10.1016/j.jep.2011.02.017] [PMID: 21349320]

[31]   Pavlatos C, Vita V, Eds. Linguistic representation of power system signals. Electricity Distribution. Springer 2016.

[32]   Liu Q, Kou JP, Yu BY. Ginsenoside Rg1 protects against hydrogen peroxide-induced cell death in PC12 cells via inhibiting NF-κB activation. Neurochem Int 2011; 58(1): 119-25.
[http://dx.doi.org/10.1016/j.neuint.2010.11.004] [PMID: 21078355]

[33]   Zhang L, Liu X, Jiang Y, Guo P, Sha L, Li Y. Effect of notoginsenoside-Rg1 on the expression of several proteins in the striatum of rat models with Parkinson's disease. Chem Res Chin Univ 2006; 22(2): 139-44.
[http://dx.doi.org/10.1016/S1005-9040(06)60063-9]

[34]   Guo S, Yan J, Yang T, Yang X, Bezard E, Zhao B. Protective effects of green tea polyphenols in the 6-OHDA rat model of Parkinson's disease through inhibition of ROS-NO pathway. Biol Psychiatry 2007; 62(12): 1353-62.
[http://dx.doi.org/10.1016/j.biopsych.2007.04.020] [PMID: 17624318]

[35]   Anandhan A, Tamilselvam K, Radhiga T, Rao S, Essa MM, Manivasagam T. Theaflavin, a black tea polyphenol, protects nigral dopaminergic neurons against chronic MPTP/probenecid induced Parkinson's disease. Brain Res 2012; 1433: 104-13.
[http://dx.doi.org/10.1016/j.brainres.2011.11.021] [PMID: 22138428]

[36]   Rojas P, Serrano-García N, Mares-Sámano JJ, Medina-Campos ON, Pedraza-Chaverri J, Ögren SO. EGb761 protects against nigrostriatal dopaminergic neurotoxicity in 1-methyl-4-phenyl-1,2-3,6-tetrahydropyridine-induced Parkinsonism in mice: role of oxidative stress. Eur J Neurosci 2008; 28(1): 41-50.
[http://dx.doi.org/10.1111/j.1460-9568.2008.06314.x] [PMID: 18662333]

[37]   Li X, Matsumoto K, Murakami Y, Tezuka Y, Wu Y, Kadota S. Neuroprotective effects of *Polygonum multiflorum* on nigrostriatal dopaminergic degeneration induced by paraquat and maneb in mice. Pharmacol Biochem Behav 2005; 82(2): 345-52.
[http://dx.doi.org/10.1016/j.pbb.2005.09.004] [PMID: 16214209]

[38]   An H, Kim IS, Koppula S, et al. Protective effects of *Gastrodia elata* Blume on MPP+-induced cytotoxicity in human dopaminergic SH-SY5Y cells. J Ethnopharmacol 2010; 130(2): 290-8.
[http://dx.doi.org/10.1016/j.jep.2010.05.006] [PMID: 20470875]

[39]   Li X, He G, Mu X, et al. Protective effects of baicalein against rotenone-induced neurotoxicity in PC12 cells and isolated rat brain mitochondria. Eur J Pharmacol 2012; 674(2-3): 227-33.
[http://dx.doi.org/10.1016/j.ejphar.2011.09.181] [PMID: 21996316]

[40]   Zhang H, Li C, Kwok ST, Zhang QW, Chan SW. A review of the pharmacological effects of the dried root of *Polygonum cuspidatum* (Hu Zhang) and its constituents. Evidence-Based Complementary and Alternative Medicine 2013; 2013

[41]   Jin F, Wu Q, Lu YF, Gong QH, Shi JS. Neuroprotective effect of resveratrol on 6-OHDA-induced Parkinson's disease in rats. Eur J Pharmacol 2008; 600(1-3): 78-82.
[http://dx.doi.org/10.1016/j.ejphar.2008.10.005] [PMID: 18940189]

[42]   Geng X, Tian X, Tu P, Pu X. Neuroprotective effects of echinacoside in the mouse MPTP model of Parkinson's disease. Eur J Pharmacol 2007; 564(1-3): 66-74.
[http://dx.doi.org/10.1016/j.ejphar.2007.01.084] [PMID: 17359968]

[43]   Zhao Q, Gao J, Li W, Cai D. Neurotrophic and neurorescue effects of Echinacoside in the subacute MPTP mouse model of Parkinson's disease. Brain Res 2010; 1346: 224-36.

[http://dx.doi.org/10.1016/j.brainres.2010.05.018] [PMID: 20478277]

[44]   Cao BY, Yang YP, Luo WF, *et al.* Paeoniflorin, a potent natural compound, protects PC12 cells from MPP+ and acidic damage via autophagic pathway. J Ethnopharmacol 2010; 131(1): 122-9.
[http://dx.doi.org/10.1016/j.jep.2010.06.009] [PMID: 20558269]

[45]   Zhang ZJ, Cheang LCV, Wang MW, *et al.* Ethanolic extract of fructus *Alpinia oxyphylla* protects against 6-hydroxydopamine-induced damage of PC12 cells in vitro and dopaminergic neurons in zebrafish. Cell Mol Neurobiol 2012; 32(1): 27-40.
[http://dx.doi.org/10.1007/s10571-011-9731-0] [PMID: 21744117]

[46]   Zhang X, Xiong J, Liu S, *et al.* Puerarin protects dopaminergic neurons in Parkinson's disease models. Neuroscience 2014; 280: 88-98.
[http://dx.doi.org/10.1016/j.neuroscience.2014.08.052] [PMID: 25218963]

[47]   Lahaie-Collins V, Bournival J, Plouffe M, Carange J, Martinoli MG. Sesamin modulates tyrosine hydroxylase, superoxide dismutase, catalase, inducible NO synthase and interleukin-6 expression in dopaminergic cells under MPP+-induced oxidative stress. Oxid Med Cell Longev 2008; 1(1): 54-62.
[http://dx.doi.org/10.4161/oxim.1.1.6958] [PMID: 19794909]

[48]   Zhang Z, Wu L, Wang J, *et al.* Astragaloside IV prevents MPP+-induced SH-SY5Y cell death via the inhibition of Bax-mediated pathways and ROS production. Mol Cell Biochem 2012; 364(1-2): 209-16.
[http://dx.doi.org/10.1007/s11010-011-1219-1] [PMID: 22278385]

[49]   Liu HT, Du YG, He JL, *et al.* Tetramethylpyrazine inhibits production of nitric oxide and inducible nitric oxide synthase in lipopolysaccharide-induced N9 microglial cells through blockade of MAPK and PI3K/Akt signaling pathways, and suppression of intracellular reactive oxygen species. J Ethnopharmacol 2010; 129(3): 335-43.
[http://dx.doi.org/10.1016/j.jep.2010.03.037] [PMID: 20371283]

[50]   García E, Villeda-Hernández J, Pedraza-Chaverrí J, Maldonado PD, Santamaría A. S-allylcysteine reduces the MPTP-induced striatal cell damage via inhibition of pro-inflammatory cytokine tumor necrosis factor-α and inducible nitric oxide synthase expressions in mice. Phytomedicine 2010; 18(1): 65-73.
[http://dx.doi.org/10.1016/j.phymed.2010.04.004] [PMID: 20576415]

[51]   Ye M, Chung ES, Lim SJ, *et al.* Neuroprotective effects of Cuscutae semen in a mouse model of Parkinson's disease. Evidence-Based Complementary and Alternative Medicine 2014; 2014
[http://dx.doi.org/10.1155/2014/150153]

[52]   Kim IS, Ko HM, Koppula S, Kim BW, Choi DK. Protective effect of *Chrysanthemum indicum* Linne against 1-methyl-4-phenylpridinium ion and lipopolysaccharide-induced cytotoxicity in cellular model of Parkinson's disease. Food Chem Toxicol 2011; 49(4): 963-73.
[http://dx.doi.org/10.1016/j.fct.2011.01.002] [PMID: 21219959]

[53]   Palkovits M, Deli MA, Gallatz K, Tóth ZE, Buzás E, Falus A. Highly activated c-fos expression in specific brain regions (ependyma, circumventricular organs, choroid plexus) of histidine decarboxylase deficient mice in response to formalin-induced acute pain. Neuropharmacology 2007; 53(1): 101-12.
[http://dx.doi.org/10.1016/j.neuropharm.2007.04.001] [PMID: 17544458]

[54]   Wang P, Niu L, Guo XD, *et al.* Gypenosides protects dopaminergic neurons in primary culture against MPP+-induced oxidative injury. Brain Res Bull 2010; 83(5): 266-71.
[http://dx.doi.org/10.1016/j.brainresbull.2010.06.014] [PMID: 20615455]

[55]   Mohanasundari M, Srinivasan MS, Sethupathy S, Sabesan M. Enhanced neuroprotective effect by combination of bromocriptine and *Hypericum perforatum* extract against MPTP-induced neurotoxicity in mice. J Neurol Sci 2006; 249(2): 140-4.
[http://dx.doi.org/10.1016/j.jns.2006.06.018] [PMID: 16876826]

[56]   Zhang L, Ding W, Sun H, *et al.* Salidroside protects PC12 cells from MPP+-induced apoptosis via activation of the PI3K/Akt pathway. Food Chem Toxicol 2012; 50(8): 2591-7.

[http://dx.doi.org/10.1016/j.fct.2012.05.045] [PMID: 22664423]

[57]   Tian LL, Wang XJ, Sun YN, *et al.* Salvianolic acid B, an antioxidant from *Salvia miltiorrhiza*, prevents 6-hydroxydopamine induced apoptosis in SH-SY5Y cells. Int J Biochem Cell Biol 2008; 40(3): 409-22.
[http://dx.doi.org/10.1016/j.biocel.2007.08.005] [PMID: 17884684]

[58]   Zhou HF, Niu DB, Xue B, *et al.* Triptolide inhibits TNF-α, IL-1 β and NO production in primary microglial cultures. Neuroreport 2003; 14(7): 1091-5.
[PMID: 12802209]

[59]   Pérez-H J, Carrillo-S C, García E, Ruiz-Mar G, Pérez-Tamayo R, Chavarría A. Neuroprotective effect of silymarin in a MPTP mouse model of Parkinson's disease. Toxicology 2014; 319: 38-43.
[http://dx.doi.org/10.1016/j.tox.2014.02.009] [PMID: 24607817]

[60]   Roghani M, Niknam A, Jalali-Nadoushan MR, Kiasalari Z, Khalili M, Baluchnejadmojarad T. Oral pelargonidin exerts dose-dependent neuroprotection in 6-hydroxydopamine rat model of hemi-parkinsonism. Brain Res Bull 2010; 82(5-6): 279-83.
[http://dx.doi.org/10.1016/j.brainresbull.2010.06.004] [PMID: 20558255]

[61]   Chandrashekhar VM, Avinash SP, Sowmya C, Ramkishan A, Shalavadi MH. Neuroprotective activity of *Stereospermum suaveolens* DC against 6-OHDA induced Parkinson's disease model. Indian J Pharmacol 2012; 44(6): 737-43.
[http://dx.doi.org/10.4103/0253-7613.103275] [PMID: 23248404]

[62]   Ramagiri S, Taliyan R. Neuroprotective effect of hydroxy safflor yellow A against cerebral ischemia-reperfusion injury in rats: putative role of mPTP. J Basic Clin Physiol Pharmacol 2016; 27(1): 1-8.
[http://dx.doi.org/10.1515/jbcpp-2015-0021] [PMID: 26280168]

[63]   Calou I, Bandeira MA, Aguiar-Galvão W, *et al.* Neuroprotective properties of a standardized extract from *Myracrodruon urundeuva* Fr. All.(Aroeira-Do-Sertao), as evaluated by a Parkinson's disease model in rats. Parkinson's Disease 2014; 2014

[64]   Moraes LS, Rohor BZ, Areal LB, *et al.* Medicinal plant *Combretum leprosum* mart ameliorates motor, biochemical and molecular alterations in a Parkinson's disease model induced by MPTP. J Ethnopharmacol 2016; 185: 68-76.
[http://dx.doi.org/10.1016/j.jep.2016.03.041] [PMID: 26994817]

[65]   Swamy A, Gulliaya S, Thippeswamy A, Koti B, Manjula D. Cardioprotective effect of curcumin against doxorubicin-induced myocardial toxicity in albino rats. Indian J Pharmacol 2012; 44(1): 73-7.
[http://dx.doi.org/10.4103/0253-7613.91871] [PMID: 22345874]

[66]   Hosseini M, Rajaei Z, Alaei H, Tajadini M. The effects of crocin on 6-OHDA-induced oxidative/nitrosative damage and motor behaviour in hemiparkinsonian rats. Malays J Med Sci 2016; 23(6): 35-43.
[http://dx.doi.org/10.21315/mjms2016.23.6.4] [PMID: 28090177]

[67]   Gourie-Devi M, Ramu MG, Venkataram BS. Treatment of Parkinson's disease in 'Ayurveda' (ancient Indian system of medicine): discussion paper. J R Soc Med 1991; 84(8): 491-2.
[http://dx.doi.org/10.1177/014107689108400814] [PMID: 1886119]

[68]   Pathak- Gandhi N, Vaidya ADB. Management of Parkinson's disease in Ayurveda: Medicinal plants and adjuvant measures. J Ethnopharmacol 2017; 197: 46-51.
[http://dx.doi.org/10.1016/j.jep.2016.08.020] [PMID: 27544001]

[69]   Govindarajan R, Vijayakumar M, Pushpangadan P. Antioxidant approach to disease management and the role of 'Rasayana' herbs of Ayurveda. J Ethnopharmacol 2005; 99(2): 165-78.
[http://dx.doi.org/10.1016/j.jep.2005.02.035] [PMID: 15894123]

[70]   Nagashayana N, Sankarankutty P, Nampoothiri MRV, Mohan PK, Mohanakumar KP. Association of l-DOPA with recovery following Ayurveda medication in Parkinson's disease. J Neurol Sci 2000; 176(2): 124-7.

[http://dx.doi.org/10.1016/S0022-510X(00)00329-4] [PMID: 10930594]

[71]   Fahn S, Oakes D, Shoulson I, *et al.* Does levodopa slow or hasten the rate of progression of Parkinson's disease. Parkinson Study 2005.

[72]   Jansen RLM, Brogan B, Whitworth AJ, Okello EJ. Effects of five Ayurvedic herbs on locomotor behaviour in a *Drosophila melanogaster* Parkinson's disease model. Phytother Res 2014; 28(12): 1789-95.
[http://dx.doi.org/10.1002/ptr.5199] [PMID: 25091506]

[73]   Dhanasekaran M, Tharakan B, Manyam BV. Antiparkinson drug - *Mucuna pruriens* shows antioxidant and metal chelating activity. Phytother Res 2008; 22(1): 6-11.
[http://dx.doi.org/10.1002/ptr.2109] [PMID: 18064727]

[74]   RajaSankar S, Manivasagam T, Surendran S. Ashwagandha leaf extract: A potential agent in treating oxidative damage and physiological abnormalities seen in a mouse model of Parkinson's disease. Neurosci Lett 2009; 454(1): 11-5.
[http://dx.doi.org/10.1016/j.neulet.2009.02.044] [PMID: 19429045]

[75]   Wang J, Du XX, Jiang H, Xie JX. Curcumin attenuates 6-hydroxydopamine-induced cytotoxicity by anti-oxidation and nuclear factor-kappaB modulation in MES23.5 cells. Biochem Pharmacol 2009; 78(2): 178-83.
[http://dx.doi.org/10.1016/j.bcp.2009.03.031] [PMID: 19464433]

[76]   Du XX, Xu HM, Jiang H, Song N, Wang J, Xie JX. Curcumin protects nigral dopaminergic neurons by iron-chelation in the 6-hydroxydopamine rat model of Parkinson's disease. Neurosci Bull 2012; 28(3): 253-8.
[http://dx.doi.org/10.1007/s12264-012-1238-2] [PMID: 22622825]

[77]   Siddique YH, Faisal M, Naz F, Jyoti S, Rahul . Role of *Ocimum sanctum* leaf extract on dietary supplementation in the transgenic Drosophila model of Parkinson's disease. Chin J Nat Med 2014; 12(10): 777-81.
[http://dx.doi.org/10.1016/S1875-5364(14)60118-7] [PMID: 25443371]

[78]   Siddique YH, Mujtaba SF, Jyoti S, Naz F. GC–MS analysis of *Eucalyptus citriodora* leaf extract and its role on the dietary supplementation in transgenic Drosophila model of Parkinson's disease. Food Chem Toxicol 2013; 55: 29-35.
[http://dx.doi.org/10.1016/j.fct.2012.12.028] [PMID: 23318758]

[79]   Jadiya P, Khan A, Sammi SR, Kaur S, Mir SS, Nazir A. Anti-Parkinsonian effects of *Bacopa monnieri*: Insights from transgenic and pharmacological *Caenorhabditis elegans* models of Parkinson's disease. Biochem Biophys Res Commun 2011; 413(4): 605-10.
[http://dx.doi.org/10.1016/j.bbrc.2011.09.010] [PMID: 21925152]

[80]   Xu CL, Wang QZ, Sun LM, *et al.* Asiaticoside: Attenuation of neurotoxicity induced by MPTP in a rat model of Parkinsonism via maintaining redox balance and up-regulating the ratio of Bcl-2/Bax. Pharmacol Biochem Behav 2012; 100(3): 413-8.
[http://dx.doi.org/10.1016/j.pbb.2011.09.014] [PMID: 22001429]

[81]   Abbaoui A, Hiba OE, Gamrani H. Neuroprotective potential of *Aloe arborescens* against copper induced neurobehavioral features of Parkinson's disease in rat. Acta Histochem 2017; 119(5): 592-601.
[http://dx.doi.org/10.1016/j.acthis.2017.06.003] [PMID: 28619286]

CHAPTER 15

Systems Analysis Based Approach for Therapeutic Intervention in Mixed Vascular-Alzheimer Dementia (MVAD) Using Secondary Metabolites

Anindita Bhattacharjee[1] and **Prasun Kumar Roy**[1,2,*]

[1] *Neuroimaging Laboratory, School of Bio-Medical Engineering, Indian Institute of Technology, Banaras Hindu University, Varanasi-221005 (U.P.), India*

[2] *Centre for Tissue Engineering, Indian Institute of Technology, Banaras Hindu University, Varanasi-221005 (U.P.), India*

Abstract: Mixed dementia is a form of dementia where Alzheimer's dementia coexists with vascular dementia (VaD) in the same patient. Currently, the treatment available for mixed dementia is conventional Alzheimer's dementia therapy dispensing symptomatic relief. We aim to delineate the therapeutic possibility of some secondary metabolites, which can provide manageable intervention because of their multi-targeting and multiple pathophysiological components of Alzheimer's dementia and VaD. We performed the acquisition of relevant information and data by accessing and analyzing Pubmed, Science Direct, Google Scholar, and Scopus sources, to assess the validity of therapeutic use of secondary metabolites against mixed dementia. For the initial acquisition of data (*in vitro*, *in vivo*, and clinical), the keywords that were used were "secondary metabolites," "plant extract," "mixed dementia," "Alzheimer's disease," and "vascular dementia." All types of relevant research articles, review articles, and books were included. In our study, clinically, preclinical, *in vivo*, and *in vitro* studies of secondary metabolites are encompassed. Furthermore, we undertook the formulation of the mechanism of action of secondary metabolites in terms of systems biology-oriented analysis and signal transduction-based methodology. Firstly, the likely mechanisms through which mixed dementia can take place are identified and analyzed rigorously. Secondly, we demarcate the pharmacological actions of the secondary metabolites in treating mixed dementia by (i) Targeting acetylcholine levels, (ii) Reducing or dissociating amyloid-beta (Aβ) load, (iii) Modulating microglial activation, and (iv) Providing vasodilation concurrently with their various constituents of Alzheimer's dementia and VaD. Thirdly, we formulate how several preclinical and clinical studies furnish evidence that secondary metabolites may have efficacy in Alzheimer's patients with cerebrovascular disorders.

We formulate comprehensive evidence to substantiate the use of secondary metabolites from medicinal plants to enhance therapeutic intervention in mixed dementia.

* **Corresponding authors Prasun Kumar Roy;** Centre for Tissue Engineering, Indian Institute of Technology, Banaras Hindu University, Varanasi-221005 (U.P.), India; E-mail: pkroy.bme@iitbhu.ac.in

Surya Pratap Singh, Hagera Dilnashin, Hareram Birla & Chetan Keswani (Eds.)

Keywords: Alzheimer disease, Mixed dementia, Plant extract, Secondary metabolites.

INTRODUCTION

As the name implies, mixed dementia is the clinical situation where Alzheimer's disease (AD) and cerebrovascular disease (CVD) exist in the same demented patient. The co-occurrence of neurodegenerative and vascular diseases is more in elderly patients since both conditions are age-dependent. According to the World Health Organization (WHO), the most common form of dementia is AD, whose prevalence is approximately 60-70%, and another crucial form of dementia is vascular dementia (VaD) ($\approx$25-30%). Globally, 22% of the population exhibit coexistence of these two forms of dementia [1].

Given Alzheimer's dementia and VaD's clinical presentations overlap, the distinction between these diseases is challenging. A mixed dementia diagnosis can be made using the clinical/neuroimaging criteria of possible AD and vascular cognitive impairment (VCI) as separate entities. Alzheimer's patients with multiple vascular or ischemic brain lesions identified from autopsy studies can provide evidence for pathologic diagnosis [2]. This concomitant occurrence has neuropathological evidence delineating the connection between AD and CVD. Clinico-pathological correlation using guidelines of (i) National Institute of Neurological and Communicative Disorders and Stroke and (ii) Alzheimer's Disease and Related Disorders Association and (iii) Consortium to Establish a Registry for Alzheimer's Disease Criteria, as performed by Lim, Tsuang, *et al.*, show that 60% cases of AD patients had co-existing vascular or Parkinson's disease (PD) lesions [3].

Along with the adequate diagnosis of each type of dementia, a proper treatment schedule needs to be introduced for optimal treatment. Currently, predominant pharmacotherapy is symptomatic and preventive, often leading to several adverse effects. Secondary metabolites obtained from bacteria, fungi, or plants can provide a therapeutic regimen with lesser adverse effects. Plant metabolites used to modulate blood pressure could also be explored for mixed dementia treatment.

METHODS

Firstly, we have undertaken the acquisition of pertinent information and data by analysis of Pubmed, Science Direct, Google Scholar, and Scopus platforms. We obtained the assessment of the feasibility and validity of therapeutic interventions utilizing secondary metabolites against mixed dementia. We used the keywords "secondary metabolites," "phytochemical", "plant extract," "mixed dementia," "Alzheimer's disease," and "vascular dementia." We analyzed different research articles, review articles, monographs, books, and treatises. For data acquisition, we provided attention to a successively higher level of the investigations (molecule-based bioinformatics, cell-based *in vitro*, animal-based *in vivo*, and human-based clinical studies). Maximal studies were bound to the period between 1990 and 2020. We have queried the keywords in specific textual fields (title, abstract, and, if available, subject). The only inclusion criterion was that the investigation should be available as full text in any bibliographic or academic databases.

Secondly, we then performed an integrative analysis of the information and data available, from the framework of systems biology modulation, signal transduction pathway profiling, and general systems analysis approach. We particularly considered the input-output analysis model, where, using the signal operations framework, the successive processes are Signal Input, Signal Transmission, Signal Modulation, and Signal Output (Fig. **1**).

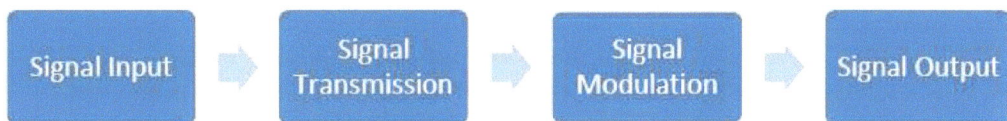

Fig. (1). The components of signal operations from the Systems Analysis framework.

Thirdly, we have thereby also proposed a likely plausible mechanism of action behind mixed vascular alzheimer's dementia, and the effects of secondary metabolites of the disease, utilizing the information accessed, analyzed, and assessed. Moreover, we have significantly validated the therapeutic interventional role of secondary metabolites in mixed dementia, including that with rigorous clinical trial data, founded on reliable *in vitro* cell line studies and *in vivo* animal studies.

PATHOGENESIS OF MIXED DEMENTIA

The pathogenesis of mixed vascular Alzheimer's dementia is unknown. However, two theories contribute to this disease state: amyloid theory and vascular theory. The amyloid theory encompasses an accumulation of amyloid-beta (Aβ) plaques in brain tissue, causing a reduction of cerebral blood flow to give rise to cognitive decline [4]. On the other hand, regarding the vascular aspect, various lifestyle diseases, such as diabetes mellitus, hypertension, cardiac ailments, and obesity can cause vascular changes, for instance, the thickening of blood vessels, causing cerebral atrophy [5]. The following vascular damages characterize the vascular theory with aging:

a. Small vessel atherosclerosis.

b. Large vessel arteriosclerosis.

c. Cortical and subcortical infarcts.

d. Lacunar infarcts with gray/white matter lesions.

e. Leukoaraiosis, amyloid angiopathy, and small brain hemorrhages.

POTENTIAL SECONDARY METABOLITES AS THERAPEUTIC AGENTS

At present, the predominant pharmacotherapy for AD and VaD [6] are acetylcholinesterase inhibitors like galantamine, donepezil, rivastigmine, and memantine for memory loss [7]. Natural alkaloid galantamine is extracted from snowdrop *Galanthus nivalis L.*, and synthetic alkaloid rivastigmine is modeled on natural physostigmine [8]. There are some adverse effects reported in standard medications used in dementia [9]. Therefore, it is necessary to evaluate their use in patients carefully. Specific groups of bacteria, fungi, plants, and animals produce a distinct natural compound known as secondary metabolites, which are biochemicals produced by organisms, as byproducts of the metabolic reactions of the cells [10 - 17]. Various ailments are treated with the secondary metabolites obtained from medicinal plants [18 - 20]. Here, we discuss some secondary metabolites obtained from medicinal plants that may ameliorate Alzheimer's dementia and VaD with less or fewer adverse effects, such as *Withania somnifera*, *Genista tinctoria*, Silybum, Curcuma longa, *Ginkgo biloba*, *Centella asiatica*, Theobroma cacao, Crocus sativus, and *Bacopa monnier*i [16, 21 - 27].

SYSTEMS BIOLOGY BASIS OF INTEGRATED MECHANISM BEHIND MIXED-DEMENTIA

Accumulation of vascular damages can cause less perfusion in cerebral blood vessels, producing neuronal death and vascular atrophy. Additionally, when amyloid load increases in the brain due to Aβ influx from the blood *via* the receptor for advanced glycation end products (RAGE), then RAGE- Aβ interaction causes the production of endothelin-1 that gives rise to vasoconstriction-mediated VaD. Since neurovascular dysfunction and Aβ load strongly correlate with each other, this suggests the possible pathology behind mixed vascular Alzheimers dementia [28]. From a systems biology framework, we find that the following successive processes enable the pathogenesis of mixed dementia. In Fig. (**2**), we have diagrammatically formulated the input-output analysis of the pathogenesis, based on the analytic formulation of Signal Operations mentioned earlier (Fig. **1**).

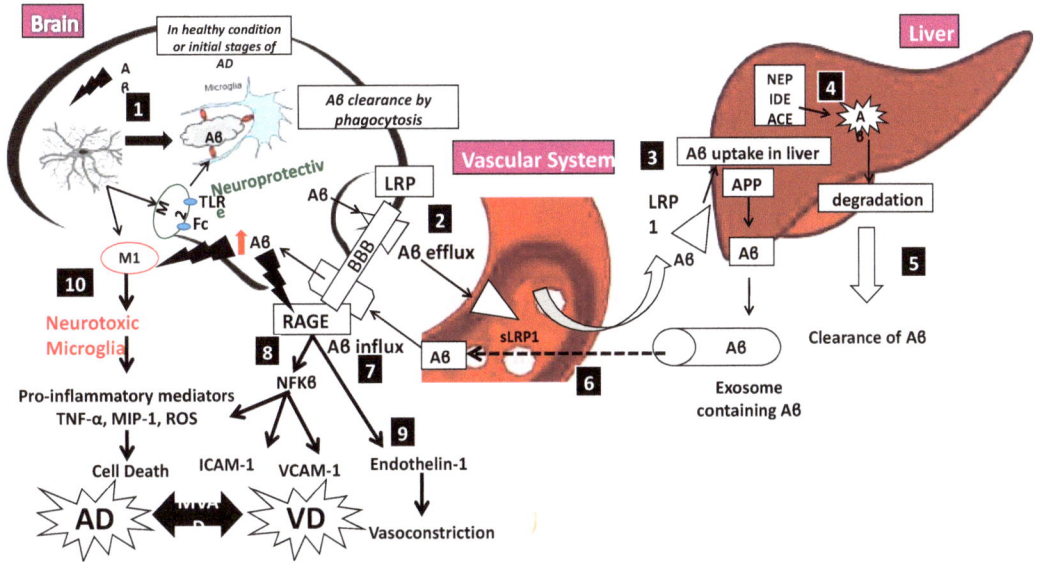

Fig. (2). Systems Approach based formulation and analysis of pathogenesis of mixed dementia showing the following processes [1]: Neuroprotective M_1 microglia-mediated phagocytosis of Aβ [2]. Low-density lipoprotein receptor-related peptide 1 (LRP1) transports monomeric Aβ [3]. Saturable uptake of Aβ by the liver *via* LRP1 [4]. Hepatic LRP1 assists in Aβ degradation [5]. Clearance of Aβ [6]. Aβ production and exsosomal transport in the liver [7]. Aβ influx *via* the receptor for the advanced glycation end product (RAGE) [8]. Interactions of RAGE with Aβ at the blood-brain barrier (BBB) [9]. RAGE-Aβ interaction actuating endothelin-1 [10]. Excessive Aβ load in brain activating neurotoxic M_1 microglia.

AMELIORATION OF MIXED DEMENTIA BY SECONDARY METABOLITES

We now delineate the mechanistic effects of secondary metabolites and the basis of therapeutic intervention for mixed dementia. We analyze and formulate the mechanisms according to the phytochemical origin.

Withania somnifera

W. somnifera (ashwagandha, family: Solanaceae) is a plant having several phytochemicals and is widely distributed in the tropical region of India, Sri Lanka, southern China, Africa, and South Africa [29]. The plant extract has been utilized in the traditional Ayurvedic system of medicine to enhance memory and improve cognition [30].

Phytoconstituents of W. somnifera

Phenolics, alkaloids, flavonoids, terpenoids, and glycosides are essential secondary metabolites obtained from *W. somnifera* [31]. Withanolide A (Fig. **3**) and withanoside IV (Fig. **3**) from WS roots were reported to have therapeutic potency in reducing the Aβ load in AD [32]. Another vital constituent is Withaferin A, obtained from leaves, which have demonstrated potent neuroprotective, antioxidant, and anti-inflammatory effects [33].

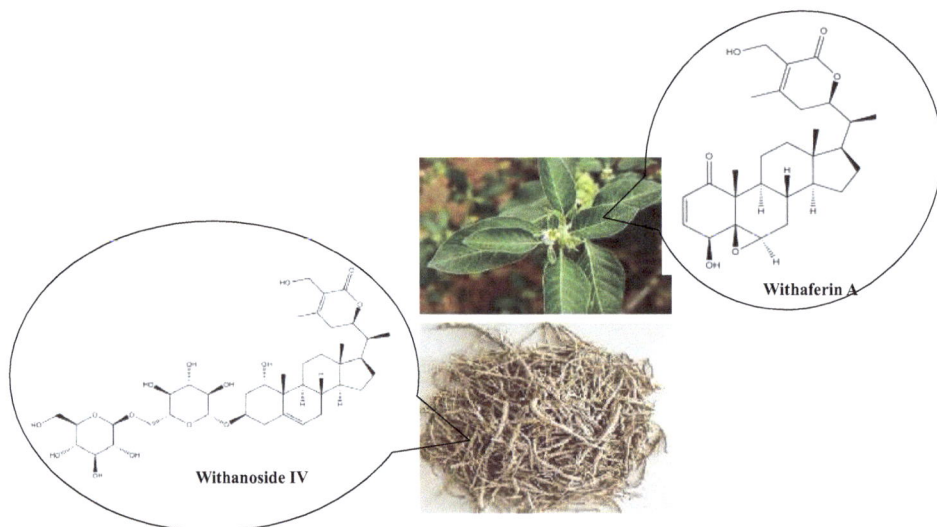

Fig. (3). Pictorial representation of *W. somnifera* (Ashwagandha) and chemical structure of its important bioactive constituents, Withaferin A and Withanoside IV.

W. somnifera in Alzheimer's Dementia

Sehgal *et al*. reported that *W. somnifera* promotes peripheral clearance of Aβ by increasing the expression of low-density lipoprotein receptor-related protein (LRP) in the brain, as well as neprilysin protease (NEP) in the liver, which helps in degrading Aβ and promoting its clearance from the liver (Fig.**15.2**). In the brain, excessive Aβ load and the consequent lipopolysaccharide stimulation can activate neurotoxic M1 microglial cells. This pro-inflammatory phenotype of microglia can cause neuronal cell death followed by cognitive decline [34]. *W. somnifera* extract also has been reported to inhibit lipopolysaccharide (LPS)-induced nitric oxide (NO) and reactive oxygen species (ROS) production in BV-2 cell, which is a type of microglial cell derived from C57/BL6 murine source [35,

36] (Table **1**).

Table 1. Significant secondary metabolites used in the therapeutic approach to Mixed Vascular Alzheimer's Dementia.

Common Name	Scientific Name	Active Secondary Metabolites	Principal Constituents	Presume Mechanical Pathway	Dose/Dose Regimen	Preclinical/Clinical Investigation	Outcome	Ref.
Ashwagandha or Indian ginseng	*W. somnifera*	Steroidal lactones, Phenolics, Alkaloids	Withanolide A Withanoside IV	Up-regulation of liver LRP promotes peripheral clearance of Aβ (Sehgal *et al.*, 2012)	300mg twice daily for eight weeks	A randomized, double-blind, placebo-controlled study conducted on 50 adults with mild cognitive impairment (MCI)	Effective (p = 0.002), in enhancing immediate and general memory in people with MCI	[30]
Snowdrop	*G. nivalis*	Isoquinoline	Galantamine	Potent antiacetylcholinesterase and promote microglial phagocytosis of Aβ	24 mg/day for 12 months	A randomized, double-blind, placebo-controlled study conducted on 55 mixed dementia patients	Effective in AD with CVD	[7]
Dyer's greenweed	*G. tinctoria*	Isoflavones	Genistein	Activates RXR/ PPARγ and upregulates ApoE expression to promote Aβ clearance	NA	*in vitro* cell line study	Genistein- O-alkylamine derivatives effective in Alzheimer's dementia	[45]
Milk thistle	*S. marianum*	Flavonoid, phenylpropane	Silibinin, Isosilibinin, Silichristin, Silidianin	Inhibit APP, prevent cholinesterase activity, attenuate microglial activation	70 and 140 mg/kg silymarin	Wistar rats	Silymarin was able to suppress APP expression.	[70]
Turmeric	*C. longa*	Polyphenols	Curcumin, demethoxycurcumin, bisdemethoxycurcumin	Antioxidant *via* reducing LPO level, scavenging ROS, inhibiting NF-κB activation	4g/day curcumin	Randomized, Placebo-Controlled, Double-Blind, Pilot Clinical Trial of curcumin in 34 patients with AD	Curcumin raised vitamin E level (P =0.01) revealing the antioxidant property	[49]
Maidenhair Tree	*G. biloba*	Flavonol, glycosides, terpenoids	Quercetin, kaempferoland, ginkgolide bilobalide	Antioxidant, decrease M1 activation, increase RBC deformability and reduce RBC aggregation, which improves blood flow	2 × 120 mg (Gingko Biloba Extract) EGb 761for 22 weeks	Double-blind trial including 400 patients with AD or VaD	Significantly superior to placebo on all secondary outcome measures, neuropsychological test battery shows a significant difference (p < 0.001)	[71]
Gotu Kola	*C. asiatica*	Triterpene	Asiatic acid, asiaticoside, madecassic acid, madecassoside	Improves synaptic plasticity by promoting dendritic growth, reducing Aβ level	60 or 120 mg/day for 2 months	A single-blind, placebo-controlled, randomized study in patients with venous hypertensive microangiopathy (VHM)	Significant improvement in VHM, useful in VaD (p < 0.05)	[72]
Brahmi	*B. monnieri*	Saponins, flavonoids, alkaloids, glycosides, sapogenin,	Bacoside A, bacoside B, bacopasaponins, D-mannitol	Antioxidant activity, increased cerebral blood flow *via* vasodilation, improving synaptic plasticity, altering ACh level, reducing Aβ load	125 mg for 12 weeks	A randomized, double-blind, placebo-controlled study in subjects with age-associated memory impairment	Efficacious in subjects with age-associated memory impairment (p < 0.05)	[73]

(Table 1) cont.....

Common Name	Scientific Name	Active Secondary Metabolites	Principal Constituents	Presume Mechanical Pathway	Dose/Dose Regimen	Preclinical/Clinical Investigation	Outcome	Ref.
Saffron	*C. sativa*	Mono-glycosyl polytene ester, carotenoid dicarboxylic acid	Crocin, crocetin, picrocrocin, and safranal	Antioxidant, prevent platelet aggregation, ameliorate inflammation	30 mg/day for 22 weeks	A randomized, double-blind, placebo-controlled study conducted on 54 adults with AD	Effective similar to standard drug donepezil in the treatment of mild-to-moderate AD ($p < 0.05$)	[69]

Galanthus nivalis

G. nivalis (snowdrop, family: Amaryllidaceae), widely distributed in northern Europe, west Spain, and east Ukraine, is reported to have therapeutic potential against Alzheimer's dementia with CVD [37]. Historically, the plant was described 2700–2800 years ago in Homer's Odyssey epic when the god Hermes gives Odysseus a herb with "a black root (snowdrop), but milk like a flower" called "moly," which helps to revive memory and fights against AD [38].

Phytoconstituents of G. nivalis

Galantamine (Fig. **4**) is an isoquinoline alkaloid isolated from the bulbs and flowers of *G. nivalis,* which proves to have anticholinesterase activities that help to increase the acetylcholine level in the synaptic cleft, thus improving cholinergic transmission and enhancing synaptic plasticity [39].

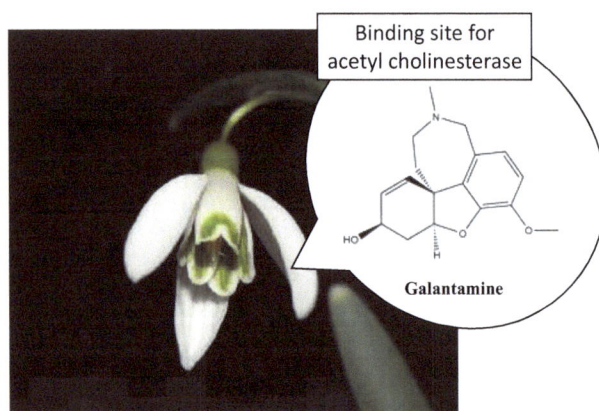

Fig. (4). Pictorial representation of *G. nivalis* (snowdrop) and chemical structure of its important bioactive constituents, Galantamine with acetylcholinesterase binding site.

G. nivalis in Mixed Dementia

Cholinergic dysfunction plays a vital role in learning and memory in patients with the coexistence of Alzheimer's and VaD. Several studies reported a significant reduction in acetylcholine levels in cerebrospinal fluid of both Alzheimer's and VaD patients [40]. Galantamine has cholinomimetic properties and acts as an acetylcholinesterase inhibitor and allosteric nicotine receptor modulator to prevent enzymatic degradation of acetylcholine and restore acetylcholine levels in dementia patients [37].

Furthermore, microglia in Alzheimer's brain also expresses nicotinic acetylcholine receptor (including the allosteric binding site recognized by the FK1 antibody), and it is known that galantamine increases microglial Aβ phagocytosis that is mediated by the combined action of competitive antagonism of acetylcholine receptor and inhibition of FK1 antibody [41]. The effective result of galantamine is that microglial activation is diminished, enhancing the neuroprotective propensity (Table **1**).

Genista tinctoria

G. tinctoria (dyer's greenweed, family: Fabaceae), widely distributed in Europe and Turkey, was found to help clear the Aβ load in an AD mouse model [42].

Phytoconstituents of G. tinctoria

More than 108 flavonoids are isolated from Genista species, and essential secondary metabolites are isoflavones which belong to the group of phytoestrogens [43] (Fig. **5**).

G. tinctoria in Alzheimer's Dementia

Genistein activates retinoid X receptor (RXR)/peroxisome proliferator-activated receptor gamma (PPARγ) to upregulate apolipoprotein E (ApoE) synthesis, which facilitates Aβ clearance [44] (Table **1**).

Silybum marianum

S. marianum (milk thistle, family: Asteraceae) is widely distributed in Europe, Asia, and North Africa from Norway and the Canary Islands to China and Maluku, and is naturalized in Australia, New Zealand, and the Americas.

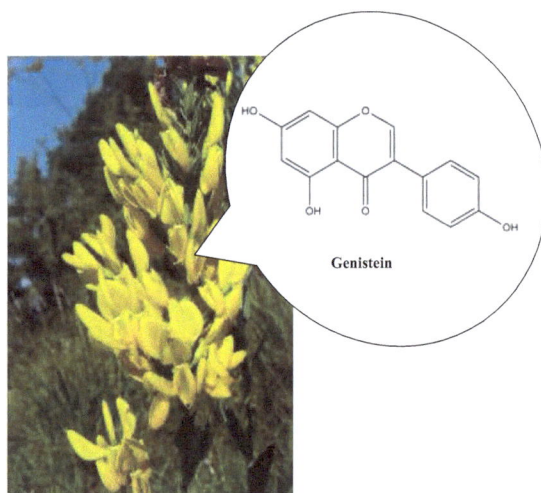

Fig. (5). Pictorial representation of *G. tinctoria* (dyer's greenweed) and chemical structure of Genistein.

Phytoconstituents of S. marianum

The principal constituent of silymarin is silibinin (Fig. **6**), a mixture of silybin A and silybin B. Milk thistle seed extract consists of a mixture of flavonoid and phenylpropane, namely silibinin, isosilibinin, silichristin, and silidianin [45]. The liver protection property of silymarin is well established.

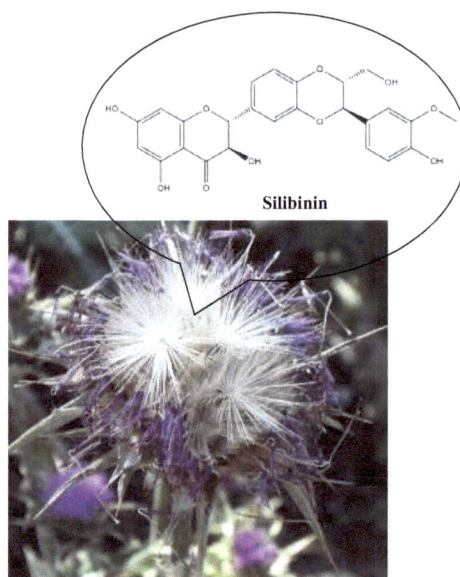

Fig. (6). Pictorial representation of *S. marianum* (milk thistle) and chemical structure of principal constituent silibinin.

S. marianum in Alzheimer's Dementia

Silymarin is reported to have some pharmacological activity in the nervous system along with its hepatoprotection property. In Alzheimer's dementia, silymarin helps to reduce Aβ production by inhibiting Aβ precursor protein (APP) and also increases acetylcholine levels by preventing cholinesterase activity [46]. Moreover, Jin *et al.* reported that silibinin intake attenuated microglial activation in the aging-accelerated mouse AD model [47] (Table **1**).

Curcuma longa

C. longa (turmeric, family: Zingiberaceae), native to South Asia and Southeast Asia [48], is traditionally well known for its anti-inflammatory effects and has been reported to have beneficial effects on atherosclerosis, arthritis, and asthma.

Phytoconstituents of C. longa

Curcumin, demethoxycurcumin (DMC), and bisdemethoxycurcumin are the three principal bioactive constituents obtained from curcumin which are polyphenolic [49] (Fig. **7**). Curcumin and DMC significantly reduced brain levels of soluble and insoluble Aβ in transgenic Alzheimer's mice [50].

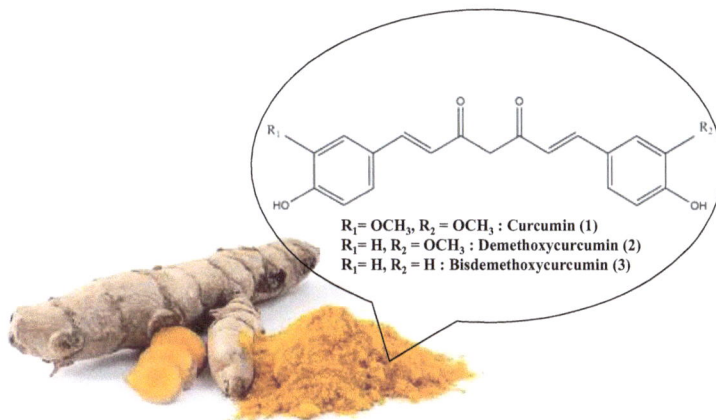

$R_1 = OCH_3, R_2 = OCH_3$: Curcumin (1)
$R_1 = H, R_2 = OCH_3$: Demethoxycurcumin (2)
$R_1 = H, R_2 = H$: Bisdemethoxycurcumin (3)

Fig. (7). Pictorial representation of *C. longa* (turmeric) and chemical structure of its important Curcumin, demethoxycurcumin, and bisdemethoxycurcumin.

C. longa in mixed Dementia

Several animal studies have reported that curcumin is effective in both Alzheimer's and VaD by targeting various pathological targets, such as inhibiting lipid peroxidation, scavenging reactive oxygen species, inhibiting NF-κB activation [51] as well as blocking Aβ fibril formation and aggregation, along with cholesterol-lowering property [11, 52] (Table **1**).

Ginkgo biloba

G. biloba (Maidenhair tree, family: Ginkgoaceae) is widely distributed throughout the world. Initially, its distribution was restricted to China. However, from 1730 onwards, human-mediated dispersal of *G. biloba* took place all over Europe, North America, and Eastern Asia due to its several therapeutic potencies [53].

6.6.1. Phytoconstituents of G. biloba

Flavonol glycosides (e.g., quercetin and kaempferol) and terpenoids (e.g., ginkgolide and bilobalide) are the principal constituents of *G. biloba* (Fig. **8**) [54]. The flavonoid derivatives of *G. biloba* have essential antioxidant properties, and the terpenoid fraction has proved to be efficacious in reducing cortical infarct volume in the cerebral stroke model [55].

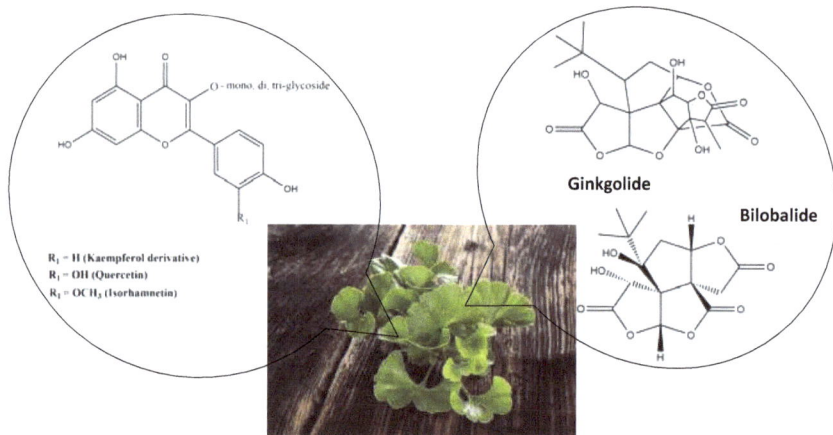

Fig. (8). Pictorial representation of *G. biloba (Maidenhair Tree)* and chemical structure of its important bioactive constituents, quercetin, kaempferol, ginkgolide, and bilobalide.

G. biloba in Mixed Dementia

G. biloba has been reported to improve cognition in patients with AD, and vascular or mixed dementia [56]. The possible mechanism of action associated with VaD is reducing oxygen radical generation, decreasing proinflammatory functions of macrophages, increasing neuronal metabolic activity by modulating glucose uptake and ATP production. Additionally, the leaf extract of *G. biloba* can increase the deformability of red blood cells and decrease RBC aggregation, promoting the improvement in blood flow which can be helpful in VaD [57] (Table **1**).

Centella asiatica

C. asiatica (Gotu Kola; family: Apiaceae) have been mentioned in the ancient Indian system of medicine (Ayurveda) as a treatment for dementia. It is native to the Indian subcontinent, Southeast Asia, and the Southeastern part of the United States [58].

Phytoconstituents of C. asiatica

The predominant secondary metabolites obtained from *C. asiatica* are triterpene derivatives, mainly asiatic acid (Fig. **9**), asiaticoside, madecassic acid (Fig. **9**), and madecassoside, which have anti-inflammatory and antioxidant properties [59].

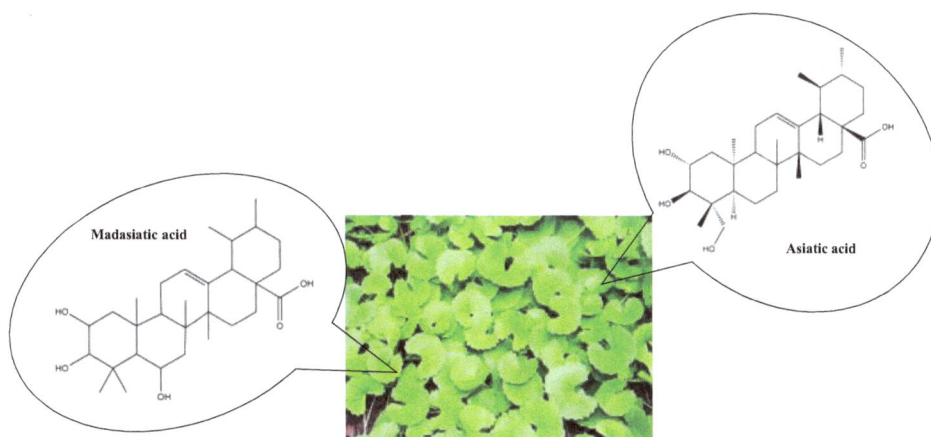

Fig. (9). Pictorial representation of *C. asiatica* (Gotu Kola) and chemical structure of its important bioactive constituents, madecassic acid and asiatic acid.

C. asiatica in Mixed Dementia

Lee *et al.* demonstrated the neuroprotective property of *C. asiatica* by exposing cultured neurons to excitotoxic glutamate [60]. The plant has a vital role in ameliorating both Alzheimer's and VaD. The fresh leaf extract of *C. asiatica* possesses hippocampal CA3 neuronal dendritic growth stimulating property in a rodent study. Augmentation of synaptic plasticity improves learning and memory, and "Gotu kola" extract also has anticholinesterase activity. Several animal studies reveal a reduction in the Aβ loads in the hippocampus and attenuation in the oxidative stress by aqueous "Gotu kola" extract. Besides, a study performed by Farhana *et al.* reported that 1000mg/day of "Gotu kola" extract could improve vascular cognitive impairment in 17 subjects [59] (Table 1).

Bacopa monnieri

B. monnieri (Brahmi; family: Scrophulariaceae), native to southern and Eastern India, Australia, Europe, Africa, Asia, and North and South America, is an Ayurvedic medicine traditionally used in cognitive decline, inflammation, asthma, and pain [61].

6.8.1. Phytoconstituents of B. monnieri

B. monnieri has several secondary metabolites, such as saponins, flavonoids, alkaloids, glycosides, sapogenin, and phytochemicals. Among these, saponins are mainly responsible for the majority of pharmacological actions. Bacoside A, bacoside B, bacopasaponins, D-mannitol, are the important saponins present in "Brahmi". Bacosides possess memory facilitating property [62] (Fig. 10).

B. monnieri in mixed Dementia

The plausible reason for *B. monnieri* can be compelling in mixed dementia because of its role in increasing cerebral blood flow *via* vasodilation [63], reducing Aβ load [62], and modulating the acetylcholine level. The principal components, bacosides A and B, reported improving learning and memory by restoring synaptic plasticity [64]. Furthermore, the metal-chelating property is attributed to "Brahmi", which proves to be effective as several metals interact with Aβ. Moreover, reduction of lipid peroxidation in the brain and scavenging the reactive oxygen species are also crucial properties of "Brahmi", which may help to retard dementia (Table 1).

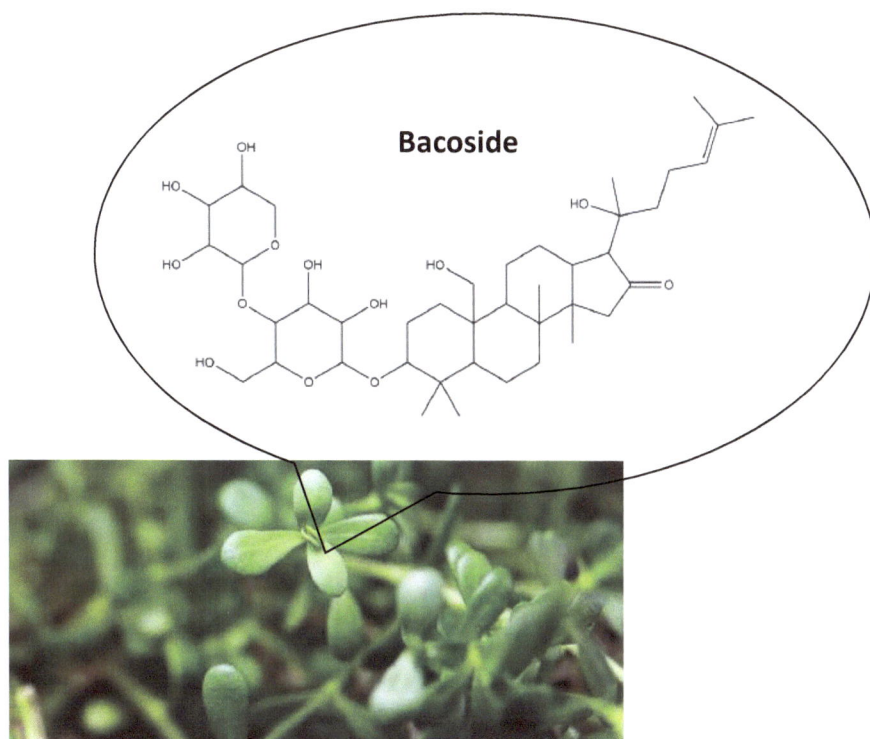

Fig. (10). Pictorial representation of *B. monnieri* (Brahmi) and chemical structure of its important bioactive constituent, Bacoside.

Crocus sativus

C sativus (saffron; family: Iridaceae) is widely distributed in South Western Asia and the Mediterranean region. In India, it is primarily cultivated in Kashmir [65]. *In vivo* and *in vitro* studies revealed the efficacy of saffron in improving learning and memory function and attenuating cerebral ischemia-induced damage in the hippocampus [66, 67].

Phytoconstituents of C. sativus

C. sativas contains four major bioactive constituents [65], such as

• Mono-glycosyl polytene ester (crocin) (Fig. **11**),

• a natural carotenoid dicarboxylic acid precursor of crocin (crocetin) (Fig. **11**),

• monoterpene glycoside precursor of safranal (picrocrocin), and safranal.

C. sativus in mixed Dementia

In vivo and *in vitro* studies in mice models demonstrate that saffron plays a vital role in increasing Aβ clearance by enhancing three mechanisms [68]

• enhancement of the tightness of blood-brain-barrier

• enzymatic degradation of Aβ

• Apolipoprotein E clearance.

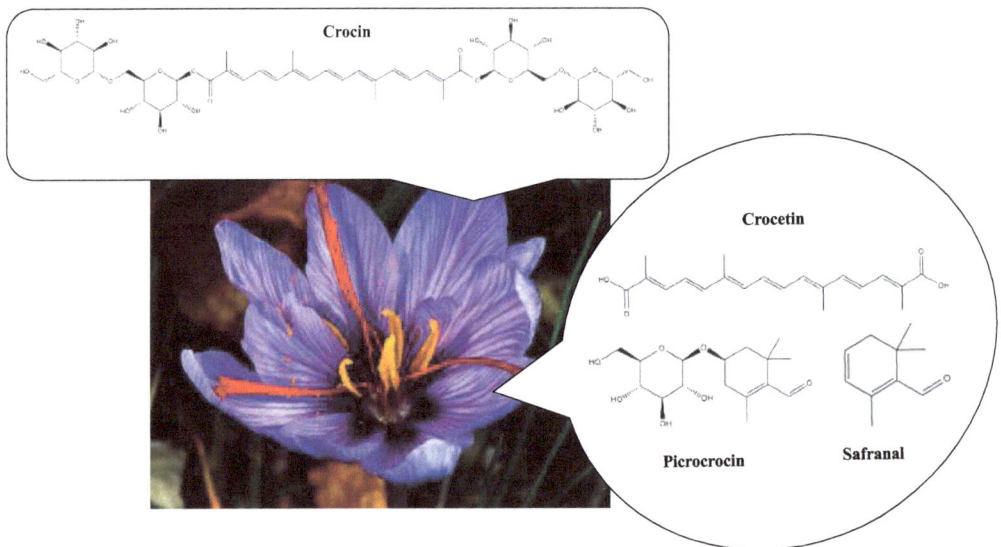

Fig. (11). Pictorial representation of *C. sativus* (saffron) and chemical structure of its important bioactive constituents, crocin, crocetin, picrocrocin, and safranal.

Recent randomized clinical trials reported saffron showed comparable results in improving cognition to donepezil, a standard drug for mixed dementia [69]. Furthermore, cerebral ischemia induces oxidative damage, which was also ameliorated by saffron in the rat hippocampus [67]. These concomitants of saffron revealed its plausible therapeutic potential in mixed dementia (Table **1**).

VALIDATION ANALYSIS OF PRECLINICAL/CLINICAL EFFICACY

We now demarcate the preclinical and clinical validation of the secondary metabolites. The detailed parameters are provided in Table **1**. Regarding the various human trials performed, the studies involve patients ranging from 35-400. All the investigations have full statistical significance, with the p-value in some clinical trials being p < 0.001. We delineate that the findings are robustly indicative of further escalation to clinical trials of Phase 3 and Phase 4 stages.

8. DISCUSSION

Among the various types of dementia, mixed dementia is reported to have less attention due to its heterogeneous neuropathological characteristics. This report has tried to unravel some of the crucial pathways through which mixed dementia occurs and the crosstalk between Alzheimer's dementia and VaD. The plausible causative interaction is from (i) Aβ influx *via* the advanced glycation end product (RAGE) receptor, and this influx produces (ii) endothelial-1 activation, which causes vasoconstriction, thereby elucidating the process of Aβ-induced VaD [1, 28, 74].

Using Systems Analysis based approach, our finding is that there is substantial experimental and clinical evidence demonstrating the efficacy of secondary metabolites from plant extract in Alzheimer's dementia, VaD, and mixed dementia. However, maximum evidence is obtained from *in vitro* and preclinical studies, which appeals for more clinical studies to obtain conclusive results. Indeed, we have identified clinical trial reports of some secondary metabolites here, showing significant efficacy in dementia, thereby suggesting therapeutic potency [43, 45, 48, 50, 59, 66]. Nevertheless, few studies have been performed to reveal the synergistic effects between the multiple active components of secondary metabolites, and to decipher the differences in effect between these multiple compounds of the same plant extract *via* [30, 38, 44, 57, 62, 64]. Each element of secondary metabolite has a discrete role in providing potency by targeting multiple numbers of pathological aspects simultaneously.

CONCLUSION

To sum up, our findings show that there is extensive indicative evidence demonstrating the potency of a single or combination of secondary metabolites in the clinical treatment of mixed vascular Alzheimer's dementia.

CONSENT FOR PUBLICATION

Not applicable.

CONFLICT OF INTEREST

The author declares no conflict of interest, financial or otherwise.

ACKNOWLEDGEMENTS

Declared none.

REFERENCES

[1]   Custodio N, Montesinos R, Lira D, Herrera-Pérez E, Bardales Y, Valeriano-Lorenzo L. Mixed dementia: A review of the evidence. Dement Neuropsychol 2017; 11(4): 364-70.
[http://dx.doi.org/10.1590/1980-57642016dn11-040005] [PMID: 29354216]

[2]   Jellinger KA. The enigma of mixed dementia. Alzheimers Dement 2007; 3(1): 40-53.
[http://dx.doi.org/10.1016/j.jalz.2006.09.002] [PMID: 19595916]

[3]   Lim A, Tsuang D, Kukull W, *et al.* Clinico-neuropathological correlation of Alzheimer's disease in a community-based case series. J Am Geriatr Soc 1999; 47(5): 564-9.
[http://dx.doi.org/10.1111/j.1532-5415.1999.tb02571.x] [PMID: 10323650]

[4]   Korte N, Nortley R, Attwell D. Cerebral blood flow decrease as an early pathological mechanism in Alzheimer's disease. Acta Neuropathol 2020; 140(6): 793-810.
[http://dx.doi.org/10.1007/s00401-020-02215-w] [PMID: 32865691]

[5]   Kalaria RN. Neuropathological diagnosis of vascular cognitive impairment and vascular dementia with implications for Alzheimer's disease. Acta Neuropathol 2016; 131(5): 659-85.
[http://dx.doi.org/10.1007/s00401-016-1571-z] [PMID: 27062261]

[6]   Román GC, Salloway S, Black SE, *et al.* Randomized, placebo-controlled, clinical trial of donepezil in vascular dementia: differential effects by hippocampal size. Stroke 2010; 41(6): 1213-21.
[http://dx.doi.org/10.1161/STROKEAHA.109.570077] [PMID: 20395618]

[7]   Auchus AP, Brashear HR, Salloway S, Korczyn AD, De Deyn PP, Gassmann-Mayer C. Galantamine treatment of vascular dementia: A randomized trial. Neurology 2007; 69(5): 448-58.
[http://dx.doi.org/10.1212/01.wnl.0000266625.31615.f6] [PMID: 17664404]

[8]   Pinho BR, Ferreres F, Valentão P, Andrade PB. Nature as a source of metabolites with cholinesterase-inhibitory activity: an approach to Alzheimer's disease treatment. J Pharm Pharmacol 2013; 65(12): 1681-700.
[http://dx.doi.org/10.1111/jphp.12081] [PMID: 24236980]

[9]   Diamond BJ, Johnson SK, Torsney K, *et al.* Complementary and alternative medicines in the treatment of dementia: an evidence-based review. Drugs Aging 2003; 20(13): 981-98.
[http://dx.doi.org/10.2165/00002512-200320130-00003] [PMID: 14561102]

[10]   Keswani C, Dilnashin H, Birla H, Singh S. Re-addressing the commercialization and regulatory hurdles for biopesticides in India. Rhizosphere 2019; 11(100155)

[11]   Rathore AS, Birla H, Singh SS, *et al.* Epigenetic Modulation in Parkinson's Disease and Potential Treatment Therapies. Neurochem Res 2021; 46(7): 1618-26.
[http://dx.doi.org/10.1007/s11064-021-03334-w] [PMID: 33900517]

[12]   Singh SS, Rai SN, Birla H, *et al.* Techniques Related to Disease Diagnosis and Therapeutics Application of Biomedical Engineering in Neuroscience. Springer 2019; pp. 437-56.

[http://dx.doi.org/10.1007/978-981-13-7142-4_22]

[13]   Zahra W, Rai SN, Birla H, *et al.* The global economic impact of neurodegenerative diseases: Opportunities and challenges Bioeconomy for Sustainable Development. Bioeconomy for Sustainable Development 2020; pp. 333-45.

[14]   Singh S, Rai S, Birla H, Eds., *et al.* Chlorogenic acid protects against MPTP induced neurotoxicity in parkinsonian mice model via its anti-apoptotic activity Journal of Neurochemistry. NJ USA.: Wiley 111 River St, Hoboken 2019.

[15]   Rai SN, Birla H, Singh SS, *et al.* Pathophysiology of the Disease Causing Physical Disability. Biomedical Engineering and its Applications in Healthcare. Springer 2019; pp. 573-95.

[16]   Rai SN, Singh BK, Rathore AS, *et al.* Quality control in huntington's disease: a therapeutic target. Neurotox Res 2019; 36(3): 612-26.
[http://dx.doi.org/10.1007/s12640-019-00087-x] [PMID: 31297710]

[17]   Keswani C. Bioeconomy for Sustainable Development. Springer 2020.
[http://dx.doi.org/10.1007/978-981-13-9431-7]

[18]   Keswani C, Singh HB, Hermosa R, *et al.* Antimicrobial secondary metabolites from agriculturally important fungi as next biocontrol agents. Appl Microbiol Biotechnol 2019; 103(23-24): 9287-303.
[http://dx.doi.org/10.1007/s00253-019-10209-2] [PMID: 31707442]

[19]   Keswani C. Agri-based Bioeconomy: Reintegrating Trans-disciplinary Research and Sustainable Development Goals. CRC Press 2021.
[http://dx.doi.org/10.1201/9781003033394]

[20]   Keswani C, Bisen K, Singh S, Singh H. Traditional knowledge and medicinal plants of India in intellectual property landscape. Med Plants Int J Phytomed Relat Ind 2017; p. 9.

[21]   Rai SN, Dilnashin H, Birla H, *et al.* The role of PI3K/Akt and ERK in neurodegenerative disorders. Neurotox Res 2019; 35(3): 775-95.
[http://dx.doi.org/10.1007/s12640-019-0003-y] [PMID: 30707354]

[22]   Zahra W, Rai SN, Birla H, *et al.* Neuroprotection of rotenone-induced Parkinsonism by ursolic acid in PD mouse model. CNS & Neurological Disorders-Drug Targets 2020; 14: 527-40.
[http://dx.doi.org/10.2174/1871527319666200812224457]

[23]   Rai SN, Zahra W, Singh SS, *et al.* Anti-inflammatory activity of ursolic acid in MPTP-induced parkinsonian mouse model. Neurotox Res 2019; 36(3): 452-62.
[http://dx.doi.org/10.1007/s12640-019-00038-6] [PMID: 31016688]

[24]   Singh SS, Rai SN, Birla H, *et al.* Neuroprotective effect of chlorogenic acid on mitochondrial dysfunction-mediated apoptotic death of DA neurons in a Parkinsonian mouse model. Oxid Med Cell Longev 2020; 2020: 1-14.
[http://dx.doi.org/10.1155/2020/6571484] [PMID: 32566093]

[25]   Zahra W, Rai SN, Birla H, *et al.* Economic Importance of Medicinal Plants in Asian Countries Bioeconomy for Sustainable Development. Springer 2020; pp. 359-77.
[http://dx.doi.org/10.1007/978-981-13-9431-7_19]

[26]   Birla H, Keswani C, Singh SS, *et al.* Unraveling the Neuroprotective Effect of *Tinospora cordifolia* in Parkinsonian Mouse Model Through Proteomics Approach 2021.

[27]   Keswani C, Dilnashin H, Birla H, Singh SP. Unravelling efficient applications of agriculturally important microorganisms for alleviation of induced inter-cellular oxidative stress in crops. Acta Agric Slov 2019; 114(1): 121-30.
[http://dx.doi.org/10.14720/aas.2019.114.1.14]

[28]   Deane R, Du Yan S, Submamaryan RK, *et al.* RAGE mediates amyloid-β peptide transport across the blood-brain barrier and accumulation in brain. Nat Med 2003; 9(7): 907-13.
[http://dx.doi.org/10.1038/nm890] [PMID: 12808450]

[29]   Kalra R, Kaushik N. *Withania somnifera* (Linn.) Dunal: a review of chemical and pharmacological diversity. Phytochem Rev 2017; 16(5): 953-87.
[http://dx.doi.org/10.1007/s11101-017-9504-6]

[30]   Choudhary D, Bhattacharyya S, Bose S. Efficacy and safety of Ashwagandha (*Withania somnifera* (L.) Dunal) root extract in improving memory and cognitive functions. J Diet Suppl 2017; 14(6): 599-612.
[http://dx.doi.org/10.1080/19390211.2017.1284970] [PMID: 28471731]

[31]   Sharma R, Chauhan A, Chaudhary P. *Withania somnifera*. Therapeutic Uses and Phyochemical Constituents 2020.

[32]   Sehgal N, Gupta A, Valli RK, *et al.* *Withania somnifera* reverses Alzheimer's disease pathology by enhancing low-density lipoprotein receptor-related protein in liver. Proc Natl Acad Sci USA 2012; 109(9): 3510-5.
[http://dx.doi.org/10.1073/pnas.1112209109] [PMID: 22308347]

[33]   Mishra L-C, Singh BB, Dagenais S. Scientific basis for the therapeutic use of *Withania somnifera* (ashwagandha): a review. Altern Med Rev 2000; 5(4): 334-46.
[PMID: 10956379]

[34]   Mosher KI, Wyss-Coray T. Microglial dysfunction in brain aging and Alzheimer's disease. Biochem Pharmacol 2014; 88(4): 594-604.
[http://dx.doi.org/10.1016/j.bcp.2014.01.008] [PMID: 24445162]

[35]   Birla H, Keswani C, Rai SN, *et al.* Neuroprotective effects of *Withania somnifera* in BPA induced-cognitive dysfunction and oxidative stress in mice. Behav Brain Funct 2019; 15(1): 9.
[http://dx.doi.org/10.1186/s12993-019-0160-4] [PMID: 31064381]

[36]   Sun GY, Li R, Cui J, *et al.* *Withania somnifera* and its withanolides attenuate oxidative and inflammatory responses and up-regulate antioxidant responses in BV-2 microglial cells. Neuromolecular Med 2016; 18(3): 241-52.
[http://dx.doi.org/10.1007/s12017-016-8411-0] [PMID: 27209361]

[37]   Small G, Erkinjuntti T, Kurz A, Lilienfeld S. Galantamine in the treatment of cognitive decline in patients with vascular dementia or Alzheimer's disease with cerebrovascular disease. CNS Drugs 2003; 17(12): 905-14.
[http://dx.doi.org/10.2165/00023210-200317120-00004] [PMID: 12962529]

[38]   Block W. Fight Alzheimer's Disease. Life enhancement 2017.

[39]   Balkrishna A, Pokhrel S, Tomer M, *et al.* Anti-Acetylcholinesterase activities of mono-herbal extracts and exhibited synergistic effects of the phytoconstituents: a biochemical and computational study. Molecules 2019; 24(22): 4175.
[http://dx.doi.org/10.3390/molecules24224175] [PMID: 31752124]

[40]   Tohgi H, Abe T, Kimura M, Saheki M, Takahashi S. Cerebrospinal fluid acetylcholine and choline in vascular dementia of Binswanger and multiple small infarct types as compared with Alzheimer-type dementia. J Neural Transm (Vienna) 1996; 103(10): 1211-20.
[http://dx.doi.org/10.1007/BF01271206] [PMID: 9013408]

[41]   Takata K, Kitamura Y, Saeki M, *et al.* Galantamine-induced amyloid-β clearance mediated via stimulation of microglial nicotinic acetylcholine receptors. J Biol Chem 2010; 285(51): 40180-91.
[http://dx.doi.org/10.1074/jbc.M110.142356] [PMID: 20947502]

[42]   Bassendine MF, Taylor-Robinson SD, Fertleman M, Khan M, Neely D. Is Alzheimer's Disease a Liver Disease of the Brain? J Alzheimers Dis 2020; 75(1): 1-14.
[http://dx.doi.org/10.3233/JAD-190848] [PMID: 32250293]

[43]   Grafakou ME, Barda C, Tomou EM, Skaltsa H. The genus *Genista* L.: A rich source of bioactive flavonoids. Phytochemistry 2021; 181: 112574.
[http://dx.doi.org/10.1016/j.phytochem.2020.112574] [PMID: 33152578]

[44]   Bonet-Costa V, Herranz-Pérez V, Blanco-Gandía M, *et al.* Clearing amyloid-β through PPAR γ/ApoE activation by genistein is a treatment of experimental Alzheimer's disease. J Alzheimers Dis 2016; 51(3): 701-11.
[http://dx.doi.org/10.3233/JAD-151020] [PMID: 26890773]

[45]   Guo H, Cao H, Cui X, *et al.* Silymarin's inhibition and treatment effects for Alzheimer's disease. Molecules 2019; 24(9): 1748.
[http://dx.doi.org/10.3390/molecules24091748] [PMID: 31064071]

[46]   Murata N, Murakami K, Ozawa Y, *et al. Silymarin* attenuated the amyloid β plaque burden and improved behavioral abnormalities in an Alzheimer's disease mouse model. Biosci Biotechnol Biochem 2010; 74(11): 2299-306.
[http://dx.doi.org/10.1271/bbb.100524] [PMID: 21071836]

[47]   Jin G, Bai D, Yin S, *et al.* Silibinin rescues learning and memory deficits by attenuating microglia activation and preventing neuroinflammatory reactions in SAMP8 mice. Neurosci Lett 2016; 629: 256-61.
[http://dx.doi.org/10.1016/j.neulet.2016.06.008] [PMID: 27276653]

[48]   Gupta SC, Sung B, Kim JH, Prasad S, Li S, Aggarwal BB. Multitargeting by turmeric, the golden spice: From kitchen to clinic. Mol Nutr Food Res 2013; 57(9): 1510-28.
[http://dx.doi.org/10.1002/mnfr.201100741] [PMID: 22887802]

[49]   Kim Y, Clifton P. Curcumin, cardiometabolic health and dementia. Int J Environ Res Public Health 2018; 15(10): 2093.
[http://dx.doi.org/10.3390/ijerph15102093] [PMID: 30250013]

[50]   Shytle R, Bickford P, Rezai-zadeh K, *et al.* Optimized turmeric extracts have potent anti-amyloidogenic effects. Curr Alzheimer Res 2009; 6(6): 564-71.
[http://dx.doi.org/10.2174/156720509790147115] [PMID: 19715544]

[51]   Wang Y, Huang L, Tang X, Zhang H. Retrospect and prospect of active principles from Chinese herbs in the treatment of dementia. Acta Pharmacol Sin 2010; 31(6): 649-64.
[http://dx.doi.org/10.1038/aps.2010.46] [PMID: 20523337]

[52]   Yang F, Lim GP, Begum AN, *et al.* Curcumin inhibits formation of amyloid β oligomers and fibrils, binds plaques, and reduces amyloid in vivo. J Biol Chem 2005; 280(7): 5892-901.
[http://dx.doi.org/10.1074/jbc.M404751200] [PMID: 15590663]

[53]   Zhao Y, Paule J, Fu C, Koch MA. Out of China: Distribution history of *Ginkgo biloba* L. Taxon 2010; 59(2): 495-504.
[http://dx.doi.org/10.1002/tax.592014]

[54]   Luo Y, Smith JV. Studies on molecular mechanisms of *Ginkgo biloba* extract. Appl Microbiol Biotechnol 2004; 64(4): 465-72.
[http://dx.doi.org/10.1007/s00253-003-1527-9] [PMID: 14740187]

[55]   Defeudis F. Bilobalide and neuroprotection. Pharmacol Res 2002; 46(6): 565-8.
[http://dx.doi.org/10.1016/S1043-6618(02)00233-5] [PMID: 12457632]

[56]   Weinmann S, Roll S, Schwarzbach C, Vauth C, Willich SN. Effects of *Ginkgo biloba* in dementia: systematic review and meta-analysis. BMC Geriatr 2010; 10(1): 14.
[http://dx.doi.org/10.1186/1471-2318-10-14] [PMID: 20236541]

[57]   Chan PC, Xia Q, Fu PP. *Ginkgo biloba* leave extract: biological, medicinal, and toxicological effects. J Environ Sci Health Part C Environ Carcinog Ecotoxicol Rev 2007; 25(3): 211-44.
[http://dx.doi.org/10.1080/10590500701569414] [PMID: 17763047]

[58]   Lakshmi Pravallika P, Krishna Mohan G, Venkateswara Rao K, Shanker K. Biosynthesis, characterization and acute oral toxicity studies of synthesized iron oxide nanoparticles using ethanolic extract of *Centella asiatica* plant. Mater Lett 2019; 236: 256-9.
[http://dx.doi.org/10.1016/j.matlet.2018.10.037]

[59]   Farhana KM, Malueka RG, Wibowo S, Gofir A. Effectiveness of gotu kola extract 750 mg and 1000 mg compared with folic acid 3 mg in improving vascular cognitive impairment after stroke. Evidence-Based Complementary and Alternative Medicine 2016.
[http://dx.doi.org/10.1155/2016/2795915]

[60]   Lee MK, Kim SR, Sung SH, *et al.* Asiatic acid derivatives protect cultured cortical neurons from glutamate-induced excitotoxicity. Res Commun Mol Pathol Pharmacol 2000; 108(1-2): 75-86.
[PMID: 11758977]

[61]   Russo A, Borrelli F. *Bacopa monniera*, a reputed nootropic plant: an overview. Phytomedicine 2005; 12(4): 305-17.
[http://dx.doi.org/10.1016/j.phymed.2003.12.008] [PMID: 15898709]

[62]   Chaudhari KS, Tiwari NR, Tiwari RR, Sharma RS. Neurocognitive Effect of Nootropic Drug Brahmi (*Bacopa monnier*) in Alzheimer's Disease. Ann Neurosci 2017; 24(2): 111-22.
[http://dx.doi.org/10.1159/000475900] [PMID: 28588366]

[63]   Kamkaew N, Norman Scholfield C, Ingkaninan K, Taepavarapruk N, Chootip K. *Bacopa monnieri* increases cerebral blood flow in rat independent of blood pressure. Phytother Res 2013; 27(1): 135-8.
[http://dx.doi.org/10.1002/ptr.4685] [PMID: 22447676]

[64]   Chowdhuri DK, Parmar D, Kakkar P, Shukla R, Seth PK, Srimal RC. Antistress effects of bacosides of *Bacopa monnieri*: modulation of Hsp70 expression, superoxide dismutase and cytochrome P450 activity in rat brain. Phytother Res 2002; 16(7): 639-45.
[http://dx.doi.org/10.1002/ptr.1023] [PMID: 12410544]

[65]   Jan S, Wani AA, Kamili AN, Kashtwari M. Distribution, chemical composition and medicinal importance of saffron (*Crocus sativus* L.). Afr J Plant Sci 2014; 8(12): 537-45.

[66]   Hosseinzadeh H, Sadeghnia HR. Safranal, a constituent of *Crocus sativus* (saffron), attenuated cerebral ischemia induced oxidative damage in rat hippocampus. J Pharm Pharm Sci 2005; 8(3): 394-9.
[PMID: 16401389]

[67]   Abe K, Saito H. Effects of saffron extract and its constituent crocin on learning behaviour and long-term potentiation. Phytother Res 2000; 14(3): 149-52.
[http://dx.doi.org/10.1002/(SICI)1099-1573(200005)14:3<149::AID-PTR665>3.0.CO;2-5] [PMID: 10815004]

[68]   Batarseh YS, Bharate SS, Kumar V, *et al. Crocus sativus* extract tightens the blood-brain barrier, reduces amyloid β load and related toxicity in 5XFAD mice. ACS Chem Neurosci 2017; 8(8): 1756-66.
[http://dx.doi.org/10.1021/acschemneuro.7b00101] [PMID: 28471166]

[69]   Akhondzadeh S, Sabet MS, Harirchian MH, *et al.* Original Article: Saffron in the treatment of patients with mild to moderate Alzheimer's disease: a 16-week, randomized and placebo-controlled trial. J Clin Pharm Ther 2010; 35(5): 581-8.
[http://dx.doi.org/10.1111/j.1365-2710.2009.01133.x] [PMID: 20831681]

[70]   Yaghmaei P, Azarfar K, Dezfulian M, Ebrahim-Habibi A. Silymarin effect on amyloid-β plaque accumulation and gene expression of APP in an Alzheimer's disease rat model. Daru 2014; 22(1): 24.
[http://dx.doi.org/10.1186/2008-2231-22-24] [PMID: 24460990]

[71]   Napryeyenko O, Borzenko I. *Ginkgo biloba* special extract in dementia with neuropsychiatric features. A randomised, placebo-controlled, double-blind clinical trial. Arzneimittelforschung 2007; 57(1): 4-11.
[PMID: 17341003]

[72]   Incandela L, Belcaro G, De Sanctis MT, *et al.* Total triterpenic fraction of *Centella asiatica* in the treatment of venous hypertension: a clinical, prospective, randomized trial using a combined microcirculatory model. Angiology 2001; 52(2_suppl) (Suppl. 2): S61-7.

[http://dx.doi.org/10.1177/000331970105202S12] [PMID: 11666126]

[73]   Singh H, Raghav S, Dalal PK, Srivastava JS, Asthana OP. Randomized controlled trial of standardized *Bacopa monnier*a extract in age-associated memory impairment. Indian J Psychiatry 2006; 48(4): 238-42.
[http://dx.doi.org/10.4103/0019-5545.31555] [PMID: 20703343]

[74]   Deane R, Wu Z, Zlokovic BV. RAGE (yin) *versus* LRP (yang) balance regulates alzheimer amyloid β-peptide clearance through transport across the blood-brain barrier. Stroke 2004; 35(11_suppl_1) (Suppl. 1): 2628-31.
[http://dx.doi.org/10.1161/01.STR.0000143452.85382.d1] [PMID: 15459432]

SUBJECT INDEX

A

Ability 10, 51, 59, 88, 127, 172, 187, 191, 200, 272, 281, 291, 292
  adhesive 51
  metal chelating 59
Abnormalities 6, 54, 288
  gait 54, 288
  neuropsychiatric 6
Accumulation 78, 83, 126, 130, 131, 136, 170, 177, 190, 198, 200, 289, 308, 317, 354
  of Lewy bodies 78, 190
  of vascular damages 354
  lipofuscin 198
  mitochondrial 83
Acetone extract 15, 344
Acetylcholine 138, 139, 152, 153, 155, 359
  breakdown 139
Acetylcholine esterase 129, 130, 132, 178
  activity 178
  inhibitor 129
Acid(s) 10, 12, 13, 16, 17, 43, 49, 50, 51, 53, 54, 55, 58, 79, 87, 89, 91, 128, 129, 130, 134, 135, 136, 137, 172, 174, 175, 176, 178, 177, 178, 197, 198, 225, 241, 242, 248, 267, 285, 302, 306, 339, 340, 341, 344, 357, 363
  aminobutyric 175
  arachidonic 241
  ascorbic 178, 344
  asiatic 43, 51, 58, 91, 128, 130, 172, 339, 344, 357, 363
  aspartic 176
  benzoic 43
  betulinic 12, 53, 128, 197
  caffeic 79, 176, 225
  caffeoylquinic 172
  catechinellagic 177
  cerebral glutamic 198
  chebulagic 134
  chebulic 134, 178
  chebulinic 134

  cinnamic 43
  docosahexaenoic 248
  eicosapentaenoic 248
  ellagic 89, 128, 134, 135, 177, 178
  folic 87, 175, 242
  gallic 43, 49, 51, 54, 134, 178, 302, 340
  glycyrrhizic 129, 136, 137
  gymnemic 225
  nicotinic 178
  octadecanoic 174
  phytic 54
  protocatechuic 10, 17, 341
  retinoic 285
  salvianic 13, 341
  salvianolic 341
  stearic 128
  tannic 177, 178
  thiobarbituric 16, 50
  uric 306
  Ursolic (UA) 55, 176
  vanillic 267
Aconitum heterophyllum 26
Action 55, 90, 130, 131, 135, 136, 140, 153, 172, 203, 215, 221, 237, 238, 261, 341,
  anti-neuroinflammatory 55
  anti-oxidative 130
  immunosuppressive 341
  insulin 215
  lipoxygenase 172
  memory-enhancing 261
  neuromodulatory 153
  neuroprotective 136, 140, 238
  nootropic 135, 203
  prophylactic 131
  protective 90, 237
  therapeutic 221
Activated 202, 309, 310, 312, 313, 316, 317
  microglia 309, 310, 312, 313, 316, 317
  NMDA 202
Activation 12, 13, 19, 47, 60, 79, 80, 83, 89, 91, 225, 285, 306, 307, 309, 313, 317, 357

C

www.ingramcontent.com/pod-product-compliance
Lightning Source LLC
Chambersburg PA
CBHW050759220326
41598CB00006B/68